DATE DUE

JAN 2 4 1995	FEB 2 5 1999
FEB 1 3 1995	SEP 29 1999
FEB 1 4 1995	DEC - 2 1999
FEB - 7 1995	MAR 2 8 2000
MAR 2 5 1995	DEC 6 2000
NOV 2 2 1995	MAR 1 6 2001
FEB 1 1996	OCT 1 8 2001
FEB 2 0 1996	NOV 2 1 2001
MAR 1 1 1996	DEC 1 9 2001
	JAN 2 2 2002
MAR 2 6 1996	FEB 2 8 2003
SEP 2 5 1997	NOV 2 1 2003
FEB - 4 1998	DEC - 5 2003
FEB 1 8 1998	
FEB 2 5 1998	
FEB 1 1 1999	

Sexual Behavior
Problems and Management

APPLIED CLINICAL PSYCHOLOGY

Series Editors:
Alan S. Bellack, *Medical College of Pennsylvania at EPPI, Philadelphia, Pennsylvania,*
and Michel Hersen, *Nova University School of Pyschology, Fort Lauderdale, Florida*

Current Volumes in this Series

ACTIVITY MEASUREMENT IN PSYCHOLOGY AND MEDICINE
  Warren W. Tryon

BEHAVIOR ANALYSIS AND TREATMENT
  Edited by Ron Van Houten and Saul Axelrod

CASEBOOK OF THE BRIEF PSYCHOTHERAPIES
  Edited by Richard A. Wells and Vincent J. Giannetti

THE CHALLENGE OF COGNITIVE THERAPY
Applications to Nontraditional Populations
  Edited by T. Michael Vallis, Janice L. Howes, and Philip C. Miller

CLINICAL PSYCHOLOGY
Historical and Research Foundations
  Edited by C. Eugene Walker

ETHNIC VALIDITY, ECOLOGY, AND PSYCHOTHERAPY
A Psychosocial Competence Model
  Forrest B. Tyler, Deborah Ridley Brome, and Janice E. Williams

HANDBOOK OF CLINICAL BEHAVIOR THERAPY WITH THE ELDERLY CLIENT
  Edited by Patricia A. Wisocki

PERSPECTIVES AND PROMISES OF CLINICAL PSYCHOLOGY
  Edited by Anke Ehlers, Wolfgang Fiegenbaum, Irmela Florin, and Jürgen Margraf

PSYCHOLOGY
A Behavioral Overview
  Alan Poling, Henry Schlinger, Stephen Starin, and Elbert Blakely

SEXUAL BEHAVIOR: PROBLEMS AND MANAGEMENT
  Nathaniel McConaghy

USING RATIONAL-EMOTIVE THERAPY EFFECTIVELY
A Practitioner's Guide
  Edited by Michael E. Bernard

A Continuation Order Plan is available for this series. A continuation order will bring delivery of each new volume immediately upon publication. Volumes are billed only upon actual shipment. For further information please contact the publisher.

Sexual Behavior
Problems and Management

NATHANIEL MCCONAGHY

Prince of Wales Hospital
Randwick, New South Wales
Australia

Plenum Press • New York and London

Library of Congress Cataloging-in-Publication Data

McConaghy, Nathaniel.
    Sexual behavior : problems and management / Nathaniel McConaghy.
        p.   cm.
    Includes bibliographical references and index.
    ISBN 0-306-44177-2
    1. Psychosexual disorders. 2. Sex. 3. Sex therapy.   I. Title.
    RC556.M394 1993
    616.85'83--dc20
                                                                92-43589
                                                                     CIP

ISBN 0-306-44177-2

© 1993 Plenum Press, New York
A Division of Plenum Publishing Corporation
233 Spring Street, New York, N.Y. 10013

Printed in the United States of America

Preface

Many issues remain unresolved in sexuality. In some cases this is because the information is not available to resolve them. In others it is, but the available conclusions the information supports block its acceptance, because they conflict with the positions of dominant groups in the politics of sexuality. Possibly the most obvious example is the determination of many theorists to ignore the evidence that while men rarely report being sexually assaulted, when questioned in community surveys, they make up a third of the victims, and a quarter of the perpetrators of sexual assault are women. These findings are incompatible with the feminist theory that sexual assault is not a sexual act, but normal male behavior motivated politically, to maintain men's dominance of women. Most research supporting the theory investigated women only as victims and men only as aggressors. Some feminists have dismissed the need for any research to support their beliefs on the ground that such research is "busy work" establishing what women already know. One belief considered not to require research is that heterosexual pornography made for a male audience increases the prevalence of rape by encouraging rape-supportive attitudes of male aggression and female submission. No criticism has been directed at the soft-core pornography of "Mills and Boon" stories written for women that promote similar attitudes. Concern not to oppose the theory that sexual assault is an expression of normal male behavior appears to have influenced the classification of sexual disorders developed by the American Psychiatric Association in the *Diagnostic and Statistical Manual of Mental Disorders*. The majority of rapists were excluded from the classification, with the implication that they were not sexually aroused by the infliction of pain on women. Yet rapists report being aroused by the thought of inflicting pain on women, as do a significant percentage of normal men, just as a significant percentage of women report being aroused by the thought of being sexually assaulted. The hostility to male sexuality expressed in much feminist theory has led to its overlooking the important role men perform in encouraging women to learn to enjoy and to maintain enjoyment of sexual activity. The presence of a sexually active male partner is the single most important factor in preserving older women's sexual interest. Health and wealth are major determinants of the presence of such a partner.

The evidence that homosexual feelings in heterosexual as well as homosexual adult males are associated with a degree of female-type behaviors (including "sissiness") in childhood, and of feeling like a woman in adulthood, is unacceptable to the ideology (a) of feminism that masculinity and femininity do not or at least should not exist, and (b) of gay liberation that homosexuals and heterosexuals differ only in their sexual preference.

In the 1970s interest in studying the sexuality of children was developing, and sexual activity between children and adults was discussed without the reaction of abhorrence that subsequently became evident. It is now widely accepted that any activities of this nature—from a single impulsive episode of brief genital fondling to violent rape—are equivalent, at least when carried out in the developed world, and almost invariably are extremely harmful to the child's subsequent development. This belief has become a tenet of victimology, an area of study developed in the 1980s, which was in part stimulated by the growth of what has been termed the child-abuse industry. Few workers appear to be prepared to examine critically the evidence supporting this belief. If it is correct, because up to 60% of women are claimed to be victims of child and adolescent sexual abuse—twice as many as men—the mental health of women should be significantly inferior to that of men. The reaction of abhorrence to any form of adult-child sexual interactions may not have reduced the likelihood of such interactions occurring. Little attention has been given the evidence that a significant percentage of otherwise normal men are capable of being sexually aroused by female children. Unless this is emphasized as part of preventative programs to minimize the incidence of child sexual abuse, many of these men will remain unaware of or deny the possibility of experiencing such feelings out of shame and guilt. They may impulsively act on them when they suddenly become sexually aroused in an unexpected situation with a female child.

Evidence that assessment of subjects' penile circumference responses to pictures of nude men and women was not able to differentiate predominantly homosexual from predominantly heterosexual men as individuals has been largely ignored, presumably motivated by professional solidarity. On the basis that this method could accurately assess the sexual orientation of individual men, it was used in single-case studies to demonstrate that a number of behavioral procedures altered the sexual orientation of the homosexual subjects treated. The findings were used to justify techniques currently employed in North America to modify the deviant urges of sex offenders. Studies using the valid penile volume assessment of responses to pictures of men and women showed that such techniques did not alter subjects' sexual orientation. Rather, these techniques gave subjects with deviant sexual preferences control over any behaviors driven by such preferences that they previously could not control. If the evidence of lack of validity of the penile circumference assessment used to determine individual subject's sexual orientation is acknowledged, the results of the single-case studies using it must also be accepted as invalid. This would mean that the deviant sexual preferences of subjects cannot be altered by the techniques currently employed, including aversive therapies using noxious gases. Instead of aiming to modify these preferences, treatment should aim to give subjects control over any unacceptable behaviors they feel driven compulsively to carry out under the influence of the preferences. Evidence is also available demonstrating the lack of validity of penile circumference assessment when used to identify individual sex offenders. This assessment continues to be used in their legal disposition and in the evaluation of their response to treatment: procedures, which in view of the evidence of the lack of validity of the assessment seem not only unscientific, but unethical.

The political motivations for the adoption of some positions are less overt—for example, the rejection of the evidence that bisexuality of feelings exists. Psychoanalytic and social learning theories that explain homosexuality as due entirely to social factors provide no adequate explanation for bisexuality. Acceptance that it exists threatens the validity of these theories and, even more significantly, raises the possibility that biological factors are involved. Theories of the causes of human behavior in America, at least since the 1920s, have had a strong commitment to the ideology that biological—including inherited—factors are not involved. If they were, they would result in people not being equal. Capitalist ideology is much more ethically acceptable if all people are intrinsically equal, and therefore equally motivated and able to seek and achieve the rewards capitalism offers. Despite evidence that acceptance that biological factors contributed to the causation of homosexuality would increase public tolerance, both the Society of Lesbian and Gay Anthropologists and the Lesbian and Gay Sociologists' Caucus consider the biological view heretical; one American social scientific journal that publishes widely on this topic refuses to publish any research that supports the biological position (Whitam, 1990).

The existence of bisexuality of feelings has been established by a number of studies carried out since the turn of the century. These studies found that a significant percentage of the population, when questioned anonymously, reported that they were aware of a degree of sexual attraction to both males and females. Where possible, these data have been ignored. Where this was not possible, because the data were too well known, they were treated with ambivalence. The Kinsey findings supporting the existence of bisexuality are referred to with admiration, although research evidence continues to be published which contradicts them. The articles reporting this evidence do not refer to the contradiction.

Reluctance to accept the existence of bisexuality may reflect a preference to regard deviant sexual behavior as categorically different from, rather than on a continuum with, normal sexual behavior. The facts that a significant percentage of heterosexual couples engage in anal intercourse, that possibly the majority of adolescents have carried out sexually offensive deviant behaviors, and that the majority of adults are sexually aroused by deviant fantasies receive little attention.

The aim of this book is to attempt to present what is currently known, and to examine critically what is believed concerning sexual behavior, where possible freeing beliefs from the effect of established political positions.

Contents

CHAPTER 1

Assessment of Sexual Activity

THE CLINICAL INTERVIEW

Most assessments of sexual activity are carried out by clinicians who treat sexual problems. Though little is published concerning the methods they use, it is apparent from discussion that the majority initiate their relationship with patients and obtain the necessary preliminary information concerning their problems by interviewing them and, if possible, their partners or other relevant persons. Usually clinicians, as part of their professional training, receive several years of training in interview techniques to enable them to establish appropriate relationships with their patients and to learn what information is required to arrive at the correct diagnosis and appropriate choice of treatment.

Unstructured clinical interviews are favored by most clinicians. The format in these is not prescribed, so the clinician is free to formulate his questions as he wishes and to introduce them in any order. This flexibility enables clinicians to assess continuously and, if necessary, to modify the nature of their interactions with patients in response to their conscious and unconscious verbal and nonverbal behavior. The clinicians can intuitively decide the most likely persona to adopt to elicit a particular patient's trust, taking into account such factors as his or her sex, age, appearance, dress, socioeconomic background, intelligence, vocabulary, level of education, ethnic origin, and moral, ethical, and sexual attitudes and values. Little research has been carried out on this aspect of the interview, but it would appear that clinicians adopt markedly different practices, presumably having learned which are most effective for them in obtaining and maintaining a working relationship with their patients. Some modify their personalities much more than others, changing their vocabulary, assertiveness, and apparent ethical value structure and social status to become the person they believe the patient would relate to best. As the interview progresses, if the patient shows signs of guilt, embarrassment, or reluctance to talk when particular topics are introduced, the clinician can respond with encouragement and support and thus elicit crucial information that may not be obtained with more structured interviews or assessment procedures (e.g., questionnaires). Patients are unlikely to reveal sensitive information unless the relationship established by the clinician is such that they are confident that it will not be disclosed, deliberately or inadvertently, without their permission.

The directivity of the interview is another aspect that can be continuously modi-

1

fied by the clinician to elicit information not easily obtained with more structured assessments. My practice in this respect is to commence nondirectively, adopting a listening approach and asking a minimum of questions in order to encourage the patient to take charge of the interview. The extent to which he or she does so allows his or her confidence, assertiveness, and dominance to be assessed, so that an initial hypothesis can be formulated as to the nature of his or her personality. As the interview progresses, I remain ready to become directive once the patient ceases to provide information that sheds further light on his or her condition or personality. Taking over direction of the interview must be done in such a way as not to threaten or antagonize assertive patients, or to allow obsessional or suspicious patients (who commonly provide excess detail) to believe the clinician is not concerned with information they consider highly relevant.

I usually begin the interview by asking the patient the nature of the problem for which he or she is seeking treatment. In asking and following up on this question, I attempt to discover not only details of the patient's complaint including its duration, but also why he or she sought treatment at the particular time. Reasons could include pressure from a partner or close contacts, or legal requirements. A woman seeking treatment to become orgasmic in sexual activity might with appropriate questioning (possibly requiring the presence of her partner) reveal that it is the partner who is distressed at her not reaching orgasms when they make love, as he finds this incompatible with his concept of himself as a lover. Discovering the reasons for patients' attendance commonly provides the initial information with which to assess their conscious and unconscious motivation for treatment. To maintain a somewhat nondirective approach, I initially respond only as much as is needed to maintain the flow of information within reasonable limits of relevance. Having determined how the patient has reacted to being given the opportunity to control the interview, I usually need to become more directive in order to obtain the information I consider relevant, using a fairly standard interview structure. Having obtained the required information about the presenting symptoms, I next inquire concerning any past history of similar problems, other illnesses, childhood and adolescent relationships with parents and siblings, social and sexual relationships, educational and work experiences, and current domestic, social, sexual, and occupational situations, including the nature and extent of recreational interests and activities.

Within a few minutes of initiating the interview, I find I have usually formulated hypotheses concerning the nature of the patient's condition and personality and, in the light of these two factors, the treatment most likely to be effective. The rest of the interview is then used to obtain data to support or reject these hypotheses, while establishing a relationship with the patient that will ensure as far as possible his or her acceptance and continued compliance with the treatment plan finally selected. I have found that the personality features most important to detect in relation to patients' responses to treatment are those indicative of psychopathy, borderline personality, and inadequate dependency.

Psychopathy is more prevalent in male patients. Its presence is suggested early in the interview by the patient's air of confidence. He may, without requesting permission, begin using the first name of the interviewer. Provided the interviewer maintains a neutral attitude, he will usually show little evidence of ethical concern or empathy concerning the effects of his behavior or sexual problems on others, particularly those emotionally involved with him. Directive questioning will reveal frequent truancy in childhood and adolescence and occasional substance abuse or other delinquent behaviors. His subsequent record of educational, occupational, social, and sexual activities demonstrates an ability to form relationships and impress others with his qualities, but an inability to persist once the activities or relationships become demanding or boring. Patients with psychopathic traits are likely to distort their accounts of their behavior (perhaps largely unconscious), minimizing features that show them in a bad light. Their compliance with treatment is likely to be poor, often demonstrated by inconsistency in keeping appointments. Nevertheless if they can be maintained in treatment, this will at times benefit both them and society—for example, as is not uncommonly the case when they report sex offenses (Chapter 8). Therefore external constraints, such as the use of probation, should be employed to maintain their cooperation where possible. When attempting to motivate such patients to become involved in therapy, its advantages to them in increasing their life satisfaction or avoiding unpleasant social consequences or incarceration should be stressed. Little is gained by attempting, at least directly, to increase their ethical values or their awareness of the distress they are causing others. Though they will be likely to respond appropriately verbally, this usually means that their dishonesty, even toward themselves, has been increased, and they will be less likely to inform the therapist of any behavioral lapses (of which they now know he or she disapproves). A therapeutic attitude of ethical neutrality makes it more likely that such patients will be truthful.

Borderline personality disorder is more likely to be shown by women. It also is commonly manifested in childhood and adolescence by truancy, substance abuse, other delinquent behaviors, and/or the initiation of sexual relationships that the subject experiences as destructive because of their transience, association with aggression, and/or resulting in pregnancy. Subjects with this personality are more likely to report being victims of incest (Chapter 6). Suicide attempts or self-mutilative acts such as cutting arms or legs are frequently repeated, consistent with the low self-esteem basic to subjects with this personality. In the interview, they are likely to present in a manner that can elicit overinvolvement from the less experienced therapist. This manner may be an initial apathy and withdrawal that the therapist feels challenged to overcome; a distressed recital of overwhelmingly tragic life-events; a report of impulses to carry out aggressive or sexual attacks on children, or an implication or claim that they have done so; or a response of intense gratitude, possibly tinged with sexual seductiveness, that for the first time in their lives they have encountered someone who is really concerned for them, who truly understands them, and to whom they have revealed information they have told no one else. Treatment of these patients is likely to be long and involved, often with an initial honeymoon period (when they appear to respond and their relationship to the therapist is positive) followed by relapse and requests for more time and attention.

This second stage may prove threatening to a therapist who has become overinvolved in response to the patients' mode of presentation and so initially gave them a great deal of attention and time. The therapist may now feel disappointed and not certain about how to continue. It is important for the therapist to recognize the possibility of this outcome and not respond with rejection (as a result of conscious or unconscious anger) if the patient now becomes critical and hostile at what she claims is the therapist's indifference. Refusal to continue to treat the patient on the grounds that she is not adequately motivated or is not likely to respond will reinforce a borderline patient's belief, based on the relationships she has previously experienced, that she is not capable or worthy of establishing a long-term relationship in which she is respected. A therapist accepting a borderline patient for treatment should immediately inform the patient that he or she will continue to provide treatment for as long as is necessary and define the amount of time he or she can give to this, so that there is no danger of giving more time in the initial stages of treatment than can be maintained indefinitely. This enables the therapist to continue to see the patient, irrespective of his or her behavior, within the limits established at the commencement of therapy. To continue to receive the interest and concern of a person they grow to respect and admire appears the major factor in the borderline patient gaining self-esteem. In view of the disturbingly high frequency with which therapists become sexually involved with patients, it is important that the therapist is aware that this response—which will totally undermine the aims of therapy—is most likely to occur with patients with borderline personalities (Gutheil, 1989).

Inadequate dependent personality results either from an inability to tolerate the anxiety and depression that is inevitable in response to the stressful events of life or from a tendency to react to such events with above-average levels of these emotions. It will be suggested in the interview by the patient's lack of confidence and evident anxiety or depression, and supported by evidence of his or her past inability to cope with the stresses of education, employment, and emotional relationships. People with this personality will have performed poorly at school, as they found examinations stressful and often avoided them. They are likely to have had several jobs, feeling forced to leave each as they encountered difficulties. Similarly, they are likely to have had several relationships, possibly until they became involved with an emotionally very supportive person or one who preferred to be involved with a dependent person. They commonly develop symptoms of illnesses that encourage such partners to remain supportive while enabling themselves to avoid stressful situations. To help these patients, the therapist will need to cater to their need for support while, without excessive optimism, encouraging them to become less dependent. Attempts should be made to engage them in activities that they enjoy and will require them to become independent of others. Their partners and friends need to be educated to gradually cease rewarding the patient's illness behaviors and begin rewarding healthy behaviors through encouragement and praise.

When it is suspected that patients have a significant personality disorder, it is imperative that attempts be made to corroborate their history by interviewing rela-tives and contacts. It is not unusual for psychopathic and borderline patients to try to prevent this by saying, for example, that they dislike their relatives too much to allow any contact. If confirmation is considered sufficiently important, it may be necessary to make treatment conditional on the patient's giving permission for such contacts. My reason for stressing the importance of personality evaluation in the assessment of sexual problems is that, in my experience, personality traits are now the major obstacle to successful treatment. Since the 1960s, the development of treatment techniques (particularly behavioral techniques) for most problems has advanced sufficiently that almost all patients who are appropriately motivated can benefit significantly from their application.

Throughout the interview, therapists must remain aware that in addition to collecting information, they are establishing the patient's confidence in their ability. At its termination, the patient should not leave feeling he or she has been asked a lot of questions or allowed to talk freely but has been given no answers. He or she should have been presented with either a treatment plan or a satisfactory explanation as to why further information is necessary before this can be done. When a treatment plan is proposed, the therapist should ensure that the patient is fully aware of what it entails and why it, rather than an alternative, has been selected. Any reservations the patient has concerning the plan should be fully dealt with so that, at termination of the interview, he or she commits either to accepting it or to making a decision within the next week (possibly in consultation with the person who referred them) that he or she will communicate to the therapist.

UNSTRUCTURED VERSUS STRUCTURED CLINICAL INTERVIEWS: RELIABILITY AND VALIDITY OF DIAGNOSES

The accuracy of the information obtained in an unstructured clinical interview depends on the ability of the clinician to assess correctly to what extent the patient's self-report can be accepted without modification and to what extent it should be regarded as distorted and in need of further confirmation. Determination of the patient's personality is of value in this regard. Patients who are seeking attention are likely to exaggerate their symptoms, those with antisocial personalities may lie concerning them, and those who are depressed (or have the high ethical standards commonly associated with obsessional features) may present them in a somewhat negative light. Though clinicians may feel confident of their ability to utilize the clinical interview to obtain information that is at least sufficiently accurate for them to treat their patients effectively, little research has been carried out to demonstrate this. Furthermore, in their own practice, clinicians tend to modify the diagnostic categories they were taught to use during their apprenticeship with their teachers. This tendency for the diagnoses of clinicians to be somewhat idiosyncratic probably does not significantly alter the type of treatment all but a few patients receive. In the few where it does, however, the clinician will believe the treatment indicated by his or her diagnosis will be more effective than the alternative treatment his colleagues making a different diagnosis would use. Again virtually no research has been carried out to justify this belief, though in my experience, if clinicians are asked to identify colleagues who have much higher than average diagnostic and treatment skills, they tend to nominate the same few people.

The increase in the number of psychiatric and psychological academics in the last few decades has been reflected in a major increase in their political power relative to that of the previously dominant clinicians. This change in the balance of power was accomplished in part by the academics critically examining and then replacing the diagnostic practices of clinicians with their own techniques. When this examination was undertaken, the question of scientific value should have been obvious: What effect do differing diagnostic practices of clinicians have on the outcomes of their patients? The answer would have provided information of practical value to clinicians while meeting the need of academics to investigate what they term the *validity* of diagnoses, or the degree to which diagnoses correctly identify the conditions from which patients suffer. In practice, the validity of most psychiatric diagnoses is impossible to establish with certainty. Unlike cancer or heart disease, where the patient's organs can be examined to determine the diagnosis, there are as yet no similar criteria to identify most psychiatric conditions. *Treatment validity* (the degree to which the diagnostic practices are associated with better treatment outcomes), however, can be assessed for psychiatric patients through a well-planned study involving the long-term follow-up of a sufficient number of patients diagnosed by different clinicians.

This truly useful research aim was largely ignored by academics. Instead, they took the easy option of investigating the reliability of clinicians' diagnoses. The *reliability* of a diagnosis is the extent to which it is consistent (i.e., the extent to which when a patient is assessed, the same diagnosis would be made by different persons, or by the same person on different occasions). Research investigating reliability merely requires investigating the level of agreement between the diagnoses made independently by two clinicians on the same group of subjects. Studies in the 1950s and 1960s revealed that this level of agreement varied from 49% to 63% for specific diagnoses (Matarazzo, 1983). Many patients given different diagnoses by different clinicians may receive the same treatment, however, so lack of reliability of diagnoses may have little clinical significance. The academics who carried out these studies did not investigate the treatment implications of the diagnoses, but concluded that this level of reliability was unacceptably low. The conclusion produced an area of research in which academics could dominate psychiatric practice: the development of assessment procedures that would have high reliability.

Concentrating on improving the reliability of an assessment procedure without incorporating safeguards to maintain its validity may impede the growth of scientific knowledge. It can be caricatured by the suggestion that schizophrenia be diagnosed in all male patients above and none below 1.8 meters (5 feet 10 inches) in height. Clearly this diagnosis would be totally reliable; used by two diagnosticians, it would diagnose the same patients with certainty. Its validity, however, would be negligible. Yet the technique advanced by academics and currently adopted widely to replace diagnosis by unstructured clinical interview in psychiatry may have produced a situation approaching the one caricatured. The technique was the development, first, of a structured interview with which all interviewers asked the same questions in the same order and manner, and second, of a set of diagnostic criteria for each psychiatric condition to apply to the patient's responses to the structured interview. The diagnostic criteria were defined sufficiently clearly that different interviewers would experience no uncertainty as to whether they were present or absent in a particular patient. Diagnoses resulting from the use of this procedure were termed *operational* diagnoses, as each operation involved in reaching the diagnosis was defined in a manner that aimed to be totally objective, requiring no judgment from the diagnosticians that could be influenced by their subjectivity. Such diagnoses should therefore be totally reliable, and indeed they are when the same structured interview is used with the same diagnostic criteria.

Two operatively defined assessment procedures have been widely used in the 1980s to diagnose patients with psychological disorders. One, developed in the United States, was the structured interview termed the Diagnostic Interview Schedule (DIS; Robins, Helzer, Croughan, & Ratcliff, 1981) to be used with the diagnostic criteria specified by the third edition of the *Diagnostic and Statistical Manual of Mental Disorders* (DSM-III; American Psychiatric Association [APA], 1980); the latter criteria have since been revised (DSM-III-R; APA, 1987). The other procedure, developed in England, was the Present State Examination (PSE), the information from which was analyzed by the CATEGO computer program (Wing & Sturt, 1978). A later study investigated the reliability of diagnoses made by the two systems (van den Brink et al., 1989). The PSE was modified so that the same interview could be used to obtain both DSM-III and CATEGO diagnoses for 175 nonpsychotic, nonaddicted psychiatric outpatients; agreement between the diagnoses made by the two systems was 58% for cases of depression and 46% for cases of anxiety. That is to say, the reliability of the diagnoses made by the two systems was of the same order as that of the unstructured clinical diagnoses by different clinicians that they were developed to replace.

An attempt was made to investigate one aspect of the validity of operational diagnoses by comparing them with more traditional psychiatric diagnoses in a population sample of 370 subjects (Helzer et al., 1985). The subjects were first interviewed by trained laypersons using the DIS and subsequently by psychiatrists who were unaware of the subjects' responses to the initial interview. The psychiatrists also used the DIS interview but were free to pursue clinical hunches and follow up on leads in an unstructured fashion. Subjects' responses to both procedures were examined to determine if they conformed to the DSM-III-R diagnostic criteria. The number of subjects whom the psychiatrists considered as having a condition diagnosed as present by the lay-administered DIS varied from a low of 3 of 29 subjects (10%) diagnosed as having obsessive compulsive disorder to a high of 42 of 57 (74%) diagnosed as having major depression. For most diagnoses, the agreement was between 40% and 50%. This low level of agreement is likely to have been significantly greater than the agreement that would have been found between lay-administered DIS diagnoses (assessed by DSM-III criteria) and the diagnoses reached by psychiatrists using totally unstructured clinical interviews, had this been investigated. It is possible that operational diagnostic procedures have sacrificed a significant degree of the validity of unstructured clinical diagnoses without obtaining a higher degree of reliability between different operational procedures. Until the treatment validity of operational and clinical diagnoses is investigated, this cannot be determined.

A further problem with operational diagnoses is that they exclude a percentage of patients as not able to be diagnosed. Matarazzo (1983), in his review of psychiatric and psychological diagnosis, praised a 1977 study of the reliability of operational diagnostic criteria as destined to become a classic. Of the 101 patients in the study, all of whom were first admitted to a medical school psychiatric service, 18% were unable to be diagnosed. In the comparison study of the PSE and DIS/DSM-III assessments discussed (van den Brink et al., 1989), all 175 outpatients had been referred by their general practitioner or medical specialist, and 80% had complaints of 6 months or longer duration. Fifty-five (31%) were unable to be diagnosed as having a current mental disorder by the PSE, 23 (13%) by the DIS/DSM-III, and 17 (10%) by both. Patients who fail to receive a diagnosis of course pose no problem in a research study, as they can be excluded; this option is not available to clinicians.

Clearly these findings do not encourage clinicians to replace their unstructured clinical interviews with structured ones. Without providing demonstrable advantages, the latter would reduce their ability to assess their subjects and reach diagnoses that they consider correct. It would prevent their using the interview flexibly to investigate the patient's personality and motivation, while establishing a relationship which would maximize the patient's likelihood of remaining in and complying with treatment. Although clinicians in the private sector need to maintain patients in treatment and produce a successful outcome at least to a comparable extent to their colleagues to retain their practice, academics and researchers have other priorities. The necessity for publication requires the latter to adopt the research methodology considered at the time to be the most appropriate; currently, this includes assessment by operational diagnosis. Because of the reliability of one particular system, the use of that system in a series of studies enables results to be compared with confidence that the subjects given a particular diagnosis in different studies are truly comparable. Some patients may not be prepared to become involved in a study when assessed by the rigid procedure of the structured interview. This could be an advantage to the researcher; such subjects are likely to be those with more "difficult" personalities who could be expected to be less compliant with and to respond less well to treatment, particularly if it is administered with the lack of flexibility required by many studies. A possible further factor encouraging the use of structured interviews and operational diagnoses is the near monopoly obtained by a few systems. This provides not only the enormous prestige of determining the psychiatric diagnoses used by academics virtually worldwide, but also the financial rewards resulting from the production of the required publications and software and their regular revisions.

The political struggle between clinicians and academics is rarely conducted openly. Currently it is being extended from the evaluation of clinicians' diagnoses to their treatment practices and may prove more effective in forcing clinicians to accept the practices of academics, as these will have demonstrated to be effective in research studies. The fact that these studies investigated the treatment of the mainly public-sector patients available to academics, and hence may not be relevant to the treatment of the private-sector patients treated by many clinicians, is likely to be disregarded. In addition, academics are increasingly dominating the training programs for clinicians. A possible consequence will be the reduction or abandonment of the apprenticeship system whereby the trainee was supervised by the clinician, and which enabled the practice of the unstructured interview to be transmitted from one generation of practitioners to the next.

BEHAVIORAL ASSESSMENT VERSUS SELF-REPORT: THE INFLUENCE OF BEHAVIORISM

In addition to the academic disquiet concerning reliability of diagnoses based on unstructured interviews, an independent dissatisfaction was expressed in the 1960s concerning the assessment of behavior using subjects' self-reports. This resulted from the introduction into psychological and psychiatric treatment of behavior modification, with its accompanying ideology. Behavior modification, developed largely in the United States, applied methods derived from the behaviorist theory of learning, which until that time had been largely restricted to the study of behavior in the psychology laboratory. In his monograph *Behavior,* Watson (1914), the originator of behaviorism, commenced the devaluation of subjects' reports of their urges and feelings as a useful source of information by advancing the belief that thoughts were implicit behaviors and that "the larynx and the tongue, we believe, are the loci of most of the phenomena" (p. 20). In his later monograph *Behaviorism* (Watson, 1925), a chapter heading read, "Do we always think in words . . . or does our whole body do the thinking?" Skinner (1966) followed this approach, criticizing those models that treated behavior as "the sign or symptom of inner activities, mental or physiological, which are regarded as the principal subject matter" (p. 213). He opposed research that was designed to test physiological, mentalistic, or conceptual hypotheses about behavior in favor of research that, without any theory, examined the frequency with which behaviors were carried out under the influence of rewards and punishments.

When behaviorism was applied to the assessment and treatment of human subjects, the emphasis put on the study of subjects' overt behaviors, rather than their mental activity, meant that information provided by self-report was regarded as of dubious value (Linehan, 1977). The aim was that subjects' self-reports should be replaced by behavioral assessments. Where possible, methods were developed to observe directly and quantify subjects' behaviors. The uncritical acceptance of such methods was evidenced by the immediate and widespread utilization in psychology departments throughout the United States of one of the earliest to be developed, the Behavior Avoidance Test (BAT). The BAT was introduced to assess snake-phobic behavior in students before and following behavioral treatment (Lang & Lazovik, 1963). The subject was requested to approach and, if possible, touch and then hold a 5-foot black snake confined in a glass case, after having seen the experimenter do so and having been assured the snake was harmless. The apparent or face validity of such a test was sufficiently powerful that its clinical significance remained unquestioned for many years until a revision occurred in the behaviorist devaluation of mental processes.

Cognitive Behavior Therapy and Self-Report

Although behaviorism in the form of behavior modification dominated the application of learning principles to treat psychological and psychiatric conditions in the United States, an alternative application was developed (largely outside the United States) that maintained the approach criticized by Skinner (1966). This alternative approach treated behavior as "the sign or symptom of inner activities, mental or physiological, which are regarded as the principal subject matter." Theories that adopt this viewpoint are termed *cognitive;* they may be physiologically oriented (when they study the brain activity related to cognitive processes) or mentalistic (when they do not). The application of the cognitive learning approach to treatment that developed outside the United States in the 1950s and 1960s was commonly termed *behavior therapy* to distinguish it from behavior modification. Behavior therapy was based on the theory of higher nervous activity developed by Pavlov (1927) from his discovery of what have been termed conditioned reflexes.

Pavlov was a physiologist with an interest in how organisms adapt to their environment. One such adaptation he studied was that of the saliva dogs produced in response to different substances put in their mouths. He found it differed, in chemical composition or degree of wateriness, to digest different foods better or to expel nonfoods, such as sand or pebbles. In the course of these studies, he noticed that the dogs salivated when they heard the sound of the food tray, before they received any food. He realized that this reflex salivation to the sound stimulus was a learned response. As it occurred conditional to the sound being followed by food, Pavlov termed it a *conditional reflex,* and the sound a *conditional stimulus.* Since food placed in the dog's mouth produced salivation unconditionally, he termed salivation to food an *unconditional reflex,* and food an *unconditional stimulus.* Administering an unconditional stimulus after a conditional stimulus (e.g., food after a sound) he termed *reinforcement* of the conditional stimulus. Other unconditional stimuli apart from food include painful stimuli (which, when administered to a limb, unconditionally produce the response of limb withdrawal) and sexual stimuli (which unconditionally produce the response of genital arousal). These responses will also be produced to conditional stimuli if the conditional stimuli are reinforced by unconditional stimuli, just as salivation was produced to the conditional stimulus of the sound of the food trays by reinforcement in the form of food. A simplified depiction of the procedure is shown in Figure 1.1.

The common use of *conditioned reflex* instead of *conditional reflex* in English indicates the interest in the English-speaking world in the use of these reflexes to "condition" or control behavior rather than understand it. Behaviorists adopted the term as *operant conditioning* to describe the technique they employed of rewarding or punishing behaviors. Behaviors that were rewarded (or "reinforced") were carried out more frequently; those that were not rewarded or were punished were carried out less frequently. Pavlov as a physiologist was interested in using conditional reflexes not to control behavior, but to study the brain activity associated with the cognitive processes whereby the organism learns to adapt to the environment. By investigating the changes in conditional reflexes in response to different strengths and types of

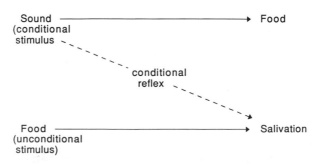

FIG. 1.1. Formation of conditional response of salivation to a sound.

unconditional stimuli used to reinforce or to cease reinforcing conditional stimuli, he advanced a theory of what he termed "higher nervous activity." His research provided evidence that cognitive activity resulted from the interactions of excitatory and inhibitory impulses in the brain brought about by conditional and unconditional stimuli. Just as the physiology of the alimentary tract adjusted its secretions to adapt to different foods or to damaging substances, so the higher nervous or brain activity adjusted behavior to adapt to different conditional stimuli that preceded and therefore predicted the arrival of unconditional stimuli. Prediction of the occurrence of unconditional stimuli (e.g., food, or painful or sexual stimuli), knowledge of which is important for the animal's survival, enabled it to take appropriate advance action, thereby increasing its chance of survival.

> In response to an unlimited number of stimuli there can be brought about in the cerebral hemispheres an activity which serves to signal the approach of the comparatively small number of agencies which are of vital importance to the organism in a favourable or an injurious sense. It is through the hemispheres that corresponding reactions are brought about, thus anticipating the actual contact or clash of the organism with those agencies. (Pavlov, 1927, p. 172)

Behavior therapy based on Pavlovian theory developed a range of inhibitory and excitatory techniques, such as the use of relaxation to inhibit fear, aversive stimuli to inhibit compulsive behaviors, or sexual stimuli to increase sexual responses, discussed here in relation to the treatment of sexual dysfunctions (Chapter 5) and minority sexual practices (Chapter 8). These techniques differed fundamentally from the operant conditioning technique of increasing or decreasing the frequency of behaviors by administering or withdrawing rewards, which was the basis of behavior modification. Clinicians who adopted a behavior therapy approach accepted the importance of mental activity and hence were prepared to use the self-reports of their patients as an important part of assessment. Most of these clinicians, however, did not adopt an ideological commitment equivalent to that of behaviorists in the United States, whose intense commitment may have resulted from the close association of their ideology with the concept, basic to capitalism, that human behavior is totally determined by rewards and punishments, and that all persons are equal. All may therefore proceed from log cabin to White House if they are exposed to the appropriate program of rewards (McConaghy, 1977a).

Most clinicians employing behavior therapy showed little interests in ideological issues. Also, unlike behaviorists, in treating patients they did not restrict themselves to the use of behavioral therapies only, but added them to the treatments they were already using in their professional practice. Nevertheless, ideological differences between behavior therapy and modification, though not spelled out, were sufficient to result in the more academic adherents of each adopting opposing research methodologies. Behavioral therapists used group designs, that is, designs developed to compare the behavior of groups of subjects, whereas behaviorists used single-case designs developed to investigate the behavior of individual subjects.

The Cognitive Reaction: Self-Report Rehabilitated

The interaction of practitioners of behavior modification and behavior therapy may have been in part responsible for the return by most practitioners of behavior modification to the commonsense awareness that cognitive factors influence observed behaviors. Commonly referred to as the "cognitive revolution" (Mahoney, 1977), this resulted in an acceptance of the usefulness of subjects' self-reports and abandonment of the assumption that behavioral assessments were inevitably superior. The role of cognitive factors in these assessments was subjected to investigation. Commenting on a finding that fearful men but not women approached a feared object, Hersen (1973) raised the possibility that when observed in laboratory situations, men felt under more pressure than women to behave in a socially desirable way. Subsequently, Lick and Unger (1977) cited evidence that subjects who showed behavior indicative of reduced fear in a laboratory test continued to behave fearfully in their natural environment. There, self-reports of their levels of fear better predicted their behavior than did the laboratory behavioral assessments. Lick and Unger also criticized role-play behavioral tests of subjects' anxiety in social situations with a person of the opposite sex, on the basis that the test situation provided only a limited range of the social situations the subjects encountered in real life. Bellack, Hersen, and Lamparaski (1979) subsequently reported poor predictability using one such test.

The original objection to clinical assessment of subjects by self-reports was to their low level of reliability, which led to questioning of their validity. When behavioral assessments were introduced, their low levels of validity was accepted without criticism:

> Concurrent validity of the behavioral ratings ranges from fair to good when compared to other behavioral ratings and observational data. For instance Lentz, Paul, and Calhoun reported correlations between .51 and .54 between the Minimal Social Behavior Scale and staff behavioral ratings. Mariott and Paul report substantial concurrent validity [no figure given] for the Inpatient Multidimensional Psychiatric Scale. (Linehan, 1977, p. 46)

Correlations of 0.51 and 0.54 mean that the scale is accounting for about 25% of the variance of the behavior validating it.

Nelson and Hayes (1981) pointed out the lack of evidence for the acclaimed relationship between behavioral assessment and improved treatment and argued that assessment decisions must be tested with data, not just logic. They continued that it could probably be said that any assessment device claiming to have applied value should be considered unproven until its treatment validity is experimentally demonstrated, and that by this standard, the applied value of virtually all of behavioral assessment is still unproven. Bellack and Hersen (1985) commented that behaviorists seem to have made a 180-degree turn on the issue of reliance on the veracity of the patient's self-report, once so hotly debated as anathema to the principles of behaviorism. More recently, they concluded (Bellack & Hersen, 1988) that the preeminence of behavioral observation is no longer accepted, and that it is now not reasonable to contrast behavioral and nonbehavioral assessment in an either-or, good-bad manner.

Despite pointing out the lack of evidence that behavioral assessments improved treatment outcome, Nelson and Hayes (1981) still believed they should be used by clinicians. Their reaction to a finding they cited—that almost half of practicing behavior therapists considered such assessments impractical in applied settings—was to recommend that forms of behavioral assessment be developed for the use of clinicians to encourage them to participate in clinical research. The alternative suggestion (that clinical assessment based on unstructured interviews should be compared with other forms of assessment to determine which is associated with a better response to treatment) does not appear to have been advanced. Addition of behavioral assessment is likely to add to the length and cost of treatment, and it may result in greater patient dropout. Appel, Saab, and Holroyd (1985) found that patient noncompliance increased with the complexity, duration, and cost of therapy. Clearly, if behavioral assessments are shown to improve outcomes of treatment, they must be used. Until this is shown, however, it would seem reasonable to consider that clinicians' judgments could be correct concerning the value of unstructured interview assessment.

It is noteworthy that several of the academic clinicians who contributed to a recent U.S. handbook of clinical behavior therapy stated that the clinical interview was their basic assessment technique, with some adding that psychophysiological assessment and formalized pretreatment behavioral avoidance measures were not useful or economically viable (McConaghy, 1988a). It would appear that a similar situation existed even when the commitment of behavior therapists to objective assessment was at its height. Swan and MacDonald (1978) cited a 1972 study that found a minimal relationship between clinical and laboratory methods in the assessment practices of 30 behavior therapy leaders. Their own survey of practicing behavior therapists also revealed a minimal relationship between the assessment techniques used by the therapists and those used in research. An additional finding of interest was that the most common intervention, employed by 58% of the therapists, was use of therapeutic relationship-enhancing methods; operant methods, the next most common, were employed by 50%.

Self-Report by Questionnaire and Rating Scale

Though a number of behaviorally oriented researchers and academics have accepted that patients' self-reports are sufficiently valid in comparison to observational or physiological data, some have preferred that the self-reports are elicited by structured rather than unstructured interviews, or by rating scales or questionnaires. Presumably this reflects the current desire of researchers to increase the reliability of assessment; increased reliability should result as structured interviews or rating scales restrict the information collected to similar areas for all subjects. There is evidence, however, that this restriction may reduce the validity obtained with unstructured interviews. A series of studies showed that psychiatrists' global assessment of patients' clinical responses based on unstructured interviews proved highly valid in comparison to that obtained by psychological tests, rating scales, and physiological measures in determining which patients had received either active treatment or placebo (Lipman, Cole, Park, & Rickels, 1965; Paredes, Baumgold, Pugh, & Ragland, 1966). Paredes et al. pointed out that in making global assessments in unstructured interviews, clinicians were sensitive to a multitude of factors. When they were limited to rating behavior on scales, they narrowed their perspective, reducing their ability to make valid intuitive judgments. A similar narrowing of perspective may occur with patients' assessments of their own responses. Women reported increased satisfaction in their sexual relationship by global assessment but decreased satisfaction when specific activities were measured by the Sexual Interaction Inventory (De Amicis, Goldberg, LoPiccolo, Friedman, & Davies, 1985).

An additional appeal to researchers of rating scale and questionnaire assessments of response to treatment is that they are usually quantified to produce a large range of scores suitable for statistical analysis, as compared with the limited range of "much improved," "somewhat improved," "no change," and "worse" usually employed in global clinical assessments. The increased range of rating scale assessments can be misleading, as a clinically trivial degree of improvement can result in a large change on the scale score. Also, if rating scales are completed by the subjects and objectively scored, it is often accepted that the resulting scores could not have been influenced by the researchers. This may not be the case. Following treatment, some patients, suspecting or knowing their self-reports of their degree of improvement will be seen by the therapist, may consciously or unconsciously distort these in a positive or negative direction, depending on their feelings toward the therapist and the degree to which, in their contacts with the therapist, the latter appeared influenced by their reports of improvement or deterioration. Enthusiastic, charismatic therapists thus could unconsciously produce major biases in their patients' self-reports. Some scales are much more reactive to such biases than others. Patients will show marked reduction in scores with minor degrees of improvement on such pencil-and-paper assessments as neuroticism questionnaires that require them to assess their degree of tension, anxiety, nervousness, and so forth on a series of scales scored from 1 to 4. Self-reports of the degree of change in their sexual behaviors are likely to reflect this much more precisely and so be less reactive to other influences.

Bias in patients' self-reports of response is likely to be maximal during or immediately following treatment, when their hopes of responding are high and they have not had sufficient time to access accurately the degree of change in their feelings and behaviors. This was shown to be the case with subjects who received 14 sessions (administered over a 5-day period) of one or other of two therapies for sexually unacceptable behaviors (McConaghy, Armstrong, & Blaszczynski, 1985). Patients completed rating scales of their expectancy of improvement and of the degree of reduction of the deviant sexual urge experienced at the end of the 1st, 8th, and 14th sessions of treatment and at 1 month and 1 year following treatment. The reported reductions in urge correlated very highly with the expectancies of response immediately following termination of treatment ($r = 0.93$ and 0.96), but significantly less so after 1 month and after 1 year. It would seem unwise to rely solely on reports of response at termination of treatment without follow-up data.

Methodological features of studies may also influence self-reports. AuBuchon and Calhoun (1985) asked 18 women to record their moods on a 16-item adjective checklist twice weekly for 8 weeks. Nine were randomly selected and informed that the study was investigating a possible relationship of mood to their menstrual cycles. Their self-report scales demonstrated a negative relationship; the scales of those not so informed did not. The authors attributed the relationship found to the social expectancy and demand characteristics resulting from the information. Patients' self-reports of their behaviors can themselves produce changes in the behaviors (LoPiccolo & Steger, 1974). These authors suggested that such changes were responsible for reducing the test-retest reliability correlations of couples' scores on a Sexual Interaction Inventory. The initial completion of the inventory would have drawn the couples' attention to the nature of their sexual interactions, and could have motivated them to change it before they completed the inventory for a second time. The possibility of such reactivity in self-reports of behavior requires control if they are to be used to assess changes in treatment. One method is to administer the inventory on a number of occasions prior to initiation of treatment until the subjects' responses stabilize. It still remains possible that there will be an element of reactivity in self-assessments while the subjects continue to use them to monitor their behavior. When they cease to do so following the final assessment, this element of reactivity will cease to operate, and so their behavior may change. This final change will not be assessed; thus their true response to the treatment will not be determined.

Just as academics have shown considerable tolerance in regard to the variable degree of reliability and lack of evidence of validity of structured clinical and behavioral assessments compared to unstructured interview assessments, they have shown similar tolerance in regard to rating scales. Conte (1983), in his review of self-report scales for rating sexual function, found several to have test-retest reliabilities in the range of $r = 0.5$. Apart from this evidence of poor reliability, he pointed out the need for studies to establish their validity. In addition, most of the scales provided no measures of such important aspects of sexual function as the frequency of sexual behaviors or subjects' satisfaction with their current sexual functioning. A review of 51 objectively scored, mainly self-rated assessments of sexual function and marital interactions reported little evidence of their validity (Schiavi, Derogatis, Kuriansky, O'Connor, & Sharpe, 1979). When validity was referred to, it was usually described as adequate or as demonstrated by the test's ability to discriminate two groups of subjects, a weak criterion that can be achieved by tests that misclassify a number of individuals in the groups.

A rating scale method frequently used to assess sexual behaviors is to ask subjects to rate their frequency daily on diary cards. Its validity was found to be low, however, when investigated by an innovative method: Patients were asked to record on diary cards their home use of relaxation audiotapes. Their use of the tapes was independently monitored, without the patients' knowledge, by incorporation of electronic devices in the tape recorders with which they were provided (Taylor, Agras, Schneider, & Allen, 1983). Comparison of the diary cards and monitoring devices revealed that 32% of patients falsely reported their use of the tapes on the cards. Wincze, Bansal, and Malamud (1986) similarly found no difference between the responses of pedophilic sex offenders receiving placebo and of those taking the male sex hormone-reducing chemical medroxyprogesterone when their reduction in frequency of urges for sexual contacts with children was assessed by diary card ratings they made daily and submitted weekly. In contrast, sex offenders' global assessments of the degree of reduction in their deviant sexual urges, self-reported at interview, were validated by the high correlations found with the degree of reduction produced by medroxyprogesterone in their serum levels of testosterone (McConaghy, Blaszczynski, & Kidson, 1988). Both patients and interviewer were unaware of the testosterone levels at the time of the assessment.

In other circumstances, diary assessments have been shown to be valid. Udry and Morris (1967) asked black women to provide written reports concerning whether they had menstruated, had coitus, and/or experienced orgasm in the past 24 hours, paying them 50 cents a day to deliver the reports and to provide first-morning urine specimens for a 90-day period. There were very few missing specimens and reports. The urine samples were examined for morphologically intact sperm, with positive sperm sightings taken as evidence that coitus had occurred in the 48 hours prior to the urine being voided. In 12 of the 15 women in whom positive sperm sightings were made, these were concordant with their reports of coitus. Before such a method were used with other socioeconomic groups, though, it would need to be established that they would be equally compliant; the effect on their behavior of a monetary reward may not be equivalent. Differences in the subjects and the behaviors investigated may result in the same assessment procedure being valid in one study, but not in another.

Rating scales that assess a limited number of behaviors (Conte, 1983) have failed to demonstrate treatment responses. This need not matter when, in addition, clinical assessments are made and their findings are given significance. This was done in a study (Becker, Skinner, Abel, Axelrod, & Treacy, 1984) of female victims of rape and/or incestuous assaults. These workers used a sexual arousal inventory developed to discriminate sexually functional from dysfunctional subjects. It did not discriminate those who on clinical assessment reported no sexual problems from those who reported one or more problems related to the assault. The authors accepted the clinical assessment finding and concluded the inventory lacked discriminative capability. Failure to accept the significance of clinical assessment when it conflicted with that by rating scale led Birk, Huddleston, Miller, and Cohler (1971) to seriously misinterpret the findings of their study. They randomly allocated 8 men seeking to control homosexual behaviors to aversive conditioning and 8 others to a control procedure. On clinical interview assessment, 5 who received conditioning and none who received the control procedure reported marked reduction or absence of compulsive homosexual urges, feelings, and behaviors. This clinically assessed improvement in the group treated by conditioning remained significantly greater than that of the control group at 1 year after treatment. Because the results were obtained by clinical assessment, however, the authors termed them "anecdotal." The patients' responses based on Kinsey rating scales altered in a heterosexual direction to a significant extent at 2 months, but not at 1 year following treatment. These results were termed "statistical" and were given major significance as compared with the clinically reported responses.

I later showed in a series of studies assessing subjects both by their self-report and penile volume responses that aversive conditioning procedures reduced homosexual urges and behaviors experienced by the subjects as compulsive, but did not alter their sexual orientation (Chapter 8). The findings of Birk et al. were similar: Their treated subjects reported marked reductions in urges, but no significant change on Kinsey scale ratings of sexual orientation. By fixating on the rating scale change and neglecting the clinically assessed response, however, Birk et al. reported a negative outcome of the treatment. Their study, published in a major American psychiatric journal, may have contributed significantly to the subsequent decade or more of neglect by American psychiatrists of behavioral interventions for compulsive sexual behaviors (McConaghy, 1977b, 1988a).

Feldman and MacCulloch (1971) also failed to take the findings of global clinical assessment into account when interpreting rating scale assessment. Though they stated that the Sexual Orientation Method (SOM) scale they used was intended to complement the clinical interview, not supplant it, they reported only SOM scores. These scores encouraged them, like Birk et al. (1971) to accept the concept that aversive therapy could be expected to produce changes in patients' sexual orientation rather than an increase in their ability to control urges experienced as compulsive. Assessment by rating scale should not be relied upon until it is established that the scale validly measures the relevant outcome. Prior to this, global assessment by unstructured interview should also be used, as it is sensitive to all possible changes in the subjects' feelings or behaviors. Without this sensitivity, as in these two studies, the actual outcome of the therapy may not be detected.

In addition to problems of interpretation attributable to rating scales not detecting the relevant behavioral changes, problems can also arise from the scales being too sensitive. Jacobson, Follette, and Revenstorf (1984) considered this one of the factors contributing to the gap between academic research and clinical practice. They pointed out that most research evaluated the outcome of different treatments by statistical comparison of the arithmetical means of rating scale measures of the responses of a group of subjects. Such ratings provided no indication of the clinical significance of the responses. If a rating scale is very sensitive to changes in behavior, differences in the mean of the scores on that scale before and following treatment can be highly significant statistically, whereas the actual changes in behavior are of trivial significance. Jacobson et al. considered that clinical evaluations, such as the number of patients rated as improved, are at least as important as group means derived from rating scales. LoPiccolo and Steger (1974) introduced the Sexual Interaction Inventory rating scale with the aim of obtaining increased reliability of assessment by replacing clinicians' global impression of changes in patients' sexual behavior as "much improved," "improved," "somewhat improved," and "no change." Again, the danger was that reliability would be improved at the expense of meaningful clinical assessment, a danger these workers showed no awareness of and suggested no precautions to avoid.

In the last decade an additional statistical technique, meta-analysis, has been introduced into academic evaluative research. It enables the results of several studies to be combined to determine the degree to which they show a treatment effect. For the findings of studies to be suitable for meta-analysis as usually practiced, they need to report the subjects' responses in terms of mean scores and standard deviations. Though (as discussed subsequently) the technique has several weaknesses, it has provided an additional area of academic research and influence and is steadily growing in popularity. It is important to the careers of researchers that their studies are quoted in the scientific literature; they are therefore under pressure to use rating scale assessments that provide means and standard deviations in order to have their studies included in meta-analyses. They may see no necessity to also include assessments that enable the responses of the subjects to be meaningful to clinicians.

Structured interviews are unlikely to be useful in obtaining information concerning sexual behaviors from patients who are illiterate, schizophrenic, depressed, or brain damaged. Also, these patients are rarely able or motivated to complete self-rating scales or questionnaires. To establish and maintain a relationship with them in which useful information can be obtained requires the more flexible approach of the unstructured interview. This is particularly relevant to the assessment of sex offenders, a percentage of whom are intellectually impaired, brain damaged, or psychotic (Chapter 8). In selecting assessments it is also necessary to take into account the likelihood of compliance of subjects without these problems, some of whom, because of their level of education, social class or personality type, may not complete procedures requiring a high degree of motivation (e.g., a series of question-naires). Reading (1983) randomly allocated paid male volunteers to report details of their sexual behavior either by interview after 1 and 3 months (N = 21); by interview after 1, 2, and 3 months (N = 18); or by the latter procedure plus diary cards completed daily and returned every 3 days (N = 29). Thirty-four percent allocated to the last form of assessment discontinued it, as compared to 14% with the first and 16% with the second. Another three subjects dropped out from the diary card assessment prior to the first month, believing that it was causing them difficulty in maintaining their sexual potency. These findings—as well as those of Taylor et al. (1983) and Wincze et al. (1986) reported earlier, which demonstrated lack of validity of reports by diary cards—indicate that it cannot be assumed that structured self-reports provide superior assessments to those obtained by unstructured clinical inter-views. Whatever assessment measures are employed in research studies, it would seem that their validity should be demonstrated for the particular subjects being investigated.

OBSERVATIONAL ASSESSMENT

The intuitive interpretation of observations of subjects' nonverbal behavior plays a major role in assessment by unstructured clinical interview. Observations of sexual behaviors currently are reported rarely, though such assessment of coital sexual activity either directly or by videotape was briefly popular in the early 1970s (LoPic-colo, 1990). LoPiccolo believed there were convincing arguments against its con-tinued employment, including that the effect of observation on patients with sexual dysfunctions would make it unlikely that their observed behaviors would be similar to their private behaviors; that the procedure would be unacceptable to the majority of couples; and that it allowed the exploitation of patients by the therapist. These issues were certainly relevant to the "sexological exam," described by LoPiccolo, in which the therapist stimulated the breasts and genitals of the opposite-sex partner to assess and demonstrate physiological responsiveness. It would seem possible, how-ever, to provide adequate ethical safeguards for videotaped observational assessment of couples' sexual interactions. With allowance for the couples to adjust to the procedure, their observed behavior could be sufficiently related to their private be-havior to be of value. This is accepted to be the case with the observational assess-ment of nonsexual behaviors (e.g., phobias) and the laboratory assessment of physio-logical evidence of sexual arousal, both of which remain widely used. It is likely that taboos concerning sexuality remain the major obstacle to observational assessment of sexual activity; such assessment, of course, plays a major role in surrogate sex therapy. Observation of erections occurring during sleep or produced by masturbation remains recommended (Karacan, 1978; Wasserman, Pollak, Spielman, & Weitzman, 1980).

Maletzky (1980a) introduced an observational assessment of exhibitionists. A comely actress, unknown to the subjects, purposely placed herself in situations in which they had previously frequently offended. This was done at the end of their treatment and a year later; the subjects had been informed that experimental and unusual procedures would be employed. Observational assessments of effeminate behavior of boys have been made by therapists (Rekers & Lovaas, 1974), teachers (Kagan & Moss, 1962), and parents (Bates, Bentler, & Thompson, 1973). The therapists observed boys playing with boys' and girls' toys through a one-way mirror. The teachers and parents were requested to complete inventories reporting the effeminate behaviors shown by their pupils or sons. Observing and quantifying the effeminate behavior of adult males has also been reported but does not appear to have been widely used, possibly because of its complexity (Schatzberg, Westfall, Blumetti, & Birk, 1975).

PHYSIOLOGICAL ASSESSMENT

Penile Tumescence Measures

The most widely used physiological assessment of sexual behavior investigates subjects' penile circumference responses (PCRs) to measure their sexual arousal. For almost 20 years I have persisted with attempts to draw attention to the lack of evidence that PCR assessment of sexual arousal has sufficient validity to justify its use in many of the situations in which it is employed, in particular when highly sexually arousing stimuli are not used to elicit the PCRs and when subjects are assessed as individuals rather than as groups. My lack of success in these attempts indicated the need for a greater understanding of the factors involved in the politics of science. When a group of academics have produced a significant body of findings based on use of a particular assessment technique, evidence of its lack of validity will be ignored for as long as possible. A large number of studies have employed PCR assessment to reach conclusions of theoretical and practical significance. These include that bisexuality of feelings does not exist, that the use of PCR assessments to identify rapists and child molesters is scientifically and ethically acceptable, and that the behavioral techniques of aversive therapy and masturbatory reconditioning are of primary value in their treatment. This body of research will be rendered valueless when the limited validity of PCR assessment is finally accepted. The longer this is delayed, the less it will threaten the position of the academics involved, as their research will have joined the vast amount of past research, accurate and inaccurate, to which little attention is paid (as, with the passage of time, what is relevant is sifted out).

Assessment of Sexual Orientation

When PCR assessment was introduced, its validity was accepted without question. This was because it was identified with the assessment of subjects' sexual orientation from their penile volume response (PVRs) to pictures of nude men and women, the validity of which had been established. PVR assessment was introduced by Freund in Prague in the 1950s. The apparatus to measure penile volume developed by Freund was cumbersome; I introduced a simpler one (Figure 1.2) and a standard film assessment. In the film, 10-second segments of movie pictures (10 of nude men and 10 of nude women) were alternately inserted into a travelogue at 1-minute intervals. Changes in each subjects' PVRs from onset to termination of each segment were measured, and Mann-Whitney U-scores were calculated for each subject's responses. A U-score of 100, indicating exclusive heterosexuality, resulted if all 10 PVRs to pictures of women were greater than any of the 10 to men; a U-score of 0 indicated the reverse (exclusive homosexuality); and a U-score of 50, indicating exact bisexuality, was obtained if PVRs to men and women were equivalent. The range of scores from 50.5 to 100 indicated increasingly predominant heterosexuality, whereas from 49.5 to 0 indicated increasingly predominant homosexuality. A number of studies by Freund and myself and colleagues (summarized in Table 1.1) demonstrated that PVR assessment was able to identify a high percentage of men on the basis of their self-assessment as predominantly heterosexual or homosexual.

At the same time, as discussed in Chapter 4, a gauge placed round the shaft of the penis that measured penile circumference responses (PCRs) was introduced to assess the degree of erections of impotent men during sleep. It was assumed that PCRs and PVRs were equivalent and that the circumference gauge could be used, instead of

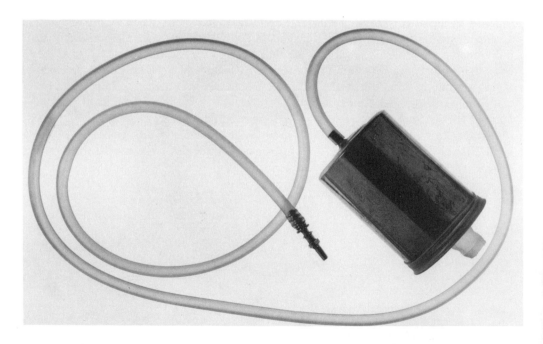

FIG. 1.2. Apparatus for measuring penile volume changes.

TABLE 1.1
Validity of Penile Volume Measures of Sexual Orientation

Homosexuality/heterosexuality

All of 65 heterosexuals classified correctly;
48 of 58 homosexuals classified correctly (Freund, 1963).

All of 11 self-reported exclusive heterosexuals classified as heterosexual;
17 of 22 men seeking treatment for compulsive homosexual feelings classified as predominantly homo-
    sexual (3 of 5 classified as predominantly heterosexual had said they were; McConaghy, 1967).

All of 18 self-reported heterosexual paraphiliacs classified as predominantly heterosexual (McConaghy,
    1976).

All of 19 self-reported predominantly heterosexual nuclear transvestites classified as predominantly
    heterosexual (Buhrich & McConaghy, 1977b)

All of 21 self-reported predominantly homosexual nuclear transsexuals classified as predominantly homo-
    sexual (Buhrich & McConaghy, 1978a).

Homosexuality/bisexuality/heterosexuality

Of 44 men seeking treatment for homosexuality:
    All 5 (100%) with PVR U-scores[a] of more than 77 had sexual intercourse with women;
    8 (50%) of 17 with PVR U-scores of 23 to 77 had sexual relations with women;
    7 (30%) of 22 with PVR U-scores of less than 23 had sexual relations with women (Barr & McConaghy,
        1971).

20 married homosexual men who reported sexual intercourse with women other than their wives obtained
    a mean U-score of 41.7;
24 married homosexual men who reported heterosexual intercourse with their wives only obtained a
    mean U-score of 19.2

58 single homosexual men who reported heterosexual intercourse obtained a mean U-score of 35;
79 single homosexual men who reported no heterosexual intercourse obtained a mean U-score of 28
    (McConaghy, 1978).

U-scores of 20 sex offenders correlated significantly with their reported ratio of heterosexual to homosex-
    ual feelings (McConaghy & Blaszczynski, 1991).

---

[a]PVR U-scores of 100 indicate exclusive heterosexuality; U-scores of 0, exclusive homosexuality; intervening U-scores
indicate varying degrees of bisexuality.

the more cumbersome apparatus required for PVR assessment, to measure changes
in the total volume of the penis.

    When PCRs were used to assess sexual arousal, the results should have led to an
immediate realization that they were not equivalent to PVRs. In reporting the PCRs
of a pedophile, Bancroft, Jones, and Pullan (1966) stated that to obtain them some
mental imagery was required, and that most PCRs occurred within 5 minutes of
exposure to the stimulus. The duration of stimuli used to elicit PVRs by Freund and
myself was 13 and 10 seconds, respectively, and mental imagery was not required.
This marked difference in the two sets of responses went unnoticed. When PCRs
became generally used in preference to PVRs, the studies validating PVR assessment
of sexual orientation were quoted to establish the validity of PCR assessment. PCR

assessment was therefore not considered to require independent validation. A possible factor in the rapid general acceptance of PCR as opposed to PVR assessment may have been the evaluation of the two measures in Zuckerman's widely cited review (1971) of physiological measures of sexual arousal. He unquestioningly accepted the belief that PVRs and PCRs were identical, to the extent of quoting results of studies using one or the other without identifying which was used. He decided the use of PCRs was preferable on the grounds that the circumference gauge was easier to apply, simpler to calibrate, and did not stimulate as large an area of the penis.

A further report (Bancroft, 1971; see Table 2) investigating the PCRs of 30 homosexual men should also have led to questioning of the validity of PCR as opposed to PVR assessment of sexual orientation, but again failed to do so. This study found that as a group, the 30 men showed mean PCRs to pictures of men that were greater than their mean PCRs to pictures of women. The number who individually showed greater responses to pictures of men than of women, however, was not reported. Only 14 of the 30 men showed PCRs to pictures of men and women that correlated significantly with their reported sexual arousal ($r = 0.65$ or more). The significance of a similar low level of validity found by Mavissakalian, Blanchard, Abel, and Barlow (1975; see Table 2) was also ignored. Like Bancroft, they investigated the sexual orientation of their subjects as groups, not individually. They found that the mean PCRs to 2-minute black-and-white videotape pictures of nude men and women engaged in sexual activity significantly differentiated 6 homosexual from 6 heterosexual men. The two groups' mean PCRs to the less erotically stimulating pictures of nude women displaying sexually provocative behavior, however, did not differ significantly. This finding was not emphasized, and its major significance was not pointed out. In a number of studies at that time, PCR measurement of individual homosexual men's responses to pictures of nude women was employed in the belief that these PCRs validly assessed the men's sexual orientation. On the basis of the belief, it was concluded that changes in their PCRs following behavioral treatments demonstrated a change in their sexual orientation to heterosexuality (Barlow & Agras, 1973; McGrady, 1973). It should have been realized that the finding of Mavissakalian et al. invalidated the conclusions of the studies; nevertheless, the studies are still cited to justify the use of aversive and other techniques in treating sex offenders (Chapter 8).

Sakheim, Barlow, Beck, and Abrahamson (1985; see Table 1.2) subsequently supported the finding of Mavissakalian et al. of low validity of PCR assessment of sexual orientation. A group of 8 homosexual men were not distinguished from a group of 8 heterosexual men by their PCRs to heterosexual, lesbian, and homosexual slides. Fifteen of the 16 were individually distinguished as heterosexual or homosexual from their PCRs to a lesbian and a homosexual erotic film; using their PCRs to a heterosexual and a homosexual film, only 12 of the 16 could be so distinguished. It would appear that it requires the more powerful stimuli of movies of same-sex couples engaged in sexual activity to distinguish individual homosexual and heterosexual men at the level of accuracy that PVR assessment achieves with stimuli of movies of individual nude men and women.

Movies of sexual activity, however, are not sufficient for PCR assessment to distinguish bisexual from homosexual men. Tollison, Adams, and Tollison (1979; see Table 1.2) were unable to distinguish groups of men who reported bisexual behavior

TABLE 1.2
Limited Validity of Penile Circumference Measures of Sexual Arousal

Sexual Orientation
Homosexuality/heterosexuality

Mean PCRs of a group of 30 homosexual men were greater to pictures of nude men than nude women. In 14 of the 30, correlations between "erection" and subjects' ratings of arousal were statistically significant (Bancroft, 1971).

Mean PCRs to 2-minute videos of sexual activity, but not to pictures of a nude young woman discriminated, as groups, 6 homosexual from 6 heterosexual men (Mavissakalian, Blanchard, Abel, & Barlow, 1975).

(No attempt in the above studies to identify individual heterosexual or homosexual men.)

PCRs to heterosexual, homosexual, and lesbian slides did not distinguish 8 homosexual from 8 heterosexual men as groups.
PCRs to lesbian (but not heterosexual) and male homosexual erotic films correctly identified 7 of 8 heterosexual and all 8 homosexual men (Sakheim, Barlow, Beck, & Abrahamson, 1985).

Homosexuality/bisexuality/heterosexuality

Mean PCRs of groups of self-reported bisexual and homosexual men to slides of male and female nudes and an explicit homosexual and a heterosexual film were almost identical (Tollison, Adams, & Tollison, 1979)

Pedophilia
Mean PCRs of groups of abusers of female children to pictures of nude female children compared to pictures of nude males and females of other ages:
were larger (Quinsey, Steinman, Bergersen, & Holmes, 1975);
were not larger (Baxter, Marshall, Barbaree, Davidson, & Malcolm, 1984; Marshall, Barbaree, & Christophe, 1986; Quinsey, Chaplin, & Carrigan, 1979).

Mean PCRs of groups of nonincestuous abusers of female children to pictures of female adults:
were smaller than those of incestuous offenders (Murphy, Haynes, Stalgaitis, & Flanagan, 1986; Quinsey et al., 1979);
were larger than those of incestuous offenders (Marshall et al., 1986).

"Pedophile aggressive index" of individual pedophiles to 2-minute audiotapes of forced and nonforced sexual activity with children:
differentiated more from less dangerous child abusers (Abel, Becker, Murphy, & Flanagan, 1981);
did not differentiate more from less dangerous child abusers (Avery-Clark & Laws, 1984).

"Pedophile aggressive index" of individual pedophiles to 4-minute audiotapes of forced and nonforced sexual activity with children:
differentiated more from less dangerous child abusers (Avery-Clark & Laws, 1984);
did not differentiate more from less dangerous child abusers (Nagayama Hall, Proctor, & Nelson, 1988).

Rape
Mean PCRs of a group of convicted rapists to individualized audiotapes of forced compared to consenting intercourse:
were larger (Abel, Barlow, Blanchard, & Guild, 1977; Barbaree, Marshall, & Lanthier, 1979);
were smaller (in much larger group; Baxter, Barbaree, & Marshall, 1986);
did not differ from those of nonrapists (Baxter, Barbaree, & Marshall, 1986; Murphy, Krisar, Stalgaitis, & Anderson, 1984)

"Rape index":
correctly identified 80% of rapists and 73% of nonrapists (Abel, Becker, Blanchard, & Djenderedjian, 1978);
failed to discriminate much larger group of rapists from nonrapists (Murphy et al., 1984).

and feelings from those who reported exclusive homosexual behavior and feelings by their PCRs to explicit homosexual and heterosexual films. On the basis of this finding, they questioned the existence of bisexuality, claiming there was to that date no physiological evidence for bisexual arousal except where this was a by-product of sexual reorientation therapy. In fact, two studies (Barr & McConaghy, 1971; Mc-Conaghy, 1978; see Table 1) had provided such evidence, demonstrating a relationship between U-scores indicative of bisexuality and degree of experience of heterosexual intercourse in homosexual men. Subsequently, the U-scores of individual sex offenders were shown to correlate with their reported balance of heterosexual to homosexual feelings (McConaghy & Blaszczynski, 1991; see Table 1.1).

Voluntary Control of PVRs and PCRs

Freund (1963) investigated the ability of subjects to fake PVRs by asking them to produce sexual arousal by using fantasies that would be erotic for them when shown pictures of members of the nonpreferred sex, and to attempt to diminish arousal to pictures of members of the preferred sex. Only 10 of 55 predominantly heterosexual men and 6 of 24 predominantly homosexual men were able to produce records that misclassified them. Laws and Rubin (1969) investigated the ability of 4 men to modify their PCRs, rejecting a further 3 who did not develop full erections to erotic films. The 4 subjects were asked to watch the erotic films on three occasions: On two they were to do nothing to modify their responses, and on the third they were instructed to avoid getting an erection by any means except not watching the film. All four were able to reduce their PCR-assessed erection to the film by at least 50%. The duration of the films was 10 to 12 minutes, and full erection in the unmodified condition was generally obtained within 3 minutes. Latency of the initial increase in their PCRs was not reported.

The subjects were then asked to produce an erection by any means except manipulating themselves, without being shown any erotic stimuli. All were able to produce partial PCR measures of erections, which reached a momentary peak of about 30% of maximum erection in 3 subjects and 90% in the other. Latency of any increase in PCRs ranged from slightly less than 1 minute to 10 minutes. Again the markedly higher percentage of subjects able to modify PCRs as opposed to PVRs escaped notice, as did the striking latency difference. Over a minute was required for subjects to produce an increase in their PCRs; PVRs occurred and were assessed within 13 seconds. Bancroft and Wu (1983) reported the mean latency for 5mm PCR increase of 8 normal men to erotic films was 56.8 sec.

The markedly longer duration of stimuli necessary for PCR assessment is likely to contribute to the greater ease with which these responses can be consciously modified. Periods of a few minutes (as compared with 13 seconds) give the subjects much greater opportunity to fantasize and, perhaps not always deliberately, to introduce stimuli into their fantasy at variance with that presented. Alford, Wedding, and Jones (1983) reported a patient who was given aversive therapy for homosexual feelings. During the treatment sessions he was asked to imagine unpleasant images while listening to audiotapes of homosexual activity; PCR assessment was used in independent sessions to determine if his arousal to the tapes had changed. The subject subsequently told the researchers he had used the unpleasant fantasies to inhibit his PCRs in the assessment sessions. On investigation, it was found that he was also able to produce 90% of full erections by using sexually evocative fantasies without any erotic stimuli being provided. The latency of his responses was not reported. The ability of some men, given sufficient time, to produce marked PCRs without exposure to erotic stimuli could explain findings that homosexual men treated by regular exposure to pictures of women developed 80% to 100% PCR-assessed erections to the pictures. These men reported no increase in their heterosexual feelings (Barlow & Agras; 1973, McGrady, 1973), another finding that should have led to questioning the validity of PCR assessment.

Direct Comparison of PVRs and PCRs

In an attempt to bring the differences in PCR and PVR assessment to the attention of researchers, two reports were published (Freund, Langevin, & Barlow, 1974; McConaghy, 1974) that directly compared the two responses. My report contained the graphs of individual subjects' PVRs and PCRs to the 10-second movie pictures of nudes in the film assessment described. Graphs were selected to show (a) that the two responses can be reasonably equivalent; (b) that they can be largely mirror images (Figure 1.3); (c) that the latency of PCRs can be much greater than that of PVRs; and (d) that the PVRs can be recorded to some stimuli—in particular, mild electric shocks to the finger—that do not appear on PCR assessment. The finding that PCRs and PVRs differed in some subjects to the extent of being mirror images was unexpected. It was explained on the basis that the rapid penile tumescence (or PVR increase) in these subjects was associated with a marked elongation of the penis, such that the increase in blood flow to maintain the elongation was not sufficient to also maintain the increase in circumference (the response measured by the PCR). The PVR increases were therefore paralleled by PCR decreases. It would appear that in their comparison of PVRs and PCRs, Freund, Langevin, and Barlow (1974) also found them to be opposed in some subjects, as they stated that they rejected responses when both did not show an increase. Presumably, they did not consider such responses could be valid.

Once the visual evidence was provided that PVRs and PCRs could differ to the extent of being opposite, I expected it would be rapidly accepted that the two types of response would no longer be treated as equivalent, or at least that immediate attempts would be made to determine if the findings that they differed were correct. In fact the findings were ignored by most researchers, who continued to treat PVRs and PCRs as equivalent. Laws (1977), in a comparison of two circumference measurement instruments, commented that there was a slight dip in the PCRs recorded by both immediately following onset of an erotic film stimulus, a phenomenon he had frequently observed in some subjects. He also suggested that this could be due to the penis increasing in length at such a rate that the circumference could not be maintained by the accompanying blood flow. He did not suggest that the finding should lead to a reexamination of the literature identifying PVRs and PCRs.

Rosen and Keefe (1978), in a review of penile assessment measures, suggested that my findings that at times PVRs and PCRs were opposed should be treated with

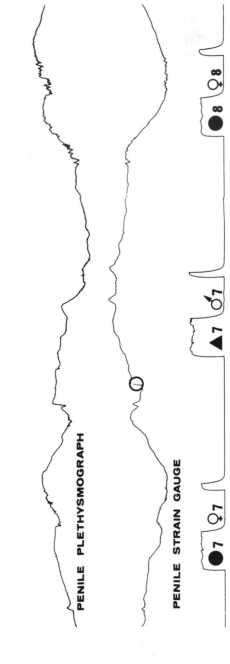

Fig. 1.3. Mirror-image penile volume (penile plethysmograph) and penile circumference (penile strain gauge) responses of a heterosexual subject to seventh and eighth presentation of films of female nudes, and seventh presentation of male nudes. The PVR was recorded at a sensitivity of 0.2 mv/cm, and the PCR at 0.05 mv/cm. The balance voltage was changed at the ringed section.

caution, because no statistical comparisons were reported and the number of subjects were small. They appeared unaware of the irony of their statement: Almost all the findings using PCRs to that date were obtained in single-case design studies in which, by the nature of this design, no statistical comparisons were reported and the number of subjects were small. No suggestion has ever been made that caution should be applied to the findings of these studies or of that by Laws and Rubin (1969), which investigated 5 subjects. Their validity remains unquestioned. As mentioned previously and discussed in more detail in Chapter 8, these single case studies continue to be cited as the only evidence to justify many of the behavioral therapies currently employed to treat sex offenders in North America. The politics of science dictates that doubt is cast only on the validity of findings that threaten current practice; as discussed subsequently, research methodology provides a number of ways in which this can be done.

Earls and Marshall (1982) investigated 6 subjects, using a transducer designed to measure changes in penile circumference and length simultaneously. They found in all subjects that in the early stages of erection to erotic photographic slides, the changes were mirror images. During erection penile length increased continually, whereas circumference decreased slightly before increasing. Despite this replication with a different instrument of my finding that PVRs and PCRs could differ, the authors did not suggest that the evidence of the validity of PVRs could no longer be used to support the validity of PCRs, and that the evidence supporting the two procedures should be treated independently. In a subsequent report of the same finding, Earls, Marshall, Marshall, Morales, and Surridge (1983) stated that PCRs provided the best single physiological index of sexual arousal, supporting the statement by citing the review of Rosen and Keefe (1978). In their review, Rosen and Keefe examined the various physical characteristics of the devices employed in PCR and PVR assessment but did not discuss the validity of the findings derived from their use.

More recently, Wheller and Rubin (1987) reported a mean correlation of $r = 0.68$ ($p < 0.01$) between the PCRs and PVRs of 6 men assessed at 30-second intervals from 1 minute before to 1 minute after three viewings of a 10-minute erotic film. On one of the three viewings the men were asked to inhibit erections by any means possible, increasing the likelihood of their showing no response. When no responses occurred, both PCRs and PVRs of course were zero, producing a perfect correlation of $r = 1.0$. As this result occurred frequently, it led to the mean correlations of the subject's responses being spuriously high. The appropriate conclusion to be made from the correlation reported is that PCRs and PVRs assess *absence* of penile responses similarly; it provided no meaningful evidence of the degree of similarity with which they assess the presence of penile responses. Apart from this issue, I pointed out that the methodology of the study was inappropriate to compare the two responses, as PVRs are used over much shorter time periods to record immediate response to erotic stimuli (McConaghy, 1977b). Nevertheless, the study has been quoted to support the equivalence of PCR and PVR assessment (McAnulty & Adams, 1992).

It would seem that for some time to come the politics of the need to maintain the validity of PCR assessment will remain a barrier to objective examination of the evidence of its inability to produce consistent data (see Table 1.2). Its validity will continue to be supported by the findings validating PVR assessment (see Table 1.1): "The assessment of male sexual arousal by direct measurement of changes in penile diameter *or volume* in response to erotic stimuli is now widely accepted as one of the most valid assessment techniques available" (Wincze & Lange, 1981, p. 313; emphasis added).

PCR Assessment of Sex Offenders

A major further reason for resistance to questioning the validity of PCR assessment was that by the mid-1970s its use was extended to sex offenders. Early studies generally of small numbers of subjects reported results supporting the validity of the investigation (Table 1.2). The mean PCRs of groups of pedophiles were larger to slides of children than of adults, and the mean PCRs of groups of rapists were larger to audiotaped descriptions of forced than consenting intercourse. A "rape index," the ratio of men's PCRs to audiotaped descriptions of forced as compared to consenting intercourse, differentiated individual rapist from nonrapists. "Pedophile aggressive index," the ratio of the pedophiles' PCRs to audiotaped descriptions of aggressive sexual assault as compared to descriptions of sexual assault in which a child is psychologically persuaded to consent, differentiated more from less aggressive pedophiles. Subsequent studies with larger subject numbers failed to replicate any of these findings (Table 1.2). As pointed out in Chapter 8, though PCR assessment continues to remain central to the investigation and assessment of response to treatment of sex offenders in many of the programs currently employed in North America, some therapists are beginning to question its usefulness. Others (McAnulty & Adams, 1992), although accepting that its ability to distinguish sex offenders from nonoffenders even as groups is limited, defended its use in their legal evaluation as individuals when the ethics of the practice was questioned (McConaghy, 1989).

PCR Assessment of Degree and Strength
of Subjective Sexual Arousal

This discussion of the validity of penile tumescence measures has dealt with their ability to determine the direction of subjects' sexual interest, that is, their sexual orientation and their deviant sexual preferences. Penile tumescence measures have also been used to assess subjects' degree of sexual arousal to sexual stimuli. As stated earlier, only 14 of the 30 homosexual men showed PCRs to pictures of men and women that correlated significantly ($r = 0.65$ or more) with their reported degree of sexual arousal (Bancroft, 1971). Wincze and Qualls (1984), however, using the stronger stimuli of erotic films, found correlations of PCRs with reported subjective arousal in 8 homosexual men of $r = 0.62$ to 0.98, the average being significant. This is consistent with findings of other studies that found higher correlations between PCRs and sexual arousal when the PCRs were larger. Hall, Binik, and DiTomasso (1985) investigated the PCRs of 20 university students who, while watching 4.5-minute audiotaped descriptions of heterosexual intercourse, continuously monitored their subjective levels of arousal by moving a dial. Correlations between the two assessments varied from $r = 0.22$ to 0.95, higher correlations ($r > 0.70$) being found in subjects with larger PCRs.

Though penile tumescence can show a strong relationship with the relative degree of sexual arousal to different stimuli, it is only weakly related to the absolute strength of sexual interest. Subjects whose absolute sexual interest and activity were reduced by administration of cyproterone showed reduction in PCRs to slides but not to erotic films; those in whom it was reduced because of their low production of sex hormone (testosterone) showed no increase in PCRs to erotic films when their blood testosterone levels were increased by administration of testosterone (Bancroft & Wu, 1983). PVRs of 20 sex offenders to movie pictures of nude men and women were unaffected when their absolute sexual interest was reduced by medroxyprogesterone (McConaghy & Blaszczynski, 1983). The validity of PCR assessment of nocturnal penile tumescence to determine whether impotence in men is organically or psychogenically caused is discussed in Chapter 5.

Female Sexual Arousal

Devices investigating a variety of genital physiological responses have been introduced to assess female sexual arousal. While the subjects were exposed to erotic stimuli, their vaginal, clitoral, or labial blood flow changes were measured either by the associated temperature changes (using a thermistor), or by vaginal color changes (using a photoplethysmograph). Clitoral responses have also been assessed by using a strain gauge. It would appear from the comprehensive review of these procedures by Rosen and Beck (1988) that photoplethysmograph assessment of vaginal pulse amplitude remains the most widely used measure of arousal and the most sensitive in distinguishing the responses of groups of women to erotic as compared to nonerotic stimuli. A number of studies found relationships between women's genital and subjectively assessed arousal to be weaker than those of men (Wincze & Qualls, 1984). Using photoplethysomography, Wincze and Qualls reported the mean maximal vaginal pulse amplitude of 8 lesbian women to differ significantly in response to five 4-minute films of varying erotic content. The greatest amplitude occurred in response to the film with explicit lesbian activity. Correlations between the vaginal responses and reported subjective arousal of the individual subjects during each film varied from $r = 0.26$ to 0.89, the average for the group not being significant. The correlations of subjective arousal and PCRs of 8 homosexual men who viewed the same films were $r = 0.62$ to 0.98, the average being significant. Hatch (1981), in his brief review, found no consistent reports of differences in physiologically assessed genital arousal to erotic stimuli of sexually functional and dysfunctional women, or of changes in the arousal of the dysfunctional women following treatment. The relatively little attention given the assessment of genital arousal of women as compared to men presumably reflects both its lower validity and the fact that the major clinical use of the assessment has been with sex offenders, almost all of whom are men.

Other Physiological Assessments

Zuckerman (1971), in his review of physiological measures of sexual arousal, pointed out that apart from penile erectile changes, those used to that time lacked specificity. This conclusion would still appear to apply, judging from the results of more recent studies included in the comprehensive marshaling by Rosen and Beck

(1988) of what must be at least the majority of studies of nongenital physiological concomitants of sexual responses. Zuckerman found that in the studies to 1971, most attention had been given to subjects' galvanic skin responses and to changes in size of the pupil of the eye; since then, these have rarely been investigated. Recent developments in physiological assessment of other aspects of sexuality are discussed in subsequent chapters. A number of measures have been introduced to determine if vascular or neurological disease contribute to individual subjects' impotence, as is discussed in Chapter 4. Hormonal influences on both normal (Chapter 2) and dysfunctional (Chapter 4) sexual behavior have been intensively studied.

METHODOLOGY OF RESEARCH ASSESSMENT

Biological and Environmental Determinants of Behavior

As discussed earlier, basic differences in the ideologies of Pavlovian and behaviorist researchers were reflected in the methodologies of their research. The conditioning process Pavlov discovered—the establishment of conditional reflexes by reinforcement of conditional stimuli with unconditional stimuli (Figure 1.1)—came to be termed *classical conditioning*. It was primarily used by Pavlov to understand how animals learned to adapt to their environment. He concluded they set up an internal reflection (or cognitive representation) of their environment in the cortex of their brains. Incoming stimuli from the animal's current environment were matched against this representation. This enabled familiar stimuli to be recognized and responded to appropriately in the light of past learning. Novel stimuli failed to be matched and so immediately produced what Pavlov termed the *orienting response,* now known to be attributable to activation of the arousal system of the brain. With the orienting response the full attention of the animal was directed to the novel stimulus, leading to its analysis, again in the light of past experience. An appropriate response was then made—withdrawal if the stimulus was assessed as threatening, approach if it was assessed as a potential source of food or sexual activity, or caution if it could not be assessed.

Pavlov considered that in men and women a second level of representation of the objects in their environment was established in the cortex of their brains, that of words. He termed this level of representation the *second signaling system.* The interaction of excitatory and inhibitory linkages in this system of words led to the development of concepts. Men and women were thus freed from the constraints of the real world by the ability to manipulate its cognitive representations in their imagination. This manipulation, interacting with behavior completion mechanisms (BCMs), resulted in the experience of what is termed free will (McConaghy, 1987a). This physiological cognitive theory of behavior will be returned to in Chapter 8, where BCMs are employed in the explanation and treatment of compulsive sexual behaviors.

Understandably in view of its emphasis of the role of physiology, Pavlovian theory accepted that neurophysiological brain processes and genetic and hormonal factors in addition to environmental stimuli were significant determinants of behavior. This contrasted with behaviorist theory, in which individual men and women were seen as biologically the same, and factors additional to rewards and punishments were not considered to influence their behavior significantly. Though the most influential modern behaviorist, Skinner, did not deny that biological factors existed, he effectively negated their role:

> Although genetic and organic factors can be efficiently evaluated only by holding environmental factors constant, and although environmental factors can be correctly evaluated only against a stable genetic and organic condition, it is probably a useful practice to explore environmental factors first to see whether any behavioral manifestations remain to be attributed to genetic and organic causes. (Skinner, 1972, p. 253)

In practice, adopting this recommendation of exploring environmental factors first allows behavior to be explained as entirely determined by these factors. This is because the human mind can readily provide plausible explanations for any set of data once they are obtained. This is sufficiently recognized that explanations developed after data is obtained are commonly objected to as *post hoc* explanations. This term is also used in the phrase *post hoc, ergo propter hoc,* which refers to the equally common methodological error of concluding that because a condition followed an event it was caused by the event (e.g., that because a disturbed adult suffered childhood trauma, his or her disturbance is attributable to the trauma). An attempt to justify post hoc explanations as valid ranks with the above quotation by Skinner as another great antiscientific statement of this century made by a major student of human behavior:

> So long as we trace the development from its final outcome backwards, the chain of events appears continuous, and we feel we have gained an insight which is completely satisfactory or even exhaustive. But if we proceed the reverse way, if we start from the premises inferred from the analysis and try to follow these up to the final result, then we no longer get the impression of an inevitable sequence of events which could not have been otherwise determined. . . . Hence the chain of causation *can always be recognised with certainty* if we follow the line of analysis, whereas to predict it along the line of synthesis is impossible. Freud (1920/1955, pp. 167–168, emphasis added)

Skinner's statement may not have been unreasonable coming from an experimenter whose major experience was in laboratory research of animal behavior, where control of the relevant variables can be virtually complete. Students of human behavior, however, should be aware how frequently conflicting explanations are advanced from different ideological viewpoints, all of which can logically account for an observation. Yet only one can be true, and possibly none are. In scientific as opposed to philosophical methodology, a theory should be accepted on the basis not of its plausibility in explaining known findings, but of its ability to explain and preferably predict findings as yet unknown. Any attempt to follow Skinner's recommendation and explore environmental factors first to account plausibly for any known behavioral manifestations is almost certain to be successful, leaving none remaining to be attributed to genetic or other biological causes. Skinner's recommendation was readily accepted in the political climate of the United States, with its emphasis on the equality of man and the importance of environmental factors—in particular, the profit motive—in determining behavior (McConaghy, 1987a). In this climate, any evidence of the role of biological factors in behavior was scrutinized intensively so that grounds were usually found, if not for rejecting it, at least for postponing its acceptance. In contrast, environmental explanations were accepted with no evidence other than their plausibility. Though this situation is changing in some areas of psychology, it remains entrenched in sociology.

Consistent with the strong empirical tradition in the United States, research in behavior focused not on understanding its underlying mechanisms as in the Pavlovian tradition, but in learning how to control it by the administration and withdrawal of rewards and punishments. This tradition was initiated in the nineteenth-century studies of the ability of animals to achieve rewards or avoid punishments by trial-and-error learning. In their investigations, behaviorists mainly utilized an operant conditioning model, studying the effects of different patterns or schedules of rewards and punishments on the frequency of responses. The aim was to use the resulting data to control behavior better, not to attempt to understand the biological mechanisms involved.

Single-Case Design

As behaviorist ideology regarded all individual animals of a species as biologically equal, a methodology termed *single-case design* was developed to study changes in behavior of a single subject, which took advantage of the further belief that the frequency of a behavior was entirely determined environmentally by the schedule of its previous reinforcement. The factor on which major weight was placed to establish that a particular schedule produced a particular effect was termed *reversal*. This was the demonstration that the effect reversed or disappeared when the schedule was withdrawn; preferably this would be shown more than once. No statistical analysis of probability was considered necessary. This methodology was ideal in the study of animal behavior, as few subjects needed to be studied, and the possibility that the effect could be attributable to suggestibility or the expectancy of the subject did not need to be considered. Human subjects could alter their behavior, however, or believe that their feelings had changed in response to a particular schedule under the influence of their expectancy that such an alteration would occur. Expectancy also could cause their behavior to reverse to its prior condition once the schedule was withdrawn.

In some studies, efforts were made to overcome this by introducing schedules that in theory should be ineffective but that the subjects could expect to be effective. It was usually not possible, however, to design schedules in which the ineffectiveness would not be obvious to the subjects by common sense. A further problem was that the study usually would employ a number of measures of the subject's response, such as physiological, behavioral, and rating scale measures as well as self-report. Recording of many such measures was not difficult when only a few subjects were studied. When this was done, though, the different measures frequently showed conflicting outcomes, allowing experimenters to emphasize the findings they considered positive while attempting to account plausibly for the opposing ones.

A number of experimenters attempting to reorient homosexual men to heterosexuality in the 1970s, published studies that explored not only these opportunities but a further and major weakness of single-case design that should be considered completely unacceptable (McConaghy, 1977b). This was to produce the appearance of reversal by withdrawing treatment once a particular response approached its maximum, then reintroducing it once the response approached its minimum. In the studies the response manipulated in this way was subjects' PCRs to slides of nude females, which were used to assess their postulated change to heterosexuality. These PCRs could fluctuate markedly without change in treatment, so that it was possible to take advantage of these fluctuations unconsciously to produce an apparent relationship between treatment and response. The treatment was introduced, and inevitably at some subsequent stage a maximum PCR would occur. The treatment was then withdrawn. In time a minimal response would occur; the treatment was then reintroduced. It would then be concluded that the treatment produced the maximal PCR to the slide of a nude female, and its withdrawal the minimum PCR to the slide—evidence that the treatment had reoriented the subject to heterosexuality. Insistence on a procedure of introducing and withdrawing the treatment at predetermined times and not according to the patient's responses would prevent this misuse of the design. The evidence cited to support many of the behavioral techniques employed in the current treatment of sex offenders (Chapter 8) was provided by studies exploiting single-case methodology in this way in addition to using invalid PCR assessment.

Group Design

The errors of reporting findings as valid when they are not can occur also with the group designs used by Pavlovian researchers. Group designs, (i.e., not the study of one or a few individuals, but the comparison of two or more groups of individuals) are considered necessary in most circumstances by Pavlovian researchers in view of their belief that individuals differ genetically and on other biological variables, and so findings on one individual cannot automatically be generalized to others. In one commonly employed group design, the response to a procedure is determined by comparing the mean change in behavior of a group of subjects before and after its administration with the change in behavior over the same period of time in a group not receiving this procedure. This form of the design does not deal with the problem of expectancy effects, discussed above, unless a different procedure can be given to the second group that matches the first in inducing the same expectancy of change in behavior, yet is designed to produce no specific change. Unlike placebo tablets, ineffective psychological procedures that subjects will believe are as likely to be as effective as the treatment being investigated are difficult to design. My personal belief is that group design treatment evaluation studies are likely to produce valid results only when two effective treatments are compared, with one administered to each of the two groups, to determine which treatment is the more effective (McConaghy, 1990a).

Type I Errors: An Inevitable Result of the Use of Statistical Significance

In groups designs, where possible, the two groups of subjects should be formed by random allocation of individual subjects. (Random allocation means that chance alone determines the membership of the two groups.) After the two groups have received different procedures, the expected change in their behavior is measured. The probability that any difference found between the behavior of the two groups could have occurred by chance is determined using a statistical test of probability. If the chance is less than an agreed figure, usually 1 in 20 (summarized when data are reported as $p < 0.05$), the difference is said to be statistically significant. The possibility that the results are attributable to chance is then rejected, and it is accepted that the difference was a true effect of the difference in procedures.

Obviously, on 1 occasion in 20, the effect will actually be the result of chance. On that occasion, rejecting the possibility that it was attributable to chance will be incorrect. There is no way of knowing on the basis of the studies themselves, however, in which one this has occurred. As that study (along with the other 19) will report its finding as statistically significant, it will incorrectly be regarded as valid. Incorrect results produced in this way are inevitable, as a consequence of this accepted methodology of using a level of significance to reject the possibility that results are caused by chance. Such errors are termed false positive, or type I, errors. For this reason it is wise not to accept a statistically significant result as valid until it is replicated (i.e., found again in one or preferably more studies carried out by different workers).

A further reason to treat the result of an initial significant finding with caution is that it is possible to increase the likelihood of its being significant after the experiment, when determining the way it is measured. For example, in some studies of PCR assessment discussed earlier, probability statistics were used to compare the mean PCRs of different groups. In one study, Avery-Clark and Laws (1984; see Table 2) attempted to replicate an earlier finding that the mean "pedophile aggressive index" of more aggressive pedophiles was significantly greater than that of less aggressive pedophiles. The PCRs in the earlier study were those occurring up to 2 minutes after the onset of audiotapes of forced and unforced sexual activity with children. Avery-Clark and Laws were unable to replicate this finding but found a significant difference in PCRs occurring up to 4 minutes after the onset of the audiotapes. This method of seeking significant findings in the results of an experiment post hoc by examining different possibilities increases the likelihood of finding results that are significant by chance (i.e., type I errors). As the mean PCRs of the two groups fluctuated over time, they could have differed sufficiently by chance to reach significance at a few points in time. By examining them at a number of different times rather than at a single predetermined time, the experimenter greatly increased the likelihood of finding a chance difference and thus reporting a type I error. In fact, in reporting their result, Avery-Clark and Laws warned that it should be treated with caution. Once in print, however, such a finding is likely to be quoted without qualification as a successful replication.

When a study is carried out to investigate an original observation and the finding is tested for statistical significance at its completion, the researchers involved are likely to examine the finding in a number of ways. The more ways that are examined, the greater the likelihood one will be found that shows a statistically significant difference by chance. Ideally, the method by which the outcome is determined and statistically assessed should be completely defined in advance of the study in order to eliminate this procedure and its increased risk of making a type

I error. It is possible the post hoc procedure was used in some of the original studies that reported positive findings with PCR assessment of sex offenders. If so, it would account for the numerous reports in Table 1.2 of failures to replicate these original studies when the original outcome measures and statistical analyses were precisely followed. Such precise replication prevents the post hoc procedure being used.

The inability to prevent the use of this procedure when original observations are made adds a further source of type I errors to those that are an inevitable consequence of the use of statistical significance. It further emphasizes the need for studies that precisely replicate the study reporting an initial finding (i.e., that do not alter any aspect of the methodology of the initial study, including the outcome measures and the means by which they are statistically analyzed). When such replicatory studies fail to confirm the original finding, however, the initial response should be to question the validity of the original finding, not to seek reasons why both sets of findings are true—as has been done (as discussed in Chapter 8) in relation to the failures to replicate findings with PCR assessment.

Type II Errors: A Further Inevitable Result of the Use of Statistical Significance

When an effect investigated in a research study fails to reach statistical significance, it is usually concluded that the study demonstrated that the effect did not occur. This conclusion can be a type II, or false negative, error. Failure of an effect to reach statistical significance means no more than that the probability of the effect occurring by chance was greater than the level of significance employed, usually 1 in 20 ($p > 0.05$). It was pointed out more than 20 years ago (McConaghy & Lovibond, 1967), taking as an example a treatment that cured 60% of subjects when 40% would recover with a placebo, that a research study in which 35 subjects were given the treatment and 35 the placebo would only have a 50% chance of finding the difference in the response of the two groups to be statistically significant at a level of $p < 0.05$. That is to say that on average, only 5 of every 10 studies with these patient numbers would find the treatment's effect to be statistically significant. Subject numbers in most treatment trials are less than 35 per condition. Even if they were tripled, though, and 105 subjects were given treatment and 105 the placebo, with the above treatment and placebo responses there would still be 1 in 10 chance that a trial would not show the treatment effect to be statistically significant. Yet the effect of curing 20 extra patients in 100 is clearly clinically very significant; to conclude on the basis of such negative trials that the treatment investigated was ineffective carries the risk of making a type II error.

As with type I errors, type II errors can be detected by replicatory studies with adequate subject numbers. In the past, it was common for academics to expect that all studies that evaluated an effective treatment should show it to produce a significant effect irrespective of the number of subjects in the studies. When inevitably some studies failed to show such an effect, academics persistently published articles criticizing clinicians for using treatments that they now accept are highly effective. Though this is now less common, it still occurs (McConaghy, 1990a).

Meta-Analysis

This situation in which academics argued whether a series of studies had or had not shown a treatment effect to be present stimulated the introduction of the statistical technique of meta-analysis, which was expected to resolve such arguments. In order to compare the results of different studies, meta-analysis abandoned the evaluation of treatment outcomes by determination of their statistical significance; instead, it relied on what was termed the *effect size* (ES) to assess this. ES was calculated by determining the difference in the mean scores of the treated group from before to after treatment and dividing the difference by the standard deviation (SD) of the treated subjects' scores. SD provides a measure of the scatter of the scores.

Division of the mean treatment responses by the treated groups' SDs resulted in the same mean response to treatment producing different ESs, depending on the nature of the group treated. The ES is larger if the subjects in the group are similar, as the scatter of their scores (and therefore their resultant SD) is small. The ES of the same mean response to treatment is smaller if the group is dissimilar, so that their scores have a large SD. Also, ESs based on a treatment response measured by a reactive outcome scale will be larger than an ES based on a scale with little reactivity. These and other problems resulted in different meta-analyses reporting different conclusions (McConaghy, 1990a). Nevertheless, as a source of academic controversy and hence of publications, use of meta-analysis is increasing. Fortunately for the careers of its proponents, it would appear to have stimulated more controversies than it has resolved.

True and Quasi Experiments: The Value of Randomization

As so many factors—environmental and biological, known and unknown—affect human behavior, when a research study attempts to determine the effect of a single factor, the effect of all the other factors cannot be determined in order to exclude them. In a true experiment, their effect is excluded by random allocation: A group of subjects are randomly allocated, half to be affected by the factor under investigation and half not (e.g., half are given a treatment and half a placebo). As stated above, random allocation guarantees that only chance determines which individuals are allocated to the two groups. Hence when random allocation is employed, apart from the treatment and the placebo, the differences in all the factors that affect the behavior of the individuals in one as compared with the other group are entirely attributable to chance. At the end of the experiment, the probability that the difference between the two groups could have been caused by these chance factors is calculated by a test of significance. If this probability can be rejected, the difference must have been the result of the treatment as compared to the placebo.

As discussed earlier, the accepted convention is that the probability that a difference is caused by chance is rejected if it is less than the selected level of statistical significance. That this convention inevitably leads on occasion to type I and type II errors, and how they are dealt with, was discussed. Strangely, a number of methodologists believe random allocation results in groups that are equal in all respects

(Cook & Campbell, 1979; Kerlinger, 1973). Some have even suggested that if following randomization the groups can be shown to differ, the randomization has been unsuccessful (J. Frank, 1959). This is not the case. Following randomization, as chance has determined the distribution of the differences in the two groups, the two groups must differ on some variables. The convention of statistical significance accepts and allows for the existence of these differences.

Research is frequently carried out to attempt to determine the effect of factors, such as child sexual abuse or sexual assault, to which individuals cannot be randomly allocated. In this situation there is no means of controlling the effect of all other variables that could also influence the outcome under investigation. Studies in which the subjects are not randomly allocated are termed *quasi experiments* to distinguish them from true experiments (in which subjects are randomly allocated; Cook & Campbell, 1979). Only in true experiments can it be argued that the factor investigated was responsible for any differences between the two groups that were not attributable to chance. In quasi experiments, the best that can be done is to form an experimental group of subjects preferably representative of all persons subjected to the factor under investigation; they are then compared in terms of the behaviors being assessed as possibly affected by the factor, with a control group of persons not subjected to the factor. To attempt to control for the influence of other factors on the behaviors being assessed, the control group is matched with the experimental group on all variables (e.g., age, sex, socioeconomic class) that it is believed might affect the behaviors. There usually remain a number of variables that could affect the behaviors, however, on which the experimental subjects cannot be matched. For example, the parents of sexually abused children could differ genetically from the parents of nonabused children. They might differ behaviorally, possibly being more aggressive or less protective. They might differ in ways as yet unknown that also could affect the behaviors being assessed. Hence, when in a quasi experiment a difference in behavior between experimental and control groups is found to be statistically significant (i.e., not caused by chance) there still remain an unknown number of factors other than that on which the subjects were selected to which the difference could be attributable. The only scientific conclusion that can be made is that the difference found is compatible with the possibility it was produced by the factor under investigation.

The statement sometimes made to emphasize the inability of quasi experiments to provide evidence of the cause of differences demonstrated is that "correlations need not be causal relations." That is to say, a correlation between childhood sexual abuse and later behavioral disturbance does not justify attributing the behavioral disturbance to the abuse. The statement could also be advanced, though, that politics make causes of correlations. As discussed in Chapter 6, the economics of the child abuse industry, the ideology of feminism, and the public abhorrence of child sexual abuse has led to the current acceptance both that the term be used for any sexual activity between a child and an adult, and that any such activity is likely to produce long-term harm to the child. The researchers who attempted until the beginning of the 1980s to examine the validity of these issues with the correct scientific methodology (Chapter 2) have become silent.

SCOPE FOR THE POLITICS OF SCIENCE TO INFLUENCE SCIENTIFIC CONCLUSIONS

As the previous discussion has revealed, current research methodology for the study of human behavior results inevitably in a percentage of incorrect findings. Assessment measures are accepted as valid on inadequate evidence. Single-case design allows manipulation of the relationship between treatment and outcome measures, and freedom to select the most useful of the conflicting findings of the many outcome measures employed to investigate the one subject. Group designs produce type I errors at a minimum probability of 1 in 20 when the usual significance level of $p < 0.05$ is used; the probability is higher when in initial studies the method of analyzing the data most likely to demonstrate significance is chosen post hoc. Type II errors are equally inevitable in group designs when results on occasion fail to reach statistical significance, which is more likely when subject numbers are not large.

Both type I and type II errors can be detected if replicatory studies are carried out. Failure of replication, however, is often not employed to question the validity of the original finding but to argue that both are correct. When the findings of a number of studies investigating a particular issue do not result in a definite conclusion, meta-analysis has been advanced as a solution. Its results, which give a spurious impression of statistical certainty, can be both unreliable and invalid in presenting trivial changes in patients' outcome as meaningful. The inability in quasi experiments to allocate subjects randomly to experiences believed to have certain effects allows correlations found between the experiences and subsequent behavioral differences to be interpreted as causal relationships according to the erroneous logic of post hoc, ergo propter hoc. The study then reports the finding as demonstrating that the experience caused the behavioral differences found.

It is not claimed that the common use of these methods to produce erroneous findings and conclusions is usually deliberate. It must be acknowledged, however, that a major source of the political power of ideologies is the apparently scientific demonstration of their truth. Inevitably their proponents will demonstrate a tolerance toward studies producing findings supporting their position, and harsh critical analysis of those producing findings that do not. The aspects of current research methodologies that have been discussed allow a broad scope for the acceptance of erroneous findings and the rejection of valid ones. That more overt pressures (e.g., intimidation of speakers, prejudiced rejection of research grant applications and refereeing of research reports submitted for publication, and impairment of opponents' academic advancement) may be employed to maintain the positions of ideologies currently dominating scientific politics does not require discussion.

CHAPTER 2

Age and Sex
Biological and Social Influences

EVOLUTION AND SEX DIFFERENCES

Throughout life, women's sexuality is more dependent on the existence and nature of a relationship with a partner than is that of men. The evidence that this is the case in adolescence, early adulthood, and middle and old age will be discussed in relation to these life stages. It may explain or result from the greater importance psychological (as opposed to biological) factors have on women's sexuality as compared to men's. Despite the overwhelming importance given in the United States to environmental as compared to biological variables in determining human behavior (McConaghy, 1987b), some of its theorists have considered the differences between the behavior of men and women to be genetically determined by the form of sexual activity selected in the evolution of human beings to enable the survival of their species (Knoth, Boyd, & Singer, 1988).

From this perspective, the likelihood that the male's genes will survive is increased if he impregnates as many women as possible, as he need take no responsibility for the care of the children produced. Evolutionary pressures should therefore preferentially select males who take every opportunity for coitus with women, particularly women who are young and healthy (and hence more likely to be fertile and to survive to take care of the child). Male sexual arousal should therefore be readily and strongly evoked by the visual cues of such women. Increased likelihood of survival of the female's genes requires that she maximize the survival of the children who result from her sexual activity. This evolutionary pressure will therefore preferentially select women whose sexual interest is directed to men who are likely to set up a committed relationship with them and who are of established politico-economic status. Women's sexual arousal should therefore be under the control much less of immediate visual cues than of the emotional relationships they establish with their partners.

Evolutionary theory would also predict that coitus would more certainly result in orgasm in the male than in the female, as male (but not female) orgasm is essential for impregnation as it accompanies ejaculation. This is consistent with the finding (Chapter 5) that unlike men, a significant percentage of women take some years to experience orgasm in their sexual activity, and possibly 5% to 10% never do. There would appear to be a weaker biological basis for female than male orgasm through-

39

out the mammalian species. Though orgasm has been observed in individual female dogs, rabbits, cats of all species, and a variety of female primates, the majority of females of these species were considered not to reach orgasm, and no evidence of orgasm was reported in any females of most infrahuman species (Kinsey, Pomeroy, Martin, & Gebhard, 1953). This could in part reflect the difficulty in recognizing the occurrence of orgasm in females by observation; some women themselves report uncertainty that they have experienced it (Sholty et al. 1984). Investigators of women's sexual behavior have commonly concluded, however, that women differ biologically in their ability to learn to reach orgasm (Mead, 1950) and that some women seem unable to do so (Kaplan, 1974).

HORMONAL DETERMINANTS OF SEXUALITY

Testosterone and Sexual Activity in Men

The suggestion that men's sexuality is more biologically determined than that of women is supported by the more consistent findings of relationships between sexual hormone levels and sexual activity in men as compared to women. This could be influenced by the fact that there is no equivalent in men to the marked hormonal fluctuations that occur throughout the menstrual cycle in women. Levels of the major male hormone or androgen, testosterone, do not vary greatly in men from day to day. Kraemer et al. (1976) estimated the testosterone levels of 20 young men between 8 a.m. and 9 a.m. every second day for 2 months. Using the standard deviation as an index of how much the levels of each subject varied, for only 1 subject was it greater than 2.0, and for 8 it was less than 1.0. W. Brown, Monti, and Corriveau (1978) reported a strong correlation ($r = 0.69$) between two testosterone levels of each of 101 healthy male students, determined from blood samples taken between 8 a.m. and 9 a.m. on two days a week apart. Most studies of men's daytime levels of testosterone take only one blood sample from each subject for estimation. Usually it is collected within a few hours of the same time of the day to allow for fluctuations that occur throughout the day; these can be substantial in some subjects (Leymarie, Roger, Castanier, & Scholler, 1974). Studies of men's testosterone levels during sleep need to take several blood samples during the night to allow for the gradual increase that takes place over this time (Schiavi, Fisher, White, Beers, & Szechter, 1984).

Kraemer et al. (1976) found that 15 of 17 men, examined as individuals, had higher mean testosterone levels during periods of orgasmic activity than of inactivity; as a group, their testosterone levels and frequency of orgasmic activity were negatively correlated. In contrast, Brown et al. (1978) found a significant positive relationship between men's testosterone levels and the number of orgasms they reached by masturbation in the previous week. Subsequently a number of studies also found a positive relationship between men's testosterone levels and various indices of their sexual activity, including frequency of total sexual outlets in adolescent boys (Udry, Billy, Morris, Groff, & Raj, 1985), frequency of orgasm in men aged 19 to 31 years (Knussman, Christiansen, & Couwenbergs, 1986), and amount of coital and masturbatory activity in healthy men aged 60 to 79 (Tsitouras, Martin, & Harman, 1982). These relationships tended to be weaker with increasing mean age of the groups of subjects investigated, suggesting that in adolescence hormone levels are a major determinant of the frequency of sexual behavior, but with experience factors such as emotional aspects of the subjects' relationships and the development of behavior completion mechanisms (Chapter 8) play an increasingly important role.

Most circulating testosterone is bound to a protein termed *sex hormone binding globulin,* with only 5% or less being unbound or free and hence able to be biologically active. Some workers (Carani et al., 1990; Davidson et al., 1983) have reported stronger correlations between men's sexual activity and their free (as compared to total) testosterone levels. Most workers who reported relationships between testosterone levels and sexual activity assumed that the higher levels produced the increased activity. Knussman et al. (1986) suggested that the higher levels resulted from prior sexual stimulation, not only from sexual activity but fantasies, reading, pictures, and the sight of attractive persons. They found the testosterone levels of 33 healthy men correlated with their reported exposure to such stimulation the day before but not the day on which the blood sample was taken. The levels correlated with frequency of orgasm on both days. Their findings require replication, as they agreed that most other studies had found no increase in testosterone levels from before to 48 hours following coitus or the watching of a sexually stimulating film. If the findings are replicated, increased sexual activity could only be responsible for part of the association between increased testosterone levels and sexual activity, as levels of testosterone have been established to affect sexual interest directly.

When men with normal levels who reported loss of sexual interest had their levels increased by administration of exogenous testosterone, their sexual interest was increased (O'Carroll & Bancroft, 1984). When sexually deviant subjects with normal levels had these reduced by androgen-suppressing chemicals, both their normal and deviant sexual interest were lowered (Kraemer et al., 1976). Chemical lowering of the deviant interest of sex offenders correlated highly with reduction of their testosterone levels, many of which remained within the normal range (McConaghy et al., 1988).

Despite the findings of the studies reviewed, most of which were carried out in the 1980s, some workers have put more weight on negative reports published in the 1970s to conclude there is no convincing evidence that levels of endogenous testosterone within the normal range are related to sexual behavior in men (Schiavi, Theilgaard, Owen, & White, 1988). None question the evidence that male sexual activity requires a certain level of testosterone and is reduced when the level is below the individual man's threshold. As pointed out in Chapter 5, when this occurs in hypogonadal or castrated men, they experience reduced sexual interest. Their interest is markedly increased when they are administered exogenous testosterone, and it is decreased when the hormone is withdrawn. The acceptance that a certain level of testosterone is required to maintain men's sexual activity is qualified. It is agreed it is necessary to maintain their sexual interest; however, some researchers argue that it is not necessary to maintain their genital erectile ability, and that this is affected only secondarily by the effect of testosterone on sexual interest (see Chapter 5).

Sex Hormones and Sexual Activity in Women

Contrary to the situation with men, researchers have argued that sex hormones do not influence women's sexual interest directly, but secondarily through their effect

on the genital organs. Perhaps the most convincing evidence that hormones do not
directly affect women's sexual interest has been the failure to find consistent changes
in their reported feelings or behaviors accompanying the major hormonal fluctuations that occur during the menstrual cycle. Following termination of the menstrual
cycle by menstruation, the level of estradiol (the major female sex hormone or
estrogen produced by the ovary) rapidly rises as the new ovum begins to develop.
This level peaks immediately before midcycle when the ovum is released to travel
down the Fallopian tube into the uterus. The area of the ovary where the ovum is
released develops as the corpus luteum, which commences to produce the hormone
progesterone. If the ovum is fertilized by male sperm, it will implant in the lining or
endometrium of the uterus, which is prepared for its acceptance under the combined
influence of the hormones of the pre- and postovulatory stages of the cycle. If the
ovum is not fertilized, the corpus luteum does not continue to develop. The consequent fall in levels of progesterone and estradiol leads to shedding of the endometrium in menstruation. Other hormonal changes that occur during the cycle include the level of the androgen testosterone, which gradually rises to peak at
midcycle and then falls to a minimum during menstruation.

Investigations of women's sexual activity during the menstrual cycle have produced markedly inconsistent findings. Seventeen studies reported it to be increased
premenstrually; 18, postmenstrually; 4, during menstruation; and 8, about the time
of ovulation (Donovan, 1985). Donovan suggested that failure to demonstrate consistent relationships could be attributable to women's sexual behavior not having
been conceptualized in a manner that allows such relationships to be observed. He
pointed out that in studying female lower primates the effects of hormones were
related to three components of sexual behavior: receptivity (preparedness to accept
the male), proceptivity (the initiating and inviting of coitus), and attractiveness (nonbehavioral features that promote a sexual approach from the male). Androgens were
considered to favor proceptivity in the monkey; estrogens, to affect all three components; and progesterone, to have inhibitory effects.

Apart from the possible effects of not conceptualizing women's sexual behaviors
appropriately, Donovan believed additional factors could have contributed to the
failure of agreement of the studies he reviewed. These included difficulty in accurately
identifying the phases of the menstrual cycle, inadequate recording of sexual behaviors, and avoidance of sexual activity by some couples during menstruation (resulting
in an increase in frequency on either side of the period of abstinence). The effects of
hormones on women's sexual organs, such as changes in degree of vasoconstriction
and sensitivity, could obscure their effects on sexual interest. Consistent with the
need suggested by Donovan for women's sexual activity to be conceptualized differently, he cited a finding by Adams, Gold, and Burt (1978) that, if valid, indicated the
importance of separating female-initiated from male-initiated behaviors. Adams et
al. reported that the former, but not the latter, peaked at ovulation in married women
who were using contraceptive devices other than the pill. These workers related the
peak in female-initiated behaviors to estrogen rather than androgen levels. Estrogen
levels peaked strongly at midcycle, and both the peak and their overall level of
secretion were greatly reduced by oral contraceptives. Androgen levels peaked only
slightly at midcycle, and their overall secretion was not decreased by oral contraceptives.

A number of studies examining women's sexuality over periods of time rather than in relation to phases of the menstrual cycle have also provided evidence that it is influenced by estrogens. Sexual activity was reduced in both young and menopausal women whose female sex hormone (estradiol) levels were below 35 to 40 pg/ml (Cutler, Garcia, & McCoy, 1987); the menopausal women were reported not to have begun to show vaginal atrophy, loss of rugae, or reduced lubrication. Twenty premenopausal and 14 postmenopausal women receiving replacement estrogen, compared to 14 postmenopausal women not receiving it, reported higher sexual arousal and greater vaginal lubrication in response to viewing an erotic videotape (Myers & Morokoff, 1986). Their vaginal lubrication correlated with blood levels of estradiol. McCoy and Davidson (1985) collected blood from 16 perimenstrual women, 1 to 5 days from the onset of menstruation, at four monthly intervals from 22 months before to 23 months after their final menstrual cycle. Correlations were found between subjects' estradiol and testosterone levels and the number of days they had engaged in sexual intercourse in the preceding 10 weeks (and in the case of testosterone, in the preceding 4 weeks also).

The finding that women's testosterone but not estradiol levels correlated with their frequency of intercourse in both the preceding 4 and 10 weeks in their study was emphasized by McCoy and Davidson (1985), consistent with the commonly stated belief that androgens are the major sex hormones that increase sexual interest in women (Donovan, 1985; Morris, Udry, Khan Dawood, & Dawood, 1987; Sherwin, Gelfand, & Brender, 1985). As discussed in Chapter 5, the belief received its major support from studies reporting loss of sexual interest in women following the major surgical intervention of adrenalectomy, with its associated fall in androgen levels, and the increased sexual interest of women with abnormally high levels of androgen attributable to its administration or to disease. A number of studies, however, failed to find the latter relationship. When it was found, it could be explained as not caused by a central hormonal effect, but as secondary to the abnormally high androgen levels producing hypertrophy and increased sensitivity of the clitoris (Donovan, 1985).

Relationships reported between androgen levels in women and their sexual activity were inconsistent, being found at different stages of the menstrual cycle. That reported by McCoy and Davidson (1985) was between frequency of intercourse in the preceding 4 and 10 weeks and testosterone levels in the first to fifth day of the menstrual cycles; that by Udry, Talbert, and Morris (1986) was between the sexual motivation and frequency of masturbation of adolescent girls, and their levels of androgen taken between the fifth and ninth days of the cycle (too few girls had engaged in intercourse for its frequency to be examined). Morris et al. (1987) replicated a relationship in healthy young married women between their midcycle peak values of testosterone and frequency of intercourse. The authors pointed out that no theoretical mechanism was self-evident to explain why the midcycle level of testosterone predicted average frequency of intercourse when baseline or average levels did not.

The failure in the many studies carried out to find consistent relationships between hormone levels and women's sexual interest suggests that if such relationships exist, they are not strong, supporting the concept that psychological and social factors are much more significant than biological urges in determining sexual activity in women as compared to men.

CHILDHOOD

For a brief period in the 1970s, it appeared that the sexuality of children was to be studied with the objectivity awarded without question to the investigation of most human behavior. Calderone (1979), writing in the American Journal of Diseases of Children, welcomed a forthcoming 3-day international symposium on childhood sexuality as indicating the coming of age of the topic. She considered that until then the sex phobias of a minority group had made it impossible to conduct adequate studies on children between the ages of 5 and 12 and looked forward to a future in which mothers would answer "fine" when asked how they felt when their child played with his penis or her clitoris, rather than "awful," "scared," "angry," "embarrassed," or "I don't know." She contrasted without disapproval the Sicilian peasant mother who took her little boy's penis into her mouth with the American mother who hesitated to even touch her child's genitalia.

Langfeldt (1981) reviewed evidence that the nonpermissive attitude to childhood sexuality characteristic of European societies had arisen only since the concept of children as innocents developed in the seventeenth century. Prior to that, a positive attitude had persisted from ancient Greek times, as it had in other advanced civilizations in the past (Quinsey, 1986). Langfeldt cited as famous a work by Beccadelli of around 1410 that treated the child as an active sexual being and advocated sexual interactions between children and adults. At the beginning of the seventeenth century, the private doctor of Louis XIII recorded his childhood sexual interactions with his sister and adults of the court; according to Aries (1973) such interactions were common at the time.

Langfeldt documented the battle against masturbation as commencing in the eighteenth century, resulting around 1800 in several countries in Europe passing laws against inducing children to masturbate. Forty-nine antimasturbatory devices were patented in the United States between 1856 and 1919. Greydanus and Geller (1980) reviewed the development of what they termed, with unconscious Eurocentricism, the strong "universal" condemnation of masturbation in the eighteenth and nineteenth centuries. They attributed the willingness of the medical profession to allow the moral tone of society to implicate masturbation as a leading cause of their then-high morbidity and mortality rate to its distracting attention from the fact that physicians could do little to correct the rate. This perhaps oversubtle explanation could be advanced to account for the readiness of contemporary mental health workers to allow the moral tone of society to dictate unquestioning acceptance of research claiming to demonstrate adverse effects of socially disapproved sexual activities on the long-term mental health of designated victims; the methodology of such research is not subjected to the rigorous criticism usual in other areas of the study of sexuality (see Chapters 6 and 7). A more likely explanation is that most mental health workers share the moral tone of society.

Ford and Beach (1951) documented the large number of non-European societies that, in contrast to those of contemporary Europe, were permissive of children's sexual activities. In some the adults participated in the sexual stimulation of infants and young children and had heterosexual intercourse with girls from the age of 8 and homosexual activity with boys from the age of 10. Langfeldt (1981) quoted from

Aries (1973) that "the physical contacts described by Heroard [Louis XIII's doctor] would strike us as bordering on sexual perversions and nobody would [now] dare to indulge in them publicly" (p. 101). Langfeldt considered that subsequent to this comment of Aries, opinion had moved in the direction of liberation of childhood sexuality. Langfeldt's own permissiveness was apparent in his statement that "even today many adults are arrested and considered as child molesters if they masturbate with someone below the age of consent. Even to teach children how to masturbate might define the adult as a child molester, or might lead him to be accused of incest" (p. 100). This permissiveness was shared at the beginning of the present decade by a number of sex researchers who were prepared to consider that some sexual interactions between adults and children might have no negative and possibly positive effects (Chapter 6).

Development of a permissive attitude to child sexuality during the 1970s was not universal. Satterfield (1975) pointed out that the most common problems parents reported concerning young children were with masturbation and nudity. She considered that though these were usually attributable to parental concern rather than abnormal behavior of the child, excessive masturbation or inappropriate nudity could be used by a defiant child to provoke the mother or be a sign of severe emotional disturbance in the neurotic, psychotic, or organically impaired child. She believed the majority of sex educators felt parental nudity was harmful if it further provoked the erotic feelings of the child toward the parent of the opposite sex, and she warned about the dangers of parents pushing the preadolescent child into precocious dating. The only study that appears to have examined some of these issues empirically is that of Lewis and Janda (1988), who found that exposure to parental nudity and sleeping in the parents' bed in childhood were positively related in university students to higher self-esteem and less discomfort about physical contact and affection.

Rather than the change anticipated by Calderone (i.e., that normal childhood sexuality would become a topic of study in the 1980s), the opposite occurred. Largely under the influence of feminist politics, virtually any sexual activities between children and adults were labeled as child sexual abuse, and these became a dominant concern of mental health workers. Such activities—when carried out in Western societies—came to be considered abhorrent, severely traumatic to the child, and requiring immediate legal intervention (Chapter 6); their persistence in non-Western societies was ignored or regarded as benign. The coercion of prepubertal boys to fellate postpubertal males among the Sambia, an isolated New Guinea tribe, was treated without approbrium as of theoretical interest in regard to its apparent compatibility with normal male psychosexual development (Chapter 3). Widespread outrage would be the only possible reaction to such activity if it was found being practiced in one of the isolated Western communities exploring alternative child-rearing patterns (Johnston & Deisher, 1973). Another apparent anomaly has been the virtual exclusion of child prostitution from the enormous attention currently given child-adult sexual activities.

To obtain information about the sexual behaviors of children, it is necessary to return to the few earlier studies. Martinson (1976) pointed out the small amount of data obtained by direct observation; most was obtained by recall. Observation revealed erections and vaginal lubrication in children at or soon after birth (Parcel, 1977), and genital play of a volitional nature in the first year of life sufficient to be labeled masturbation (Martinson, 1976). Martinson found some adults recalled discovering masturbation and the pleasures associated with it in the second or third year of life. He cited Kinsey as estimating that more than 50% of boys could achieve orgasm by age 3 or 4, and almost all by 3 to 5 years before puberty; data on girls were not adequate to make an equivalent estimation. Whitfield (1989) cited observations made in the 1970s that indicated that casual interest and exploration of the genitals could occur in both sexes from 7 months, but a more focused exploration with the aim of arousing pleasurable feelings did not begin until 15 to 18 months. Girls' behavior compared to boys tended to be delayed, was less frequent and less focused, and showed less intentionality.

Whitfield stated that it was not known whether genital self-stimulation remained a part of most children's behavioral repertoire from childhood into adolescence. She cited Kinsey et al. (1953) as reporting that by age 12, masturbation was reported in 12% of girls and 20% of boys. In Sorensen's investigation (1973) of the sexual behavior of U.S. adolescents, 7% of boys and 13% of girls reported that they had first masturbated by the age of 10 or younger. Langfeldt (1981) concluded from interviews of children and adults in Oslo that fewer than 30% of children between 2 and 7 years masturbated systematically, and even fewer reached orgasm. After 7, active teaching among boys (which sometimes involved adults) was the most common way they learned to masturbate. Girls tended to discover their first orgasms by accident—for example, while riding a horse or bicycle or sliding down a rope. Some were frightened by the experience, whereas others were pleased by their discovery. From interviews of a stratified random sample of 1,482 parents with 3- to 11-year-old children, Gagnon (1985) found that 47% of parents believed their sons masturbated, and 20% that their daughters did.

Martinson (1976) discussed the development of the child's capacity for sexual awakening in an encounter with another person, considering the infant far too young to experience the nursing experience as sexual, though mothers sometimes reported they themselves did. He quoted anecdotal data indicating that the capacity to relate to another person in an erotically intimate way is present before puberty and in many subjects before the age of 5. In addition to recalled data concerning activity between children of the same and opposite sex a few years apart in age that they found sexually and emotionally arousing, Martinson included the report of a father of a 2½-year-old girl who complied with her request to kiss her clitoris "long like you do to Mommy." She was said to have enjoyed the experience and later asked for a repeat performance. Constantine (1981) found that information concerning nonincestuous experiences was poorly represented in the nonanthropological literature.

Leitenberg, Greenwald, and Tarran (1989) reviewed studies of the sexual interactions of preadolescent children that found them to be reported by 30% to 60% of both men and women, predominantly with members of the opposite sex. Fifty percent of mothers reported they had observed one of their children engaged in such activities; exposure or manual or oral stimulation of the genitals were the most common. Kinsey et al. (1953) found that the most specific erotic activities of younger boys involved genital exhibitionism and genital contacts with other children. In other studies cited by Leitenberg et al. (1989), adults who reported such experiences in childhood showed no difference in current sexual satisfaction or experience from those who did not. In their own study, 235 (54%)of 433 undergraduate university students reported preadolescent sexual experiences with nonsiblings of either sex within 5 years of their own age. The experiences had little impact, either positive or negative, on their current sexual adjustment and behavior. Haugaard and Tilly (1988) found that 42% of more than 1,000 undergraduates reported a childhood experience with another child. Most of the encounters involved sexual kissing or exposing of the genitalia, generally with a friend. High levels of coercion from the other child and encounters with children of the same sex or who were not friends were associated with a more negative response.

Langfeldt (1981) believed that boys were sexually aroused by looking at another boy's erection, and that this could be important in creating sexual groups among boys that were common in all cultures. Often boys started their sexual activity by measuring the sizes of their erections. Langfeldt considered that because of cultural taboos, such groups showed many of the qualities of a secret society. The sexual practices varied from observing each other masturbate to mutual masturbation, fellatio, and interfemoral and anal intercourse. In the last activity, boys of similar ages usually required mutuality with respect to active and passive roles. These groups provided the only sex education most boys received about their own sexuality, that provided by schools being concerned with adult sexuality. Girls rarely formed equiv alent masturbation groups, and pair bonding was the most common situation in which their sexual interactions occurred. They seemed more occupied with caressing each other, and sexual arousal and orgasm could occur without being noticed by the partner. If girls played at intercourse, the requirement of mutual role exchange was common.

In many cases, as girls did not have words for their sexual functions, they did not interpret their sensations as sexual. Langfeldt believed that in the Victorian period a new set of words for the sexual organs and functions was developed to replace the vulgar language of the lower classes. The vulgar language was preserved in the children's culture by boys, who dominated it. This resulted in the disappearance of the female sexual vocabulary especially among girls, with the result that boys had names for penis, head, erection, masturbation, orgasm, and being sexually excited, whereas in general girls had one name for all parts of their genitals. In most Western countries, they had no names for clitoris, lubrication, hardening of the clitoris, urinary opening, vagina, masturbation, or orgasm. Langfeldt's opinion was that the sexual language of the child was a cultural inheritance passed down from older to younger children, particularly among boys.

Borneman (1983), president of the Austrian and German societies for research in sexology, reported in a presentation to the Sixth World Congress of Sexology (held in Washington, D.C.) having taped conversations with 4,367 children and juveniles, which enabled him to study "forbidden" riddles, songs, and verses. He found no evidence of reduction in sexual interest between the age of 6 and puberty, as would be expected if the psychoanalytic theory was correct that a latency period occurred in sexual development at this time. Rather, he found a high incidence of references to brother-sister incest and to parental intercourse in children aged 6 and 7. After puberty, subjects denied knowledge of sexual rhymes and activities in childhood, a denial he attributed to traumatic repression. Borneman believed that normal sexual development of mammals required observation of the mating activities of adults and that if moral laws prevented this in humans, it resulted in irreparable displacement of sexually arousing stimuli, including development of addiction to pornography. Gadpaille, in his commentary that followed Borneman's presentation, remarked that the study could become a major breakthrough in understanding of the psychosexual development of children.

Martinson (1976) suggested that the sexually repressive nature of American society resulted in a lag in sexual learning in childhood and adolescence that accounted for the failure of sex education to improve the rational use of contraceptives by adolescents. He contrasted this with the Scandinavian experience, citing a comparison of children age 5 to 15 years in Australia, North America, England, and Sweden by Goldman and Goldman (1982). This found that American children obtained the lowest scores in knowledge of the simple facts of human sexual life and in understanding of 10 sexual words. The Swedish children obtained the highest scores and were 2 years in advance of the American children. The sampling procedure employed to select the children investigated in the study, however, made it uncertain that the findings could be generalized to the total population of children in these countries. Martinson (1976) found that adults showed negative attitudes toward their recalled childhood sexual experiences, using more terms such as *embarrassed, awkward,* and *ashamed* than *excited, proud,* and *enjoyable.* He attributed this to the fact that the experiences in a sexually repressive society were by necessity furtive, accidental, and isolated.

In relation to parental attitudes to the sexual activity of their children, Martinson (1981) quoted a finding that only 2% of mothers rated themselves as "entirely permissive." He pointed out the lack of a category in the study for the mother to report that she would "actively support and encourage her child's sexual development and experience." He referred to recommendations of some social scientists at the time that parents should support and actively cooperate in the erotic experience of the child, and suggested that this category would have been included in the study if society was truly permissive. He felt safe in asserting that most parents at the time, certainly in the United States, were not convinced and did not feel comfortable or assured that they should contribute to the child's sexual-erotic learning. Calderone (1985) believed that 4- or 5-year-old children know they never get a straight answer about sex from their parents, so they give up asking and learn to keep silent and go underground about their own sexual feelings and activities. She believed the rift in family communication continued into and through adolescence. Though more than 80% of both mothers and fathers in Gagnon's study (1985) thought that most preteen children masturbated, and about 60% believed that this was all right, only about 40% wanted their child to have a positive view of masturbation. When it was observed, a third of the parents reported that they ignored it. Sons were more frequently told to do it in private, and daughters that it was harmful. Fewer than 20% of parents discussed the topic with their child; so even when parents did approve, as Gagnon pointed out, their children were unlikely to know about it.

Parcel (1977), commenting on the myth that sexuality began at puberty, referred to two situations: one of a 3-year old boy lying on top of a 3-year-old girl after both had removed all their clothes, and one of a preschool boy and girl engaged in oral-genital play. He suggested that negative reactions to these situations indicated a poor understanding of the nature of childhood sexuality. It is likely that today, behaviors of this nature between preschool children would lead to suspicion that the children involved were victims of sexual abuse. In 1985, in apparent contrast to her earlier approval (1979) of the Sicilian peasant mother taking her son's penis into her mouth, Calderone emphasized the need for careful and repeated instruction to keep all sexual activities, "sex games," and explorations to one's own age peer group, and noted that there had been an explosion of child sexual abusers. She maintained her earlier, more permissive position to the extent of including scolding and slapping the child's hand when it touched its own genitals accidentally as a form of child sexual abuse, and she referred to a finding that the apathetic, depressed child rarely masturbated, whereas the vigorous, confident child always did. She believed a child was born with a need for contact and that girls received touching much more than boys, despite equal needs. Given the evidence to be discussed in relation to sex offenses (Chapter 8) that a significant proportion of men are capable of sexual arousal toward female children, it would seem necessary to make men aware of this potential when informing them of the need to touch children. Adults instructed to encourage appropriate expressions of childhood sexuality but warned of the dangers of inappropriate adult-child interactions will understandably experience some degree of ambivalence, particularly in view of the current attention given child sexual abuse by the media, welfare agencies, and the scientific community.

PUBERTY

The development at puberty of the secondary sexual characteristics of pubic and auxillary hair and breast development results from the marked increase in male and female sex hormones that occurs at this time (Westney, Jenkins, Butts, & Williams, 1984). These authors reviewed earlier reports that African-Americans are among the earliest women to mature, and that though adolescence is commonly considered to begin at age 12, many black girls have developed early pubertal changes by age 9, with menarche occurring at an average of 12.5 years. Black boys were found to be similar to their 12- to 17-year-old white counterparts in the age of development of secondary sexual characteristics, but to be ahead of white boys and girls in preadolescent sexual activity and ahead of black girls in heterosexual behaviors. Westney et al. investigated 55 black girls and 46 black boys, aged 8 to 11 years. The girls were more advanced than the boys in physical maturation, but there was a significant association only in boys between physical maturation and heterosexual activities. More girls were involved in these activities than boys but to a less advanced degree, most being at a game-playing level. Two boys reported heavy petting, and 1 reported intercourse; no girls reported either activity. Westney et al. compared their subjects' development with earlier norms (Tanner, 1978) based on a nonblack sample. Compared with the norm for acceleration of penis growth of 12.5 years, 16%, 33%, and 60%, respectively, of the 9-, 10-, and 11-year-old black boys were at or beyond that stage.

Compared with the norm for breast development of 11 years, 18%, 74%, and 80% of the 9-, 10-, and 11-year-old girls were at or beyond that stage.

Though it is accepted, as discussed above, that some children masturbate to orgasm from an early age, the percentage who do so and the frequency of the behavior is not established. Though some studies have indicated that up to one-half of male and somewhat fewer female children masturbate, most adults report not having done so prior to adolescence (Whitfield, 1989). There is general agreement that the marked increase in sex hormones and the rapid development of sexual characteristics such as pubic hair that occur in both boys and girls at puberty (Kinsey et al., 1953) is accompanied only in boys by a dramatic increase in sexual interest and incidence of masturbation and orgasm. Kinsey et al. reported that masturbation was reported by 20% of males aged 12, but 80% of those aged 15 and 92% of those aged 20 years; equivalent percentages for girls of these ages were 12%, 20%, and 33%.

Whitfield (1989) reported similar findings from other studies. She estimated that the percentage of women experiencing orgasm increased gradually from 1.3% before 3 years of age through 2% by 5, 4% by 7, 9% by 11, and 14% by 13 years. These figures, if correct, indicate a minimal effect of puberty on the prevalence of the experience of orgasm in women; data are not available to establish if this is true also of the effect of puberty on its frequency. Whitfield pointed out the finding suggested that the sexual behavior of women as compared to men is more under social than biological control. This conclusion was also supported by the study of Knoth et al. (1988), who found that the modal age for first experiencing sexual arousal was between 11 and 12 years in boys and between 13 and 15 years in girls. The majority of girls reported that their first arousal occurred during physical contact with a male. Boys were more likely to report that it was in response to a visual stimulus. Evidence of the dependency of most women's sexuality on an emotional relationship with a male partner remains present at all stages of development after childhood.

Menarche

Whitfield (1981) reviewed studies of girls' experiences of menarche. Most found it less negative and painful than they expected, and after 3 months were talking about it with female relatives and friends, though mainly concerning related symptoms. Langfeldt (1981) reported of the Norwegian girls he studied that they were normally very proud of their first menstruation and that their talk in relation to sex was mainly about this and the growth of their breasts. One of the studies reviewed by Whitfield found that for the postmenarcheal girl, the abstract concept that menstruation was evidence of her developing maturity did not compensate for concrete concerns that she would be caught unprepared, bleed through her clothes, and be messy and unclean. In relation to such concerns, another study found that most girls were given napkins by their mothers at the time of their first period. The use of tampons had been mentioned to about half the girls by their mothers prior to or at menarche. The mothers' attitudes to their use was influential on the daughters' decisions to use them, though within 2 years most of the girls studied had used them at least some of the time. Whitfield commented on the rarity of references to virginity in the studies. She cited the belief of some theorists that tampons served a role in girls' psychosexual development, helping them to come to terms with their maturing body, to develop a positive body image, and to make a positive identification as a mature female.

Investigation of sexual feelings in relation to menarche revealed that following it, schoolgirls were more likely to perceive themselves as popular with boys and to date. McGrory (1990) considered the most interesting finding of her study of the responses to menarche of early adolescent females to be resistance of parents to their daughters' participation in the study. Of the 162 contacted, 67 refused, commonly on the grounds it was too personal a topic. Of 95 girls aged 11 to 15 years who participated, only 3 of the 31 who were premenarcheal and 22 of the 64 who were postmenarcheal answered all questions of the Menstrual Attitude Questionnaire, though they completed other scales. McGrory concluded that for early adolescent females, menstruation remains very threatening. Among the responses supporting earlier findings was that there was little difference in attitudes toward menarche of pre- and post-menarcheal girls; their overall self-esteem and physical self-esteem did not differ significantly. Consistent with the finding reported above that most girls found the onset of menstruation less negative than they expected, premenarchial girls thought it was more debilitating.

Spermarche

Gaddis and Brooks-Gunn (1985) cited Shipman as reporting in 1971 that boys experienced initial ejaculation negatively. Late adolescents reported that it scared the hell out of them, or that they thought they were ill. Only 15% of the boys investigated by Shipman understood the concept of ejaculation prior to its occurrence. Gaddis and Brooks-Gunn suggested that lack of preparation may have accounted in part for the negative reaction, as it did for that to menarche. They suggested the more positive responses reported by 11 private-school boys aged 13 to 15 were attributable to the higher number who were prepared for the experience; 6 knew a lot and 5 a little about it beforehand. Two of the latter subjects reported being very scared by it, but most of the total group reported positive feelings of excitement and being grown-up. Most had learned about ejaculation through reading, only 3 having had it explained to them. In only 1 of the 3 was this by a parent, his father. Gaddis and Brooks-Gunn commented that this was in stark contrast to girls, virtually all of them were informed concerning menarche by their mothers and also took health classes that covered menarche. Two boys found health classes an ambiguous source of information about ejaculation.

A 1975 retrospective investigation cited by Gaddis and Brooks-Gunn investigated 451 college students concerning their most frequent informational source about ejaculation. Peers were reported by 46% and literature by 26%; parents and others played an inconsequential role. None of the boys interviewed by Geddis and Brooks-Gunn talked to their friends about their first ejaculation, again in marked contrast to girls' experiences with menarche. Geddis and Brooks-Gunn suggested the conspiracy of silence concerning ejaculation could result in part from its link with masturbation, a link not present with menarche. They commented that masturbation did not seem to be discussed by girls, either.

ADOLESCENCE

As with sexuality in childhood, limited attention has been given to many aspects of adolescent sexuality. Recent adolescent psychiatry and psychology texts contained no information concerning sexual dysfunctions or sex offenses (Rutter & Hersov, 1985) or, indeed, none concerning any aspect of sexual behavior (Weiner, 1982). Contributing to this may be the marked reluctance of adolescents to reveal their sexual activity—particularly activity they regard as socially unacceptable—to clinicians and investigators. The resultant lack of knowledge concerning adolescent sexuality has proved extremely misleading. A series of studies reported that of 62 subjects exposed to increased levels of opposite-sex hormones in utero and 48 controls, only 1 had experienced homosexual feelings (see Chapter 3); about half of the subjects were prepubertal and half adolescent. These reports, grossly at variance with evidence that 20% or more adolescents are aware of some homosexual feelings, were by experienced sex researchers, and the finding was attributed major theoretical importance in refuting the theory that homosexual feelings resulted from exposure in utero to increased levels of opposite-sex hormones.

Money, Schwartz, and Lewis (1984), in a subsequent follow-up study of subjects subjected to such exposure, found that when adolescent they had treated their sexual activity as an unspeakable issue, but when adult they reported a high incidence of homosexual feelings. It was concluded that aging of these subjects brought increased sophistication and ability to talk about their sexual feelings and behavior. Schofield (1968) had earlier pointed out that boys aged 15 to 19 will not readily answer questions about homosexuality, and that such information is better obtained by asking older people to look back to the time they were teenagers. Porteous (1985) commented that when adolescents are surveyed concerning problems, they rarely mention sexual ones. A study of the 65 teenagers who committed suicide from 1979 to 1983 in Metro Dade County, Florida (Copeland, 1985), revealed that of the 80% in whom the cause was known, in 17% it was a boyfriend/girlfriend problem; in 5%, out-of-wedlock pregnancy; in 5%, a love triangle; and other sexual problems in a further 10%. Sexual problems would seem of considerable significance to adolescents, though they will not easily reveal them.

My experience with adolescent patients referred for assessment of deviant sexual activity is consistent with this conclusion. Patients with whom I believed I had established excellent therapeutic relationships have reported good response to treatment and complete control of deviant behavior, only to admit subsequently that this was not so when confronted with evidence to the contrary provided by their relatives or by legal authorities. When these adolescents were questioned as to why they found it so difficult to report their deviant behavior, many said they tried to avoid thinking about it, appearing to believe that if they could do this, it would not happen again. This led them to deny the existence of the behavior between episodes of its occurrence. In view of this reticence, in investigating and treating adolescents with psychosexual disorders it is necessary to utilize as many sources of information as possible (having obtained the patient's consent to this procedure).

The sexual activity of adolescents that is most consistently studied has been heterosexual intercourse, and in particular the age at which it was initiated. A recent monograph, "Adolescent Sexuality" (Antonovsky, Kav-venaki, Lancet, Modan, & Shoham, 1980) dealt only with heterosexual intercourse, ignoring such behaviors as masturbation, homosexuality, deviant behaviors, sexual assault, and incest. In recent years, however, a substantial literature has appeared dealing with adolescent victims of sexual assault and incest (Chapters 6, 7). The lack of interest in the broad range of adolescent sexual behaviors is perhaps evidenced by the fact that the most representative survey in the United States was carried out by Sorensen in 1973. Hopkins (1977) pointed out the sample Sorensen studied included only 47% of his original probability sample and was likely to overrepresent the most sexually aware and liberal young people.

Masturbation in Adolescence

Masturbation in adolescence has received little more attention than in other stages of life. Possibly the fact that it is usually carried out in private makes it of minimal interest to most contemporary students of behavior, who consider social factors to be the major if not sole determinant. In Sorenson's survey (1973) of adolescent sexuality, masturbation was the most common sexual outlet in males. Seventy-eight percent of boys aged 16 to 19 reported having masturbated and 72% having had heterosexual intercourse; 42% of girls aged 16 to 19 reported having masturbated and 57% having had intercourse. Of adolescents who reported having masturbated, more than 90% of boys and girls had started by the age of 14, whereas of nonvirgins only 53% of boys and 30% of girls had experienced heterosexual intercourse by that age. Also, of the group with masturbatory experience, 62% of boys and 54% of girls had such experience in the previous month; of nonvirgins, 53% of the boys and 73% of the girls had engaged in heterosexual intercourse in the previous month. In view of the difficulty many women experience in achieving orgasm, Sorensen's finding that, of adolescents with current masturbatory experience, 74% of girls masturbated without orgasm in the previous month was perhaps not unexpected. That 21% of the boys also masturbated without orgasm in this period was less so, in view of the widely held belief advanced by Kinsey, Pomeroy, and Martin (1948) that males readily reach orgasm in sexual activity.

Masturbation did not appear to be less frequent in adolescents having more regular coitus, of whom Sorensen identified two groups, the serial monogamous and the sexual adventurer. Ninety-three percent of the former and 81% of the latter had engaged in intercourse in the previous month, compared to 62% of all coitally experienced subjects; a similar percentage of the three groups (37%) masturbated over the same period. Eighty-three percent of boys and 90% of girls who masturbated fantasized some or most of the time they did so. Thirty percent of boys and 22% of girls looked at pictures some or most of the time. This practice was reported by 40% of boys aged 16 to 19, as compared to 25% of those aged 13 to 15. The reverse trend, for older adolescents to cease the behavior, was found in girls. Of girls aged 16 to 19, none reported the practice most of the time, and only 10% some of the time; of girls aged 13 to 15, 18% and 32%, respectively, reported these frequencies. Of all the adolescents who masturbated, 59% of boys and 49% of girls said they enjoyed it somewhat or a great deal.

Clifford (1978) investigated 100 undergraduate women, aged 17 to 25 years, who agreed to be interviewed on subjective aspects of sexuality (186 women were approached). Forty-nine had reached orgasm through masturbation, and a further 25 had masturbated without orgasm. Both groups remembered stimulating themselves most commonly between the ages of 12 and 15, with 7 commencing before 10 and 4 not until the age 20 years. In high school, 47 subjects had enjoyed masturbation somewhat or a good deal. Giving up masturbation was strongly related to the incidence of orgasm; 14% of those who were orgasmic gave up masturbation for a year or more, as did 56% of those who were not. Significant positive relationships were found between incidence of orgasm with masturbation and various techniques, including lying flat on the back, using several fingers, stroking around and on the clitoris, and tensing of muscles. The most common reasons given for masturbation were pleasurable sensations and physical release of sexual tension. There was no relationship between frequency of masturbation and intercourse in subjects with both types of experience. Fifteen women noted that they preferred masturbation when they specifically desired self-exploration; others preferred it when tired, suffering genital soreness, ill, or during their periods. The relationship reported by Kinsey et al. (1953) that women who masturbated to orgasm were more likely to achieve orgasm in intercourse was not found, though Clifford pointed out that her subjects (unlike those of Kinsey et al.) had intercourse irregularly.

Sorensen (1973) commented that of the sex practices he investigated, there seemed to be none about which the adolescents felt more defensive or private than masturbation. Of his sample of adolescents with masturbatory experience, 17% of boys and 13% of girls reported experiencing guilt, anxiety, or concern about the activity often, and only 17% of boys and 22% of girls never did. Sorensen opined that, if anything, the incidence of masturbation was underreported in his survey. Clark and Tifft (1966) found that 30% of 45 male sociology students underreported masturbation in an anonymous questionnaire; 95% admitted it after being given an opportunity to correct their report prior to undergoing a polygraph examination on their final responses. The percentage underreporting masturbation was higher than that underreporting heterosexual or homosexual relations. Lo Presto, Sherman, and Sherman (1985) suggested that statements by many researchers and clinicians that masturbation is beneficial to self-awareness and sexual behavior had not significantly modified the views of many young people who retained societal and religious taboos concerning it.

Adolescents continue to be exposed within their families to what must be considered at best ambivalent attitudes toward their masturbation. About 80% of Sorensen's sample (1973) of adolescents reported that their parents had never talked to them about masturbation, a similar percentage to that of parents who reported they never discussed masturbation with their preteenage children, although over 80% believed preteenage children masturbated (Gagnon, 1985). The findings of these two studies suggest there was no change in parental behavior in this respect in the intervening decade. There appears to be some community acceptance that children should be reassured that there is nothing wrong with masturbation: 62% of the 4,000 readers of *Consumer Reports* who answered a questionnaire about the quality of personal relationships believed this was needed, and only 16% were opposed (Brecher, 1984).

In view of the strong relationship between masturbatory guilt and low self-esteem widely reported throughout the literature, Lo Presto et al. (1985) attempted to reduce such guilt by a 40-minute masturbation seminar. They compared its effect with that of a discussion of homosexuality of similar duration; assessment was by the Negative Attitudes Toward Masturbation Inventory. They concluded that the masturbation seminar produced more positive attitudes toward masturbation and reduced sex myths, but did not influence guilt feelings. Reduction in negative attitudes was not expressed through increase in self-reported frequency of masturbation. Researchers into sexuality, meanwhile, have shown little interest in investigating possible long-term effects of the significant level of guilt experienced by most adolescents concerning this common sexual activity. Houck and Abramson (1986) cited a few unreplicated studies finding that the Negative Attitudes Toward Masturbation Inventory predicted diaphragm use, the effect of sex education, the experience of female orgasm, and less pelvic vasoconstriction in response to sexual stimuli.

Initiation of Heterosexual Intercourse

Consistent with the major interest of sex researchers in investigating the initiation of intercourse, it has been considered one of the most important psychological events in adolescent development, a declaration of independence and autonomy from parents, an affirmation of attainment of sexual identity, and a statement of capability of interpersonal intimacy (Hopkins, 1977). The increase in incidence of premarital intercourse and reduction in the age at which it was initiated in the United States in the 1970s were considered so great as to constitute a sexual revolution. Certainly a revolutionary change occurred in attitude to premarital coitus: In 1963, 80% of a representative national sample of adults believed it was always wrong; in 1975, 30% believed this (Rodman, Lewis, & Griffith, 1984). Hopkins (1977), however, questioned the evidence that an increase in the incidence of premarital coitus in adolescents had occurred at that time. He stated that the samples studied were not adequately representative of the total adolescent population and that the terminology used could have distorted the findings. Some younger adolescents reported having had "sexual intercourse" in the belief that it meant socializing with the opposite sex, and older adolescents varied considerably as to the meaning they attached to "loss of virginity."

Studies of college students provided more convincing evidence of change. From the mid-1960s to the mid-1970s, premarital coitus incidence figures rose from about 25% to 40% for women and from 55% to 60% for men; Hopkins (1977) pointed out the trend to intergender convergence. If initially the increased incidence of premarital intercourse was restricted to the oldest adolescents, within a few years it was present in the younger also. The marked increase in the 1970s in incidence both of sexually transmitted diseases and of pregnancy in unmarried teenagers in the United States demonstrated that a major change in adolescent sexual activity had occurred at least by the end of the 1970s.

Zelnik, Kantner, and Ford (1981) reported that of a fairly representative sample of unmarried metropolitan teenagers, 20% of girls and 35% of boys aged 15 and 45% of girls and 56% of boys aged 17 had experienced coitus. This was a striking increase in incidence when compared with the data provided over 20 years earlier by

Kinsey et al. (1948, 1953). By the 1980s, when the increase in incidence leveled off, about half of white females and three-fourths of black females were having intercourse by age 18 (Furstenberg, Brooks-Gunn, & Chase-Lansdale, 1989), as were 60% of white males by age 18 and of black males by age 16 (Brooks-Gunn & Furstenberg, 1989). The relative increase was much greater in girls than boys, demonstrating that the intergender convergence noted by Hopkins (1977) in college students had occurred in adolescents generally. These trends to earlier age of initial coitus and intergender convergence have been reported in many Western countries, including Canada (Barrett, 1980) and Czechoslovakia (Raboch and Bartak, 1980). Studies from West Germany (Clement, Schmidt, & Kruse, 1984) and Sweden (Lewin, 1982) found more young adolescent girls having begun coitus than boys. These trends may not have taken place in non-Western cultures. Of unmarried Columbian university students (mean age 22 to 23) studied from 1979 to 1981, 94% of the males reported having experienced coitus, compared with 38% of females (Alzate, 1984). Investigation of Nigerian university students (median age 22) found that 28% of women had experienced coitus by age 16 but only a further 10% by age 21, compared to 7% and 23% of men, respectively (Soyinka, 1979), suggesting a different pattern of adolescent sexual development than that in Western countries.

Brooks-Gunn and Furstenberg (1989) discussed the factors determining the age of initiation of coitus. They noted that early maturation may reduce this not only by increasing sexual interest, but by encouraging friendships with older subjects, with adoption of their patterns of smoking, drinking, and sexual behaviors. Brooks-Gunn and Furstenberg found little evidence of parental influence, pointing out that parents were often uncomfortable discussing sexual topics with their children, other than menarche, which mothers discussed with their daughters. They reported the finding of one study that whereas communication between mothers and their sons and daughters was associated with later intercourse, that between fathers and sons was associated with earlier intercourse.

Brooks-Gunn and Furstenberg suggested that commonly held beliefs about the importance of peer influence were not supported by the research data available, which indicated that adolescents' perceptions about what their peers were doing, or what was normative adolescent behavior, were more strongly associated with the subjects' sexual behavior than their peers' actual behavior. Male adolescents were found to be more likely than females to be influenced by such perceptions in Sorensen's study (1973): Of the nonvirgin adolescents, 32% of boys and 22% of girls aged 13 to 15, and 12% of boys and 5% of girls aged 16 to 19, reported having sex on one or more occasions mostly because people would have put them down if they had not. A number of the boys in Schofield's fairly representative sample (1968) of English teenagers reported that the reason for their first intercourse was to prove themselves. Muehlenhard and Cook (1988) found that peer pressure and a desire to be popular, as well as sex-role expectations, were reported as reasons why more male than female students engaged in unwanted sexual intercourse in their study. Teenagers who were not doing well in school and had lower educational aspirations were more likely to have sex during adolescence than those faring better. As school functioning was mediated by the education, job, and welfare status of the mother, children in poverty were at risk both for school failure and early sexuality.

Smith and Udry (1985) attributed the lower age at first intercourse of black as compared to white adolescents to different patterns of sexual activity. In their pro-spective study of adolescents aged 12 to 15 years, they found that the black subjects were less likely than the whites to engage in a predictable sequence of noncoital behaviors for a period of time before they commenced intercourse. White adolescents tended to progress through kissing, necking, light petting (above the waist and/or over clothes), heavy petting, and intercourse. The precoital experiences of black teenagers often involved only kissing, resulting in less delay before intercourse oc-curred in their relationships. Brooks-Gunn and Furstenberg (1989) suggested that black girls who move from necking to intercourse without intermediate steps may have less time to think about and obtain contraceptives.

Hacker (1987) advanced an alternative explanation for the earlier age of inter-course in black as compared with white teenagers. He cited evidence that the dif-ference in age was much less marked in those who attended integrated schools, and that teenage parentage was most pronounced in black girls in segregated settings, where their schools, housing, and acquaintances were almost entirely within their race. Blacks in this situation rated marriage as less important and reported a greater tolerance for sexual activity and childbearing outside marriage. Currently most black Americans live in neighborhoods that are all or mainly black, and Hacker considered this was unlikely to change, as whites tended to leave a neighborhood once the number of blacks living there rose above 8%. Residential segregation was as pro-nounced among black families with incomes over $50,000 as it was among those with lower earnings. Hacker concluded that this social and cultural isolation, more than any other single factor, encouraged the early siring and bearing of children without thought for the future. As discussed subsequently, thought for the future does appear among the majority of black mothers in adulthood.

The somewhat negative attitude toward early age of initiation of intercourse reflected in the studies discussed expresses the tendency in the United States, noted by Jones et al. (1985), to react to the high levels of extramarital teenage pregnancy by aiming to discourage teenage sexual activity; they pointed out that the U.S. govern-ment has advocated and subsidized a program intervention for this purpose. There appears little evidence that early sexual activity of itself has harmful consequences. Leitenberg et al. (1989) found that 302 (70%) of 433 undergraduate university students reported early adolescent sexual experiences with nonsiblings of either sex within 5 years of their own age and not older than 16 years. Similar to their finding concerning preadolescent sexual interactions, there was no relationship between the occurrence of the experiences and the students' current sexual adjustment and behav-ior. This was true also of the 38 subjects (of whom 19 were female) for whom the experiences included intercourse. Furstenberg et al. (1989) commented that most efforts to influence teens' postponement of sexual activity, such as school-based health clinics, are recent and innovative, and their impacts have yet to be fully evaluated. The governments of the other developed countries Jones et al. investigat-ed—in particular, Canada, England and Wales, France, the Netherlands, and Swe-den—directed their policies at reducing not teenage sexual activity but pregnancy levels, by deliberately encouraging the use of contraception. In these countries, apart from Canada, the percentage of teenage girls having intercourse by age 17 was comparable with that in the United States; the percentage in Sweden was higher at all ages. Their levels of adolescent pregnancies, however, were markedly lower.

In contrast to the number of studies investigating age at initiation of intercourse, Weis (1985) commented on the lack of empirical evidence concerning the subjective reactions of women to this experience. He found that the belief was widely held that pain was a central feature, citing as sources Deutsch, Freud, and popular sex books, of which the most recent was published in 1973. Weis reported the responses of 130 college women who had experienced coitus to an anonymous questionnaire. One-third experienced severe pain, two-fifths moderate pain, and a quarter no pain. On a series of affective dimensions, 58% reported high levels of nervousness; 38%, romance and excitement; 34%, fear; and 24%, guilt. Women who experienced coitus at an early age, who did not expect pain, and who experienced little pleasure and high levels of guilt, anxiety, and a sense of exploitation were most likely to experience pain.

Though Weis referred to the earlier study of Sorensen (1973), he did not discuss the disparity in their findings. One question asked in Sorensen's study of a more representative sample of U.S. adolescents aged 13 to 19 years was which of a list of possible responses represented their feelings the first time they had sex with a member of the opposite sex. Only 25% of the girls reported "hurt" as one of them. Otherwise, like the women investigated by Weis, their most common responses were negative; 63% were afraid, and 31% to 36% were worried, guilty, and embarrassed. The male adolescents' most common responses were positive; 40% to 46% were excited, happy, satisfied, and/or thrilled. In Schofield's study (1968) of a representative sample of English teenagers, less than half the boys and one-third of the girls said they liked their first experience of intercourse. It is possible, though unlikely, that as many U.S. as English teenagers reported negative feelings in the two studies. Sorensen did not report the total number of boys whose responses were positive; if the 40% to 46% of boys who reported the different positive responses in his study were the same boys, the majority may not have liked the experience.

Brooks-Gunn, Boyer, and Heim (1988) also pointed out the lack of information concerning aspects of the sexual behavior of adolescents other than their age at initiation of heterosexual coitus. Additional data were needed to understand the possible spread of human immunodeficiency virus (HIV) infection, including the percentage of adolescents who had intercourse only once, the number of their partners, and whether they were in relationships with their first partners. Brooks-Gunn et al. cited Sorensen's identification (1973) of two types of adolescents, the serial monogamous and the sexual adventurer. The latter, who composed 41% of the sexually experienced males and 13% of sexually experienced females in his study, had an average of 3.2 partners in the month preceding their interview. A 1987 national survey Brooks-Gunn et al. also cited found that 39% of male and 17% of female unmarried 18- to 24-year-old subjects had intercourse with three or more partners in the previous year. Brooks-Gunn et al. suggested that more than 10% of adolescent males probably had some same-sex experience; homosexuality in adolescence is discussed in Chapter 3.

Sexually Transmitted Diseases

The increase in sexual activity of teenagers up to the early 1980s was accompanied by a marked increase in incidence in sexually transmitted diseases (STDs).

From 1960 to 1981, the incidence of gonorrhea in the United States rose from 15 to 25 per 100,000 for boys and 25 to 75 per 100,000 for girls aged 10 to 14 years, and from 490 to 1,000 per 100,000 for boys and 350 to 1,400 per 100,000 for girls aged 15 to 19 (Howard, 1985). While reporting that rates had remained relatively stable since 1975, Mascola, Albritton, Cates, and Reynolds (1983) believed that twice as many cases in adolescents remained unreported and pointed out the significance of such future complications in the infected girls as infertility and ectopic pregnancies. They attributed the increased incidence not only to increased sexual activity but also to a change in contraceptive methods less protective against STDs. Similarly, Brooks-Gunn and Furstenberg (1989) implicated early age of intercourse and no or irregular contraceptive use. They cited 1985 reports that apart from homosexual men and prostitutes, female teenagers had the highest rates of gonorrhea, cytomegalovirus, chlamydia cervicitis, and pelvic inflammatory disease of any age group. A similar trend was evident in England where the incidence of new cases of gonorrhea per 100,000 of the population was 145 and 79, respectively, for men and women of all ages, but 277 and 390 for men and women aged 16 to 19 (Peters, 1989).

The appearance of HIV infection, with its associated likelihood of producing the acquired immune deficiency syndrome (AIDS), added a further health risk to sexual activity. Brooks-Gunn and Furstenberg (1989) pointed out that though few adolescents have been reported to have AIDS, the number has been doubling in recent years. Also, one-fifth of all cases have occurred in 20- to 29-year-olds; in view of the long incubation period of the virus, many of these individuals were likely to have been infected in late adolescence. Brooks-Gunn and Furstenberg concluded that if the proportion of cases increases significantly in the heterosexual population, adolescents may be at relatively high risk, given their current rates of other STDs and their poor use of contraception. Brooks-Gunn et al. (1988) pointed out that as of May 1988, there were 705 AIDS patients (1% of all cases) aged 13 to 21 years, of whom compared to the adult patients, a greater percentage were female (14% vs. 7%), members of minority rather than nonminority groups (53% vs. 38%), and infected by heterosexual rather than homosexual transmission (9% vs. 4%). Heterosexual contact accounted for 46% of the female adolescent cases.

Twenty percent of the adolescent AIDS patients were in New York City. There the sex ratio was 2.9 males to 1 female, in contrast to the 7 to 1 ratio for adults; and heterosexual transmission accounted for 52% of the adolescent female patients (Brooks-Gunn et al., 1988). These authors pointed out that as of 1987, only a small percentage of teenagers had received formal instruction about AIDS in school, though the vast majority desired this. Subsequently, more than half of the large urban schools initiated AIDS education, although the programs tended to be short and nonspecific. Studies revealed that some teenagers reported changes in casual behavior, such as "avoiding gays," but few reported changes in most sexual behaviors that transmitted the virus: 10% used condoms, and 10% abstained from sex.

Male–Female Differences in Sexual Motivation

Studies of male and female adolescents found differences in their motivation for becoming involved in sexual activity that have remained unchanged over the past few decades. Skipper and Nass (1966) concluded from their study of dating behavior of student nurses, medical students, interns, residents, and college males that the females' primary motivation was courtship (i.e., selecting a mate whom they might marry); the males' was primarily recreation (i.e., a source of entertainment and immediate enjoyment). Of the fairly representative sample of English teenagers aged 15 to 19 studied by Schofield (1968), approximately half of both males and females agreed with the statement that a girl is usually looking for a man to marry, but a boy is usually looking for sex. Asked the reason for their commencing coitus, boys were most likely to report they were impelled by sexual desire; girls, that they were in love. Though more boys than girls enjoyed their first experience of coitus, following it they were more likely to seek a new partner; girls were more willing to try again with the same partner. In Sorensen's investigation (1973) of U.S. adolescents, 65% of girls but only 49% of boys reported they wouldn't want to have sex only for the physical enjoyment; 76% of girls and 47% of boys wouldn't want to have sex with someone they didn't love, and similar percentages wouldn't want to have sex with someone who didn't love them. Boys appeared to recognize the importance girls placed on the love relationship. Eighteen percent of those aged 16 to 19 would tell a girl he loved her when he didn't; only 2% of girls would tell a boy she loved him when she didn't. Of adolescents who reported they were having sex mostly or only with one partner, 60% of the girls aged 13 to 15 and 50% of those aged 16 to 19 planned to get married to him; 4% and 25% of boys in those age ranges planned to get married to their partner. The most common description of the first person they had intercourse with, in the case of girls, was a boy they were going steady with and planned to marry (36%); in the cases of boys, a girl they knew well and liked a lot, though they weren't going together (31%).

Carroll, Volk, and Hyde (1985) investigated a random sample of 130 male and 119 female college students aged 18 to 23 by questionnaire. Forty-five percent of the women and 8% of the men reported that an emotional involvement was a prerequisite for participating in sexual intercourse. The authors concluded that the men's motives for intercourse were pleasure, fun, and physical satisfaction; the women's were love, commitment, and emotion. Thirty-eight percent of the women and 16% of the men believed the male should be more the initiator in a sexual relationship; 3% of the men and no women thought the women should be. Wilson (1987) cited a finding with children raised on an Israeli kibbutz, in what he termed a sex-blind highly permissive environment, that 12% of the boys but only 2% of the girls agreed with the statement that it doesn't matter with whom one has coitus. Randolph and Winstead (1988) reported an analysis of the questionnaire responses of 79 female and 135 male unmarried students aged 19 or more that revealed that men were more likely to show a desire to have sex with a great many partners and to engage in sex because of their interest in the partner's good looks or "great body" or because they saw sex as a challenge; females endorsed items indicating that they formed a sexual relationship because they were interested in what their partner felt and thought, because they were in love, because they valued their partner, and because they wanted a mutually satisfying relationship.

Townsend and Levy (1990) investigated the significance of socioeconomic status (SES) in relationships of college students. In addition to finding that women as compared to men were more likely to prefer that coitus took place in relationships that involved affection and marriage potential, women also placed more emphasis on the partners' higher SES. Townsend and Levy cited studies that reported that this emphasis did not change as the women's SES increased; rather, their economic standards for male partners tended to increase accordingly. Townsend and Levy pointed out that their findings were more consistent with the evolutionary theory of determination of men and women's sexual interest (discussed at the beginning of the chapter) than the idea that the differences were solely the result of differential access to resources and differential socialization.

Though initiation of coitus in a relationship appears more motivated by enjoyment in the male and the need to love and be loved in the female, it appears that it is important to the male that his partner enjoys the experience. Of the nonvirgin boys in Sorensen's study (1973), 64% of those aged 13 to 15 and 83% of those aged 16 to 19 reported that it bothered them a lot if they had sex with a girl and she didn't seem to be completely satisfied. Interestingly, the equivalent question was not asked of nonvirgin girls, who instead were asked was it very important to them when they had sex that they reached a climax or orgasm; 60% of those aged 13 to 15 and 45% of those aged 16 to 19 stated it was. This is consistent with the data, discussed in Chapter 5, that indicated that it is more important to the male than the female partner than the woman experiences orgasm in coitus.

Despite differences in male and female expectations of sexual relationships, both male and female adolescents appear to share similar attitudes toward male coercion. In Sorensen's study (1973), 26% of boys and 25% of girls agreed that if a girl had led a boy on, it was all right for the boy to force her to have sex. Goodchilds and Zellman (1984) concluded from interviews of 432 California adolescents that the norms of the earlier era were still operative. Males were expected to be sexually aggressive, whereas females had to control sexual behavior, be responsible for sexual outcomes, and maintain positive affect despite rejecting the advances of the male. The subjects were asked if it was all right for a boy to hold a girl down and force her to have sexual intercourse in the following circumstances: (1) he spends a lot of money on her, (2) he's so turned on he can't stop, (3) she is stoned or drunk, (4) she has had sexual intercourse with other guys, (5) she lets him touch her above the waist, (6) she says she's going to have sex with him and then changes her mind, (7) they have dated a long time, (8) she's led him on, or (9) she gets him sexually excited. Two-thirds thought force was definitely contraindicated in the first circumstance, but less than one-third considered this for the ninth. One-third of the subjects who thought it was justified in some of the circumstances were girls. The ordering of the behaviors was essentially the same for boys and girls. The authors commented that what was most sobering was the finding, repeated in several shades and nuances, that both males and females accepted as the norm an essentially adversarial cross-gender relationship regarding sexual issues, and that efforts to change these patterns must be more sweeping than anyone had imagined.

Adolescent Pregnancy

As Brooks-Gunn and Furstenberg (1989) pointed out, the tension between sexuality as pleasure and as reproduction results from the need of all societies to manage sexuality in order to regulate fertility, and political and economic considerations are evident in discussions of the societal and individual cost of adolescent pregnancy and parenthood. By the 1980s, the greater incidence of adolescent pregnancies in the United States compared to other nations was being identified as having reached epidemic proportions (Beck & Davies, 1987), with more than a million 15- to 19-year-olds pregnant (one-tenth of all women in this age group) and 30,000 girls younger than 15 becoming pregnant annually (Rodman, Lewis, & Griffith, 1984). Rodman et al. cited data from Zelnik and Kantner's surveys of metropolitan-area teenagers that showed an increase in premarital pregnancies in women aged 15 to 19 from 9% in 1971 to 13% in 1976 and 16% in 1979. This increase could be largely attributed to the increased number of unmarried adolescents who were sexually active rather than to reduction in effective contraceptive practices, given that the increase in pregnancies in those sexually active over the same period was much less (from 28% to 30%). It would appear that the use of contraception remained at much the same level of relative inadequacy among the unmarried throughout the 1970s.

Twenty percent of teenagers who experienced an unwanted pregnancy repeated the experience at least once (Byrne, 1983). Of those who gave birth, one of four became pregnant again within a year (Sugar, 1984). The ratio of first pregnancies in 15- to 19 year-olds that were terminated by abortion almost doubled from 17% in 1971 to 30% in 1976. Annually, however, more than 200,000 adolescent pregnancies resulted in out-of-wedlock births, and about 100,000 in what were considered hasty, unanticipated marriages that disrupted the mothers' educational and vocational plans (Byrne, 1983). Sugar (1984) pointed out that most unmarried upper- and middle-class girls opted for abortion, whereas lower- or working-class girls kept their babies in about 95% of cases. Flick (1986) interpreted data from the late 1970s to conclude that 50% of females 15- to 19-year-old were sexually active, and 33% of these became pregnant. Of the 33%, 14% had a miscarriage or stillbirth, 38% an abortion, and 49% delivered a baby (which 90% reared and 10% had adopted out). Hence 1 in 6 adolescent girls aged 15 to 19 years had been pregnant, and 1 in 14 were raising a child premaritally conceived.

A mid-1980s National Research Council study (Hacker, 1987) found that 40% of black and 20% of white teenagers became pregnant, approaching half the number who were sexually active, which indicates no improvement in the use of contraception. Differences in the outcome of the pregnancies of the black and white girls were not great. Respectively, 35% and 40% arranged abortions and 51% and 46% delivered the baby, and of the latter, 99% and 92% subsequently reared the child—a pattern similar to that of the earlier cohort described by Flick. The annual birth rate per 1,000 unmarried girls aged 15 to 19 was 87 for blacks and 19 for whites, giving the United States the highest rate of developed countries for out-of-wedlock childbirth, even among the white teenagers (Hacker, 1987). It also had one of the highest rates of abortions for adolescents (Furstenberg et al., 1989).

In an attempt to find reasons for the high adolescent fertility of U.S. teenagers, Jones et al. (1985) obtained relevant data from 37 countries. They pointed out that the high level of fertility of younger teenagers in the United States fell between that in Romania and Hungary, which would suggest that the United States had a pronatalist fertility policy, high levels of maternity leaves and benefits, and a low minimum age of marriage; in fact, it had none of these. The United States did fit the general pattern of high as opposed to low teenage fertility countries in that it was less open about sexual matters, and a relatively small proportion of its total income was distributed to the poorest 20% of the population. Lack of openness about sexuality may have been attributable to the level of religiosity in the United States, which was the highest of the 13 countries for which there were data. Other possibly relevant differences discovered by Jones et al. are discussed in relation to contraception.

Adolescent Parenthood

Sugar (1984) reported that of married women giving birth before age 16, nearly one-third lived in poverty, and the marriages of one-third ended in separation or divorce. Of married women first giving birth after age 22, one-tenth lived in poverty, and one-tenth suffered marital breakup. Deliveries in teenagers were associated with a high risk of obstetric complications (Halperin, 1982), and teenage mothers had a high rate of child abuse and a suicide rate 10 times that of the normal population (Byrne, 1983). Their children had lower birth weights and the problems associated with this, including increased incidence of mental retardation and cerebral palsy (Halpern, 1990). Two percent of children born to parents younger than 17 died in their first year of life, twice the rate of children in other families (Robinson & Barrett, 1985). Furstenberg et al. (1989) cited what they termed a monumental review by the National Research Council documenting a host of negative consequences of early childbearing on the educational, economic, and marital careers of young mothers. They believed that the effect of the many ameliorative programs, other than those providing prenatal care, had been modest. A number of hospital- and school-based prenatal programs reached teenagers who otherwise would not have sought this care. Those who obtained it were more likely to have healthy babies than those who did not; Furstenberg et al. emphasized that a significant number did not. With the exception of alternative schools designed specifically for pregnant teenagers, few programs exclusively promoted educational or occupational advance for adolescent parents.

More positively, Furstenberg et al. pointed out that though adolescent mothers were very likely to become dependent on welfare for a considerable period, the majority entered the labor force when their youngest children reached school age and staged a recovery in later life that diminished, though it did not eliminate, the economic gap between them and later childbearers. Young mothers who succeeded in educational achievement, fertility control, and marriage appeared indistinguishable from older childbearers; those who failed in all three were likely to become chronic welfare mothers with a number of children and few prospects of future betterment. They were more likely to be black women. In 1976, one-third of a sample of metropolitan black teenage girls thought 18 years was the ideal age to have a first baby, though only 6% of white girls did so (Zelnik et al., 1981).

A mid-1980s survey showed there were approximately the same number of black and white single mothers with incomes below the poverty line—1,383,000 and 1,322,000, respectively—although blacks made up only 12% of the population (Hacker, 1987). Among the white mothers, 46% had only one child; 71% of the black mothers had two or more. Hacker commented that if more black mothers were poor or on welfare, it was because more started having children earlier, often leaving school or jobs to do so. Also, because more had never been married, it was harder for them to make claims on the fathers of their children. Hacker pointed out that 60% of black infants were born outside wedlock, that almost 60% of black families were headed by women, and that the majority of black children lived only with their mothers. The figures were three to five times those for white Americans. By age 18, 25% (and by their early 20s, 40%) of unmarried black women were mothers, and virtually all chose to keep their babies. Nevertheless, in later adulthood the majority of black teenage mothers master the three hurdles of educational achievement, fertility control, and marriage. Unlike adolescent black and white females, who are equally likely to terminate pregnancies by abortion, black women in their late 20s are much more likely than white women to do so. From the ages of 25 to 29 years, the ratio of abortions to births for black women was 591 per 1,000; that for white women was 185/1,000 (Hacker, 1987). According to Hacker, this suggested that at least half of young black women had no wish for early motherhood. He reported a follow-up study of 330 black inner-city unmarried teenage mothers that found that in their early 30s, 71% had completed high school, 76% had married (though most of the marriages did not last), and whereas 70% had been on welfare at one time, only 29% were still receiving public funds.

As discussed in Chapter 1, when associations are found between preceding and subsequent events in quasi experiments (those in which subjects are not randomly allocated to the conditions studied), it cannot be concluded that the preceding event caused the subsequent event until all other possible explanations are excluded. Hence, it is not justified to accept that motherhood in adolescents is responsible for all the negative features found associated with it in research studies. This is commonly done, and the need for preventative programs for adolescent motherhood is generally unquestioned (Flick, 1986). Only recently has parenthood been considered a problem for women aged under 18; paradoxically, the concern accompanied a decline in its incidence. In 1957 the annual birthrate among teenagers was 97 per 1,000; in 1974, it was 59 per 1,000 (Cvetkovich & Grote, 1983). Despite an enormous expansion in the size of the teenage population, the total number of births to teenagers also declined, though only slightly. What did increase was the proportion of these births that were to unmarried teenagers; these were 15% in 1960 but more than 25% in 1970. As stated earlier, in the mid-1980s the annual birth rate for unmarried girls aged 15 to 19 was 87 per 1,000 for black and 19 per 1,000 for white girls.

Furstenberg (1976) provided an interesting discussion of the social, political, and ideological factors that appeared to produce the recent negative appraisal of teenage pregnancy. He pointed out that the percentage of adolescents who married and became mothers following World War II was unusually high. In previous decades, 50 to 60 15- to 19-year-old girls per 1,000 annually had given birth; in the 1950s, the figure peaked at over 90. By the early 1960s the terms *premature parents,* school-age mothers, and *high-risk adolescent mothers* were liberally sprinkled throughout social work and educational journals. Furstenberg believed that there was no single explanation for this appearance of a negative attitude toward adolescent pregnancies. Possible factors that contributed were the diminution of job opportunities for teenagers and the accompanying expansion of educational training following World War II, producing an awareness that teenagers needed increased education to obtain white-collar jobs and enter the middle class; a general apprehension about overpopulation that emerged in the 1960s; the higher percentage of births to teenagers that were out of wedlock, particularly as the appeal of early marriage diminished; and the attention paid by government officials in the 1960s to issues of racial and economic inequality, which singled out promiscuous sexual behavior, illegitimacy, and early marriage as contributing to the cycle of poverty and led in the early 1970s to a growth of programs for school-age mothers that was "nothing short of spectacular" (p. 11). Furstenberg cited as evidence of the change in attitude toward adolescent pregnancy the shift in public sentiment from strong opposition in the early 1960s to approval in the early 1970s of provision of contraception to teenagers who requested it.

In an attempt to provide evidence to support a causal connection between adolescent motherhood and the negative conditions found associated with it, Furstenberg (1976) compared mainly black low-income adolescent mothers with their classmates. He found that the latter, particularly those who did not become pregnant premaritally during the 5 years of the study, had a far better record of achieving their marital, educational, and occupational objectives. A sizable proportion of the young mothers, however, by successful marriage or by restricting further childbearing, making child-care arrangements, and resuming their education, were coping as well as their former classmates by the end of the 5-year study. As comparison of the family backgrounds of the adolescent mothers and their former classmates revealed mainly only minor differences, Furstenberg considered the classmates to be an appropriate comparison group and that the worse outcome of the adolescent mothers as a group could be accepted as a consequence of their motherhood.

As this was a quasi experiment, from a scientific viewpoint this evidence can only be regarded as suggestive, not conclusive. Though only minor differences were found between adolescent mothers and their classmates, it was not possible to compare them on all possibly relevant variables. Significant differences in such variables could therefore have existed between the two groups prior to the members of one group becoming pregnant; the most obvious differences would be personality variables that could not easily be assessed in routine studies. More recently, Furstenberg et al. (1989) concluded that it was difficult to sort out the effects of early childbearing from the selective factors that led some young girls to become parents. They suggested that low academic ability could account for both early childbearing and low achievement in later life.

Furstenberg et al. (1989) also reviewed evidence that children of teenage mothers, particularly sons, were likely to show developmental disadvantages compared to children born of older mothers. As preschoolers, they were more active, more aggressive, and less self-controlled. By adolescence their school achievement was markedly lower, and their misbehavior higher. The authors considered only environmental factors as possible causes for these differences, ignoring biological factors such as genetic differences or brain damage in childbirth or from physical abuse.

With the aim of providing information to reduce the prevalence of adolescent motherhood, Flick (1986) reviewed the research concerning the four decisions made, or not made, by adolescent mothers—becoming sexually active, failing to use adequate contraception, not obtaining an abortion, and not arranging adoption. Little evidence was available concerning the last decision, but the other three all correlated with lower socioeconomic status, lower educational attainment, and membership of large families. Younger age was associated with less adequate contraception, but increased likelihood of abortion rather than delivery. These findings demonstrated that pregnant adolescents who became mothers differed as a group from those who did not on variables existing prior to the pregnancy, confirming that it was not possible to compare the two groups meaningfully in quasi experiments, at least not without matching them individually on these variables. This renders more powerful the methodological criticism of the assumption that negative factors associated with adolescent motherhood were produced by it. In view of the major social consequences involved if adolescent motherhood does produce even some of the negative factors, however, until it is established whether it does or not, it would seem wise governmental policy to allow for the possibility that it does.

Flick (1986) pointed out that despite poverty being associated with early sexual activity, less use of contraception, and lower abortion rates, numerous studies had found no relationship between availability of welfare support for single mothers and increased sexual activity or adolescent pregnancy. The developed countries comparable to the United States studied by Jones et al. (1985) provided extensive benefits to poor mothers that the authors considered more generous than those provided under the U.S. Aid to Families with Dependent Children program. All had teenage pregnancy rates markedly less than those of the United States. Though the evidence is not yet available that adolescent motherhood contributes significantly to the cycle of poverty, there is equally no evidence to justify failure to alleviate the poverty with which it is strongly associated.

A recent attempt to reduce this poverty and other negative factors associated with adolescent motherhood was by introduction of programs aimed at helping teenage fathers remain more involved with their children and more supportive of the mothers (Robinson & Barrett, 1985). These workers concluded that many teenage fathers went through the same emotional struggle and confusion that young mothers did; they often faced unbridled hostility from their girlfriends' families. Furstenberg et al. (1989) commented that services for the fathers were still in the experimental stage and focused on males who elected to remain involved with the mother and child. Such studies could not establish whether educational assistance and training in work or fathering skills would increase their commitment to their offspring. Furstenberg et al. found, not unexpectedly, that young fathers seemed less adversely affected by early parenthood than young mothers. They cited studies, however, that indicated that the fathers' educational careers were negatively affected by the occurrence of an early birth even if they did not marry their pregnant partner.

Furstenberg et al. did not discuss the possibility that the adolescent fathers' increased rate of high school dropout compared to that of nonfathers may have been associated with their likelihood of fathering a child, rather than a result of it. Elster and Peters (1987) found that 98 (51%) of 192 fathers of children born to adolescent mothers had committed a legal offense prior to the pregnancy. Robinson and Barrett

(1985) reported that teenage fathers had been involved in problem behaviors at school and with drinking; those who attempted to provide financial support to the mothers of their children tended to cease the support within a year. Hacker (1987) cited a mid-1980s National Research Council study finding that 20% of black and 45% of white teenage mothers received some child support from the fathers. States in the United States varied in their efforts to collect child support for women under 18, and in general, fathers' child-support payments to women were extremely low, the average annual award being $2,460 (Furstenberg et al., 1989). These authors concluded that it was likely payments to never-married adolescent mothers were lower.

Contraceptive Use

In their investigation of possible factors explaining the much higher number of adolescent pregnancies in the United States compared with other developed countries, Jones et al. (1985) found that differences in sexual activity were insufficiently marked to be a significant factor. They suggested that the major cause was the low level of use of contraceptives (and, in particular, the contraceptive pill) by U.S. teenagers compared to those in the other countries. Byrne (1983) found regular use of contraception reported by less than one-third of sexually active unmarried female university students, a frequency of use not much superior to that of all sexually active female adolescents, 30% of whom used no, 10% irregular, and 10% ineffective contraception. As quoted above, a National Research Council study in the mid-1980s found that 40% of black and 20% of white teenagers became pregnant, approaching half the number who were sexually active, and thus indicating no improvement in the effective contraceptive use by adolescents at this time (Hacker, 1987).

Brooks-Gunn and Furstenberg (1989) reported that about one-half of all teenagers did not use contraceptives the first time they had sexual relations, and younger as compared to older subjects were much less likely to do so. Male methods were the overwhelming choice of those who used them, according to both girls and boys. Brooks-Gunn et al. (1988) pointed out that these methods had the advantage that condoms acted as a barrier against HIV infection. Reasons given for not using contraceptives included that they were not available, that intercourse was not planned, and that pregnancy was not thought possible. Brooks-Gunn and Furstenberg (1989) pointed out that failure to use contraception wasn't a one-time event. The percentage of teenagers who continued to have intercourse with no or inconsistent contraception was such that one-half of all first pregnancies occurred in the first 6 months following initiation of intercourse. The only group who commenced contraceptive use within the first or second month in large numbers were white teenagers aged 18 and 19; this might reflect a concern to avoid HIV infection rather than pregnancy. Black women were reported to wait longer than white women after beginning coitus before they initiated contraception; they comprised 52% of all women in the United States with AIDS. Almost one-third acquired the infection through heterosexual activity (Fullilove, Fullilove, Haynes, & Gross, 1990).

Brooks-Gunn et al. (1988) suggested that ignorance about the range and effectiveness of contraceptives was common, particularly in younger, educationally and economically disadvantaged adolescents. Jones et al. (1985) believed an important factor in U.S. teenagers' reluctance to use contraception was the mixed messages they received about sex. Movies, music, radio, and TV told them sex was romantic, exciting, and titillating but also sinful and dirty. Premarital sex and cohabitation were visible features of the adult way of life, yet teens were told that good girls should say no. They received almost no information about contraception or the importance of avoiding pregnancy. Jones et al. believed that in European countries, matter-of-fact attitudes toward sex seemed more prevalent. The openness about sex they noted in these countries (and attributed to their lesser religiosity compared to the United States) was mentioned previously. Jones et al. also commented on the central role of the contraceptive pill everywhere outside the United States, noting that when U.S. teenagers did use contraceptive methods, they used less effective ones. In all countries the authors' research teams visited, they were told the medical profession accepted the pill as highly appropriate and usually the most suitable method for adolescents. In many countries a pelvic examination was not necessary before it could be prescribed, whereas medical protocol required this in the United States. The authors commented that young girls could find this procedure daunting.

Jones et al. believed there was a good deal of ambivalence in the United States about use of the pill, on the part of both the medical profession and potential users. Media publicity given to claimed adverse effects of both the contraceptive pill and intrauterine devices was considered responsible for a marked decline in their use as a first method from 1976 to 1979 (Kulig, 1985). Kulig pointed out that the mortality attributed to pregnancy and childbirth in 15- to 19-year-olds was 12.9 deaths per 100,000 live births, whereas mortality rates attributed to contraception included 0.3 deaths for nonsmokers on the pill, 2.2 deaths for smokers on the pill, and 0.8 deaths for IUD users per 100,000 users per year. Also, studies had found noncontraceptive health benefits with oral contraceptives. At the time Jones et al. and Kulig were writing, the advantage of condoms in reducing transmission of HIV as well as other STDs was presumably not recognized. Jones et al. (1985) pointed out that the postcoital contraceptive pill that was available at many family planning clinics in the United Kingdom, the Netherlands, and France had not been approved for use in the United States by the federal Food and Drug Administration (FDA), and no plans existed to market it; it was available in some college health clinics and rape treatment centers. The FDA had also not approved medroxyprogesterone acetate as a contraceptive, despite its being the only effective method for some adolescents (in particular the retarded) and its excellent safety record with extensive clinical use.

Reluctance by members of the medical profession, especially psychiatrists, to become actively involved in encouraging contraceptive use may have resulted from their accepting what Rodman et al. (1984) labeled a clinical myth prevailing from 1945 to 1964: the psychoanalytically based theory that many unmarried women did not use effective contraception because they unconsciously desired pregnancy. Rodman et al. argued that before the early 1970s, the most commonly available contraceptive was the condom—which was primarily under the control of men, who were less motivated to use contraception. When effective methods under women's control became available, many women, including teenagers, rapidly took advantage of them. In fact, as pointed out earlier, there appears no consistent evidence that contraceptive practices of sexually active single girls significantly improved in the 1970s.

Supporting this label of clinical myth, Furstenberg et al. (1989) stated that surveys and qualitative case studies revealed that most teenagers did not deliberately plan to become pregnant. Those who decided to deliver their child became increasingly committed to the decision as the pregnancy proceeded, however, and their family and friends, though initially disappointed, eventually provided social support and encouragement. Thus it would seem to observers who interviewed these adolescent girls late in their pregnancies that they were highly motivated to become pregnant, when earlier they may have voiced considerable misgivings. Furstenberg et al. also pointed out that studies that examined only adolescents who become parents exaggerated their motivation for early childbearing by omitting the 40% who terminated their pregnancies by abortion.

Rodman et al. (1984) believed that an important reason for failure of adolescents to employ contraception was to preserve a "good girl" image—that being contraceptively ready implied that they expected to be sexually active. Zelnik et al. (1981) pointed out that the sexual activity of teenagers is irregular, episodic, and unplanned; factors not conducive to efficient contraception. Nevertheless, as Jones et al. (1985) emphasized, the evidence from Sweden demonstrated that teenagers can commence sexual activity at a younger age than their U.S. peers and maintain much more effective use of contraception.

Sex Education and Sex Clinics

The 1970s saw the widespread introduction of sex education programs in the United States, many of which were directed at adolescents and aimed at prevention of unwanted pregnancies and of sexually transmitted diseases. Kilmann, Wanlass, Sabalis, and Sullivan (1981) reviewed 33 studies assessing the effectiveness of such programs. Almost all investigated programs for college or university students, lacked follow-up, and rarely examined behavioral change. Kilmann et al. stressed the need for systematic investigation of programs for younger adolescents. Howard (1985) commented of a more recent study of exemplary sex education programs in the United States that teenagers experienced knowledge gains but showed little change in behavior. Cvetkovich and Grote (1983) found no difference in sex or contraceptive knowledge between good and poor contraceptive users in their study of white, mainly middle-class high school students aged 16 to 18, almost all of whom had attended a health course that included birth control information. The conclusion of Rodman et al. (1984) that the results then available were promising enough to warrant developing and evaluating programs of education in human sexuality seemed questionable. Durant, Jay, and Seymore (1990) subsequently reported further negative findings concerning the association between birth control knowledge and use.

There appears to be no consistent evidence that sex education alone has had a significant effect on teenage pregnancy levels in the United States. This could in part be attributable to such education being a community option (so that frequently parents excuse their children from it) and to some courses not addressing decision making about sexuality, nor providing adequate information about contraception (Brooks-Gunn et al., 1988; Jones et al., 1985). Acceptance of an educative role concerning these two issues has been resisted by the media (Brooks-Gunn & Furstenberg, 1989). Public service announcements concerning them that were not associated with disease prevention were rejected by the three major television networks.

Introduction of sex education in Sweden was deliberately linked with the establishment of clinics for adolescents in which school nurses dispensed nonprescription contraceptives (Jones et al., 1985). This link was made in the hope of preventing the liberalization of abortion laws, carried out at the same time, from resulting in a sharp rise in teenage abortions. It was apparently effective, as adolescent abortion rates declined dramatically; those for adults did not greatly change. P. Brown (1983) believed that the decline in both adolescent pregnancy and abortion rates in Sweden resulted from the establishment of the clinics, which occurred in 1975, rather than the introduction of the improved sex education, which commenced in 1977.

Introduction of services similar to those of the Swedish youth clinics into U.S. high schools were also followed by falls in pregnancy rates (Brooks-Gunn et al., 1988; L. Edwards, Steinman, Arnold, & Hakanson, 1980). Few such clinics, however, were available for adolescents. Jones et al. (1985) pointed out that though family planning clinics were reasonably accessible and were required to serve adolescents to receive federal funding, many adolescents avoided them, believing they were only for welfare clients because they were developed as a service for the poor. Brooks-Gunn and Furstenberg (1989) found adolescents also avoided them because they believed incorrectly that their parents would need to be informed of their visit. They pointed out that this underscored the lack of communication between parents and children about sexuality. Brooks-Gunn and Furstenberg also criticized the lack of effort to involve male teenagers, reporting that men made up less than 1% of the clinics' clients. This meant that male methods of contraception, with their advantage in reducing HIV transmission, were not usually prescribed.

Abortion

The failure of U.S. adolescents to employ adequate contraception as they became sexually active at a younger age resulted in the percentage of those pregnant who relied on abortion increasing from 23% in 1971 to 33% in 1976, 37% in 1979 (Rodman et al., 1984), and 40% in the mid-1980s (Furstenberg et al., 1989). At the last date, adolescents received more than a quarter of all abortions performed. Furstenberg et al. cited studies indicating that pregnant teenagers who chose abortion were more likely to be educationally ambitious and good students, to come from higher socioeconomic backgrounds and less religious families, to have mothers and peers with a more positive attitude toward abortion, and to be less likely to have friends or relatives who were teenage single parents. A sparse literature suggested that teenagers who had their children adopted were more similar to those who chose abortion than those who kept their children. Flick (1986) found that younger as compared to older adolescents were more likely to have abortions. Forty-five percent of teenagers having abortions did not inform their parents (Rodman et al., 1984), a further indication of the failure of communication between children and parents concerning sexuality.

Two laws before the U.S. Supreme Court required parents of unmarried girls under 18 to be notified that their daughter was having an abortion before the operation was performed (Halpern, 1990). One effect would be to delay their obtaining it; when one of the laws was temporarily made operative in 1981, an increase in the number of adolescents requesting second-trimester abortions increased. Deaths resulting from abortion increase approximately 20% for each week of gestation from the 8th to the 15th week of pregnancy, and 50% thereafter. Understandably, therefore, 82% of abortion services will not provide abortions after the first trimester. In relation to the possibility that other recent state laws will limit the access to abortion of adolescents who cannot afford high fees, Halpern commented that even with the access available the majority of the children of teenage mothers are fed, housed, and clothed primarily by state and federal welfare, at a cost in 1987 of $19.27 billion. She further commented that as poverty had become feminized, it had become a teenage wasteland, and that girls refused access to abortion will be largely black (of whom 70 per 1,000 obtained abortions, compared with 36 per 1,000 whites).

Romans-Clarkson (1989) pointed out, in reviewing the scientific literature concerning the psychological sequelae of induced abortion, that it took on the quality of a debate reflecting the deeply held religious, political, social, and philosophical beliefs of the participants. Publications from the 1930s to the 1950s tended to share a psychoanalytic perspective and viewed abortion as a tremendous threat to the ego structure. By the mid-1950s, psychiatric opinion was swinging away from the expectation that abortion was invariably followed by deleterious psychological effects. Romans-Clarkson related this to a 1955 study by Ekblad of 479 Swedish women who had received abortions. Ekblad found that 11% of the women reported severe and 14% mild self-reproach, but only 1% showed psychic sequelae severe enough to produce work impairment.

Romans-Clarkson conducted a literature search that produced little research of the issue published in the last 10 years. Studies in the intervening period showed a remarkable consensus: Apart from single-case studies, all concluded that induced abortion did not cause deleterious psychological consequences. Religion was found to be unrelated to guilt in four of the five investigations that examined this variable. Women refused abortion had a worse outcome than those granted abortion, despite the refusal being on the grounds that they were less psychiatrically disturbed. Little data were available on the outcome of illegal abortions, with one author pointing out that unlike legal abortions, criminal abortions had never been indicted as a possible cause of female neurosis or guilt. Romans-Clarkson cited the comment of Illsley and Hall (1976) that as guilt is deliberately induced as part of a traditional system of social control, it is superfluous to ask whether abortion patients experience guilt; it is axiomatic that they will.

Prostitution

It would seem excessively cynical to believe that the economic basis of adolescent prostitution was a significant factor in its failure to attract strong legal sanctions against its adult organizers or clients equivalent to those against adults involved in noncommercial heterosexual activities with adolescents. In New York, where both prostitution and patronizing a prostitute are crimes, arrests of prostitutes are 100 times more common than arrests of clients. When clients were arrested, it is a common practice to have them testify against the prostitutes so that charges against them are dropped (Rio, 1990). Rio cited an estimate that the prostitution business in the United States grossed $7 to $9 billion a year. To determine the degree to which sex crimes against children and adolescents were investigated, questionnaires were sent to 2,383 law enforcement agencies, of which 832 (35%) responded (D'Agostino et al., 1985). Thirty-two percent of the responding agencies had investigated child sexual assault cases, and 20% child prostitution cases. The mean ages of the youngest girl and boy prostitutes per agency were between 13 and 14 years. More than 50% of the agencies that investigated child or adolescent prostitutes cases had made no adult arrests.

Female Prostitutes

Gibson-Ainyette, Templer, Brown, and Veaco (1988), in discussing adolescent female prostitutes in the United States, reported that from 1967 to 1976 there was a 240% increase in their number; that of the estimated 2 million prostitutes, 600,000 were under the age of 18 years; and that the average age for the beginning prostitute was 14, 2 years after her initial experience of coitus. Schaffer and DeBlassie (1984) stated that the average age of prostitutes in Boston was 20, and in Miami, 18. Neither study discussed how the data were obtained, nor the likelihood of their accuracy. Brecher (1984) believed that men's sexual contacts with prostitutes were currently much less frequent than in Victorian times, in part because they were then deemed less dangerous to the male body and soul than masturbation. Passage of a law in 1918 authorizing the military to declare towns off-limits if they harbored prostitutes led to the suppression of "red-light districts" in most towns in order to retain the patronage of free-spending soldiers. As a result, although the same proportion of men continued to have sex with prostitutes, their frequency of contacts was drastically reduced. Brecher cited Kinsey (Kinsey et al., 1948) as stating that following 1918, one-third to one-half of the intercourse men used to have with prostitutes was diverted to premarital activity with other girls. In view of the intergender convergence in the age at which male and female adolescents begin coitus since Kinsey's 1948 report, it would be expected that males have further reduced their number of contacts with prostitutes.

The claimed marked increase in the number of adolescent prostitutes in the last few decades, if valid, may be attributable to a majority being involved briefly rather than for some years. Potterat, Woodhouse, Muth, and Muth (1990) attempted to calculate the number of female prostitutes in the United States by extrapolating from their investigation of the 1,022 known to their health department in Colorado Springs, where there were several military institutions. They suggested that the military presence combined with the town population produced a prostitution marketplace characteristic of both large and small communities, and hence could be typical enough to represent the national mean. They supported the suggestion by the gonorrhea rate, pointing out this was higher in large and lower in small population centers; in Colorado Springs, it was virtually identical to the national mean. Potterat et al. believed that sustained monitoring both by their health department and the police enabled them to obtain an accurate estimate of the number of prostitute women in the town, of whom they saw about 80%. The median age of the prostitutes was 22 years, with almost three-quarters under 25 years and only 2.3% over 34 years at their first visit. Fifty-two percent were involved in prostitution for 30 to 40 days and 12% for several months in any year; 35% were involved continuously for several years.

From this data, Potterat et al. calculated that during the 1980s there were an average of 84,000 women working as prostitutes yearly in the United States. They supported their estimate with FBI reports that from 33,153 to 83,777 women were arrested annually for violation of prostitution laws between 1970 and 1987. These figures were considered to provide a conservative estimate on the basis that though some prostitutes would have been arrested more than once, the wiser and more clandestine would not have been arrested at all. As further support, the authors quoted a 1987 National Opinion Research Center (NORC) investigation of a probability sample of 843 women, of whom 443 were in what they termed the high-risk years for prostitution 18 to 44. None of the women in the NORC study reported any sexual partnership for payment. Potterat et al. considered this to be consistent with their estimate that 1 woman in 260 in the United States exchanged sex for payment sometime during that year; they did not discuss the possibility that some women in the NORC study may not have wished to report paid sexual activity. Their other conclusion was that most female prostitutes remain in the profession only a short time, about 4 to 5 years for long-term prostitutes. Potterat et al. made no mention of male prostitutes, which suggests that their sample may not have been representative of prostitutes in large cities.

Gibson-Ainyette et al. (1988) reviewed evidence indicating that female adolescent prostitutes tended to be from broken homes where they often experienced emotional and physical abuse and early sexual exploitation, at times including incest; that they were often runaways and had a history of school absenteeism and dropping out; and that in some instances drug use started them in prostitution. Gibson-Ainyette et al. found that research studies showed the attitude of adult female prostitutes toward their clients and men generally was varied, not uniformly negative as clinical studies reported. In their own study, they compared adolescent delinquent prostitutes, adolescent delinquent nonprostitutes, and high school students using a number of rating scales. They found the prostitutes to show a very negative attitude toward men, which they related to beatings, disfigurations and at times murders committed by clients, as well as beatings, cheating, and exploitation by pimps. The prostitutes also showed cynicism, alienation, and nonconformity, with a veneer of adequacy.

Rio (1991) criticized the tendency to classify all prostitutes within one deviant culture. She found that earlier reports that they were addicted to alcohol and psychologically abused, with resulting deficiencies, were based on studies of those of low socioeconomic level, primarily streetwalkers, soon after arrest, while in prison, or soon after release. When these individuals were compared to the general female population, such findings were inevitable. More recent studies that Rio cited found the major difference between prostitutes and controls matched for age, education, marital status, and paternal socioeconomic status was that prostitutes earned more. Personality differences between call-girls and in-house prostitutes and their controls were minimal, and it was concluded that these prostitutes showed no evidence of pathology. Some deficits were found between streetwalkers and controls, and greater deficits between controls and housewife and drug-addict prostitutes. Rio (1991) opined that theories that prostitutes entered the profession following childhood abuse, broken homes, and early sexual activity (including incestuous encounters) were derived from studies on lower-class streetwalkers who were prone to arrest. These factors were also found in nonprostitute matched controls, but not among call-girl and in-house prostitutes, who advanced more middle-class explanations for their entry (e.g., independence and realistic attitudes about morality). The one factor that cut across socioeconomic lines and appeared to be almost every prostitute's primary, if not sole, motive was economic. All classes of prostitute had higher annual incomes than the nonprostitute controls. Rio recommended, however, that the study of juveniles be separated from that of adult prostitution, and appeared to suggest that virtually all juvenile prostitutes were in the lower-class streetwalker category.

Savitz and Rosen (1988) pointed out that earlier beliefs that female prostitutes were sexually unresponsive or lesbian were impressionalistically based and not supported by research. They interviewed 46 street prostitutes assigned to probation after conviction. The percentages who enjoyed various sexual acts with customers all or most of the time were 70% for receiving and 56% for giving oral sex, 39% for intercourse, 17% for anal sex, and 30% for administering and 9% for receiving sadomasochistic activities. The percentage enjoying these activities to the same extent with current lovers were 100% for oral sex and intercourse, 58% for anal sex, and 39% for sadomasochistic activities. Receiving oral sex was the most enjoyable activity with lovers and customers, all the prostitutes achieving orgasm all or most of the time with lovers, and 75% of the time with clients. Fifty-seven percent of the women labeled themselves as completely and 24% as predominantly heterosexual, and 11% as equally hetero- and homosexual.

Male Prostitutes

As with females, the number of male adolescent prostitutes in the United States is commonly stated to be high; Deisher, Robinson, and Boyer (1982) cited an estimate of 300,000. Strommen (1989) claimed there had been a dramatic rise in teenage male prostitution in the United States, which he attributed in part to the casting out of homosexuals by their parents. Pleak and Meyer-Bahlburg (1990), in a study of young Manhattan male street prostitutes, had to extend the age range from 14–22 years to 14–27 years, as they found too few subjects under the age of 19. They commented that this was particularly the case in bars and theaters, but also on the street where more young hustlers were observed during the study planning stage than during recruitment, and that a similar change was observed in other U.S. cities over the same period. As Schaffer and DeBlassie (1984) pointed out, the greatest difference between male and female prostitutes was that the paid contacts of the males were mainly homosexual, including those of the males who identified themselves as heterosexual. These authors suggested that like the females, most male prostitutes had been abused or neglected in childhood, but that there were fewer supports for them, whereas the females on the streets formed an elaborate social network.

As Rio more recently concluded of female prostitutes, Allen (1980) found in a study of 98 male prostitutes contacted through their personal network that there was no specific type. The mean age of those investigated was 16.6 years, ranging from 14 to 24. Twenty-three were full-time and 48 were part-time prostitutes who mainly made contacts in street or bars; 13 were involved as part of a peer-delinquent subculture in threatening, assaulting, or blackmailing vulnerable male homosexuals, as well as in other criminal activities; 14 were call or "kept" boys. By age 18, 35% of the total group had engaged in intercourse with a female. The peer delinquents were the only group considered predominantly heterosexual, whereas call and kept boys were the most homosexually oriented. The part-time prostitutes had the highest percentage of intact families, and the full-time prostitutes the lowest. Part-time prostitutes also had the least involvement with heavy use of drugs and alcohol, and at average follow-up of 1 year continued to have the highest educational and work status. They usually worked only when they needed money for some specific purpose, such as a date with a girlfriend or boyfriend. Allen commented that because of this and their loner status, part-time prostitutes were the most difficult to identify and interview, adding that because of their successful overall adjustment, there was less need to study them. These comments may also apply to and explain the little attention given males who are paid for companionship, social or sexual, by women.

In their study of young Manhattan male prostitutes, Pleak and Meyer-Bahlburg (1990) excluded escort-service men, call boys, cross dressing street prostitutes, and boys under 13, who they stated were predominantly involved in sex rings under the control of pimps. The final sample of 50 had a mean age of 20.7 years and had commenced prostitution at a mean age of 17.6; 25 were from the street, and 25 from bars and theatres. None had been involved in sex rings or had pimps. Their mean number of male clients was 495, and their mean number of male partners for pleasure was 109. The largest percentage of street subjects described themselves as heterosexual; the bar and theater subjects, as homosexual. Sixteen had been involved in heterosexual prostitution, with a mean of 3.4 female clients. All but one had engaged in heterosexual intercourse with a woman, with a mean of 42 partners. Of all sexual encounters with clients, 86% involved masturbation; 71%, fellatio, (22% of the prostitutes fellated clients); and 17%, anal intercourse (4% of the prostitutes were receptive).

Earls and David (1989) compared 50 male street prostitutes with 50 males recruited in shopping malls who denied ever engaging in prostitution. The mean age of both groups was 21.5 years. Thirty percent of the prostitutes and all the controls considered themselves to be heterosexual. Both groups had attained similar levels of education, and they did not differ in the number coming from broken homes or their age at leaving home. More of the nonprostitute group regularly consumed alcohol, and more of the prostitute group used cocaine, marijuana, or hashish. The prostitutes were more likely to report violence between their parents, alcohol and drug problems in family members, and sexual relations with a family member; however, they did not perceive their family backgrounds as traumatic. Their first sexual experiences were more often with a male, at a much earlier age, and with a person considerably older compared with those of the nonprostitutes, which were exclusively with females. The most common reason prostitutes gave for their involvement was financial gain; their mean reported weekly income was $562 weekly, whereas that of the nonprostitutes was $194. A number of the prostitutes scored high on the Beck Depression Inventory. Eighty-six percent of the prostitutes had a regular sexual partner outside of prostitution, with whom their sexual contacts were much more enjoyable.

The authors believed that these findings rendered hypotheses of involvement in prostitution for sexual release or to establish affective relationships implausible for the majority. They pointed out the need in future research for a control group matched on sexual orientation, but they did not comment on the possibility that the answers of the control group were biased in the direction of social desirability. The study, together with that of Rio, suggests that a number of male and female prostitutes may not show significant evidence of traumatic childhood experiences or current psychological disturbance when compared with socioeconomically matched controls. Factors additional to monetary gain appear to influence the professional activity of male street prostitutes; most of those interviewed in a number of cities in the United States and Canada preferred younger clients and expressed a general contempt for the older (Visano, 1991).

HIV Infection and Prostitution

Fifty-eight percent of the prostitutes and 48% of the control males interviewed by Earls and David (1989) reported changes in sexual practices attributable to awareness of AIDS; those who reported no changes had generally refrained from behaviors associated with a risk of contracting HIV infection. There was no significant difference in AIDS awareness of the prostitutes and controls. Forty-two percent of the prostitutes and 15% of the controls had contracted STDs. Pleak and Meyer-Bahlburg (1990) cited a number of recent studies investigating the prevalence of HIV infection in male prostitutes. Twenty-five percent of 194 male street prostitutes in Atlanta were HIV positive. Infection was not associated with sexual orientation; of those positive, 44% identified themselves as heterosexual, 27% as bisexual, and 29% as homosexual. Of males attending a New York STD clinic, 17 (53%) of 32 who admitted to prostitution with men were seropositive; none of the 17 admitted to IV drug use. Five (10%) of 52 who admitted to prostitution with women were seropositive; 1 of the 5 was using IV drugs, and 3 had engaged in homosexual activity. Ten percent of street prostitutes and 23% of call men in San Francisco were seropositive.

The Manhattan bar/theater and street prostitutes investigated by Pleak and Meyer-Bahlburg (1990) used condoms on 16% and 37%, respectively, of their occasions of heterosexual intercourse, but on 80% and 100%, respectively, of occasions of receptive anal intercourse, whether for money or pleasure. In active anal intercourse, bar/theatre subjects used condoms on 25% of occasions with women partners for pleasure, 82% with male partners for pleasure, and 90% with male partners for payment; comparable percentages for street subjects were 6%, 4%, and 89%. In receptive fellatio, bar/theatre subjects used condoms on 21% of occasions for pleasure and 64% of those for payment; street subjects used them in 66% and 59% of these situations, respectively. The authors commented that the patterns of higher condom use with clients or casual partners than with lovers, and lower use with female than male partners, have been observed in other studies within and outside the United States. It would appear that the prostitutes investigated took significant precautions to avoid HIV infection, particularly from receptive anal intercourse. Those who became infected, however, posed a very high risk to their women partners. The authors suggested that the intervention programs most likely to succeed in increasing the safety of male prostitutes' sexual practices were those using selected male prostitutes (or former ones) trained to educate their colleagues.

Adolescent Clients

Regular clients of female prostitutes would appear to include a significant number of adolescent males in some cultures, as Primov and Kieffer (1977) found in Peru. In the United States, they are mainly men aged 30 to 60 years (Rio, 1991). There is no information to determine whether a significant percentage of male adolescents in the United States continue to have infrequent contacts. Seven percent of 15-year-old and 49% of 21-year-old males in Kinsey's (1948) sample reported one or more experiences with prostitutes.

Sexual Problems of Adolescence

Male adolescents provoke and female adolescents suffer from a significant percentage of problems associated with sexuality. The majority of sex offenders are male and, apart from those who molest female children, begin their deviant activity in adolescence (Chapter 8). The majority of their victims are female (Chapters 6 and 7). Of 45 men who sought treatment for compulsive sexuality other than homosexuality (McConaghy et al., 1985, 1987), 6 were adolescent. A further 21 reported that their sexually deviant behavior had commenced and was usually repeated fairly regularly in adolescence. This trend for early commencement was particularly marked in the 5 fetishists, 3 of whom showed a marked, though apparently not sexual, interest in the fetishistic object some years prior to puberty; in a fourth, the fetishistic interest commenced at age 13. Twelve of 19 exhibitionists, 7 of 11 homosexual pedophiles, and 2 of 3 voyeurs also reported that their behavior started in adolescence. Heterosexual pedophiles did not show this trend strongly, only 2 of 7 reporting the behavior in adolescence. Five of the 6 sexually deviant adolescents were referred following convictions—2 for homosexual and 1 for heterosexual pedophilia, and 2 for sexual assault. The sixth, a fetishistic transvestite, was brought by his parents, having stolen clothes from schoolmates. One-third of the adult sex offenders or deviants, mainly pedophiles, sought treatment voluntarily and had no prior convictions; no adolescents sought treatment voluntarily.

It is noteworthy that none of the subjects who reported exposing regularly in adolescence were referred for treatment or charged with this offense until adulthood. As it is the most common sexual offense in adults and begins in adolescence, it must be carried out regularly by a significant number of adolescents. Presumably, victims do not regard exhibitionism by adolescents as justifying a report to the police. Groth, Longo, and McFadin (1982) commented on the unfortunate frequent dismissal of sexual offenses by adolescents—in particular, rape and child molestation—as sexual curiosity or experimentation, or with the diagnosis of adolescent adjustment reaction. In the studies by McConaghy et al. (1985, 1987), the sex offenses of the adolescent subjects showed a trend to be more resistant to treatment than those of adults. Three of the 6 adolescents, but only 6 of the 44 adults, required treatment additional to the initial course.

Victims in the National Crime Survey reported that adolescent males were responsible for 15% of forcible rapea in 1978 and 21% in 1979 (Ageton, 1983). As discussed in Chapter 7, the rapes recorded in this survey are substantially less than those that are unrecorded. How many of the latter are carried out by adolescents who do not differ in personality or degree of emotional disturbance from those who are charged cannot be determined. Sorensen (1973) reported that two basic categories of masturbatory fantasies in his sample of male teenagers were sex with someone who was forced to submit, and varying degrees of violence to the other person. Rape may usually be less a result of male pathology than of the lack of social concern to proscribe it effectively. At present, a high percentage of adolescent girls are required to cope with varying degrees of physical pressure for intercourse from male acquaintances (Chapter 7) with minimal advice or information from parents or society.

As discussed subsequently, 50% of adolescent girls do not experience orgasm in sexual relations. Of the girls who reported its absence in Sorensen's sample (1973), one-third considered it very important to them that they had this experience, and one-half stated that they didn't get as much physical satisfaction out of sex as they thought they should. The latter statement was endorsed by only 16% of the girls who had orgasms frequently. Intercourse characterized by pain of psychological origin is usually established in adolescence, but rarely causes the sufferer to seek treatment until adulthood. An interesting but unexplored statistic in Sorensen's study (1973) was that 21% of adolescent males with masturbatory experience reported masturbation without orgasm in the previous month, 12% on five or more occasions. No data were given concerning the incidence in males of coitus without orgasm, nor the percentage who had difficulty reaching orgasm. Certainly some adolescent males must experience these conditions, as adults seeking treatment for them usually report they were present since adolescence. Also, men who develop impotence in middle age and in whom a contributing organic factor is commonly found not infrequently report difficulties in attaining or maintaining erections dating back to their initial experiences in adolescence. These usually were resolved sufficiently with further sexual experience at that time, so that treatment was not then sought. Adults with premature ejaculation also usually date its onset from their earliest sexual relationships. Despite awareness of the number of adolescents who have commenced sexual intercourse, there appears to be a preference to know as little as possible about any difficulties they may experience concerning it.

ADULTHOOD

Male-Female Differences in Sexual Motivation

The greater motivation of males to indulge in sexual activity for its own sake, and of females to incorporate it in an affectionate relationship, is also found in young adults. In M. Hunt's questionnaire investigation (1974) of American adults, 60% of men and 37% of women considered premarital coitus acceptable for men where no strong affection existed; 44% of men and 20% of women considered it acceptable for women under the same circumstances. Of U.S. couples asked whether they needed to be in love to have sex, wives said yes more than husbands, and lesbians more than gay men (Blumstein & Schwartz, 1983). Blumstein and Schwartz suggested that the report by lesbian (compared to heterosexual) couples of reduced frequency of genital sexual relations and the greater value given nongenital contacts of hugging and cuddling could reflect the sexual interest of women as compared to men. They quoted women in heterosexual relationships as saying that their partner misinterpreted their wishes to cuddle or kiss as initiations of intercourse.

Byers and Heinlein (1989) found in their study of heterosexual couples that not only did more men initiate sex, more thought about initiating it. They pointed out their findings required modification of the sociological theory of behavioral scripts. This theory provided an alternative to the biological theory that more men than women initiated sex because men had stronger sexual urges. The theory of scripts proposed that both men and women were conforming to a socially determined script in which men take the role of initiator for the couple. To explain the findings of Byers and Heinlein, the script must also call for men to take responsibility for thinking about whether to initiate sex. In their study, no women reported considering initiating sex but not doing so because they were waiting for their partner to make the first move or for fear of a negative partner reaction, as had been suggested by Blumstein and Schwartz.

Mancini and Orthner (1978) asked a stratified area probability sample of middle class married couples to indicate and order the 5 activities they enjoyed most of a list of 96 possible leisure activities. Forty-five percent of husbands and 26% of wives selected sexual or affectional activities as one of the five. It was the most preferred activity of the men and the second most preferred of the women, 37% of whom selected reading as the first. Wilson (1981) analyzed the questionnaire responses of British men and women; the mean age of the 1,862 men was 30, and of the 2,905 women, 28. The men were about three times as likely as the women to seek sex at the first possible opportunity; the women were three times as likely to wait until there was some commitment to a steady relationship. Fifty-five percent of the men and 41% of the women were not getting enough sex; the ideal of 62% of these women, and 37% of the men, was more of the same type of sex with their steady partner. The ideal of the majority of the men was more exciting variations with the partner, or more different partners. Wilson found little differences in the responses of the men and women above and below the age of 30, which he pointed out indicated a lack of change between two generations.

Clark and Hatfield (1989) reported an experimental investigation of male-female differences. Four men and five women aged about 22 years were instructed to approach members of the opposite sex individually on the campus of Florida State University and say, "I have been noticing you around campus. I find you to be very attractive." Then they asked, according to a randomized procedure, one of three questions: "Would you go out with me tonight?", "Would you come over to my apartment tonight?", or "Would you go to bed with me tonight?" Fifty percent of both men and women approached agreed to the request to go out; no women, but

69% of men agreed to the other two requests. The men were reported to be at ease with those requests, saying, "Why do we have to wait till tonight?" or "I can't tonight, but tomorrow would be fine." Men who refused gave apologies (e.g., "I'm married," or "I'm going with someone"). The women's responses to the latter two requests were, "You've got to be kidding," or "What is wrong with you? Leave me alone." The study was carried out in 1982, before there was concern about HIV transmission, and the authors reported a similar one had been carried out in 1978 with almost identical results. They pointed out that the interpretation that men were more interested in sex and women in a relationship was not the only one possible. Both men and women might have been equally interested in sex, but the men may have felt there were fewer risks in accepting a sexual invitation.

Sexual Activity in Cohabitation and Marriage

Blumstein and Schwartz (1983), in their study of American couples, found the frequency of sexual relations was less in married than cohabiting couples, 45% of the former compared to 61% of the latter having relations three or more times a week in their first 2 years together; the equivalent figures were 27% and 38%, respectively, for the subsequent 8 years. The authors suggested that the presence of children may have been a factor in the reduced frequency in married couples. Cohabitation was primarily a childless life-style; 72% of the cohabiting heterosexual couples did not have children living with them. Men were three times more likely than women to initiate sexual relations among married couples and twice as likely among cohabiting heterosexual couples. In about one-third of the two types of couples, both partners were equally likely to initiate intercourse; this was also the case in one-third of gay males and lesbian couples. Sixty-two percent of the heterosexual males and 48% of their partners wanted sex a good deal more often than they were currently having it.

Byers and Heinlein (1989) reported an investigation of 22 male and 55 female psychology students, of mean age 29.6 years; 65% were married and the remainder cohabiting. Half had children. Eighty-three percent scored in the nondistressed range on the Dyadic Adjustment Scale measure of the quality of their relationships. More initiations of sexual activity were reported by couples who were younger, cohabiting, had been romantically involved for a shorter time, were more satisfied with the relationship, and reported greater sexual satisfaction. Having children had an insignificant negative effect on initiations. Men initiated sexual behaviors twice as often as women, but younger and more sexually satisfied subjects reported a higher percentage of initiations by women compared to the remainder. Rejections of initiation were associated with less sexual satisfaction for men and women, and lower relationship satisfaction by men.

The mean frequency of sexual interactions of 2.6 a week reported by Byers and Heinlein's subjects was similar to that found by Hunt (1974) in his married group of comparable age (2.55 in those aged 25–34). This would suggest there has been no significant change in this frequency in the 1980s. Hunt believed a significant increase had occurred in the years prior to his study. He found the range of weekly frequencies of marital intercourse decreased from 3.25 in subjects aged 18–24 to 1 for those aged 45–54, an appreciable increase compared to the weekly frequencies reported by Kinsey (a decrease from 2.45 to 0.85 over the same age range).

Reduction in the frequency of coitus following marriage, particularly in the first year, has been reported in numerous studies (W. James, 1981; Udry, 1980). Mancini and Orthner (1978) found that the proportion of husbands and wives who preferred sexual or affectional to other leisure activities declined steadily in both husbands and wives with duration of marriage (from 0–5 to 36–50 years). At all durations, more husbands than wives preferred sexual and affectional activities. James suggested the marked decline in the first year was attributable to the wearing off of a honeymoon effect. He compared the reduction to sexual satiation with a specific partner noted in male lower mammals; following satiation with one partner, the male could ejaculate with a different partner.

Edwards and Booth (1976) found in a study of married couples mainly aged 20 to 39, with one or more children, that their marital intercourse tended to be discontinuous. When asked if coitus had ever ceased for any reason other than pregnancy, one-third responded affirmatively. The median length of the period reported was 8 weeks, and the reason most often given for cessation was marital discord. Subjects who gave decreased sexual interest as the reason were on average 3 years older than those who gave other reasons; for them, the cessation had lasted 3 months or more. The authors concluded that because the median length of all cessations was 8 weeks, coitus might be highly discontinuous for many married couples. Thirty three percent of Swedish women aged 37–46 years, of whom 91% were in stable sexual partnerships, reported periods without sexual relationships of 2 to 3 months, and a further 37% of half a year or longer (Hagstad & Janson, 1984). The reasons given were as follows: 41%, pregnancy or childbirth; 26%, no partner; 10%, lack of desire; 8%, illness; and 3%, stress and lack of time. Relationship discord was among the other reasons accounting for the remaining 12%. Hunt (1974) believed the duration of sexual foreplay by Americans in the 1970s had increased from that of the previous generation. Compared to the median duration of foreplay of 12 minutes reported to Kinsey by women in the 1950s, women in Hunt's study reported a median duration of 15 minutes. Kinsey found that the duration among less educated men was brief, but the college-educated subjects had prolonged it to 5–15 minutes; in Hunt's sample, the duration was 15 minutes for both noncollege and college men. In regard to the duration of coitus, Hunt pointed out that Kinsey had not presented detailed data but had offered the much-quoted estimate that perhaps three-quarters of men reached orgasm in 2 minutes or less after intromission. Hunt opined that sexual liberation had led to most men prolonging coitus, not only for the woman's sake but also for their own. In Hunt's married white sample, the median duration of coitus was about 10 minutes, with no tendency for it to be shorter in noncollege and blue-collar men than the remainder. It was longer in younger subjects. Byers and Heinlein (1989) reported that the average lovemaking of their college sample lasted 36 minutes, ranging from 5 minutes to 2 hours; intercourse lasted 14 minutes, ranging from 2 minutes to 1.25 hours. If their subjects and the college students in Hunt's study were comparable and representative of the general population, the increase in duration of coitus and particularly of foreplay noted by Hunt has continued into the 1980s.

Hunt (1974) reported evidence that married couples at the time of his study used more positional variations in sexual activity than did those a generation previously. Almost three-quarters of his sample used the female-above position at least occasionally, whereas one-third had in Kinsey's time. Comparisons of the two sets of data for other positions were as follows: on the side, over one-half versus over one-quarter; sitting, over one-quarter versus one-twelfth; and rear-entry vaginal intercourse, four-tenths versus one-tenth. Hunt said that Kinsey had found variations in positions to be more widely used by college-level subjects; Hunt found that during the following generation, subjects of lower socioeconomic level had adopted the use of varied sexual positions, as with many other aspects of sexual behavior previously limited to those of higher level.

Female Orgasm

Little attention has been given the male experience of orgasm in comparison to that of women, reflecting the importance of the latter in the politics of sexuality. In psychoanalytic theory, the experience of vaginal rather than clitoral orgasms identifies the mature feminine woman. The theory states that in early childhood, girls' genital excitement is experienced in the clitoris, and at that stage their emotional and sexual feelings, like those of boys, are most strongly directed toward their mothers. Once they discover and resent the fact that, unlike boys, they do not have a penis, they blame their mothers (concluding she has castrated them) and thus turn to their fathers as love objects. The boy's attachment to his mother, with resulting jealousy and fear of his father, was termed the Oedipus complex; the girl's hostility to her mother and resultant attachment to her father was termed the Electra complex. It was believed that her shift from mother to father was accompanied by a shift in experiences of genital excitement from the "masculine" clitoris to the feminine vagina, and from active to passive sexual urges. If the girl clung to her threatened masculinity, hoping for a penis, she would continue to experience clitoral rather than the only true and mature vaginal orgasm (Morokoff, 1978).

No experimental data were provided for these beliefs, which perhaps today seem ludicrous to many analysts. As they postulate that woman is destined to be passive and receptive by her anatomy, however, they continue to fuel dispute concerning the nature of women's orgasms. For some, the issue was resolved when Masters and Johnson (1966) reported from laboratory studies that whether women's orgasms were produced by clitoral or vaginal stimulation, the physiological responses that accompanied them were the same. Singer and Singer (1978), however, believed that this research investigated just one type of female orgasm, that which involved vulval contractions. They suggested the emotional differences that characterize different forms of orgasm may not be experienced when subjects know they are being observed in a laboratory, and the fact that Masters and Johnson never reported data for women who distinguished between their clitoral and vaginal orgasms may have indicated this major limitation of their methodology. They cited the finding of one researcher who questioned couples about woman's orgasms that more than one-third of the women answered in ways that left the questioner unsure whether they actually referred to orgasm. This reaction could also be provoked by the description Singer and Singer

(1978) quoted from Doris Lessing's *The Golden Notebook:* "A vaginal orgasm is emotion and nothing else, felt as emotion and expressed in sensations that are indistinguishable from emotion. The vaginal orgasm is a dissolving in a vague, dark generalized sensation like being swirled in a warm whirlpool."

The clitoral orgasm was described as having a sharp violence, and Singer and Singer believed it was associated with apnea and laryngeal displacement. Simple hyperventilation was typical of the vulval orgasm. Lightfoot-Klein (1989) questioned the acceptance in Western sexological literature that the clitoris must be stimulated to produce orgasm. The author interviewed 300 Sudanese women and 100 Sudanese men over a 5-year period concerning the sexual experience of circumcised and infibulated women. Sudanese circumcision involved excision of the clitoris, the labia minora, and the inner layer of the labia majora and infusion or infibulation of the bilateral wound. The majority of women subjected to this extreme sexual mutilation were reported to experience sexual desire, pleasure, and orgasm in spite of their being culturally bound to hide these experiences.

The limitation of verbal descriptions of orgasms was suggested by an interesting study of Vance and Wagner (1976) that does not appear to have been followed up by other researchers. They asked 70 judges—medical students, obstetricians, and psychologists—to attempt to identify male from female college students' written descriptions of intercourse. They were unable to do so at levels better than chance. Vance and Wagner eliminated wording that was sex identifying, substituting *genitals* for "penis" or "vagina." Though clearly this was essential for the purposes of the study, it may have allowed some unconscious bias to operate. If adequate replication confirms the finding, it would seem unlikely that the issue of whether vaginal orgasms differ from clitoral orgasms can be solved by use of women's verbal descriptions of the experiences, given that they do not distinguish either from penile orgasms.

Lack of conceptual clearness concerning the emotional and cognitive concomitants of orgasm seem unlikely to account for the different durations reported in laboratory and clinical studies. Two laboratory studies investigated womens' vaginal blood flow while they masturbated, using a heated oxygen electrode attached to the vaginal wall. Seventeen American women aged 23 to 46 years, half of whom used a vibrator, were studied by Amberson and Hoon (1985). Their subjectivity reported duration of orgasm ranged from 30 to 120 seconds, with a mean of 48 seconds. Of the women, 8 masturbated to orgasm in succession twice; 4, three times; 3, four times, and 1, seven times. It was not stated that they were a specially selected group. The mean subjectively reported duration of orgasm of 26 Danish women whose mean age was 27 (SD = 4) was 20 seconds (SD = 12); two of the Danish women used a vibrator (Levin & Wagner, 1985).

The mean durations of orgasm found in these two studies, though differing considerably, were longer than the estimates reported by clinicians that were cited by Levin and Wagner; in these, the duration varied from a few seconds to rarely more than 20 seconds. Levin and Wagner also assessed the duration of orgasm by vaginal blood flow and found it to be significantly longer than that reported by the subjects, a finding they interpreted as indicating a lack of validity of the subjective estimate. They supported their conclusion by citing the finding of another study that the mean duration of orgasms of 11 women, determined from records of their vaginal and anal contractions, was 35.6 seconds (SD = 24.5).

The Grafenberg Spot and Female Ejaculation

Sholty et al. (1984) questioned 30 undergraduate and graduate students about their sexual behaviors. Thirty-nine percent reported they had experienced orgasms at only the clitoral or the vaginal site; the remainder reported they had experienced them at both, often in a blended form. Most of the women who had experienced blended orgasms preferred them. One woman reported what could be called an ejaculation, the release of significant amounts of fluid at orgasm. Sholty et al. cited reports by other workers that some women are capable of ejaculation, provided the Grafenberg spot in the anterior wall of the upper vagina is properly stimulated. The existence of this spot, claimed to be a well-delimited erogenous zone that swells with strong tactile stimulation, is also disputed.

Alzate (1985) reported finding more than one erogenous zone in many of the 27 women whose vaginas he stimulated manually. When he found a region of erotic sensitivity, he used increasing rhythmic pressure until they reached orgasm or his fatigue caused him to stop. All subjects reported erotic sensation on either or both vaginal walls (85% on the posterior, and 74% on the anterior wall). In the 24 women who experienced orgasm, the area of maximal sensitivity was more frequently on the lower part of the posterior wall and/or the upper part of the anterior wall. Nine of the 27 subjects reported the impression of having expelled a fluid through the urethra at the moment of orgasm in the past, but this was not observed in those reaching climax during the study. He believed that they confused urethrai fluid with vaginal lubrication or stress urinary incontinence. One who was particularly emphatic that she often ejaculated was invited to stimulate her clitoris to orgasm, at which point 5–10 ml of fluid was expelled through the urethra. It was chemically indistinguishable from urine. Most of the women were overt or covert prostitutes; in regard to this possibly rendering them inappropriate as subjects, Alzate commented that it was unlikely they were atypical as regards psychophysiological responses to sexual stimulation.

Alzate (1990) was critical of a study by Darling, Davidson, and Conway-Welch (1990) that reported responses of the half of more than 2,000 professional health workers who completed questionnaires. Forty percent reported having experienced ejaculation at the moment of orgasm: 35% of these believed its primary source was the vaginal walls; 18%, the urethra; and 27% were uncertain. The remainder attributed it to either Bartholin glands, Grafenberg spot, cervical glands, bladder or skene glands. Seventy percent perceived a sensitive area in the vagina, stimulation of which produced pleasurable feelings; 72% of these subjects reported that stimulation of the area during sexual arousal produced orgasm, and 80% were stated to have experienced ejaculation. As 80% of 70% is 56%, and only 40% of the entire sample reported ejaculation, this last claim must have been an error. Alzate believed research investigating the existence of the Grafenberg spot and the nature of women's orgasmic ejaculation required physiological investigation. The question of ejaculation in women has provided a further area of sexual politics; some feminists have considered it an unwarranted and undesirable biological analogy between women and men (Darling et al., 1990).

Prevalence of Orgasm

The number of women who are unable to achieve orgasm falls steadily from adolescence until middle age. Whereas over 50% of adolescent girls rarely or never reached orgasm in sexual relations in one study (Sorensen, 1973), this was true of only 25% of women in the first year of marriage, and 11% in the twentieth year, in another (Kinsey et al., 1953). A similar percentage of adolescent girls may not reach orgasm with masturbation as with sexual relations; 74% of those in Sorensen's study had masturbated in the previous month without reaching orgasm. Of 100 female undergraduates aged 17 to 25, 74 reported they had masturbated, 25 without reaching orgasm (Clifford, 1978). The increasing ability of women to reach orgasm appears to come to an end in middle age. Hallstrom (1979) investigated the sexual behavior of 800 Swedish women (aged 38, 46, 50, and 54 years) who made up 89% of a representative sample. Of those who were married or cohabitating, total inability to reach orgasm in sexual activity was reported by just under 10% of the women aged 46. It was reported by just over 10% of women aged 38, 15% of women aged 50, and 25% of women aged 54. Hunt (1974) found the regularity of orgasm in women of 55 and over to be considerably lower than that of the younger women, though he qualified this by pointing out that 13% of the older women said they had no marital coitus in the previous year, and another 17% did not provide information concerning this.

Communication of Sexual Needs

It would appear that effective communication of sexual needs between partners is often markedly inadequate. Couples' lack of sexual satisfaction has been consistently found to be related to problems concerning the emotional tone of their sexual relations rather than physical difficulties in performance (Chapter 5). The emotional problems included the partner choosing an inconvenient time, too little foreplay, and too little tenderness after intercourse. These problems would seem to be able to be corrected readily if they were appropriately communicated to the partner. I have gained the impression that there is a resistance to communicating sexual needs verbally that seems qualitatively different from the resistance to communicating other needs, and I have commented to students that people do not rub against the refrigerator when they wish to inform their partner they are hungry.

Byers and Heinlein (1989) in the study referred to earlier, obtained descriptions of subjects' initiations and responses over a 1-week period. Initiations that were nonverbal only were slightly more common, whereas those that were ambiguously or directly verbal only or both verbal and nonverbal were about equal. Nonverbal initiations included nonsexual touching, looks, kissing, and sexual fondling. The nature of the initiation did not influence the proportion of positive or negative responses, and most respondents were satisfied with how sex was initiated. The majority of positive responses were indicated nonverbally, with the noninitiator continuing the sexual contact started by the partner. Sixty percent of rejections were verbal, with the remainder being equally verbal and nonverbal, or nonverbal only. Disagreements lasted a median of 2 minutes, with a range of less than 1 minute to 60 minutes. In 60% of these, the couples mutually agreed not to have sex, but 7 subjects (18%) reported changing their mind: 4 because they got turned on, 2 for the partner's sake, and 1 was verbally convinced. Of those who did not have sex at the time, 30% reported it was initiated again later that day, in 80% of cases by mutual consent. Overall, 80% were satisfied with how the disagreement was resolved. Rejections of responses made verbally were resolved more satisfactorily.

Byers and Heinlein suggested that it may be easier to say no to or accept refusal of a verbal request than it is to do the same in the case of physical sexual advances. If so, it would seem that one factor in reducing the prevalent coerciveness of sexuality could be the encouragement of more verbal communication concerning sexual needs. Nonverbal communications can be misinterpreted; as reported earlier and subsequently, both young adult and older women in heterosexual relationships report that at times their partner misinterpreted their wishes to cuddle or kiss as initiations of intercourse (Blumstein & Schwartz, 1983; Hagstad & Janson, 1984).

The most disturbing evidence of poor communication in sexual partnerships was the finding that at least 10% of married women have been sexually assaulted by their current or former spouses by the threat or use of force (Yllo & Finkelhor, 1985, Chapter 7). In a study investigating less physically coercive methods of sexual assault, 26% of women and 24% of men assaulted reported being victims of spouses or lovers (Sorensen, Stein, Siegel, Golding, & Burnam, 1987). Both forms of sexual assault were perpetrated less frequently by strangers.

Masturbation and Oral and Anal Erotic Activities

Masturbation is continued by the majority of subjects in adulthood. Hunt (1974) reported of the young married subjects in his sample that 68% of the women and 72% of the men masturbated, at mean frequencies of 10 and 24 times a year, respectively. The percentages of both men and women who did so were about twice those reported by Kinsey. Relief of sexual tension was the most common reason given for masturbation by the subjects in Hunt's study, though some did so to relieve general tension. He found that men and women without college education were more apt to be distressed by their desires to masturbate, and regularly churchgoing women (but not men) were less likely to have masturbated than irregular or nonattenders. A sample of London men aged 20 to 35 who were in stable relationships reported reaching orgasm by masturbation a mean of 5 times, and by activities with a partner a mean of 13 times, in the previous 4 weeks (Reading & Wiest, 1984).

Hunt (1974) believed the most dramatic changes in sexual activity that had occurred in the years prior to his study were in the formerly all-but-unmentionable oral-genital acts, which were still classified as punishable crimes against nature in most of the United States. In Kinsey's study, 15% of men who had been educated to high school level included oral-penile and oral-vaginal contacts in their marital sexual activities; in Hunt's study, the figure was 55%. Equivalent changes in college men were from 40% to 60%, in women educated to high school level from 48% to 55%, and women educated to college level from 55% to 72%. In Blumstein and Schwartz's study (1983), about 30% of the heterosexual couples engaged in oral-penile and oral-vaginal sex usually or always, and a further 43% sometimes, when they had sex; only 10% never did. Frequency of these contacts were higher in lesbian and higher still in gay male couples. Of the British men and women surveyed by Wilson (1987), 88% of the men and 89% of the women reported having experienced oral sex. On a scale from −5 to +5, men rated it +4.25 on extent of enjoyment, and women +3.4. It would appear oral sexual activities may have become even more popular since the time of Hunt's study.

As Bolling and Voeller (1987) have pointed out, though anal intercourse was considered to play a major role in the transmission of the HIV in the homosexual population of the developed countries, most physicians, unlike sex researchers, were unfamiliar with the data that about one-fourth of American women occasionally engaged in anal intercourse, and about 10% did so regularly for pleasure. The authors stated they found most women only revealed this after repeated personal interviews and development of strong trust in the interviewer, so that it would be unlikely to be revealed in standard medical or field interviews. In fact, such inter-views have revealed an incidence not far below that these authors reported from their personal interviews. In the Kinsey studies, though few of the total number of subjects were questioned concerning it, about 4% of college level educated men and 9% of college level educated women said they had experienced anal intercourse pre-maritally more than rarely; half those numbers had experienced it more than rarely in their first marriage (Gebhard & Johnson, 1979). In Hunt's possibly more represen-tative sample (1974), about 20% of single men and women under 25 years who had ever had coitus had tried anal intercourse, 9% of men and 6% of women having used it at least occasionally in the previous year. Nearly a quarter of married subjects under 35 had also used it in the previous year, rarely in most cases but sometimes or often for more than 5%. Nine percent of 240 women, whose mean age was 37 years, attending a medical clinic in Sydney reported practicing anal intercourse occasionally (McLaws, Cooper, Leeder, & Chapman, 1988).

Bolling (1977) reported that of the gynecologic patients he interviewed, 15% acknowledged erotic feelings with anal stimulation, and most of these used oral-anal contacts for pleasure. Eight percent reported regular use of anal intercourse with pleasurable sexual responses, minimal or infrequent pain, and participation for their own enjoyment; almost half of this group were orgasmic with anal intercourse episodes. Thirty-seven percent of women and 34% of men surveyed in Britain by Wilson (1987) reported having experienced anal sex; men rated their enjoyment of it as +2.11, women as −0.56. The form of the anal sex was not specified.

Little data have been collected about the use of other anal erotic activities in heterosexual relationships. Half the younger married couples in Hunt's study (1974) indicated they would find manual-anal foreplay either as an active or passive partici-pant acceptable with someone they loved, and more than one-third indicated they would find oral-anal foreplay in either role acceptable under the same circumstances. Hunt did not inquire if they had carried out any of these practices in the past year, but well over half the under-35 men and women had experienced manual-anal foreplay at some time, and more than one-quarter had experienced oral-anal foreplay. As his sample of single subjects reported much lower incidences, Hunt concluded most of the married subjects' anal erotic experiences had occurred within their marriages rather than before. At most, only half the married subjects over 35 years old had such experiences; 11% of the women and 13% of the men reported ever having been active in oral-anal foreplay.

Padian et al. (1987) reported what they claimed was the first study apart from a case history to find an association between anal intercourse and HIV infection among heterosexuals. They investigated 97 female partners of seropositive men; those who had anal intercourse were 2.3 times as likely to become infected compared to those who did not. No association was found with oral intercourse. Of the 22 women who became seropositive, half reported never having engaged in anal intercourse. Padian et al. concluded that the transmission had occurred in these women through vaginal intercourse, as no association was found in their or other studies with HIV transmission and oral intercourse. It is not clear if they inquired about oral-anal activities.

Bolling and Voeller's belief (1987) that sex workers were aware of the incidence of heterosexual anal erotic practices may not be correct. Gagnon and Simon (1973) did not appear to be when they advanced the script theory that sexual behaviors are determined not by biological factors, but by subjects putting into practice the descriptions, or scripts, of behaviors they learned about in social experiences. Gagnon and Simon suggested that mouth-genital contact was perhaps the most tension-producing technique in sexual experimentation, given the definitions that the penis and vagina had in terms of odor, taste, and cleanliness. As mouth-anus contact would seem rather more tension producing in these terms, presumably Gagnon and Simon were unaware of it as a sexual practice. This must have meant that its performance was not revealed at the time in most people's social experience. If this was so, one-quarter of married men and women under 35 had performed the activity (Hunt, 1974) without a script, causing doubt on script theory as explanatory of the production of sexual behavior.

Pregnancy, Parturition, and Child Rearing

Moderate reduction in frequency of couples' sexual relations during the first two trimesters of pregnancy and marked reduction in the third has been consistently reported (Bogren, 1991; Robson, Brant, & Kumar, 1981). The reduction in frequency paralleled the reduction in desire reported by women; men reported little reduction in desire in the first two trimesters, but marked reduction in the third. Bogren related the marked reduction in desire of both men and women at this time to the worry they experience about the birth of the child. Reamy and White (1985) found that more women reported painful intercourse as pregnancy progressed. Understandably, those who reported pain also reported less frequent coitus, and 40% of the total sample ceased coitus in the third trimester. Women who derived little or no pleasure from sex prior to the pregnancy were those most likely to cease in the first trimester (Robson et al., 1981). Reamy and White found that 4%, 11%, and 22%, respectively, of those who continued intercourse experienced pain on at least 25% of occasions in the first, second, and third trimester. Possible causes of the pain suggested included vaginal congestion, vulvar varicosities, hemorrhoids, and deep pelvic congestion. Though Reamy and White mentioned the possibility that in late pregnancy, weight of the partner on the gravid uterus could be a factor, they did not report investigating the use of different coital positions. Initial pregnancy, unhappiness about being pregnant, and fears about delivery were associated with painful coitus.

In Robson et al.'s study (1981) of women having their first child, about one-third resumed intercourse by the sixth week, and almost all by the twelfth week following delivery. This would appear consistent with Reamy and White's report (1987) that the tiny superficial vaginal tears and lacerations resulting from childbirth that are too small to require suturing heal by the sixth week. Grudzinskas and Atkinson (1984) reported that the use of episiotomy to reduce the likelihood of lacerations that are difficult to heal was not associated in spontaneous deliveries with delay in resumption of coitus.

Robson et al. (1981) found that in the year following delivery, the mean frequency of coitus in their subjects remained lower than it was prior to the pregnancy. Persistent discomfort and pain with coitus were still present in 40% of subjects at 3 months, in 18% at 6 months, and 8% at 1 year later. These feelings were usually attributed to soreness at scar sites, or the impression of being sewn up wrongly. Throughout the year following parturition, women said that tiredness interfered with their sex lives. Very few mentioned sexual difficulties to their family doctors, though at 3 months after delivery, 30% thought sexual counseling would have been beneficial. If the common belief is correct that women are mildly to moderately depressed for weeks to months following childbirth, this could contribute to their reduced sexual interest. Gitlin and Pasnau (1989), however, pointed out that studies reporting this did not use comparison groups. Puerperal women were not found to be more depressed when compared with nonpuerperal women, or with their husbands (Richman, Raskin, & Gaines, 1991).

Blumstein and Schwartz (1983) concluded that having dependent children in the home had a big impact on sexual relations as experienced by husbands. Though the frequency was not affected, husbands in their study complained of a marked change in their quality because of the presence of children, whereas wives did not believe they caused any sexual problems. Blumstein and Schwartz supported their conclusions with statements from husbands (the first below with a recently born child, the second with older children):

> We are so tired, we just think of it too late to do anything about it. She is also tender, she tells me. But I am afraid she is also less interested. It's been four months and she puts so much into the kid that I feel she's more maternal than sexy.
> As soon as the children were born, I was a second-class citizen. (p. 204)

One of my women patients reported her husband as saying, "You tell the kids you love them every night, you never tell me"; she added, "It's true, but I feel differently about my kids, of course."

Nettelbladt and Uddenberg (1979) found in a study of Swedish married men that those reporting sexual dissatisfaction considered that their relationships with their wives had deteriorated since the birth of the first child, and they felt neglected at this point in time. They also reported a negative attitude toward the child. Blumfield and Schwartz concluded that women accepted the disruptions caused by children much more readily than fathers and did not feel less sexually satisfied when they had children, and that this difference could cause serious marital conflict.

Brecher (1984) reported anecdotal evidence from older married couples that suggested that both men and women went to considerable lengths to conceal their sexual activity from their children. This continued into the children's adulthood, leading Brecher to describe an "empty nest honeymoon"—the experiences of couples who became more free in their sexual activity when their children left home. He found 87% of couples without (as compared to 80% of those with) dependent children living at home reported being happily married. He concluded that he found little evidence of the "empty nest syndrome" invoked by health professionals to explain a variety of problems experienced by women whose children have left home. Before the syndrome is dismissed as another example of faulty post hoc, ergo propter hoc reasoning, however, it needs to be considered that Brecher's conclusion may be relevant only to the socioeconomically advantaged subjects he studied. They were readers of *Consumer Reports* aged over 50 and were above average in education, health, and income. Less educated women might obtain more of their satisfaction in life from their children, and hence experience more dissatisfaction when they leave home.

Middle Age

Male Clients of Prostitutes

Of the males investigated by Kinsey et al. (1948), about 7% had one or more experiences with prostitutes by age 15, 49% by age 21, and 69% by age 45. Twenty-two percent of the extramarital sex of men aged 55 was with prostitutes. Men of lower socioeconomic class and less education were more likely to have this experience. The 2,402 male readers of *Consumer Reports* aged over 50 who completed questionnaires in Brecher's investigation (1984) were above average in education, health, and income; 34% reported experiences with a female prostitute prior to age 50, and 7% since. Of the 86 who reported any homosexual activity since age 50, 17 (20%) reported experiences with a male prostitute. Women respondents were not asked concerning activities with prostitutes; several said they sometimes fantasized themselves in that role. Twenty-six percent of men and 1% of women who responded to questionnaires in Britain reported experience with prostitutes (Wilson, 1987).

Surveys of U.S. clients of female prostitutes found them to be predominantly white, middle-class married men between the ages of 30 and 60 (Rio, 1991). They were not psychologically disturbed. The reasons they gave for paying for sexual services were numerous: guaranteed sex, elimination of the risk of rejection, companionship, undivided attention of the prostitute, no other easy access to sexual activity, ability to engage in sexual activity partner does not accept, sexual therapy for impotence, temporary absence of partner, adventure, curiosity, and limitation of partner choice as a result of physical or mental disability.

Male clients' experiences with male prostitutes appear less positive than those with female prostitutes. Most male street prostitutes in cities in Canada and the United States investigated by Visano (1991) reported that 70 to 80% of their clients were over 40 years of age. Clients interviewed believed that 95% were over this age. Visano reported that most of the clients were gay and straight men who preferred boys. The older clients were devalued by the prostitutes, who commonly subjected them to considerable psychological, emotional, or physical abuse to establish control. Visano commented that older clients also devalued themselves, responding passively and at times deferentially to the abuse.

Menopause

Menopause contributes independently of age to decline in women's sexual interest and activity. The sexual interest of Swedish women aged 46, 50, and 54 was lower in those who were experiencing menopause than among those of the same age who were not (Hallstrom, 1979). In a longitudinal study, McCoy and Davidson (1985) found that menopause was associated with reductions in both sexual interest and frequency of intercourse in 16 perimenstrual women, independent of their age. The reductions were noted after the final menstrual cycles of the women, who were followed up from 22 months before to 23 months after their final cycles. This postmenopausal reduction, however, was not as great as that which occurred over the period preceding the women's final cycles. The women investigated showed relatively high postmenopausal hormonal levels and had less difficulty with menopause than 23 women who were excluded (mainly because it was not possible to investigate the relationship of their sexuality to the menopause over time because they required replacement hormone therapy). The 16 women investigated reported on average fewer sexual thoughts and fantasies, lack of vaginal lubrication during sex, and less satisfaction with their partners as lovers in the postmenopausal period. Their mean levels of estradiol and testosterone in this period were significantly lower than their mean levels in the premenopausal period.

McCoy, Cutler, and Davidson (1985) reported a close association in 43 perimenopausal women, probably many of those in the study just discussed, between increasing irregularity of menstrual cycles, hot flashes, declining estradiol levels, and declining frequency of intercourse. Explanations they suggested included that discomfort from hot flashes and other symptoms reduced interest in sexual activity, that sexual activity protected against hot flashes by releasing hormones, and that reduction of estrogens associated with the menopause resulted in hot flashes and reduced sexual interest. Myers and Morokoff (1986) found vaginal lubrication and sexual arousal to an erotic film to be significantly greater in premenopausal women and postmenopausal women receiving replacement estrogen than among postmenopausal women who were not. Degree of both responses to the film were significantly related to the estradiol levels in the total sample.

Some workers have held that vasomotor symptoms (hot flashes and sweating) and atrophic vaginitis are the only true symptoms of menopause (Dennerstein & Burrows, 1982). Chakravarti, Collins, Thom, and Studd (1979) investigated middle-aged women still having menstrual cycles who sought treatment for symptoms generally associated with menopause; they compared 40 who reported hot flashes with 42 who did not. Other symptoms of the women with hot flashes were mainly headaches (70%) and insomnia (77%), although 22% experienced loss of sexual interest associated with painful coitus. Those without hot flashes complained mainly of depression (85%); however 45% experienced loss of sexual interest without painful coitus. Estradiol levels in the women with hot flashes, but not those without, were significantly lower than normal; the testosterone levels of both groups were not. The women with hot flashes as compared to the remainder, showed a markedly better response to administration of estrogen in regard to most symptoms, apart from loss of sexual interest. Only one-third of both groups of women with this symptom reported that it improved. These findings, suggesting that depression and reduced sexual interest in women of menopausal age are not produced by the hormonal changes of menopause, was supported by the finding by Hunter (1990), discussed subsequently, of relationships in menopausal women between depression and psychological and social factors, but not hormone levels.

Opposing conclusions were reached by Brincat et al. (1984) in a study of menopausal women randomly allocated to receive implants of estradiol and testosterone or placebo. Those who received the hormones reported significant improvement at 2 and 4 months on a wide range of symptoms compared to those given the placebo. The symptoms responding included depression, palpitations, irritability, and loss of concentration, as well as hot flashes, palpitation, headaches, insomnia, painful coitus, and loss of sexual interest. The apparent conflict between the findings of this and those of the study by Chakravarti et al. (1979) may be due to the different assessment methodologies used. Patients in the study by Brincat et al. scored the intensity with which they experienced all the symptoms investigated on an assessment sheet that they completed at each bimonthly visit. When confronted with a list of all possible symptoms, patients who improved on some may have reported some degree of improvement on all (a "halo effect"). The changes in intensity of symptoms determined in this way could have been statistically but not clinically significant, as discussed in Chapter 1. Changes in symptoms volunteered by patients in a clinical interview, the method used by Chakravarti et al., may have produced more valid findings.

The findings of the studies discussed suggested that the lowered estrogen levels accompanying menopause were responsible for the hot flashes, genital changes of reduction in vaginal lubrication and vaginal atrophy, and, either directly or secondarily to the genital changes, reduction of sexual interest. Leibeum, Bachmann, Kemmann, Colburn, and Swartzman (1983) reported contrary findings emphasizing the role of androgens. Unlike the women in the previous studies, who were perimenstrual, the 52 in the Leibeum et al. study were investigated 6.75 years after menopause. No relationship was found between frequency of coitus and estradiol or androgen levels, but testosterone levels correlated negatively with vaginal atrophy. Those who had less atrophy were more sexually active. Liebeum et al. concluded that sexual activity reduced the degree of vaginal atrophy, though they did not consider the alternative possibility that women with atrophy would be less likely to be sexually active. They stated the less sexually active women had not decided to stop sexual activity but that the decision was made for them by circumstances, such as lack of functional partners. This would not explain the lower frequency of masturbation reported by the less active women; Leibeum et al. suggested that masturbation might be helpful in maintaining the condition of the vagina in lieu of intercourse.

A problem in interpreting their findings is that virtually no estradiol is produced by the ovaries after 4 years (Rosen & Beck, 1988). It is possible that sexual activity present 6 years following menopause was established in the immediate postmenopausal years under the influence of the hormonal levels then present, which included estradiol. Subsequently it might be maintained by other factors such as psychological or social influences, or physiological processes such as the behavior completion mechanisms discussed in Chapter 8. Walling, Andersen, and Johnson (1990) pointed out that the severity of menopausal symptoms is related to the length of time since menopause, with vasomotor symptoms declining in severity while genital symptoms such as atrophic vaginitis worsen.

Investigations of the sexual activity of women during and following natural menopause appear to have provided little support for the widely accepted belief that androgens rather than estrogens are the major determinants of women's sexual interest. In most studies, reduction in interest among menopausal women, along with vasomotor symptoms and atrophic vaginitis, responded to administration of estrogen alone (Dennerstein & Burrows, 1982). A few studies reported a positive effect of addition of androgen, however, when sexual interest remained low (Sherwin & Gelfand, 1987). As discussed in Chapter 5, a similar finding of increased sexual interest and activity following administration of combined androgen and estrogen (as compared with estrogen alone) was reported in some but not all studies of women whose menopause resulted from surgical removal of the ovaries. When this response was reported, it was associated with production of androgen blood levels above normal. It is possible that such high levels resulted in clitoral hypertrophy and increased sensitivity, thus producing increased sexual interest in this way rather than directly by a central nervous system effect. As Walling et al. (1990) pointed out in their review of this literature, it is now accepted that addition of a progestin to estrogen treatment of postmenopausal women with intact uteri is indicated on medical grounds to prevent the increased incidence of uterine endometrial hyperplasia and adenocarcinoma when estrogen alone is used.

A number of workers have attributed the reduction in sexual interest reported by many menopausal women to negative psychological reactions, such as feelings of reduced sexual attractiveness or of loss of biological or social roles. Similarly, the maintained sexual interest of some menopausal women was attributed to positive psychological reactions (e.g., reduced anxiety concerning the possibility of pregnancy). Though little evidence has been advanced to support these beliefs, the contribution of other psychological and social factors has been demonstrated. Dennerstein and Burrows (1982) cited findings of associations in menopausal women between decline in sexual interest and level of depression and introversion, as well as between maintenance of interest and higher socioeconomic class and being employed. These findings were consistent with the relationships reported by Hunter (1990) in a study of women during and following menopause. She found that the presence of negative stereotyped beliefs concerning the effects of menopause, previous episodes of depression, unemployment, and lower social status were related to increased depression in

ıereas hormone levels and vasomotor symptoms were not. Hunter
ıot all studies found an increase in depression to be associated with

As pointed out earlier, the difficulty in consistently demonstrating that sex hormones act directly on women's sexual activity, rather than indirectly through effects on the genitalia, suggests that if direct effects exist they cannot be strong in the majority of women.

DECLINE IN SEXUAL ACTIVITY IN MIDDLE AND OLD AGE

George and Weiler (1981) cited the Kinsey et al. (1948, 1953) studies as the earliest to examine the relationship between age and sexuality; a general decline in all measures of sexual activity was found to be associated with increased age across the entire adult range. Similar findings continue to be reported. Mulligan and Moss (1991) surveyed by questionnaire approximately half of a random sample of registered veterans in Richmond, Virginia, aged 30 to 59 years. The average frequencies of their sexual activities were reported separately for the three age groups (30–39, 40–49, and 50–59). Frequencies were as follows: for touching or caressing, weekly for all three groups; for intercourse, weekly for the two younger groups and monthly for the 50–59 group; for oral sex, monthly for the 30–39 group and yearly for the two older groups; and for masturbation, yearly for the three groups. Their erectile ability expressed as a percentage of their prior best erection was 78%, 75%, and 53%, and the percentages of their ability to reach orgasm on a regular basis were 82%, 84%, and 72%, respectively for the three groups.

Though women's frequency of coitus decreases over the adult range, their sexual interest and ability to reach orgasm increases until they reach middle age. Hagstad and Janson (1984) reported the questionnaire responses of 77% of a representative sample of Swedish women aged 37 to 46 years. All but 4% had a sexual partner. Only 3% reported a frequency of coitus of once a day or every other day; in 74% it was at least once a week. More than one-third of the 32% having coitus 2 to 3 times a week or more considered this to be too often. The majority of the women believed their sexual interest had remained unchanged over the previous 5 years; one-quarter thought it had increased. Only one-third of the women who experienced a decreased interest in sex considered this decrease to be negative. Forty-one percent of the women aged 37 to 41, but 19% of those aged 42 to 46, reported an increased capacity for orgasm.

The authors concluded from their data that women's sexual interest and capacity for orgasm reached a maximum around the age of 40. Ninety-six percent of the women had experienced orgasm during intercourse, which could include clitoral stimulation by hand or otherwise; one-half usually and one-fifth always did. Sixty-four percent admitted experiences with masturbation, but in the majority these were infrequent. Only 8% masturbated once a week or more. Ninety-seven percent felt that the desire for sex was entirely or partly associated with the desire for a certain person. In response to the question whether they thought there were differences between female and male sexual needs and interests, 42% felt there were, along the usual lines that women wished for more tenderness and emotional response, whereas men had a stronger desire for sex. A few complained of men's inability to caress without coitus as a consequence. The greater need for women to have sex in a committed relationship was found to persist in Brecher's study (1984) of subjects 50 to 70 years and over. Fifty-one percent of women and 17% of men disagreed with the statement that sex without love was better than no sex at all.

Little data are available concerning the prevalence of orgasm in middle and old age. It was investigated by Hallstrom (1979) in 89% of a representative sample of married and cohabiting Swedish women. Total inability to reach orgasm in sexual activity was reported by just under 10% of the women aged 46, 15% of those aged 50, and 25% of those aged 54. Hunt (1974) found the regularity of orgasm in women of 55 and over to be considerably lower than that of the younger women. In the socioeconomically advantaged subjects aged 50 to 70 years and over investigated by Brecher (1984), the percentages who seldom or never experienced orgasm in sexual activities with a partner were 19% for women aged 50 to 59, 22% for those aged 60 to 69, and 28% for those 70 and over; for men in these age ranges, the figures were 1%, 4%, and 10%, respectively. Equivalent percentages for those seldom or never experiencing orgasm with masturbation in these age ranges were 7%, 10%, and 14% for women and 4%, 7%, and 13% for men.

These studies reporting decline in sexual activity with age were cross-sectional rather than longitudinal in nature—that is, they examined the relationship in subjects of different ages at one point in time. In cross-sectional studies, the effects of aging are confounded with the effects of belonging to a particular age group or cohort. Findings of such studies cannot exclude the possibility that the sexual activity of older subjects had always been less than that of younger subjects because, for example, of such factors as different socialization experiences and religious and moral values. In an early study, Pfeiffer, Verwoerdt, and Davis (1972) attempted to examine the age effect in isolation by asking subjects if they were aware of a change in their sexual interest and activity. Their report was part of an investigation of the effects of aging conducted at Duke University Medical Center at Durham, North Carolina. The subjects were 261 white men and 241 white women, aged 45 to 69 at the commencement of the study. They were chosen randomly from membership lists of the local medical group, so that they were broadly representative of the middle and upper socioeconomic levels of the community.

The number who reported awareness of a decline in sexual interest and activity increased with age, the sharpest reduction being found between subjects in the 46–50 and 51–55 age groups. Decline in interest was reported by 58% of women aged 46 to 50, 78% of women aged 51 to 55, and 96% of women aged 66 to 71, as well as by 49% of men aged 46 to 50, 71% of men aged 51 to 55, and 88% of men aged 66 to 71. Cessation of intercourse was reported by 14% of women aged 46 to 50, 38% of those aged 56 to 60, and 76% of those aged 66 to 71, and also by 0%, 7%, and 24% of men in the same age ranges. Eighty-sex percent of the women attributed responsibility for stopping intercourse to their spouse's absence as a result of death, separation, or divorce, or of his illness or inability to perform sexually. Seventy-one percent of the much smaller number of men who reported cessation of intercourse reported that they were responsible because of illness, loss of interest, or inability to perform sexually. Despite their considering the absence of an effective partner to be responsible for cessation of intercourse, women reported a much greater reduction of sexual interest in relation to their age than did men. One-quarter of women in their 50s and 50% of those in their 60s reported no sexual interest; corresponding figures for men in these two age ranges were less than 5% and 10%, respectively.

Regression analysis revealed that in men a number of factors were associated with reduced current activity (Pfeiffer & Davis, 1972). These included less past sexual activity, age, poor health status, lower social class, taking of antihypertensive medication, and reduced life satisfaction. A much smaller number of factors were associated with reduced sexual activity in women. They were principally no intact marriage and age; small contributions were made by postmenopausal status and less education. It would seem that in the absence of a partner, women may cease all sexual activity. The percentages of married women who were sexually active in Brecher's study (1984) were 95%, 89%, and 81%, respectively, for the age ranges 50–60, 60–70 and 70 and over; those for unmarried women of the same ages were 88%, 63%, and 50%. Pfeiffer and Davis pointed out that with advancing age, fewer women have a sexual partner available, and they believed the remedy to lie in efforts to prolong the vigor and life span of men. Turner and Adams (1988) cited U.S. Bureau of the Census figures that 75% of men but only 37% of women over 65 are married. In addition, as Brecher (1984) pointed out, more unmarried men than women (57% compared to 37% in his study) are in an ongoing sexual relationship, and more (10% compared to 1% in his study) consider themselves homosexual. This resulted in there being five unattached heterosexual women for every unattached heterosexual man among those over 50 years old.

Longitudinal studies (i.e., studies following up the same subjects over time) are methodologically the most appropriate to investigate age independently of cohort effects. Two such studies that followed up the subjects over a 6-year period restricted their investigation to those who were married. The findings, even more than those of the earlier studies, established the importance of the presence of a partner for women's sexuality. The married women did not show the marked decline in sexual activity in middle age found in the cross-sectional studies of married and single subjects. George and Weiler (1981) investigated the frequency of sexual relations of the subjects in the Duke University study of Pfeiffer et al. (1972); Hallstrom and Samuelsson (1990) studied the sexual interest of 497 Swedish women. No change was found over 6 years in the aspects of sexual activity assessed in more than 55% of the women aged 65 or less at the start of the Duke University study, and in 50% of those aged 54 to 60 at the start of the Swedish study. In the Duke study, cessation of sexual intercourse was reported by 10% of the women initially aged under 56, and by 28% of those initially aged 56 to 65. Reduction of sexual interest was reported by 26%, 31%, and 37% of those initially 46, 50, and 54 years old, respectively, in the Swedish study.

The authors of the Duke study tended to emphasize the lack of change in the majority of subjects, and those of the Swedish study the reduction in the minority, though in almost all cases it was slight. The Swedish authors also found a reduction in the number of women who experienced strong sexual desire, with none reporting this after the age of 50. Hypoactive sexual desire disorder (i.e., absence of sexual desire) was reported by 3% of those aged 34 to 46, 9% of those aged 50, and 29% of those aged 60. The women in the Swedish study were representative of all married women in the community, whereas the women in the Duke study were of good health and mainly of medium or high income and educational attainment.

It would seem that though older middle-aged women report less sexual interest and activity than younger ones, the difference in the majority is not great. The healthy and socially advantaged can expect their sexual interest and frequency of coitus to remain relatively unchanged until their 60s provided they have an active sexual partner, though some will experience a reduced ability to reach orgasm. The decline in frequency of coitus that follows the 60s is likely to be significantly influenced by the reduced interest of the male partner. A possible index of women's sexual interest that is uninfluenced by relationship factors is frequency of masturbation: Brecher (1984) found that the percentage of women who masturbated in the 50–60, 60–70, and over-70 age groups declined from 47% to 37% and 33%, respectively; the mean frequency of masturbation in those who continued it remained the same (0.7 times per week). The percentage of men who masturbated in these three age groups declined from 66% to 50% and 43%; the mean frequency also declined, from 1.2 to 1.0 and 0.7 times per week. Biological factors may play a larger role in the decline in male sexuality with age.

George and Weiler (1981) also followed up the married subjects in the Duke University study of Pfeiffer et al. (1972) for 6 years. Again, frequency of sexual relationships remained stable over the 6 years in the majority of men who were aged 65 or below at the commencement of the study. The frequency was reduced in about 10%, however, and sexual relations ceased in 5% of men initially aged 56 and under and 16% of those initially aged 56 to 65. Only a minority (42% of men and 33% of women) of those over 66 at the commencement of the Duke University study maintained the same frequency of relations over the following 6 years. The remaining 66% of women and 30% of the men ceased relations. As the follow-up was only over 6 years, the marked reduction in sexual activity in these subjects may have been in part a cohort effect, in which case it may not be shown to the same extent by younger subjects as they age. More recently, Weizman and Hart (1987) found a decline in frequency of intercourse and increase in frequency of masturbation in married men aged 66 to 71 as compared to those aged 60 to 65. Coitus was reported by all 64% of the total sample who were potent, and masturbation by 59%. The relationship of the use of masturbation and impotence was not reported. Pfeiffer et al. (1972) pointed out the importance of not extrapolating the finding of mean reduction in sexual interest and activity of a total sample of older subjects to the individuals in the sample, a number of whom may show no change.

Bretschneider and McCoy (1988) investigated upper-middle-class subjects living in retirement facilities for the healthy elderly, none of whom were taking regular medication, including aspirin or vitamins. One hundred white men and 102 white women, aged from 80 to 102, completed anonymous questionnaires. Fifty-three percent of the men and 25% of the women said they had a regular sex partner; 29% of the men and 14% of the women were married. Eighty-eight percent of the men and 71% of the women fantasized or daydreamed at least once a year about being close, affectionate, and intimate with the opposite sex. Touching and caressing without sexual intercourse was the most common activity for men (82%) and women (64%), followed by masturbation (72% and 40%, respectively) and sexual intercourse (63% and 30%). Forty-seven percent of the women and 22% of the men considered sex to be of no importance. Many of the subjects did not answer questions concerning masturbation, and so the percentage reported was based on the answers of those who did. The sexual activity of these healthy and upper-middle-class 80- to 102-year-olds was not consistently reduced compared to that of the unmarried 50- to 70-year-olds investigated by Brecher (1984). They were also of above average in income and health. Fifty-seven percent of the men and 33% of the women had a regular sex partner; 62% of the men and 54% of the women were currently masturbating; and 34% of the men and 13% of the women had engaged in sex with one or more casual partners in the previous year. The unmarried women's regular male partners were mainly married or much older or both; the unmarried men tended to seek much younger women.

In contrast to these physically and economically advantaged subjects, the majority of whom enjoyed sexual activity, C. White (1982) found that 91% of 250 residents of nursing homes in Texas were sexually inactive, that is, they hadn't masturbated or had intercourse in the previous month. Their mean age was over 80 years, and about two-thirds were women. Seventeen percent of those sexually inactive said they would be interested in being sexually active but lacked opportunity, having no partner or a lack of privacy. A possibly more representative sample of men up to the age of 95 was reported in a Danish community study (Hegeler & Mortensen, 1978). Only 3% of those in their 90s reported having coitus, though about 30% had partners. The reduction in coitus appeared to increase more rapidly after the age of 70. Decline in frequency of masturbation was slower; it was reported by 60% of men aged 51 to 55 years, and 23% of those aged 90 to 95 "confessed" they still did. A further 31% in that age group did not answer the question; the authors interpreted comments made as indicating that a lot of guilt still existed about masturbation. This was also suggested by Brecher's finding (1984) that 19% of the women and 28% of men in his study who considered masturbation as not being proper for older people reported that they masturbated.

Bretschneider and McCoy (1988) concluded, on the basis of a comparison of their data with that of Pfeiffer et al. (1972), that there was a small steady increase in the number of men losing interest in sex and ceasing intercourse from their late 40s to the 90s. The majority of healthy men in their 90s, however, maintained both behaviors. They further concluded that the increase in number of women losing interest in sex and ceasing intercourse did not continue after women reached the age of 80. They suggested the major decline in sexual activity that occurred in women in their late 50s and early 60s could be related to menopause and the associated fall in hormone levels. These conclusions, based on socioeconomically advantaged and healthy subjects, ignored the findings of much greater decline in the disadvantaged and in women without healthy partners. More longitudinal studies over the entire range of middle and old age are required to exclude cohort effects and to examine the influence of health and socioeconomic and relationship status before such conclusions can be supported.

Martin (1981) investigated possible reasons for the different levels of sexual interest and activity in 188 married men, aged 60 to 79 years, who had volunteered for a Baltimore study of aging. Twenty-six percent had ceased coitus. When masturbation, nocturnal emissions, and homosexual activity were included in his measures, Martin found the frequency of all sexual behaviors assessed was independent of marital adjustment, sexual attractiveness of wives, and sexual attitudes, but strongly related to the subjects' reported frequency of sexual behaviors from the age of 20. Men who were less than fully potent were virtually free from performance anxiety, feelings of sexual deprivation, and loss of self-esteem, which he considered consistent with his belief that lack of motivation was responsible for their lower sexual functioning. Lack of dissatisfaction with the reduced sexual activity associated with aging was also found by Schiavi, Schreiner-Engel, Mandeli, Schanzer, and Cohen (1990) in a study of married men aged 45 to 74 and of higher socioeconomic class. Despite the presence of erectile difficulties in the older subjects, their enjoyment of marital sex and their satisfaction with their own sexuality did not change with age. As pointed out in Chapter 5, there is little relationship between sexual dysfunctions and satisfaction in younger men investigated in community studies.

Davidson et al. (1983) stated that a decline in testosterone levels was commonly found to occur with aging and could in part be responsible for the associated reduced sexual activity. They studied 220 men, aged 41 to 93 years, who attended a hospital clinic; they found weak but significant correlations between free testosterone levels and sexual activity, in particular difficulty in achieving erections and orgasms rather than reduced libido. This finding appeared to conflict with Davidson's belief (see Chapter 5) that testosterone maintains libido but not potency. Davidson et al. pointed out that studies that had not found a decline in testosterone with age were all of men highly selected for health criteria. They considered their subjects, though attending a clinic, to be of average health, as most had come for routine checks. They attached sufficient weight to their findings to suggest that treatment with androgen could be indicated for the subgroup of older men with both sexual dysfunction and the desire to correct it. As few of the subjects had testosterone levels below the normal lower limit of 3 ng/ml, they suggested that an altered threshold of the androgen-sensitive elements maintaining sexual function might occur in aging men.

Tsitouras et al. (1982) found no reduction in total testosterone levels but the usual reduction in sexual activity with increased age in healthy married men. They investigated 183 men, aged 60 to 79 years, who were part of the Baltimore longitudinal study on aging; it is probable they were largely the same subjects reported upon by Martin (1981). A relationship was found between the subjects' testosterone levels and their sexual activity, but not their potency. Tsitouras et al. pointed out that their sample was not representative of U.S. older males but were of higher than average social and economic success, good general health, and greater than average concern for health issues. They cited other studies that found no reduction in testosterone levels of healthy older men and suggested that when it was found it was attributable to such accompanying factors as obesity, alcoholism, chronic disease, and stress, all of which were known to affect the level of the hormone. Chambers and Phoenix (1982) pointed out that the decline in the sexual performance of aging males is a general phenomenon found in several different mammalian species, including rodents, farm animals, and nonhuman primates as well as human beings. They noted that the decline in aged rhesus monkeys could not be attributed to reduction in testosterone levels, as there is no change in these levels with age.

George and Weiler (1981) commented that both men and women in their longitudinal study overwhelmingly attributed cessation of sexual relations to the attitudes or physical condition of the male partner. They believed this testified to the importance of the man's role as initiator of sexual behavior among current cohorts of middle-aged and older adults. The data reported earlier indicate the situation is the same among younger cohorts. Given the wealth of information concerning frequencies of sexual activities in the elderly, it is disappointing that there is so little concerning the communication between sexual partners, and whether (and if so, how) they deal with the problems connected with the increase in frequency of men's erectile problems with age and the dependence of women's sexual activity on the presence of an active partner. Brecher (1984) quoted a 66-year-old husband as saying, "Most partners go through life playing a guessing game. By the time they really know what turns each other on, it's turn-off time" (p. 95).

CHAPTER 3

Homosexuality/Heterosexuality
Sissiness and Tomboyism

PREVALENCE OF HOMOSEXUAL FEELINGS AND BEHAVIORS

Throughout this chapter, the term *homosexual/heterosexual ratio of feelings* will usually be employed in preference to *sexual orientation,* as common usage has caused the latter term to carry the implication that subjects' sexual orientation can only be one of three categories (heterosexual, homosexual, or bisexual). Evidence will be advanced that such feelings are distributed not categorically but dimensionally in the population. Marked resistance has been shown not only by the general public but also by sex researchers to accepting the evidence that the majority of the population who are or have been aware of homosexual feelings are predominantly heterosexual (McConaghy, 1987a).

It would appear that the first study that provided evidence of a significant prevalence of homosexual feelings and behaviors was that carried out by Schbankov and Iakowenko in Moscow in 1907. Davis (1929/1965) drew attention to the study, pointing out that most of its data were destroyed after confiscation by the Russian government. The remaining data included the questionnaire responses of 324 female university students; 169 (52%) stated they had experienced intense emotional relationships with other women, which in 16% of the cases had included overt homosexual practices. Davis obtained comparable data in her own study of U.S. female college graduates carried out in 1929. Fifty percent of 1,200 single and 30% of 1,000 married subjects reported experiencing intense emotional relationships with women. Over half of both groups who reported these relationships recognized them as sexual in character and usually expressed them in sexual activities such as mutual genital contact or masturbation.

It is noteworthy that these studies by women researchers received little attention, in marked contrast to those of Kinsey and his colleagues that reported similar findings, initially in men. Hunt (1974), in his survey of sexual behavior in the 1970s, stated that prior to Kinsey's work the only quantitative estimates of homosexual behavior dealt only with males and were based on wholly inadequate samples. Kinsey et al. (1948) found that 50% of white males interviewed in the United States said that they had experienced erotic responses to males, and 37% that they had at least one experience of homosexual arousal to orgasm. Subsequently, Kinsey et al.

(1953) reported that 28% of women similarly interviewed said they had experienced erotic responses to females, 20% specific homosexual contacts, and 14% homosexual arousal to orgasm. The findings of all these studies were at variance with the popular view that only a small percentage of the population are homosexual or bisexual and the rest exclusively heterosexual. Kinsey had in fact questioned this concept as early as 1941, believing that the picture was one of endless intergradation between every combination of homosexuality and heterosexuality. Despite the intense media attention given the findings of Kinsey's studies both within and outside the United States, a curious ambivalence has been demonstrated toward them. They are often quoted as accepted; at the same time studies in total contradiction to them continue to be published without any attempt being made to resolve the contradiction or even to acknowledge that it exists.

Gonsiorek (1982) stated that Kinsey's "notion of a heterosexual-homosexual continuum revolutionized theorizing about sexuality and challenged the dichotomous, either-or view of sexual orientation. The concept remains controversial in some quarters to this day, but it has gained acceptance over the years" (p. 59). A reviewer for a leading U.S. psychiatric journal identified by the editor (personal communication, 1990) as a most eminent and competent investigator in the field made the following statement, with which the editor agreed: "My impression is that most people [i.e., sexuality research workers and theorists] from Freud or Kinsey to the present look on these qualities [heterosexual and homosexual impulses and behavior] as ranging along a continuum rather than being absolutes." If these statements are correct, most sex researchers would believe that homosexual feelings are experienced to various degrees by a significant proportion of the population. The following studies by leading sex researchers all reported data that, to be valid, required that only a very small percentage of the population experienced homosexual feelings. None of the studies made reference to the fact that their findings and those of the Kinsey group could not both be correct.

Absence of homosexual feeling was reported in all of 42 girls exposed to excess androgen in utero and 26 matched controls (Ehrhardt & Baker 1974; Ehrhardt, Epstein, & Money, 1968; Ehrhardt & Money, 1967). Of twenty 16-year-old boys exposed prenatally to female hormones and 22 matched controls, only 1 of the controls was reported to show some degree of homosexuality (Yalom, Green, & Fisk, 1973). None of 10 teenaged children or young adults raised by transsexual or female homosexual parents were reported to have experienced any homosexual fantasies (Green, 1978). Thirty-four control males aged 13–23 years reported no homosexual behavior, and only 2 reported slight homosexual fantasies (Green, 1985). The validity of the reported incidence of homosexual arousal in these studies was of major theoretical importance, being crucial to the investigators' aim of supporting or refuting theories concerning the etiology of homosexuality. Most of these investigators' ideological orientation was toward considering that social factors determined sexual orientation. It is perhaps more surprising that workers (Doerner, Rohde, Stahl, Krell, & Masius, 1975; Gladue, Green, & Hellman, 1984; Gooren, 1986) who considered biological factors of importance also treated heterosexuality and homosexuality as categories rather than as dimensionally distributed, in view of the fact that most biological variables tend to be dimensionally rather than categorically distributed. As recently as 1991 the *Archives of Sexual Behavior,* possibly the leading international journal of sexuality research, published an article reporting an investigation of the sexual arousal patterns of normal men that described 95% of the male undergraduates they studied as exclusively heterosexual (Templeman & Stinnett, 1991).

As none of these workers discussed the issue, it is impossible to know how they interpreted the marked disparity between their findings and those of Kinsey and his colleagues. Though I drew attention to it on several occasions (McConaghy, Armstrong, Birrell, & Buhrich, 1979; McConaghy, 1984, 1987b), to my knowledge no other reference has yet been made to it in the literature, indicating the widespread acceptance of the findings of these researchers that only a small percentage of the population are aware of homosexual feelings. It is possible that the researchers considered the Kinsey findings invalid but did not wish to point this out.

The Kinsey and the earlier studies, which demonstrated a dimensional distribution of subjects' ratio of heterosexual/homosexual feelings with a significant percentage of the population aware of some homosexual feelings, were open to the criticism that the subjects were volunteers who might not be representative of the total population. This methodological weakness was understandable. Saghir and Robins (1973) suggested that because of the social and legal stigmata attached to homosexuality, it was not possible to obtain relevant data from representative samples drawn from the normal population. A possible solution would be to obtain data anonymously from representative samples of a number of different subgroups of the population concerning the degree to which they were aware of both heterosexual and homosexual feelings. If the data from all samples were reasonably congruent, this would indicate their validity. This method was initiated by the author (McConaghy et al., 1979).

Eighty-five percent of all students enrolled in the second-year medical course (*N* = 232) at the University of New South Wales anonymously completed a questionnaire (McConaghy, 1988b) as one item of which they rated the degree to which, until the age of 15 years and also currently, they felt sexually attracted to members of the same and opposite sex on the following relative scale:

to opposite sex	0	10	20	30	40	50	60	70	80	90	100
to same sex	100	90	80	70	60	50	40	30	20	10	0

where

$$\frac{0}{100} = \frac{\text{not attracted to opposite sex}}{\text{exclusively attracted to same sex}} \quad \text{and} \quad \frac{100}{0} = \text{the reverse}$$

The study was replicated in 2 subsequent years. Over the 3 years, 51% to 63% of the men and 60% to 69% of the women reported they had been aware of some degree of homosexual feeling by the age of 15 years. From 33% to 45% of the men and 44% to 51% of the women were currently aware of some degree of homosexual feelings (McConaghy, 1987a). The ratio of heterosexual to homosexual feelings currently experienced by these students is shown in Figure 3.1. It will be noted that the majority of both men and women who reported awareness of some homosexual feelings were aware of predominant heterosexual feelings. These reports, from almost

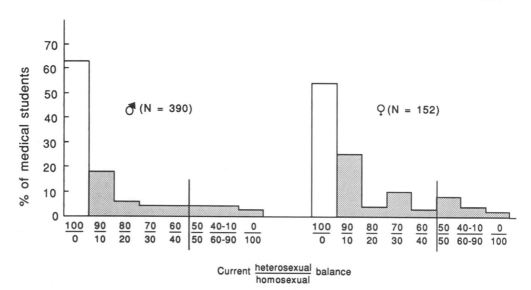

FIG. 3.1. Percentage of male and female medical students reporting different balances of heterosexual to homosexual feelings. Reprinted with permission from McConaghy (1981).

all second-year students in the medical school, were compatible with the incidence of homosexual feelings reported by Schbankov, Davis, and the Kinsey group.

It could be argued that medical students were markedly different from the rest of the population in regard to their ratio of homosexual/heterosexual feelings. The same questionnaire was completed by 411 of 606 men on the Australian NHMRC Twin Registry (McConaghy, Buhrich, & Silove, 1993). Twenty percent reported awareness of some homosexual feelings in adolescence, and 12% were currently aware of such feelings. It was considered that these figures might underestimate the prevalence of homosexual feelings in the total sample, as some subjects with homosexual feelings may have failed to complete the questionnaire out of concern that their anonymity might be breached. Again, the majority of subjects reporting awareness of some homosexual feelings experienced predominantly heterosexual feelings.

If 20% or more adolescents and young adults are aware of some homosexual feelings, how has the community view been established that only a small percentage of the population are homosexual and the rest are exclusively heterosexual? Perhaps more importantly, how has this view come to be accepted by almost all sex re-searchers? The community view reflects the inevitable effect of the marked societal discrimination against homosexuality. As a consequence, subjects with homosexual feelings deny these to others—and, in some cases, to themselves. The strong approval of heterosexual and disapproval of homosexual activity results in subjects aware of homosexual as well as heterosexual feelings being under pressure to express only the latter in sexual behaviors.

The significant percentage of the population who are aware of some homosexual but predominantly heterosexual feelings could therefore be expected to engage ex-clusively or almost exclusively in heterosexual behavior, at least following adolescence. Fay, Turner, Klassen, and Gagnon (1989) published an analysis of data from a 1970 study of a U.S. national probability sample, emphasizing that though approximately 20% of the male adults reported that they had had sexual contacts to orgasm with another man, no more that 6.7% had such contacts after age 19, and in half of the 6.7% they were infrequent. The authors considered that because of societal intolerance, there could have been some degree of underreporting. As discussed below, the original Kinsey data—usually considered to inflate the incidence of homosexuality—indicated that at most 6% of men and 2% of women engaged in significant homosexual activity in adulthood. In the data analyzed by Fay et al., 14% of the men and 10% of the women believed that sex with a person of the same sex offered them some possibility of enjoyment, and 12% of the men and 14% of the women felt that sex with a person of the opposite sex offered them no possibility of enjoyment (Klassen, Williams, & Levitt, 1989).

It is probable that most persons with nonpredominant homosexual feelings identify themselves publicly and also internally as exclusively heterosexual. The majority of medical students in the studies discussed above who anonymously reported such homosexual feelings identified to their colleagues as heterosexual. When asked to volunteer for penile assessment of their homosexual/heterosexual ratio of feelings, few of these students did so, unlike those who reported exclusive heterosexual feelings. Presumably, they feared their anonymity would not be maintained in the assessment process (McConaghy & Blaszczynski, 1991).

A significant percentage of subjects with predominant homosexual but some heterosexual feelings also express mainly or exclusively heterosexual feelings in their sexual activity, at least for significant periods of their adult lives, and identify themselves publicly as exclusively heterosexual. Probably some of these subjects deny the sexual aspects of their interest in members of the same sex and also identify to themselves as heterosexual. Forty-four of 181 men who sought treatment for homosexual urges they experienced as compulsive were married and identified publicly and usually to their wives as heterosexual (McConaghy, 1978). Most of these men reported experiencing predominant homosexual interest; this report was confirmed by their penile volume responses to pictures of nude men and women (Table 1.1). One form of uncontrollable urge these men commonly reported was to frequent public lavatories for homosexual contacts. Humphries (1970) investigated men who showed this sexual behavior and found that about half were married and identified socially as heterosexual. One half of the 3.3% of U.S. men who in the study by Fay et al. (1989) reported more than infrequent homosexual contacts were currently or previously married.

Almost all subjects who as adults express homosexual feelings to a significant degree in their sexual behavior and identify to themselves as bisexual or homosexual must, therefore, be those who experience very predominant or exclusive homosexual feelings. A percentage of these self-identified homosexuals identify as homosexual publicly to some or all of their acquaintances. As the majority of subject with homosexual feelings behave in their overt sexual activity and identify as exclusively heterosexual, and as only a small percentage identify publicly as homosexual, the common perception of heterosexuality/homosexuality as dichotomously distributed with only a small percentage of subjects having homosexual feelings is inevitable. It will presumably remain until the evidence to the contrary is accepted by sex researchers and subsequently disseminated by the media. Strangely, limited consideration has been given to the influence of societal prejudice and guilt on the expression of homosexual feelings in behaviors. Altshuler (1984) argued that "if the heterosexual-homosexual range were truly a continuum, bisexuals at the midpoint should (show) equal frequency and pleasure with either sex, and therefore an equal preference and relatively random choice in the sex of their partners." In criticizing the naïveté of this believe, it was pointed out (McConaghy, 1987b) that it would be equivalent to arguing that for a person to like herrings and cavier equally, he or she must eat equal quantities of both.

The reason the majority of sex researchers have accepted the public perception of the distribution of sexual orientation could be related to their belief that sexual orientation is determined totally by social factors. This belief has dominated thinking concerning not only sexual but all human behavior for several decades, particularly in the United States (McConaghy, 1987a). From this perspective, the only sexual behaviors of interest are those carried out in a social context. This interest in public behavior rather than private feelings was evidenced in the sociological study of homosexuality by Gagnon and Simon (1973). In discussing its incidence, they examined the data from the college-educated sample interviewed by Kinsey et al., as they considered that sample most free from possible volunteer bias. They pointed out that though 30% of the 2,900 men in the sample reported at least one homosexual experience in which they or their male partner had reached orgasm, in the majority of these (25% of the total sample) the homosexual experiences were confined predominantly to adolescence or to isolated experiences in early adulthood. Of the remaining 5% to 6% of the total sample, 3% had only homosexual experiences throughout their lives, and 3% had substantial homosexual as well as heterosexual experiences.

From the Kinsey data for college-educated women, Gagnon and Simon concluded that 4% of the total sample had homosexual experiences limited to early adolescence with a few scattered experiences later in the teens, with only 2% having any significant homosexual experience and less than 1% being exclusively homosexual in behavior. Gagnon and Simon attached little significance to homosexual behavior occurring in adolescence, possibly influenced in part by a psychoanalytic view that all adolescents pass through a bisexual phase (Mullaly, 1970) and in part by the view that adolescence is a developmental period characterized by transient acting-out or experimental behaviors of no long-term significance. By totally ignoring the issue of feelings and treating homosexual activity in adolescence and early adulthood as insignificant, Kinsey's data were interpreted by Gagnon and Simon (1973) as conforming to the popular view that homosexuality and bisexuality were categorical conditions shown by a small minority of the population, the rest of whom were exclusively heterosexual.

Without referring to the study of Gagnon and Simon, Van Wyk and Geist (1984) used a similar procedure to reach the same conclusion. They also reanalyzed the Kinsey data, excluding subjects they believed may have biased the results. They computed ratings of each subject's degree of homosexuality/heterosexuality by separately summing frequencies of his or her heterosexual and homosexual behavior from age 18 to age at interview or to age 40, whichever occurred first. Sexual behavior in early adolescence and later adulthood was thus excluded from consideration. Total homosexual behavior was divided by the sum of total heterosexual and homosexual behavior to obtain each subject's rating. Of the sample of 3,392 women and 3,849 men, 94% of the women and 86% of the men obtained scores of 0 to 0.004, "the exclusive heterosexual end of the distribution," and 1.8% of the women and 4.7% of the men obtained scores of 4.01 to 6, the homosexual end. Nevertheless, 3.4% of the women and 8.4% of the men obtained scores of 0.005 to 1.99, indicating predominantly heterosexual but also some homosexual behavior.

Thus the subjects' homosexual and heterosexual behaviors between the ages of 18 and 40 years were not dichotomously distributed. Homosexual behavior was reported by almost twice as many subjects who reported predominantly heterosexual behavior as by subjects who reported predominantly homosexual behavior. In conflict with this evidence from their own analysis, Van Wyk and Geist stated that the distribution was extremely bipolar, and that it would appear that the popular conception of heterosexuality and homosexuality as polar extremes was quite accurate. In addition to the scores not being bipolar, the prevalence of homosexual behavior found (6% of women and 14% of men) was higher than that given significance by Gagnon and Simon (1973), presumably because Van Wyk and Geist included homosexual activity after the age of 18 years.

Unlike Gagnon and Simon, Van Wyk and Geist (1984) computed scores for the subjects' sexual feelings as well as their behaviors. Indicative of the lack of significance attached to feelings, however, they gave no details concerning how this was done, nor did they provide the distribution data for these scores. Correlations were reported for the relationships between the scores for the subjects' feelings and their overt behaviors. These were $r = 0.83$ for the male and $r = 0.54$ for the female sample, accounting for 69% and 29% of the variance, respectively. Many more subjects, particularly females, could therefore have reported homosexual feelings than homosexual behaviors. It is likely that the scores of sexual feelings not provided by Van Wyk and Geist would have demonstrated a less dichotomous distribution than the behavior scores in regard to the subjects' ratio of homosexuality/heterosexuality.

The lack of interest shown by the majority of sex researchers in homosexual feelings as opposed to homosexual behaviors is of considerable significance in relation to theories of etiology of sexual orientation. If biological factors contribute to this, they would do so by influencing the subject's homosexual/heterosexual ratio of feelings. Whether the subject expressed the feelings in behaviors would depend largely or entirely on social variables. By ignoring feelings, the role of biological variables could be overlooked. A further obstacle to the awareness that sexual orientation was distributed dimensionally was created by biological research that attempted to investigate the distribution of male subjects' heterosexual and homosexual feelings. As discussed in Chapter 1, this was done this by assessing their penile circumference responses (PCRs) to pictures of male and female nudes. In choosing this method, the researchers ignored the evidence that only subjects' penile volume responses (PVRs) to these pictures could identify most subjects who reported they are heterosexual or homosexual; for PCRs to do so required the more powerful stimuli of videos of homosexual and lesbian activity.

This difference in the sensitivity of PCRs and PVRs has remained unacknowledged. The failure of PCR assessment to differentiate subjects who reported bisexuality from those who reported homosexuality (Table 1.2) was therefore accepted as evidence that bisexuality did not exist. The findings, using PVR assessment, that subjects could be distinguished on the basis of their dimensionally reported ratio of homosexual to heterosexual feelings (Table 1.1) was ignored. As it remained widely accepted, covertly if not overtly, that heterosexuality and homosexuality were categorical entities, no interest was shown in the possibility that the opposite-sex-linked behaviors reported by homosexual men could be distributed dimensionally in the total population, including that portion of the population who were predominantly heterosexual.

SEX-LINKED BEHAVIORS: SISSINESS AND TOMBOYISM

Sex-linked behaviors are behaviors that are shown significantly more frequently by members of one as compared to the other sex. The related term *cross-gender behaviors* tends to be restricted to behaviors known generally to be associated with the opposite sex, such as wearing the clothes of the opposite sex (cross-dressing or transvestism). Sex-linked behaviors such as interest in music and performing (statistically more common in women) and in sport (statistically more common in men; McConaghy, 1982; McConaghy & Zamir, 1992a) are usually not regarded as cross-gender behaviors. Also, as Maccoby (1980) pointed out when justifying her decision not to use the term *gender,* some workers use it for behaviors that they believe are entirely socially determined, so that its use prejudges the issue as to whether biological factors could contribute. The term *sex-linked behaviors* implies nothing about etiology.

A few decades ago, it appeared generally accepted that young boys who showed extreme opposite-sex-linked behaviors would become homosexual in adulthood. They were commonly labeled as effeminate or sissy by the lay public, and as homosexual by clinicians (Bakwin & Bakwin, 1953; Bender & Paster, 1941). The boys studied by clinicians were described as dressing in female clothes at every opportunity, using cosmetics, and posturing like girls. Subsequently, a number of workers (Bakwin, 1968; Green, 1985, 1987; Money & Russo, 1979; Zuger, 1966, 1978, 1984) followed up groups of boys who showed these marked opposite-sex-linked behaviors. In all studies, the majority in adulthood identified to themselves and to the researchers as homosexual. Bakwin and Bakwin (1953) believed that the families of these effeminate boys were not unusual and that this and the early age at which the behaviors appeared suggested that the effeminate behaviors were biologically determined.

These data and conclusions were generally ignored, being incompatible with current sociological ideology concerning members of minority groups, particularly discriminated-against minorities. This ideology required that behaviors of members of minority groups that could disadvantage them be attributed to the discriminatory treatment they received. Evidence that the behaviors might be innate or not reversible with appropriate modification of the minority members' social environment was unacceptable. This attitude was reflected in a popular 1950s Broadway play, *Tea and*

Sympathy, admired at the time for its liberal values. (Following the rise of gay liberation, it would now be considered reactionary.) In the play, the nonmasculine behavior of the sensitive adolescent hero provoked fears and taunts that he was homosexual. These were dispelled by the timely dispensation of tea, sympathy, and seduction by the wife of his schoolteacher. Such liberally approved beliefs resulted in a covert censorship that led pediatricians and child psychiatrists at that time to disregard transvestism and effeminate behaviors in male children and offer troubled parents the unfounded reassurance that the boy would grow out of them (Bakwin, 1960; Green & Money, 1961).

Clinicians appear still to be insensitive to opposite-sex-linked behaviors in boys. Of one hundred 5- to 12-year-old boys referred for outpatient psychiatric evaluation, 30% to 50% were reported to score within the clinical range on two scales assessing cross-gender behavior (Pleak, Meyer-Bahlburg, O'Brien, Bown, & Morganstein, 1989). The authors commented on the clinicians' lack of alertness to the boys' degree of cross-gender behavior, a lack that they considered as possibly attributable to the boys' concomitant psychopathology and masculine behavior. The authors thus implied that inability to accept that sex-linked behaviors were distributed dimensionally impaired the clinicians' judgment; they did not notice the opposite-sex-linked behaviors because the boys also showed same-sex-linked behaviors. This tendency to ignore or attribute little significance to opposite-sex-linked behaviors presumably accounts for their presence in boys and girls when not extreme remaining unnamed scientifically. Lay terms continue to be used, "sissiness" for boys and "tomboyism" for the equivalent, much less studied condition in girls.

The term "gender identity disorder of childhood" is restricted to the presence of extreme opposite-sex-linked behaviors (i.e., in boys dressing in female clothes; using cosmetics, jewelry, and handbags; and showing markedly feminine postures and gait). The lay use of the term sissiness is much broader. Boys who avoid rough-and-tumble play, sport, and fighting and who show interest in behaviors considered feminine (e g , house work, sewing, cooking, or artistic activities) are likely to be labeled as sissies. Sex researchers did not appear to consider that such behaviors could be dimensionally distributed and hence on a continuum with the extreme effeminate behaviors they studied. The few who did rejected the idea. Zuger and Taylor (1969) compared the incidence of feminine behaviors in 95 schoolboys and 26 patients who showed the marked effeminacy usually studied; overlap in the frequency of the behaviors occurred with six schoolboys and one patient. Zuger and Taylor decided that the patient may have been incorrectly diagnosed, enabling them to conclude that the behavior of the patients was clearly differentiated from that of the school boys. Though their results indicated that one-quarter of the school boys showed some feminine behaviors, they did not attribute any significance to this. They thus retained the accepted belief that opposite-sex-linked behaviors of interest to sex researchers were extreme and categorical, being present in only one or two boys in a thousand, rather than varying in intensity and dimensionally distributed in 20% or more of the population. My attempts to challenge this belief have been ineffective. It was maintained without discussion in the recent monograph *The "Sissy Boy Syndrome" and the Development of Homosexuality* (Green, 1987). To add to the confusion, the term "sissy boy syndrome" was used instead of "gender identity disorder of childhood," for the extreme effeminate syndrome. No reference was made to the less extreme and more common opposite-sex-linked behaviors usually referred to as sissiness.

Several studies additional to that of Zuger and Taylor have found that a percentage of normal children show some degree of opposite-sex-linked behaviors. Fagot (1977) reported a "moderate" level of opposite-sex-linked behaviors in 6.6% of 106 preschool boys and 4.9% of 101 preschool girls. Criterion for the moderate level was that preference scores for opposite-sex-linked behaviors were at least one standard deviation above the mean of the opposite sex, and that preference scores for same-sex-linked activities were at least one standard deviation below the mean of their own sex. Kagan and Moss (1962) investigated the opposite-sex-linked behaviors considered sissy or tomboyish, in the lay sense, in 45 girls and 44 boys when they were 0–3, 3–6, 6–10, and 10–14 years of age. Involvement in athletics, in competitive activities, and with mechanical objects was regarded as masculine; involvement in gardening, music, cooking, and noncompetitive activities was considered feminine. Individual boys and girls showed varying degrees of involvement in these activities, the degree remaining constant from the age of 3 to 14. Reduced involvement in same-sex-linked behaviors in boys but not in girls was associated with avoidance of heterosexual erotic behavior in adulthood. The incidence of subjects' homosexual behavior in adulthood was not investigated, and its possible relationship with the opposite-sex-linked behaviors they studied was not discussed by Kagan and Moss.

Retrospective evidence of a relationship between the milder sissy behaviors in the lay sense in boys and their adult sexual activity was provided by a series of studies comparing adult males who identified as homosexual with males who identified as heterosexual. In all studies, the homosexual men reported that as children they were significantly more likely to be fearful of physical injury and to avoid fights and involvement in competitive sports. The subjects included psychiatric patients (Bieber, 1962); prisoners (Holemon & Winokur, 1965); members of a homosexual organization compared with volunteers for a cardiac study (Evans, 1969); and homosexuals from organizations, or who responded to word-of-mouth requests, compared to heterosexual volunteers (Saghir & Robins, 1973). Whitam (1980) reported that nonpatient male homosexuals in the United States, Guatemala, and Brazil reported similar incidences of opposite-sex-linked behaviors in childhood. Saghir and Robins (1973) were among the few workers who studied the relationship in women. They reported that more than two-thirds of lesbians reported tomboyish behavior, as compared with 16% of women who identified as heterosexual.

The consistent evidence from the prospective studies of markedly effeminate boys and the retrospective studies of adult homosexuals suggested the possibility that degree of opposite-sex-linked behaviors in childhood and adolescence and likelihood of identifying as homosexual in adulthood were dimensional and related. The more marked the subject's opposite-sex-linked behaviors, the stronger would be the homosexual feelings he or she would experience. This led to investigation of this relationship in the studies of medical students discussed earlier (McConaghy et al., 1979). It was considered that if the relationship was found, this would support the validity of the students' reports of the ratio of their homosexual/heterosexual feelings.

It would also provide evidence that like such feelings, sex-linked behaviors were also distributed dimensionally rather than categorically. The questionnaire that students were asked to complete contained, in addition to the items on which they reported their sexual orientation assessed dimensionally, items investigating dimensionally their degree of involvement during childhood and adolescence in sex-linked behaviors such as sports, fighting, music, and avoidance of being hurt (McConaghy, 1988b). Items investigating their desire to be of the opposite sex, the intensity of their feelings of identity as members of the same or the opposite sex, and the quality of their relationships with their parents in childhood and at present were also included.

Over 3 years, consistent relationships were found in the male students between the intensity of opposite-sex-linked behaviors in childhood and adolescence and current degree of homosexual as compared to heterosexual feelings (McConaghy, 1987b). The criticism that it may not be appropriate to generalize from the reported behaviors of medical students to the male population in regard to the relationship between sex-linked behaviors and reported ratio of homosexual/heterosexual feeling can be rejected; relationships of similar strength were found in the 411 men on the Australian NHMRC Twin Registry who answered the same questionnaire (McConaghy et al., 1993). Relationships between opposite-sex-linked behaviors and ratio of homosexual to heterosexual feelings were much less consistent in female students, paralleling the findings of Kagan and Moss (1962). Even so, desire to be of the opposite sex, feeling they had effeminate (if male) or butch (if female) traits, feeling that others thought they had behavioral traits of the opposite sex, and degree of opposite-sex identity all correlated with degree of homosexual feelings in both men and women (McConaghy, 1987b).

This pattern of correlations (i.e., that apart from opposite-sex-linked behaviors the other variables tended to correlate with degree of homosexual feeling in both men and women) was found again in a more recent study of medical students (McConaghy & Silove, 1991). The authors pointed out the apparent contradiction between the responses of the women with a homosexual component—that they and others thought they had behavioral traits of the opposite sex, yet they did not report more opposite-sex-linked behaviors than did their exclusively heterosexual peers. It was suggested that the opposite-sex-linked behaviors investigated might be more appropriate for males, and that other behaviors might be more relevant to the study of female sex-linked behavior. Sex-linked behavior has been studied mainly in males. A recent study (McConaghy & Zamir, 1992a), however, found the relationship to be more complex. Women with masculine psychological traits as assessed by the Bem Sex-Role Inventory (Bem, 1974) reported marked levels of the opposite-sex-linked behaviors investigated, but no increase in awareness of homosexual feelings.

This series of studies demonstrated that male subjects' degree of sex-linked behaviors correlated with their degree of homosexual feelings, thus establishing that sex-linked behaviors are dimensionally distributed. It would seem unlikely that the marked effeminate behaviors in the boys studied by clinicians and diagnosed as showing gender identity disorder of childhood are categorically different from the less marked sissy behaviors referred to in the lay use of the term. The marked behaviors would be at the extreme end of the continuum, and so would be shown by subjects who would later develop a high homosexual-to-heterosexual ratio of feelings. Most such subjects would identify as homosexual in adulthood, consistent with the results of the follow-up studies of extremely effeminate boys.

Zuger (1988) continued to regard both effeminate behavior in childhood and homosexuality in adults as categorical conditions, and suggested that effeminate behavior in childhood be regarded as the earliest stage of homosexuality. This suggestion needs to be interpreted in the light of the data that up to 30% of adolescents and young adult men show some degree of opposite-sex-linked behaviors associated with some awareness of homosexual feelings, and that most of them will identify as heterosexual in adulthood and be mainly or exclusively involved in heterosexual activity. Effeminate behavior in childhood is the earliest stage of homosexual feelings, but these feelings are usually not predominant. The significance of these data in relation to the therapy of subjects confused about their sexual orientation will be discussed subsequently. It also has implications for the classification of psychiatric disorders. Sreenivasin (1985) investigated the degree of effeminacy in one hundred 6- to 12-year-old male psychiatric out-patients. She found that 15 boys showed a high degree and 39 a moderate degree of effeminacy. The study lacked a healthy control group, and the author treated effeminacy as pathological, suggesting that all the subjects with high and some of those with moderate scores could be coded as having atypical gender identity disorder.

Management of Gender Identity Disorder of Childhood

DSM-III-R (APA, 1987) emphasized the categorical nature of gender identity disorder of childhood stating that it is not merely a child's nonconformity to stereotypic sex-role behavior (as, for example, in "tomboyishness" in girls or "sissyish" behavior in boys), but rather a profound disturbance of the normal sense of maleness and femaleness. The terms *tomboyishness* and *sissyish* were presumably used in the wider lay sense. It could be argued that it is both "childhoodist" and irrational that the DSM-III-R classifies effeminate behavior in childhood as a gender disorder when its adult expression as homosexuality, with its associated variable degree of opposite-sex-linked behaviors, is accepted as a normal behavioral variant. The reactions of peers (as well as some older subjects) to boys and girls who show marked opposite-sex-linked behaviors can cause them marked distress, however, so that therapy to aid them minimize the behaviors would appear justified.

Bakwin and Bakwin (1953) recommended in the management of effeminate boys that the dominating mother be curbed, the passive father encouraged to be actively involved with the child, and the child encouraged in behavior characteristic of his sex, with clarification of his confusions about sex. Coercion, teasing, and shaming were to be avoided. Green, Newman, and Stoller (1972), using this approach to modify the attitudes of parents, reported reduction of opposite-sex-linked behaviors in 5 effeminate boys. Similar results were obtained without parental involvement by Greenson (1966), who acted as a male role model, teaching an effeminate boy who cross-dressed to swim and reinforcing his masculine behavior and interest in games they played together. Myrick (1970) reported a marked favorable response of an effeminate boy to treatment by two women teachers advised by the school counselor. The boy was tutored in touch football and was sat next to and therefore involved in many activities with the most popular boy in the class, who was also the best athlete. Though prior to treatment the subject played with girls 57% of the time and spent his lunchtime with them, he may not have been extremely effeminate, as Myrick commented that effeminate boys can be found in almost every school and could benefit from additional attention by their teachers and counselors.

Rekers and Lovaas (1974) reported a single-subject study of a 5-year-old effeminate boy who in treatment sessions sat at a table on which were boys' and girls' toys. His mother was instructed by earphones to reinforce masculine play with smiles and complements and to ignore feminine play by reading a book. During reversal sessions, she attended to all his behavior indiscriminately. During baseline assessment prior to treatment, his play was almost exclusively feminine. Masculine play increased when it was differentially reinforced and decreased during initial but not later reversal sessions. Subsequently, the mother was trained to reward masculine behaviors and ignore feminine behaviors at home. It was reported that 2 years later, the boy looked and acted like any other boy.

The authors' conclusion that there was no doubt the treatment was responsible for the change would appear to be true of the immediate change, but possibly not of that in the long term. Bakwin (1960) reported the disappearance in 2 years without specific treatment of opposite-sex preference, cross-dressing, and opposite-sex-linked behaviors in a boy aged 5 years, and in 3 years in a girl aged 11 years. Bakwin may have recommended to the parents that they reward same-sex- and discourage opposite-sex-linked behaviors. This advice was given by Zuger (1966) to the parents of effeminate boys, of whom he commented that with time, the telltale symptoms of effeminacy were suppressed as a confirmed orientation toward homosexuality was taking place. Kosky (1987) reported that cross-dressing and other opposite-sex-linked behaviors that had been shown for several years by 7 boys and 1 girl disappeared within weeks of their admission to a child psychiatric unit, without attempts being made to encourage same-sex behaviors. Money and Russo (1979) followed up 5 effeminate boys into adulthood. They were interviewed annually and on demand with what was termed a minimal form of treatment, in which the interviewer was totally nonjudgmental. Opposite-sex preference disappeared in all subjects and cross-dressing in all but one, who cross-dressed for costume parties. Effeminacy was restricted to subtle bodily movements, minimal in four and a little more obvious to an educated observer in the fifth.

THE ETIOLOGY OF HOMOSEXUALITY/HETEROSEXUALITY

If homosexuality and heterosexuality are distributed dimensionally on a continuum, it would not seem possible to discuss the etiology of homosexuality independently from the etiology of heterosexuality. This was possible while they were regarded as categorical entities, and psychoanalysis adopting this perspective provided the first generally accepted theories of the etiology of homosexuality. These theories regarded homosexuality as attributable to a deviation from the normal pattern of psychosexual development that resulted in heterosexuality. Evidence to support the theories was provided by clinical interpretations of case histories of homosexual subjects seeking treatment, and as such was subject to possible bias by the clinician. Freud concluded that both constitutional and experiential factors contributed to the development of homosexuality (Bieber, 1962). Bieber believed that experiential factors—exposure to highly pathological parent-child relations and early life situations—were alone responsible. He was the first analyst to provide research data to support his theory. He examined the case histories of 106 homosexual men and 100 male controls, all of whom had sought treatment with 77 therapists. He did not, however, attempt to remain unaware which subjects were homosexual and which were not as a method of excluding possible bias.

Bieber concluded that the mothers of homosexuals tended to establish a closely binding, often explicitly seductive relationship with their sons, producing sexual overstimulation and intense guilt and anxiety about heterosexual behavior and thus promoting compulsive homosexual activity. The fathers of homosexuals were detached, hostile, and rejecting, so that they did not act as male models to protect their sons from demasculinization. Bieber reported that in comparison to controls, significantly more homosexuals in childhood were fearful of physical injury, avoided fights, played predominantly with girls, and avoided participation in competitive sports. Bieber attributed this behavior to maternal overprotection. Bene (1965a) pointed out that a number of investigations of male homosexuals found the presence of poor relationships with their father to be more common than undue attachments to their mothers, and she provided further data to support this finding. In a subsequent study (Bene, 1965b), she found that homosexual women reported similar parental relationships. She concluded that the role of the father was more important than that of the mother in the genesis of homosexuality.

The development of learning approaches provided an alternative source of theories of etiology of homosexuality. The earliest of these attributed its development to conditioning. McGuire, Carlisle, and Young (1965) suggested that an initial deviant sexual experience supplied the basis for subsequent fantasies accompanying masturbation. The regular temporal association of the deviant stimulus (in the case of homosexuality, members of the same sex) with sexual arousal would by conditioning cause the subject to become sexually aroused in the future by the deviant stimulus, both in fantasy and reality. Concurrently, his or her arousal by heterosexual stimuli would be extinguished through lack of reinforcement. This theory provided no explanation for the association of predominant homosexual activity in adulthood with opposite-sex-linked behaviors in early childhood. Also, though it could explain the development of exclusive homosexuality, it did not easily account for the presence of a homosexual component in the larger percentage of the population who are predominantly heterosexual. This was also true of the theory advanced by some psychoanalysts, as well as learning theorists, that fear and consequent avoidance of heterosexuality were major determinants of homosexuality (Barlow, 1973).

Stoller and Herdt (1985) recently criticized the conditioning theory of the etiology of homosexuality on the basis of anthropological evidence concerning the psychosexual development of male members of the Sambia, an isolated New Guinea tribe. In this tribe, prepubertal boys fellate postpubertal males as a phase in initiation, being told that they need to ingest semen to become masculine adults. The postpuberal males enjoy being fellated and only experience heterosexual activity when they marry in their late teens or early 20s. "Only a few mature men ever again sample the boys" (p. 401) and most "love their lust for women" (p. 401), a lust Stoller and Herdt noted that the behavioristic theory predicted should not exist.

They gave an account of one aberrant case who in adulthood was indifferent to hunting, not a fighter, and preferred gardening (an activity of women and older men). Prepubertally, he had wished to be born a girl, and though he feared and resisted initiation, he rapidly began to enjoy performing fellatio. Following puberty, he enjoyed being fellated. He failed to consummate his marriage and continued to use boys, harboring taboo wishes to fellate them. Herdt and Stoller attributed his aberrant development to his unusual childhood. His mother was rejected by his father, and he was told his father was dead. His mother became bitter to all men and withdrew from community life, including contact with men. Stoller and Herdt believed that the unavailability of the father as a man worthy of identification prevented adequate resolution of the oedipal situation, so that the subject remained excessively identified with his mother.

Baldwin and Baldwin (1989) reanalyzed the subject's development from a social learning perspective, pointing out the need to include social and cognitive factors in addition to direct conditioning experiences. They considered that the heterosexual development of most Sambia boys could be attributed to their thinking about attaining the high status of manhood while fellating postpubertal males, thus interfering with the conditioning of homosexual arousal. Also, as the boys were initially coerced into fellatio, their negative reactions could cause them to fantasize doing something else, again interfering with conditioning. Baldwin and Baldwin pointed out that the aberrant case was socially isolated and in addition experienced aversive socialization: "Humiliation, banishment and bastardization dominated [his] childhood" (p. 26). They suggested that his reported enjoyment of fellating postpubertal boys could be the result of the experience being his first truly rewarding social interaction. This positive response could therefore cause him to experience sexual arousal, which by conditioning would produce his later homosexual feelings.

Both Stoller and Herdt's and Baldwin and Baldwin's accounts are typical of psychoanalytic and social learning explanations of human development. Both plausibly account for the case material with which they deal, but make no attempt to deal with relevant additional data. Neither of the accounts refer to the evidence demonstrating that homosexuality is preceded by opposite-sex-linked behaviors in childhood. Dislike of fighting and interest in women's activities were reported in the aberrant case in his adulthood. It might be expected that evidence of these as well as other sex-linked behaviors would have been sought in his childhood in addition to his reported wish to be a girl. Such behaviors, if present, would have suggested that he was predisposed to experience marked homosexual feelings prior to his initiation. Both approaches also demonstrated no awareness that a theory is not scientifically acceptable merely because it plausibly accounts for certain data. It is necessary that it also provides reasons to reject other equally plausible theories. One is reminded of Freud's statement, quoted in Chapter 1, that although psychoanalysis cannot predict an event, after the event it can explain it with certainty.

Purely environmental theories have some difficulty dealing with the extensive data demonstrating an association between opposite-sex-linked behaviors and male homosexuality, in view of the early age at which such behaviors have been reported to appear. Zuger (1966) opined that the marked effeminate behaviors he studied began in many of the subjects almost as soon as their motor and speech development allowed their manifestation. This early development could not be explained in terms of inadequate resolution of the oedipal situation, as this situation does not develop until after 3 years of age. Social learning accounts would need to postulate that the boys became effeminate by adopting the behavior of the significant role models to whom they were exposed in their first 3 years, presumably their fathers. No relationship has been found, however, between the sex-linked behaviors of children and their parents (Maccoby, 1980).

Also clinicians' impressions concerning the families of effeminate boys have varied widely. Green and Money (1961) considered a lack of forceful paternal dominance, greater maternal concern about their sons' behavioral anomalies, and the relatively fragile build of many of the boys to be important factors producing their effeminacy. Stoller (1970) believed that the preschool effeminate boy's parents found his femininity most endearing and encouraged it. Zuger (1966) suggested that the closeness of effeminate boys with their mothers was secondary to their femininity, rather than responsible for it. As pointed out earlier, Bakwin and Bakwin (1953) found that the families of effeminate boys were not unusual and concluded from this and the early age at which the behaviors appeared that the latter were biologically determined.

Further data concerning sex-linked behaviors that theories of the etiology of homosexuality/heterosexuality need to take into account are those indicating that the behaviors are in part under prenatal hormonal control. This was initially demonstrated in a number of mammalian species by altering the level of sex hormone to which the mammal was exposed while in utero or, in the case of some species, shortly after birth. Females were exposed to increased levels of testosterone in utero by administration of the hormone to the pregnant mother. Males were exposed to reduced effective testosterone by administration to the mothers of antiandrogens (hormones that reduce testosterone activity) or by castration within a few days following birth. In response, the mammals showed not only opposite-sex-linked behaviors but some features of opposite-sex activity (Reinisch, 1974). As these changes were not produced by subsequent equivalent alterations in the mammals' hormone levels in their later life, these data provided convincing evidence that critical periods exist in the development of their central nervous systems during which the ratio of sex hormones to which they are exposed permanently determines aspects of their later sex-linked and sexual behaviors.

One of the most definitive sex-linked behaviors in the primate group of mammals that includes man is the increased initiation of and persistence in rough-and-tumble play shown by male as compared to female juveniles (Hutt, 1972). Whiting and Edwards (1973) concluded from its presence in diverse human cultures throughout the world that it seemed the best candidate for a sex-linked behavior that was biologically determined. Harlow (1965) demonstrated in the rhesus monkey that this sex-linked behavior occurred in the absence of social influences from older primates. It was shown by infant monkeys reared with inanimate (wire model) surrogate mothers and deprived of the company of other monkeys except for brief periods when they could mix with similarly reared peers. Female offspring of pregnant rhesus monkeys injected with male hormone during the appropriate critical period showed as juveniles levels of rough-and-tumble play approaching those of males.

In human subjects, as discussed previously, degree of rough-and-tumble play in childhood has been found to be related to their later ratio of homosexual/ heterosexual feelings. Lack of participation in rough games and contact sport in men consistently, and tomboyish behavior in women less consistently, correlated with increased homosexual feelings or behaviors. Evidence has been advanced (Ehrhardt & Baker, 1974; Ehrhardt et al., 1968; Ehrhardt & Money, 1967) that tomboyish behavior in girls is in part under hormonal control. Girls exposed prenatally to excess male hormones, either as progestins administered to their mothers or produced by hyperplasia of their own adrenal glands, showed as children significantly more tomboyish behavior than did controls. The evidence that reduced same-sex-linked behaviors is produced in males by exposure in utero to alterations in their hormonal environment is less conclusive (Meyer-Bahlburg, Grisanti, & Ehrhardt, 1977), though a recent study (Sandberg, Meyer-Bahlburg, Rosen, & Johnson, 1990) found that boys exposed to methadone in utero showed increased feminine behaviors, an effect attributed to methadone altering their intrauterine hormonal environment.

The only theory currently advanced that accounts for all the above data is that subjects' ratios of homosexual/heterosexual feelings and associated sex-linked behaviors are determined in utero by the sex hormone ratio operating at critical periods of brain development for these feelings and behaviors. The association of homosexuality with poor parental, and particularly paternal, relationships would be accounted for by parents responding negatively to homosexual subjects' childhood "sissy" and "tomboyish" behaviors. Such negative parental relationships were experienced by subjects who reported these opposite-sex-linked behaviors (McConaghy & Silove, 1992). The negative maternal relationships were accompanied in men but not women by some degree of maternal overprotection, consistent with the findings of Bieber (1962).

Two sets of findings are not immediately compatible with this theory that homosexual/heterosexual feelings and sex-linked behaviors are established by sex hormone levels in utero. Animals and humans showing opposite-sex-linked behaviors produced by prenatal exposure to altered levels of sex hormones also showed alterations of genital morphology toward those of the opposite sex. Ward (1972, 1984), however, reported that stressing pregnant rats resulted in their male offspring when adult showing the feminization of sex-linked and sexual activity similar to that produced by exposure to reduced level of male hormone in utero, but without change in genital morphology. Compared to controls they demonstrated little or no copulatory behavior with females, and if castrated and given estrogen and progesterone in doses sufficient to activate estrous behavior in female rats, they showed an increased lordosis (female) sex response when tested with stud males. If given testosterone daily for 6 weeks, a greater number responded with the lordosis pattern to vigorous stud males. These changes were associated with a lowering of the fetal rats' plasma levels of testosterone on days 18 and 19 of gestation. Ward (1984) cited replicatory studies that found similar behavioral changes in the male offspring of females stressed during pregnancy by social crowding, malnutrition, or conditioned emotional responses. These findings indicate that it is possible for alterations in sex hormone levels to occur in mammals during the critical periods for the development of ratio of sex feelings and sex-linked behaviors, but not during the earlier period when genital morphology is established.

The second set of findings that appear incompatible with this etiological theory of sexual orientation are those of early studies that followed up human subjects exposed prenatally to altered levels of sex hormones (Ehrhard & Baker, 1974; Ehrhardt et al., 1968; Ehrhardt & Money, 1967; Yalom et al., 1973). The female subjects exposed to increased levels of male hormones were reported to show increased opposite-sex-linked behaviors, but no evidence of increased homosexual feelings or behaviors. Of the 62 subjects and 48 controls, only 1 (a control) reported some degree of homosexual feelings. About half the subjects in these studies were prepubertal; the rest were adolescent. In view of the evidence discussed that up to 30% of adolescents experience homosexual feelings, the validity of the non-anonymous reports of the adolescent subjects of these studies that only 1 in more than 50 experienced homosexual feelings must be questioned. It was suggested (McConaghy, 1982) that the adolescents in these studies had denied experiencing homosexual feelings or behaviors, consistent with the experience of myself and others (Schofield, 1968) that adolescents are very unlikely to admit to any socially disapproved sexual feelings or behaviors they have experienced. This suggestion has been confirmed; Money et al. (1984) reported that girls exposed in utero to increased male hormones as a result of hyperplasia of their adrenal glands treated their sexual activity as an unspeakable issue when they were adolescent. When followed up into adulthood they reported an increased incidence of homosexual feelings compared to controls. Money et al. commented that aging of these subjects led to increased sophistication and the ability to talk about their sexual feelings and behavior.

Ehrhardt et al. (1985) asked 76 women prenatally exposed to the synthetic estrogen diethylstilbestrol to consent to investigation. This hormone has a masculinizing effect on brain development. Fifty-four of the women, aged 17 to 30 years, agreed. Bisexual or homosexual responsiveness (Kinsey scales 2 through 6) was reported in the preceding 12 months by 21% and throughout their lives by 24%; equivalent figures for their matched controls were 3% and 0%. Ehrhardt et al. commented that unlike women with adrenal hyperplasia, their subjects did not show an association between increased homosexual feelings and marked childhood tomboyishness. This is consistent with the finding that women show a weaker association than men between opposite-sex-linked childhood behaviors and degree of homosexual feelings in adulthood (McConaghy & Zamir, 1992a).

This finding has interesting implications for the theory that prenatal exposure to opposite-sex hormones results in an increase in both opposite-sex-linked behaviors and homosexual feelings. If the theory is valid, the critical periods in intrauterine brain development for the establishment of sex-linked behaviors and the ratio of homosexual/heterosexual feelings must overlap more completely in males than in females. In women, adrenal hyperplasia would produce exposure to increased androgen throughout both periods. It would be expected, as Ehrhardt et al. (1968) and

Money et al. (1984) found, that these women would show both increased homosexual feelings and tomboyism. Women whose mothers received diethylstilbestrol at varying periods during the pregnancy would be exposed to the hormone over different periods of their intrauterine development. In some this would affect the critical period for only one of the two sets of behaviors, that is, either sex-linked behaviors or sexual feelings. These women would not show an association between tomboyism and increased homosexual feelings, consistent with the finding of Ehrhardt et al. The conclusion of the earlier studies that women exposed in utero to increased levels of masculinizing hormones showed increased opposite-sex-linked behaviors in childhood and adolescence, but no increased incidence of homosexuality, can now be rejected.

If subjects' ratios of homosexual/heterosexual feelings are determined by alterations in the level of sex hormones to which they were exposed during a critical period in their uterine development, what determines the alterations in these levels? Evidence has been advanced that genetic factors play a role. Kallmann (1952) reported 100% concordance for homosexuality in 37 monozygotic (identical) male twins (i.e., if one monozygotic twin identified himself or herself as being homosexual, so did the other). Kallmann found the concordance in 26 dizygotic (nonidentical) male twins to be only 12%—3 of the 26 twins of self-identified homosexuals identified as homosexual. As almost all monozygotic twins have the same genetic structure, this finding suggested that homosexuality was determined entirely genetically.

A number of studies, however, subsequently reported monozygotic twins who were discordant for homosexuality (McConaghy & Blaszczynski, 1980); Kallmann later suggested the high concordance he found may have been an artifact of his method of sampling. Heston and Shields (1968) determined the presence of homosexuality in the male twins on the register of twins admitted to the Maudsley Hospital, London, from 1948 to 1966. Concordance was between 40% and 60% for monozygotic and 14% for dizygotic twins. These figures indicate that genetic factors play a significant but not total role in the etiology of homosexuality. If genetic factors are involved in the etiology of homosexuality, they could operate by influencing the ratio of same- and opposite-sex hormones subjects produced during their intrauterine development.

As about 50% of monozygotic twins in Heston and Shield's study did not both report homosexuality, environmental factors must also be involved. It could be postulated that all monozygotic twins have the same ratio of homosexual/heterosexual feelings, but in some twins differing environmental factors influenced one but not the other to identify as homosexual. This can be ruled out as a total explanation; at least in one pair of monozygotic male twins discordant for homosexuality, their reports that one experienced predominant homosexual and the other predominant heterosexual feelings were confirmed by their penile volume responses to pictures of nude men and women (McConaghy & Blaszczynski, 1980). In reporting this finding, these authors reviewed the studies of other male twins discordant for homosexuality. In all cases, the twin who identified as homosexual was reported to show increased opposite-sex-linked behaviors—in particular, reduced rough-and-tumble play in childhood—compared to the twin who identified as heterosexual. This suggests that the homosexual twin was exposed to a higher level of female hormones in his uterine development than was the heterosexual twin. Monozygotic twins share the same placenta; in 15% to 30% of cases, this results in a transfusion syndrome that impairs their blood circulation. As a consequence, monozygotic twins have about twice the number of congenital malformations and three times the fetal death rate of dizygotic twins or single births (Campion & Tucker, 1973). Homosexuality in one monozygotic twin could therefore be attributable to the transfusion syndrome or other factors differentially stressing that twin, thus altering its (but not its co-twin's) sex hormone levels at the appropriate critical period.

Independent evidence that genetic factors can in part determine homosexual interest was provided by a study of 16 subjects with the chromosomal abnormality XXY who were identified among 4,139 men tested (Schiavi, Theilgaard, et al., 1988). Compared with matched normal chromosomal XY male controls, the XXY subjects reported significantly less pleasure in gymnastics and less interest in boys' games and were judged as significantly less masculine by an interviewer blind to their chromosomal condition. Significantly more reported having engaged in homosexual activities. The authors commented that no significant familial or early environmental differences were identified between the subjects and controls.

Further evidence consistent with a role for biological determinants of male subjects' ratio of homosexual/heterosexual feelings is the inability of treatment to alter homosexuals' penile volume responses to pictures of nude men and women. It was argued from conditioning theory that if a subject regularly experienced sexual arousal in association with heterosexual stimuli, his or her heterosexual arousability would be increased (Marquis, 1970). This concept, however, has not been supported. Subjects with a homosexual component who were married and had experienced regular and satisfying heterosexual intercourse with their wives showed no evidence of increased heterosexual arousability, as measured by penile volume plethysmography, compared with those with no experience of heterosexual intercourse (McConaghy, 1978). As discussed in more detail in Chapter 8, following various forms of aversive therapy claimed to modify subjects' sexual orientation, 135 male patients showed no meaningful change in their homosexual/heterosexual ratio of feelings as measured by penile volume plethysmography (McConaghy, 1976). No evidence has been advanced by other workers that any form of treatment has altered subjects' homosexual/heterosexual ratio of feelings as measured by a valid physiological assessment.

SURVIVAL VALUE OF HOMOSEXUALITY/HETEROSEXUALITY: MASCULINITY, FEMININITY, AND ANDROGYNY

When genes determine a condition that appears to impair the likelihood of its bearer having children, explanations are commonly sought as to why the genes do not die out. One suggestion is that partial expression of the genes in the subject's relatives may enhance their survival and hence the likelihood of their transmitting the genes. The classic example in humans is sickle-cell anemia. Few individuals with the complete expression of the condition survive to reproduce. Its partial expression, however, is maintained at a relatively high frequency in some African populations and among African Americans. This high frequency appears because of the subjects with the partial expression being more resistant than subjects without it to a form of malaria prevalent in certain parts of Africa (Plomin, De Fries, & McClearn, 1980). It was suggested that the genes for schizophrenia may persist because in less extreme form they are expressed as allusive thinking, a form of cognitive thinking that enhances certain types of creativity (McConaghy, 1960, 1961; Tucker, Rothwell, Armstrong, & McConaghy, 1982). This could either increase the individual's ability to procreate or the likelihood of survival of the individual's community and hence of the individual and his or her children. The association of homosexual feelings with opposite-sex-linked behaviors may explain their persistence as in part genetically determined.

Controversy exists concerning the range of sex-linked behaviors. Maccoby and Jacklin (1974) tended to limit differences between men and women to the presence of higher levels of overt aggressiveness and visual-spatial and mathematical ability in men and of verbal ability in women. Hutt (1972) argued for much broader differences, adopting an evolutionary perspective to relate man's hunting activities to his developing a sense of direction, agility, strength, aggression, and ability to enjoy male company and to function in a hierarchical team in cooperative activity. Women, remaining within their home territory to rear the young, developed nurturant skills and interest in social interactions. Hutt quoted evidence than women had greater aesthetic, social, and religious interests; men, political and theoretical interests. Her generalizations included that boys are object oriented and have better-differentiated concepts with respect to impersonal matters; girls, being person oriented, differentiate more subtly along social and emotional dimensions.

Possibly the truth lies somewhere between these views of Hutt and Maccoby and Jacklin, and a number of important behaviors in addition to interest in sports, fighting, and music may be both sex-linked and related to subjects' homosexual/heterosexual ratio of feelings. If so, a variable degree of bisexual feelings in a significant percentage of the population would result in a degree of flexibility of sex roles, rather than all men being stereotypically masculine and all women feminine. This flexibility could be desirable in the complex human societies which with their ability to greatly increase food production by cultivation and improve public health, have resulted in the enormous increase in human population. Compared to the earlier hunter–gatherer societies such societies require men and women to adopt a wide variety of roles both occupationally and socially and to interact with varying degrees of intimacy. A prospective study (Mussen, 1971) provided data consistent with this speculation. Boys aged 17 to 18 years who had more masculine interests and more instrumental than emotional-expressive characteristics showed at that age evidence of better social adjustment and a relaxed, happier attitude than did those with the opposite characteristics. In their early 30s, the more feminine group showed greater leadership ability, social initiative, and sense of personal worth. Different social qualities would appear to be required in different circumstances.

If Hutt is correct, evolutionary pressures resulted in important behaviors being linked to the biological mechanism that determines sexual orientation. As a result, societies in whose members these linkages occurred would be more likely to have flourished and moved on from the simpler hunter-gatherer economy to one requiring more complex abilities from both its male and female members. At this stage of societal development, it could have been advantageous that not all the members were sterotypically male and female in their sex-linked characteristics. If so, evolutionary pressures would favor those societies that contained members with different degrees of sex-linked characteristics. As these characteristics were linked to sexual orientation, this would result in societies in which the members showed differing degrees of heterosexual and homosexual feelings. If this concept is correct, the dimensional distribution of homosexual/heterosexual feelings has resulted as a by-product of the need in complex human communities for men and women with different degrees of the same- and opposite-sex-linked behaviors.

Masculinity-Femininity

The concept that a combination of male and female attributes could be advantageous to the possessor has been advanced in an independent area of research, initiated by attempts to assess "masculinity-femininity" (M-F) from a trait psychology perspective. Terman and Miles (1936) developed a scale to measure M-F, which they considered to be a central personality trait. In an impressive critical review of M-F research, Constantinople (1973) pointed out the lack of a satisfactory theoretical definition. Items, mainly psychological characteristics, were taken as indicators of M-F if in that particular culture at that particular time they differentiated men from women; no attempt was made to assess the centrality of the item to an abstract definition of M-F.

The sex-linked behaviors Ehrhardt and her colleagues had shown in the studies reviewed earlier to be under the control of prenatal sex hormones would seem prime candidates for enduring culture-free items that differentiate men from women. It appears surprising that Constantinople ignored these studies, particularly as she said it was assumed that M-F was in part biologically determined. M-F and subsequently sex-role studies, however, have continued to ignore this research investigating relationships between sex-linked behaviors, biological factors, and homosexual/heterosexual feelings. Another criticism made by Constantinople was the lack of a reliable empirical approach to the measurement of M-F. When various measures of M-F were used to assess the same population, agreement between the measures was not high.

In the 1970s, in the context of feminist theory, the concept of M-F was largely replaced by that of sex roles. Heilbrun and Thompson (1977) stated that sex roles were behaviors that were culturally prescribed as appropriate for males and females and were transmitted and maintained by reinforcement. Heilbrun and Thompson regarded subjects' sexual orientation as part of their sex role; thus, by definition, sex-role theory rejected the possibility that biological factors influenced sex roles or sexual orientation. This resulted in only social factors being considered worthy of study.

The consequent failure to acknowledge research that did not adopt the perspective of sex-role theory presumably explains the otherwise astonishing statement of Heilbrun and Thompson that few researchers have chosen to examine the relationship between sex-role deviation and homosexuality. Pleck (1981), another sex-role theorist, repeated the statement. The numerous prospective and retrospective studies reviewed earlier that demonstrated a relationship between homosexuality and opposite-sex-linked behaviors did not use sex-role questionnaires but relied on descriptions of actual behaviors. It would appear that sex-role theorists considered that subjects' assessments of the degree to which they showed various M-F psychological characteristics provided the only valid measure of their sex roles. The theorists were thus able to conclude that "masculinity and femininity are culturally defined attributes. . . . They have no demonstrable correlation with sexual orientation" (Katchadourian, Lunde, & Trotter, 1979).

Constantinople (1979) much less critically reviewed theories of sex-role acquisition. She no longer required demonstration of the centrality of the items assessing sex role, or agreement between various measures used on the same population. Initially sex roles like M-F were treated as dichotomous; subsequently, considerable attention was given the "iconoclastic idea . . . that masculinity and femininity are not opposite poles but . . . two separate, orthogonal, and equally important aspects of human personality; [and] that individuals . . . can be androgynous, [that is,] both masculine and feminine" (p. 704) (Lenney, 1979). A number of androgyny scales were developed and used to demonstrate that androgynous compared to nonandrogynous subjects were more psychologically healthy or otherwise advantaged. These data have been the source of considerable controversy, with Lenney (1979 warning against their resulting in the value statement that androgyny is the ideal of mental health being "carved in granite" (p. 706).

Researchers who agreed that M and F were independent personality dimensions disagreed concerning how these dimensions combined to determine androgyny. Holmbeck (1989) pointed out that Spence considered individuals androgynous if they scored above the median on both M and F, and that though Bem later endorsed this approach, she originally maintained that those individuals were androgynous who obtained equivalent scores on M and F whether the scores were low or high. Lubinski, Tellegen, and Butcher (1981) argued that androgyny should be assessed as a distinct and intrinsically interactive variable, rather than as merely the sum of its masculine and feminine comonents. Depending on the approach used, the same data could indicate the androgynous person was advantaged or disadvantaged on some positively valued dependent variable. Holmbeck (1989) also criticized the faulty use and interpretation of statistical analyses in androgyny research.

Taylor and Hall (1982) and Whitley (1983) pointed out that the proposed relation between androgyny and psychological well-being was called into question by findings suggesting that the relation was primarily attributable to the masculinity component of androgyny, and that the influence of the femininity component on measures of well-being was negligible. Whitley supported this conclusion by meta-analysis of studies investigating the relationship of androgyny and self-esteem. If androgyny and self-esteem are related through the high masculinity component of androgeny, the validity of the relationship can be further questioned, as the scales for both masculinity and self-esteem share similar items (Nicholls, Licht, & Pearl, 1982). Whitley pointed out, as did Lenney, that the different scales employed to measure androgyny lacked reliability. Examined by median split, the proportion of subjects classified differently on the different scales was very high (Lenney, 1979). One of the best-known scales, the Bem Sex-Role Inventory (Bem, 1974) asked subjects to indicate how well each of 60 masculine, feminine, and neutral personality traits described them. The traits were those previously judged by undergraduates to be more desirable in American society for one sex than for the other. Whitley pointed out that sex-role scales assessing only desirable traits could also be measuring self-esteem. When Spence, Helmreich, and Holahan (1979) added scales of negative masculinity and femininity to their sex-role instrument, they found that in both men and women, self-esteem was positively related to desirable but unrelated to undesirable masculine characteristics and negatively related to undesirable feminine characteristics.

In a society in which sexually stereotyped behavior is under attack, individuals who assess themselves as androgynous might be saying more about their social skills and adaptability than their masculinity or femininity. In conformity with this view, Spence (1985) suggested the androgyny scales were not measuring masculinity or femininity but personality characteristics. Bem (1981), operating within the ideological constraint that sex roles were established by schemata (i.e., sociologically determined beliefs and values about M and F), subsequently decided that the concept of androgyny was insufficiently radical from a feminist perspective. It was to be replaced by the feminist prescription, not that the individual be androgynous, but that society be aschematic. The feminist ideology of which she was the spokesperson had ruled that masculinity and femininity were no longer to exist. To advance such views, it is necessary to believe that sexual behavior is virtually entirely determined by the political conflict between men and women.

Bem was not alone in ignoring the evidence that other factors than politics are involved. Pleck (1981), operating within the same ideology, argued that masculinity is a myth, ignoring the data accumulated since the early study of Kagan and Moss (1962) that the sex-linked behaviors of male children are major determinants of their adult heterosexual behaviors and the lack of evidence that these behaviors are influenced by the power struggle between men and women. More recently, McConaghy and Zamir (1992a) carried out the first study to examine the relationship between subjects' sex-linked behaviors and their M and F scores as measured by the Bem Sex-Role Inventory. Women's opposite-sex-linked behaviors, or tomboyishness, showed significant relationships with their M scores, but only weak relationships with their sexual orientation. As discussed earlier, there is significant evidence that sex-linked behaviors are determined at least in part by the balance of sex hormones to which the individual was exposed during his or her intrauterine development. This balance of sex hormones may therefore also contribute to women's M scores. Whether or not this proves to be the case, the existence of these relationships between sex-linked behaviors and M sex roles in women and sexual orientation in men would seem to establish that, when appropriately assessed, masculinity is no myth.

Maccoby (1987) more recently has emphasized the need to discriminate the various meanings of M-F, pointing out that at least three are in current usage. One is based on the degree to which subjects show behaviors empirically demonstrated to be shown more often by members of one as compared to the other sex (i.e., sex-linked behaviors). The second is based on the degree to which subjects show behaviors socially expected or required to be shown by members of one as compared to the other sex (i.e., sex-role behaviors). The third is based on the degree to which subjects show behaviors the are sexually attractive to the opposite sex (e.g., wearing sexually appealing clothes, being flirtatious, and in boys, being good at sports). Maccoby pointed out that the three meanings were not isomorphic. Rough-and-tumble play is masculine, according to meanings one and two. The increased spatial ability demonstrated to characterize males, however, is masculine only according to meaning one. In all cultures, nurturance is consistently found to be associated with femininity in its first and second meanings. Teenage girls, at the time they become most actively interested in behaving in ways that are sexually attractive to males (i.e., feminine according to the third meaning), show a drop in their responsiveness to babies.

HOMOSEXUAL BEHAVIOR AND IDENTITY

The etiology of homosexuality was discussed in relation to the ratio of subjects' homosexual and heterosexual feelings. Much less information is available concerning the factors that determine the degree to which subjects express these feelings in behaviors at different periods of their lives, and the degree to which they identify to themselves and others as bisexual or homosexual. The factors must include the intensity of the subjects' sexual feelings, the nature of their chance encounters with significant individuals, and the influence of family, peer, and community attitudes. Bell and Weinberg (1978) reported that of a San Francisco sample of self-identified homosexuals, 14% of the white males but 26% of black females believed they had a substantial or predominant degree of heterosexual feelings. A possible explanation of the difference is that more subjects with a homosexual component who are discriminated against by society on other grounds than their homosexuality identify as homosexual, either feeling they have less to lose or as a form of protest. If community prejudice against homosexual behavior lessens, it could be expected that more subjects with a significant degree of homosexual feelings would express these in behaviors; it was suggested this was occurring in the United States in relation to lesbian behavior (Van Gelder, 1982). The subsequent awareness of the association between homosexual behavior in men and increased risk of infection with human immunodeficiency virus (HIV) would be expected to have the opposite effect.

Adolescent Homosexuality: "Coming Out"

As evidence discussed earlier revealed, 20% to 30% of adolescents are aware of a degree of homosexual feeling, and a similar percentage of boys but fewer girls have expressed them in behaviors. There is little information concerning the degree to which they are anxious or guilty about these feelings and experiences. The small number involved in homosexual activity who were available for investigation were found to show significant problems. Roesler and Deisher (1972) investigated 60 such adolescent males aged 16 to 22, most of whom were introduced through acquaintances. Sixty percent had at least one experience to orgasm with a female, and 22% had extensive heterosexual experience. The authors considered that these males were in various stages of development of a homosexual identity and that "coming out" was significant in this development.

Coming out is the term used in the homosexual subculture to designate the event or time of introduction of a person to that culture as a potential member. To the question, "Have you come out yet?" 44 of the 60 answered yes, 8 said no, and 8 didn't recognize the term sufficiently. Of those who had come out more than a year previously, 27% thought there was a good or fair chance eventually they would "go straight" (become heterosexual), as did 44% of those who had come out in the last year and 61% of those who had not come out. In terms of self-identification, of those who had come out for more than a year, 26 considered themselves homosexual, 6 considered themselves bisexual, and 2 were undecided. Of those who had come out less than a year, the equivalent figures were 6, 4, and 0; respectively; and of those who hadn't come out, 5, 9, and 1, and 1 considered himself heterosexual; Coming out could therefore not be equated with adopting a homosexual identity. Of the 60, 29 had consulted a psychiatrist at least once, most with problems related to their sexuality; 19 had made what they considered a significant attempt on their lives, half on several occasions. Roesler and Deisher's study demonstrates the difficulty in determining an adolescent population that can be defined as homosexual, and also that some adolescents who do not identify as homosexual are sufficiently distressed by homosexual feelings or experiences to seek psychiatric help.

Rates of professional consultations and suicide attempts similar to those found by Roesler and Deisher were also reported in a more recent study of 29 males aged 15 to 19 who were involved in homosexual activity, recruited through gay media and a health department clinic (Remafedi, 1987a,b). Thirteen had a history of sexually transmitted diseases, and 17 met DSM-III criteria for substance abuse. Half had been arrested or appeared in juvenile courts at least once, mainly for substance abuse, truancy, prostitution, or running away for home. At most, 6 of their mothers and 3 of their fathers responded or were expected to respond supportively to disclosure of their homosexuality. Eight were victims of gay bashings, 2 of sexual assaults, and 16 of regular abuse from classmates. Six wished to be heterosexual. Ten reported a steady male partner at the time of interview, the relationships being less than a year's duration, except in one case. The partners' mean age was 25 years, and the mean number of male partners in 1 year was 7. Fifteen of the adolescents had heterosexual experience during the previous year, with a mean of six partners. Five admitted accepting money for sex at least once. Remafedi believed it was unlikely the sample was biased by selection toward dysfunctional adolescents, as they were recruited from a wide variety of sources. It would seem likely that the majority of adolescents involved in some homosexual activity would not be prepared to be interviewed about this activity, however, and may well show less pathology.

Homosexual experience in adolescence makes the adoption of a homosexual identity more likely, particularly in males. In the study by Saghir and Robins (1973), 82% of self-identified homosexual adult men reported experiencing homosexual activity by age 15, compared with 23% of heterosexual men. Only 53% of homosexual women had such experience by age 19. Nevertheless, as Remafedi (1985) commented, to date no investigator has identified variables that can accurately predict a young person's ultimate behavioral sexual orientation. A percentage of the extremely effeminate boys in the studies discussed earlier identified as heterosexual in adulthood.

ADJUSTMENT OF HOMOSEXUALS

The most significant recent change in attitudes toward homosexuality was the rejection of the earlier belief held by most psychiatrists and psychologists that it was a form of mental disorder. Hooker (1957) quoted a statement of the Group for the Advancement of Psychiatry that "when . . . homosexual behavior persists in an adult, it is then a symptom of a severe emotional disorder." In a major British textbook, *Psychological Medicine* (Curran, Partridge, & Storey, 1980), homosexuality was classified among the disorders of personality and intelligence. These attitudes could be considered liberal, given the long history of the moral belief that homosexuality was unnatural, the legal belief that it was criminal, and the poorly substantiated but commonly cited historical belief that it was prevalent among societies in decay. The decision of the American Psychiatric Association in April of 1974 that homosexuality would no longer be listed as a mental disorder in its classification was virtually revolutionary. Apart from the ideological and political factors that determined the decision, studies demonstrating that homosexuality was not invariably associated with other evidence of personality or social maladjustment must have been of significance.

Hooker (1957) published data that, as she pointed out, questioned the then-current psychiatric view that homosexuality was a mental disorder. She believed the view was based on experience with homosexuals seeking help or found in mental hospitals or prisons. She investigated 30 relatively exclusive male homosexuals who were members or friends of the Mattachine Society. They were matched for age, education, and IQ with 30 exclusively heterosexual men from community organizations. All completed Rorschach projective tests, along with other measures; two judges expert in Rorschach analysis could not differentiate the protocols of the two groups. Hooker's reliance on projective tests might now be questioned. She concluded cautiously that homosexuality may represent a severe form of maladjustment to society in the sexual sector of behavior, but this need not mean that the homosexual is severely maladjusted in other sectors of his or her behavior.

Subsequently, a number of studies compared groups of nonpatient homosexuals with heterosexuals matched on various variables, using clinical impression or a variety of tests to assess the subjects' adjustment. Results of the studies of female homosexuals conflicted, with some finding their adjustment superior, some no different, and some inferior to that of heterosexual women. In their review, Hart et al. (1978) commented concerning these conflicting findings that the homosexual subjects were usually employed women living independent of their parents, whereas the heterosexual controls were often either married women who were financially and socially dependent on their husbands or college students who were dependent on their parents. They considered that the findings favoring homosexual women could be attributable in part to the failure to control for financial and social independence. In contrast to the findings with women, the adjustment of homosexual men enrolled in such studies was more consistently found to be inferior to that of the heterosexual controls. The homosexual group commonly reported higher levels of tension, depression, and suicidal behavior; obtained higher neuroticism scores; and were more likely to seek psychiatric treatment (Bell & Weinberg, 1978; Saghir & Robins, 1973).

The greater maladjustment of male homosexuals could result from the greater social proscription of male as compared to female homosexuality. Differing life-styles could also contribute. In the studies by Schaefer (1977) and Bell and Weinberg (1978), unlike female homosexuals, half or more of the males had most of their sexual contacts with partners they saw only once. This could have contributed to the finding of the latter study that homosexual as compared to heterosexual men reported greater loneliness; homosexual and heterosexual women reported no difference in loneliness. The transient sexual experiences of these self-identified male homosexuals differed markedly from the stereotypic idealized heterosexual love relationship with which they are socially confronted. It makes understandable Saghir and Robins's finding (1973) that they experienced shame and guilt commonly and for much longer periods of their lives than did female homosexuals. The search for transient contacts in public lavatories or by cruising beats in parks or secluded streets also renders homosexual men liable to gay bashings. The frequency and severity of such bashings have rarely been investigated, presumably because of the reluctance of most victims to report them. Deaths established as the result of gay bashings made up 5% of all murders in the state of New South Wales, Australia, in 1990 (Goddard, 1991).

Bell and Weinberg (1978) commented of their survey findings that they would have been forced to conclude that homosexual adults tended to be less well adjusted psychologically than heterosexuals but for the fact that two subgroups of homosexuals (the "close-coupled" and the "functionals") were virtually as well adjusted as the heterosexual controls. These two subgroups made up only about a third of the total group of homosexuals studied. Both subgroups had been selected from the total group because of their low number of sexual problems and, in the case of the "functionals," because they scored low on regret over their homosexuality. Loney (1972) had previously commented that the use of special normalizing criteria for selecting homosexual subjects would seem to cripple arguments about their essential normality. She recommended against adopting a theory requiring either that homosexuals were superpathological or supernormal.

The criteria for selection of homosexual subjects in the studies discussed varied markedly. Hooker (1957) excluded those with a history of either considerable emotional disturbance or heterosexual experience. Saghir and Robins (1973) excluded those who had been hospitalized for psychiatric reasons or who were nonwhite, but not those who had heterosexual experience. Fifty-nine percent of the male and 49% of the female homosexuals they studied gave a history of a heterosexual romantic attachment; 60% and 70%, respectively, of sexual arousal in heterosexual physical contact; 48% and 79% of heterosexual intercourse (10% and 9% currently): and 53% and 44% of a sustained heterosexual relationship. Bell and Weinberg (1978) selected their homosexual subjects from a larger group of volunteers recruited from gay bars, baths, organizations, and personal contacts in San Francisco to form groups representative of recruitment source, age, educational level, sex, and race. Heterosexual intercourse had been experienced by 64% of the white and 73% of the black male homosexuals, and 83% of the white and 88% of the black female homosexuals. The percentages of these groups who reported heterosexual intercourse in the previous year were 14%, 22%, 24%, and 33%, respectively; those who reported predominant or substantial heterosexual feelings were 14%, 24%, 22%, and 26%, respectively. As the heterosexual controls were drawn from different sources in these studies, it is likely that they differed from the homosexual subjects on a number of variables apart from homosexuality.

In a recent study (Atkinson, Grant, Kennedy, Richman, Spector, & McCutchan, 1988), the 56 homosexuals investigated were subjects who had joined a study of health outcome. It is possible that they considered themselves at risk of HIV infection because of their life-style, and so were not representative of all identified homosexuals. Forty-five of the 56 were seropositive for HIV. They were matched for age and demographic features with healthy heterosexual controls from a service organization. The homosexual subjects were found to have higher lifetime rates of alcohol or nonopiate drug abuse, generalized anxiety disorder, and major depression that often preceded medical illness or knowledge of their HIV infection. In discussing their findings, the authors indicated that the two groups might not be comparable. Nevertheless, they concluded that the data suggested a higher prevalence of anxiety and major depression in homosexual as compared to sociodemographically matched heterosexual men. This conclusion was reported in the article's summary without any qualification concerning the high likelihood that the control group was supernormal (to use Loney's term) in relation to the homosexual group.

Stall and Wiley (1988) suggested that the increased rates of alcohol and drug use often reported in homosexual men (Saunders & Valente, 1987) could be attributable to reliance on what they termed "convenience" samples that overrepresented bar patrons. Stall and Wiley investigated a random household sample of homosexual and heterosexual men in San Francisco. They found few differences in drinking patterns or the prevalence of weekly drug use, but did report a finding of major interest, if replicated—that older homosexuals, unlike heterosexuals, were more likely to persist with the heavier intake of alcohol both groups showed when younger.

In attempting to determine whether there is an association between homosexuality and psychiatric disorder, it is necessary to take into account the fact that some subjects, because they are homosexual, are subjected to pressure from relatives to seek psychiatric consultation. A history of such consultation is commonly used as an index of psychiatric disorder. Another index of psychiatric disorder is subjects' scores on neuroticism scales; commonly, though, the same items are scored as neurotic on neuroticism scales, and as feminine on femininity scales. This results in masculine women scoring as somewhat less neurotic, and feminine men as somewhat more so.

As long as it remains impossible to obtain representative samples of all self-identified homosexuals in the community and appropriately matched control groups, definitive research cannot be carried out to establish whether self-identification as homosexual has a specific association with personality disorder or emotional maladjustment. It would seem unlikely that the prejudice against homosexuality would not produce some negative features in the adjustment of many homosexuals. The fact that a significant percentage in the studies discussed showed no evidence of negative features, however, has doubtless contributed to the increasing acceptance of the view that homosexuality is not necessarily associated with significant personality or social maladjustment.

A variability similar to that which characterizes findings on maladjustment of homosexuals is found in investigations of homosexuals' dissatisfaction with their sexual orientation. Loney (1972) reported that of self-identified homosexuals drawn from friendship networks, almost half the men but only 10% of the women were not satisfied with their homosexuality. About a third of both men and women would have liked to be heterosexual if that could be accomplished without much effort, but many seemed to prefer themselves as they were. In Bell and Weinberg's San Francisco study (1978), if a magic heterosexuality pill were available, about 25% of men and 15% of women would have accepted it when they were born, and 14% of men and 5% of women would have done so at their current age. About 25% of men and 27% of women reported that they would be upset to some or a marked extent if a child of theirs were to become homosexual. Homosexuals who are not maintaining a lifestyle that makes them available for interview may report a different degree of dissatisfaction; knowledge of their life-styles, is of course, limited by their lack of availability.

RELATIONSHIPS OF HOMOSEXUALS

The most consistent finding of studies comparing sexual life-styles of heterosexuals and the homosexuals available for research is that homosexual men have sexual relationships with a much greater number of partners, and the relationships of male and female homosexuals with one partner are significantly briefer than those of heterosexuals. In Loney's study (1972), the homosexual men had an average of 194 male and 1.3 female partners, the women an average of 3.7 female and 5.3 male partners. In Saghir and Robins's study (1973), more than three-quarters of the homosexual men had more than 30 male partners; none of the heterosexual controls reported as high a number of female partners. The difference in number of partners of the preferred sex was much less between homosexual and heterosexual women. Sexual relationships lasting more than 6 years were uncommon in both male and female homosexuals; however, this would appear to be true also of heterosexual couples who are in relationships of cohabitation rather than marriage. Blumstein and Schwartz (1983) reported in their study of American couples that although they found many cohabitation relationships that lasted 5 to 8 years, fewer than 2% lasted 10 years. Approximately the same percentage of cohabiting heterosexual, gay male, and lesbian couples in relationships of 2 years or less duration had broken up at follow-up 18 months later.

Blumstein and Schwartz found a major difference between heterosexual and homosexual cohabiting couples in the frequency of their sexual activity. In the first 2 years, this was three times a week or more in 67% of gay male couples and 61% of heterosexual cohabitators, but only 33% of lesbian couples. In the third to tenth years, the equivalent figures were 32%, 38%, and 7%, respectively. The reduction in frequency of sexual relationships in the gay male couples was balanced by an increase in sex with other men, which was found in many cases not to damage the relationship. The low frequency of sexual relations in lesbian couples was not balanced by sex outside the relationship. Blumstein and Schwartz found, however, that lesbians valued nongenital contacts—cuddling, touching, and hugging—probably more than other couples, considering them as ends in themselves rather than as foreplay to genital sex. Blumstein and Schwartz stated that it was almost unheard of for a woman to have sex with someone whose name she didn't know or whose face she hadn't seen. In both Bell and Weinberg's study (1978) and Schaefer's study (1977) from West Germany, at least half of the male homosexuals had most of their sexual contacts with partners they saw only once. This could explain the significant amount of time devoted to "cruising"—seeking a sexual partner in public places—by most male homosexuals in such studies. A number of the men who "cruised" were concurrently involved in a longer-term relationship. Bell and Weinberg reported that a third of the male homosexuals in their study were involved both with a male partner and in a high level of cruising behavior. Saghir and Robins (1973) commented that "infidelity" was characteristic of the majority of homosexual males who reported prolonged homosexual relationships.

OLDER HOMOSEXUALS

One group of subjects about whom little is known is that of older homosexuals. Harry (1983) pointed out that all the major studies of homosexual men seriously underrepresented this group if it was assumed that the age distribution of adult homosexual men approximated that of the general male population. He attempted to overcome this bias by adding a sample from a gay organization for men over 40, but was only able to obtain 62 subjects with a mean age of 50.3 years, the mean age of the other 1,494 (obtained through a major Chicago gay newspaper) was 29.7 years. Of readers of *Consumer Reports* aged 50 or more who answered a questionnaire, 56 (2.3%) of the 2,402 men and 9 (0.5%) of the 1,844 women considered themselves homosexual; 86 (3.6%) of the men and 25 (1.4%) of the women had one or more homosexual experiences, and 5% of both sexes had been sexually attracted to a person of their own sex since the age of 50 (Brecher, 1984). As with adolescents and younger adults, the majority of these older subjects who were recently aware of homosexual feelings did not regard themselves as homosexual. Brecher considered the number of avowed homosexuals too small to permit statistical analysis, and so their adjustment compared that of the remainder was not reported.

Little data are available to investigate the common belief that "the gay man in particular dreads growing old, wrinkled and sexually unattractive. The potential rupture in social ties associated with aging is especially frightening. The gay man or lesbian often lacks the stable permanent couple or family relationship that most people turn to as they grow older" (Saunders & Valente, 1987, p. 10). If this view is correct, it would be expected that older homosexuals would be overrepresented among the elderly depressed. This does not seem to have been noted by psychiatrists, and it has not been my experience.

Contrary to Saunders and Valente's statement, I have found many that older homosexuals report a wide network of supportive homosexual friends. This was also reported of a group of 14 homosexual men aged from 55 to 81 years (Kimmel, 1979-1980); only 3 reported they did not have a number of long-term friends. Kimmel pointed out the lack of attention to aging homosexual men and women in gerontological research. He concluded of his subjects that their homosexuality did not appear to have had a negative effect on their adjustment to aging or satisfaction with life, and that though they could not be considered representative of all aging homosexual men, they did demonstrate that growing old as a homosexual man does not necessarily lead to despair, loneliness, or the other negative stereotypes attached to this group.

HOMOSEXUAL PARENTS

In addition to aging and adolescent homosexuals, another group considered to have particular problems are separated homosexual parents. It is reported that courts have consistently been concerned that negative effects would result from placing children with a homosexual parent (Kleber, Howell, & Tibbits-Kleber, 1986). The concern was thought to stem particularly from psychoanalytic and social learning/modeling theories of the etiology of homosexuality, despite findings that children reared by homosexual parents showed no evidence of aberrant sexual identity, social development, or sexual object choice compared to children reared by single heterosexual parents (Golombok, Spencer, & Rutter, 1983). Lesbian mothers felt more oppressed than single heterosexual mothers in relation to not only child custody but housing and employment; they used a variety of "passing" techniques to avoid revealing their homosexuality. It has been reported that homosexual men as compared to women have found it more difficult to acknowledge their homosexuality to their children, but in most cases, the children's responses were minimal or understanding (Bozett, 1989). Homosexual fathers also reported more difficulties in adjusting to the gay world, as the male gay world's youth orientation made establishing relationships after age 35 difficult. If achieved, the relationships were likely to be transient compared to lesbian relationships. The fathers felt constrained in terms of finance, time commitment, and living arrangements in contrast to homosexuals without children, who were considered to view children as a stigma, so that few were willing to couple with a homosexual father.

TREATMENT IN HOMOSEXUALITY

Parent-Child Problems

Parents who have learned that their adolescent child has had homosexual relations often persuade the child to attend a therapist in the hope that he or she can be reoriented to heterosexuality. In this situation, I first attempt to discover the adolescents' motivation for attending. If they have already identified themselves as homosexual and wish to maintain this identity, I believe my first responsibility is to support their decision. If they are uncertain about their identity, I attempt to aid them come to terms with this uncertainty, on the basis that there is no need for them to decide at this (or indeed, at any) stage in their development to commit themselves to being either heterosexual or homosexual.

I then provide them with the information I consider appropriate, from that reported in more detail subsequently, in relation to the counseling of men seeking to alter their sexual orientation from homosexual to heterosexual. This includes that a significant percentage of adolescents, most of whom are predominantly heterosexual, are aware of some homosexual feelings; that some adults in whom these feelings are strong adopt a heterosexual life-style; that, as Remafedi (1985) commented, to date no investigator has identified variables that can accurately predict a young person's ultimate sexual preference; that there is no treatment that will alter the ratio of a subject's homosexual to heterosexual feelings; and that there are treatments that can enable them to become sexually aroused in situations where their anxiety may have prevented this, as well as to control compulsive sexual urges and fantasies if these are distressing. That is to say, I encourage them to accept that though their balance of homosexual and heterosexual feelings cannot be altered, they still have considerable flexibility as to how they express these feelings in sexual behaviors.

I find the same information of value in aiding their parents. In providing it, it is necessary to be empathic to their reasons for being distressed at the possibility of their child adopting a homosexual identity. They are understandable; a quarter of the homosexual men and women in Bell and Weinberg's San Francisco study (1978) reported they would be upset if a child of theirs were to become homosexual. At the time of presentation, the level of family discord may be high, particularly if the adolescent insists that the parents accept as final the decision that he or she homosexual. For the well-being both of the parents and the adolescent, every effort needs to be made to keep the family together. It has been suggested that expulsion of homosexual children from their homes results in some becoming prostitutes (Strommen, 1989).

In my experience, parents can usually be encouraged to accept the situation if they are persuaded that though their child is presenting the decision as final, it may not be. It is important that this information is given to the parents in such a way that they will not use it to harass the adolescent into seeking treatment to modify his or her orientation. At the same time, there can be a role for behavioral treatment to help adolescents who for religious or other reasons cannot come to terms with aspects of their homosexuality that they experience as compulsive. This is more likely to be those who have a significant or predominant heterosexual component, and whose awareness of their homosexual component may become minimal with increasing age (McConaghy, 1987a).

More attention is being paid to the need for supportive counseling of overt adolescent male homosexuals with obviously effeminate behavior, who are commonly treated negatively at school by both staff and other students (Price, 1982; Tartagni, 1978). Eighty percent of teenagers in Sorensen's study (1973) considered two boys having sex together to be abnormal or unnatural, a marginally higher percentage than thought this of parent-child incest (78%) and of two girls having sex together (76%). Seventy-eight percent of boys and 72% of girls considered two men having sex together to be disgusting—a question not asked concerning incest or female homosexuality. Martin (1982) pointed out the difficulties that adolescents aware of a significant homosexual component encounter in their socialization because of a lack of appropriate role models and of acceptable situations in which to learn homosexual courting behavior. These difficulties appear significantly greater for males. Little disapproval, or indeed a positive attitude, is frequently shown toward tomboyism in teenage girls, presumably because it is associated with a much lower incidence of homosexual activity and possibly with greater success in life in view of its relationship with high sex-role masculinity.

Requests for Sexual Reorientation

The evidence discussed indicating that male as compared to female homosexuals are less well adjusted and more discontented with their sexual orientation is consistent with the fact that subjects who seek treatment to alter homosexual feelings or behaviors are almost always male. Some wish to control homosexual activity that has become compulsive, such as seeking contacts on "beats" or in lavatories, because of the associated increased risk of HIV infection or because they are in a heterosexual (or, less commonly, a homosexual) relationship. The alternative behavior completion or medroxyprogesterone therapy for other compulsive behaviors (discussed in Chapter 8) is usually effective in enabling these subjects to cease unacceptable sexual behaviors while not altering their enjoyment of acceptable behaviors, whether heterosexual or homosexual. For those whose heterosexual partner is aware of the subjects' homosexual interest or behavior, joint counseling may be indicated (Wolf, 1988).

In addition to men who wish to control compulsive homosexual behaviors, some seek to lose their homosexual feelings and become exclusively heterosexual. It is first necessary to establish that they are in their customary state of mental health and are not suffering a psychiatric disorder (e.g., depression following the breakup of a relationship. In this case, any decision about treatment in relation to their sexual orientation should be postponed until they have returned to their normal emotional state. If no such disorders are present, their reasons for seeking to lose their homosexual feelings or behaviors should be discussed. The most common reasons for concerns about the social unacceptability of homosexuality, guilt as a result of religious beliefs, inability to accept a homosexual life-style, and/or desire for a heterosexual life-style, including marriage and fathering children.

With these subjects, I attempt to determine the ratio of their homosexual/heterosexual feelings. Though (as discussed in Chapter 1) this can be done with a high degree of accuracy by use of penile volume plethysmography, it is rarely necessary. This ratio can be estimated in most subjects by asking them the degree to which they are aware of sexual attraction to males as compared to females they see casually (e.g., while walking in the street) and to the male versus the female nude body. Occasionally subjects say that they are interested in the male nude body not because they are sexually attracted to it, but because they have concerns about their own physique and wish to compare it with those of other men. In my experience, both from use of penile plethysmography and follow-up of these subjects, it almost invariably becomes apparent that this interest is an expression of homosexual feelings they are unable to accept. Details of the subjects' sexual fantasies accompanying masturbation and their sexual experiences with men and women provide additional relevant information in making this decision concerning the ratio of their heterosexual and homosexual feelings.

I then discuss the conclusion I have reached from my experience and research in treating problems associated with subjects' sexual orientation: that I do not believe it is possible to change subjects' basic ratio of homosexual/heterosexual interest, as expressed physiologically in men by their penile volume reactions to male and female nude bodies. (The evidence on which this conclusion is based is discussed in the Chapter 8.) I then point out that a significant proportion of the population have some homosexual feelings, though most, particularly after adolescence, identify themselves as exclusively heterosexual. Subjects who experience predominantly heterosexual feelings but are concerned by homosexual feelings or behaviors (though they do not experience these as compulsive) may find this information, given in the context of a few counseling sessions, sufficient to resolve their concerns.

In subjects with a significant homosexual component who have had no (or at best unsatisfactory) heterosexual relationships, I attempt to clarify why they are not satisfied to express their homosexuality. If they wish to establish or already enjoy homosexual relations but are unwilling to adopt the life-style associated with identifying as homosexual, they may be encouraged to do so by counseling based on what has been termed the affirmative model of homosexuality (Gonsiorek, 1982). Heterosexually identified therapists might find it difficult to take a positive view of such aspects of the male homosexual life-style as cruising for brief casual sexual relationships in bars, baths, and public lavatories; those who feel this is the case could suggest referral to an identified homosexual therapist. Alternatively, if the subject's rejection of homosexuality is associated with reduced self-esteem and lack of social skills, cognitive-behavioral therapy of these conditions can be considered.

Subjects with significant homosexual feelings who for religious or other reasons are totally unwilling to accept a homosexual adjustment continue to present for treatment seeking help to live as heterosexual. Though this is obviously more possible and probably more satisfactory when the subjects' heterosexual feelings are predominant, a number of men with predominantly homosexual feelings appear to maintain satisfactory heterosexual relationships. Most subjects seeking to change their sexual orientation who have not had heterosexual experience are unaware of the findings of the studies revealing that the majority of self-identified homosexuals have experienced heterosexual emotional attachments and intercourse. I discuss these, pointing out the likelihood that men with predominantly homosexual feelings will not experience the same degree of sexual excitement in response to the psychic stimuli associated with heterosexual as compared to homosexual activity (i.e., to fantasies or to the sight of a nude female as compare to a nude male). Some report, however, that they enjoy both the love relationship and the physical experiences of heterosexuality more. Indeed, some state they have never been in love with a man, although most or all of their sexual partners have been male.

With subjects seeking to become heterosexual who are aware of only minimal or no heterosexual interest, where appropriate I discuss the treatments based on conditioning that are claimed to increase subjects' inherent ability to be aroused by heterosexual stimuli (Chapter 8). I state my belief that such ability, like their homosexual arousability, is established prior to birth and subsequently is not modifiable by psychological techniques. I next point out that if this is correct, it is only possible to increase their awareness of their innate heterosexual arousability by reducing any anxiety they may have concerning its expression, as well as any competing preoccupations with homosexual or other fantasies or behaviors that they experience as compulsive. Reduction of such preoccupations can be achieved by alternative behavior completion therapy (Chapter 8). After this treatment, the subjects are likely to still feel the same initial physical attraction to men they encounter causally as they did in the past; but where previously they remained preoccupied with fantasies concerning these men, they will now be able easily to dismiss them. The treatment will also enable them to stop sexual behaviors, such as cruising, if before treatment they were unable to control them. Though other workers use aversive therapy (in particular, covert sensitization) to produce this reduction in homosexual compulsions, it has been shown to be less effective than alternative behavior completion (previously termed *imaginal desensitization;* McConaghy, Armstrong, & Blaszczynski, 1981).

Reduction of anxiety concerning the expression of heterosexual feelings is achieved by the treatment used to treat the same condition in heterosexual men (discussed in Chapter 5). I have found referral to a female surrogate therapist the most effective treatment for reducing men's anxiety concerning heterosexual physical relationships. It also gives them the opportunity to explore their ability to become aroused heterosexually. Surrogate therapy is also effective for men who report reluctance to form heterosexual friendship relationships either from lack of social skills or because they are anxious that their female partner will immediately expect them to be active sexually. They commonly fear they will be impotent, and that this will reveal they are homosexual. When surrogate therapy is suggested to homosexual men, some refer to negative experiences they have had with female prostitutes. It is necessary to emphasize that the surrogate will initially establish a warm, supportive relationship with them in which physical intimacy will be introduced in a gradual and non-threatening manner, similar to the procedure employed in the treatment of men with psychological impotence.

Other workers use social and dating skills or assertiveness training to increase the heterosexual ability of homosexual men. I have rarely found this to produce significant changes in their behavior, though many report improvement in their feelings. This is consistent with the findings of S. James (1978). She treated male homosexuals with social skills training, sex education and training in dating behavior, and interpretation of women's nonverbal communication in addition to electric-shock aversive therapy. Subjects' response to treatment was not as good in terms of the reduction of homosexual outlets they sought or of ability to develop heterosexual relationships compared with the response of subjects treated with the aversive procedure alone in an earlier study (S. James, Orwin, & Turner, 1977). Of the 20 patients in James's study who received the additional training, 2 at most had experienced successful heterosexual intercourse at 2-year follow-up.

The rare women who seeks treatment to reorient sexually to heterosexuality usually reports anxiety or aversion concerning such activity. In my experience, they are reluctant to accept male surrogate therapy, but fortunately, like heterosexual women with aversion to sexual activity and unlike men (Chapter 5), if they do not have a partner of the opposite sex they respond to systematic desensitization in imagination to situations of increasing heterosexual intimacy. I usually point out to both men and women seeking to improve their heterosexual relations that their initial sexual attraction to potential heterosexual partners may not be strong, and that they should aim to find a partner for whom they feel a strong friendship and degree of compatibility rather than rely on feelings of sexual attraction as the main motivation. Men with predominantly homosexual feelings who are in heterosexual relationships not infrequently report they are in love with their partner and are sexually aroused by fantasies of her, though they are not aware of sexual attraction to other women. These love relationships seem usually to have been initiated in the context of a close friendship.

Some therapists (Davison, 1977; Silverstein, 1977) have argued that subjects seeking treatment to reduce awareness of or to control homosexual feelings, or to increase their potential for heterosexual relationships, should be denied this treatment on the grounds that treating them helps to maintain society's attitude that homosexuality is a disease. They also considered that homosexuals seeking these changes were acting under the coercion of societal prejudices and were not in a position to exercise freedom of choice. I argued against these views (McConaghy, 1977a), pointing out that treatments are provided for conditions that are not diseases in order to relieve the patients of difficulties in adjusting to societal demands. Most of the opponents of this treatment for homosexuals, in my experience, approve of termination of pregnancy for the women requesting it. This does not mean that pregnancy is regarded as a disease. Though many women seeking termination have been coerced by societal prejudices and pressures to adopt this solution, it is not suggested that they are unable to exercise freedom of choice. To regard homosexuals who wish to adopt a heterosexual life-style as not capable of an informed choice, and therefore to deny them treatment to help them fulfill their wish, seems a return to the concept that homosexuals are severely maladjusted.

It is disappointing that the proponents of the view that homosexuals should be offered only treatment to maintain a homosexual adjustment have failed to produce evidence of the success of this approach with subjects seeking reorientation to heterosexuality. In my experience, a number of patients with this aim, in the course of receiving treatment to aid their heterosexual adjustment, abandon it and decide to accept their homosexual feelings and behaviors. They usually report appreciation of the therapist's willingness to support their changed decision. I believe such patients benefit from the opportunity to explore the heterosexual option and become more confident and less guilty in accepting their homosexual identification. Had they initially been offered only treatment for the option they finally adopted, many would have refused it, with resultant feelings of rejection and depression. Silverstein (1977) reported this response in a clergyman whom he denied help to reduce his homosexual concerns, and who departed "still in that limbo state of humiliation and low self-esteem."

Apart from this ethical objection, some therapists would disagree with the management I have outlined for different reasons. Hammersmith (1988) stated of adolescents who were confused because they felt both homosexual and heterosexual attractions or were capable of both types of sexual experience that the Kinsey Institute research indicated that homosexuality would be their enduring orientation in adulthood. Using the term *homosexual* in a categorical sense, she was critical of homosexual men and women entering heterosexual marriages, suggesting that such marriages were likely to end in unhappiness and eventual divorce. Writing in the same volume as Hammersmith, however, Kirkpatrick (1988) reported of lesbian and heterosexual women in heterosexual marriages that the marriages of the two groups were no more conflicted and endured for the same length of time. Comparable data do not seem available for males. Wolf (1988), from his experience with group therapy for bisexual men and their wives, adopted a positive view of their relationships. He reported data suggesting that as many as 10% of married men might be dealing with some aspect of homosexual behavior. Sophie (1988) rejected "the dichotomous view we commonly hold of sexual orientation" (p. 58) and pointed out that the client may be neither homosexual nor heterosexual but some combination of both. She recommended that in counseling subjects with concerns about their sexual orientation, the therapist initially leave the question of identity open.

Sexual Dysfunctions

Subjects who seek treatment for sexual dysfunctions in their homosexual relations respond to the treatments discussed in Chapter 5. Masters and Johnson (1979) treated 56 male and 25 female couples, of whom 57 men and 27 women were identified as having sexual dysfunctions. The men all suffered primary or secondary impotence, and 4 also had sexual aversion. The women all were anorgasmic, and 6 also had sexual aversion. Treatment was by counseling and desensitization to situations of increasing sexual intimacy. A further 2 male couples, one of each of whom suffered from premature ejaculation, were treated by brief counseling and explanation of the penile squeeze technique (Chapter 5). All but 4 of the impotent men and 2 of the anorgasmic women responded to treatment. After 5 years, 2 men and 1 woman had relapsed, and 3 men and 1 woman were not available for assessment.

Masters and Johnson believed it was easier to treat impotence and anorgasmia in homosexuals than in heterosexuals, as ability to achieve penetration in anal intercourse was not a requirement of successful treatment of impotence in male homosexuals, and female homosexuals did not need to achieve orgasm by the act of intercourse. It would seem that none of their male patients sought to be successful insertors or insertees in anal intercourse, nor did any complain of failure of ejaculation. This is considerably at variance with my experience with homosexual subjects reporting sexual dysfunctions in Australia. The fact that Silverstein and White (1977) in *The Joy of Gay Sex* discussed techniques for overcoming anxiety in insertees of anal intercourse suggested that the desire for this form of intercourse was not uncommon in U.S. homosexuals also, at least at that time.

In Bell and Weinberg's study (1978) of San Francisco area self-identified homosexuals, anal intercourse was performed once a week or more by 22% of white and 42% of black males, and more than a few times in the past year by 40% of white and 37% of black males. Blumstein and Schwartz (1983) reported of the gay American couples they investigated that 19% engaged in anal sex usually or always, and 50% occasionally.

In my experience subjects seeking treatment for difficulties with being penetrated anally, usually responded to desensitization in sexual situations (with their partner initially employing digital anal dilation). Erectile dysfunction or failure of ejaculation in anal insertors responds to the treatments used for the equivalent conditions in heterosexual intercourse (Chapter 5). Homosexual men with these problems require a cooperative partner; many, however, are not in a relationship that provides this. Of the 485 acknowledged male homosexuals investigated by Bell and Weinberg (1978), 298 were without partners. For such men who have sexual dysfunctions, referral to a male surrogate is often the only treatment likely to be successful. In addition to desensitization to sexual situations, bibliotherapy with such books as *The Joy of Gay Sex* (Silverstein & White, 1977) or the equivalent volume for women, *The Joy of Lesbian Sex* (Sisley & Harris, 1977), appears at times to be of value.

AIDS-RELATED PROBLEMS

A recent major concern of health workers has been to modify the behavior of male homosexuals who are practicing "unsafe sex" (sexual behaviors that put them at increased risk of HIV infection). A variety of educational campaigns have been instituted to educate sexual partners to avoid activities that lead to the transfer of semen, blood, and possibly saliva from one to the other. Receptive anal intercourse was identified as the highest-risk activity, and subjects who continued it were encouraged to ensure that the insertive partner wore a condom. The evidence from the Pittsburgh Multicenter AIDS Cohort Study (Kingsley et al., 1990) that in homosexual relations hepatitis B is transmitted more than eight times more efficiently than HIV and that insertive—not receptive—anal intercourse was the major risk factor identified for hepatitis B transmission might prove useful in media campaigns to encourage the use of condoms by the insertive partner. Education concerning condom use would seem advisable in the light of reports that 4% to 8% of condoms tore or slipped off during anal intercourse (Golombok, Sketchley, & Rust, 1989; van Griensven, de Vroome, Tielman, & Coutinho, 1988).

Reduction in the number of casual sex partners and in the frequency of unprotected anal intercourse have been reported of male homosexuals studied in several countries (Bennett, Chapman, & Bray, 1989). Evidence of the validity of these reports is the marked change in incidence of other sexually transmitted diseases. New problem visits to the public sexually transmitted diseases (STD) clinic in King County, Washington, fell from 4,124 in 1980 to 509 in 1988, but then rose to 937 in 1989 and 527 in the first half of 1990 (Handsfield & Schwebke, 1990). These authors reported also that the combined cases of gonorrhea in homosexually active men treated at the STD clinic and private-sector cases of rectal gonorrhea in men fell from 955 in 1982 to 33 in 1988, then rose to 102 in 1989. Similar changes were noted in the incidence of several other STDs, and the authors found that the trends were reported from other STD clinics. They concluded that there had been a substantial reduction in the frequency of unsafe behavior over most of the 1980s, followed by an increased frequency of unsafe behavior after 1988.

Attribution of the reduction to changes in sexual practices consequent on awareness of the risk of HIV infection was supported by reductions in infection rates of gonorrhea and syphilis in subjects attending a STD clinic in Sydney, New South Wales (Peters, 1989). From 1983 to 1987, these rates changed from 16.6% to 3.4% and 3.2% to 1.8%, respectively, in male homosexuals and from 4.6% to 3.8% and 0.5% to 0.7% in male and female heterosexuals. The major fall was in homosexual subjects, who were considered and presumably considered themselves at much higher risk of developing HIV infection than heterosexuals. Though changes in homosexual behavior appear to have occurred through most of the developed Western world, it has not been established what type of educational program has been effective in producing the changes. It was reported from London that the greatest alteration occurred before the government information campaign began in 1986 (Evans et al., 1989; Johnson & Gill, 1989). These workers also pointed out that half the subjects studied in 1987 were continuing sexual activity with casual partners.

Other studies have also reported that the adopting of safe-sex behaviors by men involved in homosexual activity was far from total. A significant percentage had not changed their behaviors at all, and the majority of the rest only reduced the frequency of (rather than ceasing) unsafe practices even though they were aware of the risk involved (Becker & Joseph, 1988). Becker and Joseph suggested that it is not information but attitudes or other factors that need to be targeted in future interventions. Change has been less common in homosexuals who could be presumed to have less access to information—for example, men living in smaller cities (St. Lawrence, Hood, Brasfield, & Kelly, 1989); bisexual men who make contacts mainly through going to beats and avoid involvement in the homosexual community (Bennett et al., 1989); and men who were younger, of lower socioeconomic class, and from racial minorities (Linn et al., 1989).

The recent reversal in reduction of STDs noted by Handsfield and Schwebke (1990) in the United States was also observed in Amsterdam by van den Hoek, van Griensven, and Coutinho (1990) in relation to number of new cases of gonorrhea, syphilis, and HIV infection in 1989. van den Hoek et al. drew attention to a similar "rebound" effect observed in Seattle. Both groups of workers believed that an increase in high-risk behavior was responsible and that maintenance of sexual safe practices required urgent attention in educational campaigns and sociological research. The management of HIV-infected subjects known to be continuing unsafe sexual behaviors is another area of concern (Carlson, Greeman, & McClellan, 1989).

The need for psychosocial support for AIDS sufferers, their families, and their friends has been identified by health workers as a significant problem; the development of grief recovery groups was one response (Klein & Fletcher, 1986). Many homosexual AIDS patients have not identified to their families as homosexual, and face the possibility of rejection if they do so. Hostile community attitudes both to homosexuals and to HIV-positive subjects have appeared. Some health workers refused to treat HIV-positive subjects, threatened by the danger of infection despite evidence that transmission is only by bodily fluids and that seroconversion even following needle-stick injuries is rare (Ratzan, 1988). In reaction to these negative responses, a federal law has been requested barring discrimination against persons infected with HIV (Blendon & Donelan, 1988). Members of homosexual communities have to cope with the prolonged and debilitating illness, followed by death, of close friends, at times knowing they are themselves at risk and often feeling unable to communicate the fact to heterosexual colleagues that they are grieving.

Twelve of 3,828 New York resident men with AIDS committed suicide, a rate 36 times that of comparably aged male residents (Marzuk et al., 1988). In discussing these findings, Glass (1988) considered that the presence of psychiatric symptoms and absence of physical wasting argued against these suicides being rational decisions by terminally ill patients. Most occurred within 6 months following diagnosis. Glass suggested that the suicides should be considered an untoward outcome and that efforts at suicide prevention were appropriate. Three of the 12 committed suicide by jumping from the window of a medical unit, and 5 had seen a psychiatrist in the preceding 4 days, with 2 having just been released from a psychiatric hospital. These figures suggest that therapy aimed at suicide prevention may not be highly effective. Perry, Jacobsberg, and Fishman (1990), however, found that high-risk subjects given 1-hour sessions of individual counseling by a psychiatric nurse prior to HIV testing and again when notified of the test result showed a decrease in suicidal ideation at 2 months following HIV testing, whether or not they were found to be seropositive. Those randomly allocated to more intensive counseling did not show further benefits on the assessments used; the authors warned their results might not apply to HIV testing in other contexts.

Education of gay men concerning HIV may have led to neglect of the risk of other serious infections. McCusker, Hill, and Mayer (1990) reported inadequate perception of risk of hepatitis B and knowledge of the availability of an effective vaccine among homosexual male clients of a Boston community health center. The awareness of homosexuals who practice active or passive anal intercourse or oral-anal contacts of the consequent increased risk of acquiring enteric diseases such as giardiasis, salmonellosis, and shigellosis (Sohn & Robilotti, 1977) does not appear to have been investigated.

It appears a tragic irony that so soon after it seemed possible that for the first time in history society might treat homosexuality as not immoral, unnatural, or illegal, it became identified with an epidemic that, though minor in the developed world compared to epidemics of the past, has been accepted as their equivalent. Equally ironically, if the public awareness of homosexuality required for its acceptance had not been developed, this identification may not have occurred. The spread of syphilis in Renaissance Europe resulted in it being identified with its postulated country of origin as the English, Spanish, or Italian disease; there appears to be no evidence it was linked with homosexual activity. Yet it would seem likely that such activity played a major role in its transmission, unless men's heterosexual activity then involved the large number of partners that homosexual activity does today (and presumably did then).

CHAPTER 4

Transvestism and Transsexualism
Sex Identity Disorders

DSM-III-R (APA, 1987) uses the term *gender identity* rather than *sex identity* for what it states is the sense of knowing to which sex one belongs. In fact, it is the sense of feeling to which sex one belongs. As Maccoby (1980) pointed out when justifying her decision not to use the term *gender,* a number of workers define gender behaviors as entirely socially determined, so that use of the term prejudges the issue as to whether biological factors also contribute. The alternative name, *sex identity,* implies nothing about etiology. The concept of sex identity was initially advanced in relation to the condition of transsexualism, recognition of which resulted from the development of the surgical procedure for converting male to female genitalia. Prior to its development the existence of cross-dressing, termed *transvestism* by Hirschfeld (Benjamin, 1954), had been noted in many societies dating back to antiquity (Buhrich, 1977b; Gilbert, 1926).

When surgical sex conversion became possible, an increasing number of men and a smaller number of women who cross-dressed requested and, in the case of the men, often demanded the procedure (Worden & Marsh, 1955). Though such subjects remain relatively small in total number, in view of the controversial nature of the operative procedure their condition attracted and continues to attract considerable attention. It became apparent that it differed markedly from that of men who cross-dressed but had no strong desire for sex conversion; the term *transvestites* was restricted to the latter. Though Benjamin (1954) considered the condition of those who requested sex conversion an extreme degree of transvestism, he termed it *transsexualism* "because a transformation of sex is the foremost desire." Benjamin pointed out that the transsexual always seeks medical aid, whereas the transvestite as a rule merely asks to be left alone. Benjamin's belief that there was no sharp separation between the two conditions but that one merged into the other was rejected by many workers who decided that the two conditions were completely separate clinical and psychopathological entities (Barker, 1966). Others agreed that transvestites could develop into transsexuals (Freund, 1974). As the majority of transvestites (unlike transsexuals) do not present for treatment, they have not been readily available for investigation of these beliefs.

143

Transvestism: Transvestic Fetishism and Gender Identity Disorder of Adolescence or Adulthood, Nontranssexual Type

DSM-III-R separated transvestism into two conditions. *Transvestic fetishism* was classified as a paraphilia characterized by recurrent, intense sexual urges and sexually arousing fantasies, of at least 6 months' duration, involving cross-dressing. The person had acted on these urges or was markedly distressed by them. While cross-dressed, he usually masturbated and imagined other males being attracted to him as a woman in his female attire. The DSM-III-R account stated that the condition had been described only in heterosexual males, consistent with most workers' experience. The only recent account of its occurrence in women appears to be that of Stoller (1982), who cited a 1930 report by Gutheil of a 34-year-old unmarried woman for whom the putting on of men's clothes was associated with a tense anticipation of pleasure, which subsided in relief and gratification once the behavior was completed. She identified the pleasure as sexual, stating that putting on a suit could provoke orgasm and that she experienced lustful satisfaction in dreams of cross-dressing. The behavior commenced when she was about the age of 14 years. Stoller reported two further cases: One was an unmarried woman in her 30s who a few years previously had begun to experience sexual feelings and marked excitement when wearing male clothes. The other was a thrice-divorced woman in her 40s, who experienced sexual excitement from the age of 11 years when wearing men's denim jeans. All three women apparently had both heterosexual and homosexual desires.

The DSSM-III-R account of transvestic fetishism continued that in some people the sexual arousal by clothing tended to disappear, although the cross-dressing remained as an antidote to anxiety. In such cases the specified diagnosis was to *gender identity disorder of adolescence or adulthood, nontranssexual type* (GIDAANT). DSM-III-R stated that the essential features of this disorder were persistent or recurrent discomfort and sense of inappropriateness about one's assigned sex and persistent or recurrent cross-dressing in the role of the other sex, either in fantasy or in actuality, in a person who has reached puberty. It differed from transvestic fetishism in that the cross-dressing was not for the purpose of sexual excitement, and from transsexualism in that there was no persistent preoccupation (for at least 2 years) with getting rid of one's primary and secondary sex characteristics and acquiring the sex characteristics of the opposite sex. Only some subjects with GIDAANT once had transvestic fetishism, the rest being homosexuals who cross-dressed and female impersonators, among whom GIDAANT was common. DSM-III-R also stated that GIDAANT was more common in men, implying that it could occur in women. These DSM-III-R accounts of transvestic fetishism and GIDAANT reflect the poor understanding of the natural history of transvestites resulting from the infrequency with which a significant number have been available for investigation.

Prince and Bentler (1972) reported findings from 504 anonymous questionnaires returned from 1,300 sent to subscribers of *Transvestia,* a magazine for heterosexual cross-dressers. The authors commented that the magazine rather explicitly avoided catering to individuals interested in homosexuality, sex conversion, sadomasochism, or pure fetishism. Buhrich and McConaghy (1977a) took the opportunity offered by a transvestite club to investigate its membership, which consisted exclusively of males. The guidelines of the club stated that it was dedicated to the needs of heterosexual transvestites who had become aware of the other side of their personality, and that the areas of homosexuality, bondage, domination, or fetishism were left to others. Subjects who identify as heterosexual transvestites appear to consider themselves distinct from primarily homosexual subjects who cross-dress and from female impersonators. No members belonging to either of these groups were identified among the club membership. Croughan, Saghir, Cohen, and Robins (1981) interviewed 70 male members of two national organizations of cross-dressing clubs or subjects referred by them. Homosexual drag queens and subjects who had received sex conversion operations were excluded. The numbers of these subjects and the criteria used to exclude homosexual drag queens were not reported.

Homosexuals Who Cross-Dress

Little information is available concerning homosexuals who cross-dress. Person and Ovesey (1984) cited White as stating that "drag" (dressing as a girl) was once a major gay pursuit throughout the country. In its place an increasing masculinization of gay life has recently occurred, with a preoccupation with leather, sadomasochism, and the insignia of violence. Person and Ovesey distinguished homosexuals in whom cross-dressing played a central role in their psychological life from those who cross dressed rarely for a lark (e.g., to attend a masquerade party, or to see how it felt). Cross-dressing was considered to be shown almost exclusively by homosexuals at the extremely effeminate end of a gradient of sex-role behavior. It was distinguished from transsexualism and transvestism, which the authors identified as heterosexual fetishistic cross-dressing. Homosexual cross-dressers were considered to have a much less insistent compulsion to cross-dress, so that usually they were able to do so or not at will; they could have periods, however, in which it was compulsive. Some developed transsexual impulses and underwent sex conversion. Person and Ovesey investigated 19 adult and 6 adolescent subjects, presumably all male. Five of the adults were termed homosexual transsexuals.

Two major personality types were distinguished: passive-effeminate homosexuals with hysterical personalities, and hyperaggressive effeminate homosexuals with narcissistic personalities (who were labeled "drag queens"). Some subjects were intermediate, and it was stated that any could move from one type to the other. All as children showed the "sissy" opposite-sex-linked behaviors found to correlate with degree of homosexuality (see Chapter 3). They began to cross-dress then, with fantasies of impersonating females, and showed what the authors termed a "mimetic hunger"—a theatrical flair shared within their families, where it was viewed as charming and precocious. During their adolescence mannerisms emerged, such as archness, facetiousness, sarcastic wit, and bitchiness, which Person and Ovesey commented were associated in the popular mind with "queens," but which permeated a sizable part of the gay community. In adulthood they remained children of fantasy, being movie buffs with a love of theater, music, and dance. Some placed a premium on refinement and sensitivity with an abhorrence of male crudeness and violence; some were preoccupied with royalty; and some were "slut queens," quick to anger, flamboyantly vulgar and aggressive, and intent on shocking their companions. Some reported they readily learned to project a more masculine facade after a traumatic event, an ability Person and Ovesey considered to underline the enormous power of mimicry available to the homosexual cross-dresser. They did not experience cross-dressing as sexually arousing, though one reported sexual arousal to male under-pants. Person and Ovesey commented that the fetishistic cast to the interest among the gay community in leather, buttocks, and uniforms was widely acknowledged.

The findings of Person and Ovesey suggest that homosexuals who cross-dress are toward the exclusively homosexual end of the dimension of sexual orientation and hence would show marked "sissy" behaviors in childhood, with strong wishes to be of the opposite sex. It could be expected that exclusive homosexuals who in addition have marked narcissistic personalities would respond to environmental experiences that reinforce cross-dressing behaviors by showing these behaviors to a much more pronounced extent than other men who identify as homosexual. There is little data investigating the prevalence of cross-dressing in adult homosexuals. Whitam (1977) reported that 44% of exclusive and 37% of nonexclusive homosexual men reported liking as children to dress in women's clothes more than other boys; 20% of nonexclusive and no exclusive heterosexual men reported this. The condition of homosexual cross-dressers appears sufficiently different from that of men who identify as heterosexual transvestites and who experience the urge to cross-dress as compulsive that it seems inappropriate to include both groups in a single category of GIDAANT. Indeed, given that homosexuality is no longer considered a disorder in DSM-III-R, it is not clear why those who cross-dress in the absence of evidence of pathology should be regarded as having a disorder of sex identity. This would also seem true of professionals who cross-dress, about whom there appears no evidence that they suffer significant psychological disturbance.

Self-Identified Heterosexual Transvestites

Members of the club for subjects who self-identified as heterosexual trans-vestites and who invited Buhrich and McConaghy (1977a) to investigate their condition met once a month in one of their homes, conforming to a club rule that they cross-dress in taste. When cross-dressed, they addressed each other by their chosen feminine names, frequently a modification of their first name (e.g., Paula for Paul, and Wendy for Warren). They spoke to each other in their normal masculine voices, though some softened them; otherwise they attempted to appear convincingly as women. They usually wore semiformal clothes (e.g., cocktail gowns with female accessories including necklaces, brooches, and wrist watches), possibly appearing somewhat overdressed. No attempt was made to parody women or to titillate or behave seductively toward others present, male or female. Wives of members, and at times their children, were encouraged to attend.

Thirty-five of 50 club members agreed to investigators' request to be interviewed at length, to complete forms, and to undergo penile volume assessment. The ages of the 35 ranged from 21 to 73 years, with a mean of 39 years. Twenty-six were currently married or cohabiting with a member of the opposite sex. All but one had experienced sexual arousal to female clothes in adolescence, when they would have been diagnosed as transvestic fetishists according to DSM-III-R. Their behavior at that stage would seem identical with that of adolescents with fetishes for female clothes who occasionally are compelled to present for treatment after having been discovered using the clothes of female relatives, or having been charged with stealing female clothes. In my exprience such adolescents initially agree that they used the clothes for sexual arousal with masturbation, at which point they would be diagnosed by DSM-III-R as showing fetishism. In response to further sympathetic questioning, however, almost all reveal that at times they wore the clothes when masturbating and when doing so to some extent felt like a girl. They would then be diagnosed as showing transvestic fetishism. There seems to be no prospective studies following up such adolescents to determine how many become transvestites in adulthood.

Thirty-one of the 34 transvestite club members who reported sexual arousal to cross-dressing stated that its frequency and intensity had diminished with age. Nine reported that they had not experienced it in the preceding 6 months; over that period, 12 had masturbated to fantasies of being partially or fully cross-dressed (Buhrich & McConaghy, 1977b). Club members were asked what the primary sensations were that they experienced while cross-dressed, both in adolescence and currently (Buhrich, 1977a). In adolescence, 50% had experienced feelings of relaxation, and 50% sexual arousal. Currently the majority reported their primary sensations were feeling relaxed, relieved of responsibility, and/or sensual, elegant, and beautiful, only 10% considered sexual arousal primary.

Arousal was not always sought or enjoyed. Comments of subjects included, "When I ejaculate it is an accident and undesirable," "I can manage to 'dress' now and not have an erection," and "I masturbate to get rid of the erection so I can get on with dressing." Blanchard, Clemmensen, and Steiner (1987) commented on the marked tendency of heterosexual male cross-dressers to minimize this feature of their history. Many showed penile volume response evidence of sexual arousal to fantasies of cross-dressing, though they denied awareness of ever having been aroused by the activity. Of 504 heterosexual cross-dressers investigated by questionnaire, only 12% looked upon themselves as men with just a sexual fetish for feminine attire (Prince & Bentler, 1972); 69% felt they were men who had a feminine side seeking expression, and 12% felt themselves to be women trapped in a man's body. In answer to a separate question, 78% considered themselves to be a different personality when cross-dressed, and 20% felt they were just themselves dressed up. The number who had ever experienced sexual arousal to cross-dressing was not reported by Prince and Bentler, who commented that because fetishism was often thought to be a concomitant of transvestism, it was interesting to note that only 12% of the sample looked upon themselves in this way.

No differences were noted by Buhrich and McConaghy (1977b) between subjects who remained aware of fetishistic sexual arousal and those who did not, so that the separate categorizations of the former as transvestic fetishists and the latter as showing GIDAANT seems unjustified. Blanchard and Clemmensen (1988) stated that in view of the number of heterosexual male cross-dressers who continue to experience sexual arousal to the activity, the criterion for GIDAANT should be modified to include this experience. Little support has been reported for the DSM-

III-R statement concerning GIDAANT that when sexual arousal to clothing disappeared, cross-dressing continued as an antidote to anxiety. Of the transvestites studied by Buhrich and McConaghy (1977a), 15 reported an increased and 5 a decreased frequency of cross-dressing when under stress; 14 considered it was unaffected. Croughan et al. (1981) reported that tension or conflict increased the urge to cross-dress of only 15% of their 70 subjects. Less than 6% said desire for sexual arousal or relief was a motive.

The number of dresses subjects owned largely depended on their economic situation and the degree of acceptance of their wives (Buhrich, 1977a). All had at least one full female outfit that included accessories; five owned over 20. They gave much more care to their female than male clothes. Self-grooming behavior appeared a significant factor: Most of the subjects investigated by Buhrich and McConaghy took more than 1 hour (and 10 took 2 hours or more) to apply makeup and cross-dress. All reported that they spent some time examining themselves cross-dressed in a mirror; this was also noted by 4 of 7 female partners of transvestites interviewed by G. Brown and Collier (1989).

In terms of the degree of compulsiveness of the urge to cross-dress, 6 subjects investigated by Buhrich (1977a) reported it was present all the time and 18 that it occurred at least once a day. In some, it was in partly under stimulus control in that it was precipitated by seeing an attractively dressed girl, or women's clothes in a shop window or a magazine. Croughan et al. (1981) reported a similar finding. Buhrich found the compulsiveness of the subjects' urges was also demonstrated by the failure of their attempts to cease cross-dressing because of feelings of guilt or shame. Twenty-one (60%) had discarded all their female clothes on at least one occasion; 13 of the 21 had done so more than once. This usually occurred in adolescence or prior to marriage; almost all began cross-dressing again within a few months. Of the transvestites investigated by Croughan et al. (1981) and Prince and Bentler (1972), 80% and 70%, respectively, reported discarding their female clothes at least once. Prince and Bentler reported that currently 22% of their subjects reported some guilt or shame after cross-dressing, 32% that they were substantially free of guilt, 21% that transvestism had made a valuable contribution to their lives; and 20% some combination of the latter two attitudes. Only 1% wished to stop their cross-dressing; 22% expected to continue as they were, and 72% hoped to expand their activities and develop their feminine self more fully. It would appear that with the passage of time, most transvestites adjust to their behavior and lose their feelings of guilt. This renders questionable the DSM-III-R statement that an essential feature of GIDAANT is a persistent or recurrent discomfort and sense of inappropriateness about one's assigned sex. It would seem that a significant percentage feel appropriate in their male and female roles but wish to experience both. Forty-four of the subjects in Prince and Bentler's study preferred their masculine self to their feminine self.

Nuclear and Marginal Transvestites

Of the 34 club members investigated by Buhrich and McConaghy (1977b) who reported current or previous sexual arousal to cross-dressing, 20 had no desire to alter their bodily appearance by taking female hormones or having surgery, though 9 of the 20 had considered either or both of these procedures in their late adolescence. Six of the remaining 14 were taking female hormones prior to the investigation, and 7 requested them when interviewed. One did not want hormones, as he feared his potency would be impaired, but he as well as 11 of the 14 desired surgical intervention. Eight wanted complete and 4 partial sex conversion (e.g., silicone breast implantation while wishing to retain their penis). At least 3 of those desiring full sex conversion said they would not seek it because of their family responsibilities. Of the 504 heterosexual cross-dressers interviewed by questionnaire (Prince & Bentler, 1972), 5% were taking female hormones, and 50% indicated they would like to; 14% indicated they would have a sex conversion operation if it were financially possible and legal, and 34% indicated they would have had one when they were younger.

A number of significant differences in the clinical features of the transvestites demonstrated that those desiring physical sex conversion had a stronger feminine sex identity and homosexual interest than those not desiring it (Buhrich & McConaghy, 1977b). It was suggested that those desiring sex conversion be classified as *marginal transvestites* (MTVs), and those not desiring it as *nuclear transvestites* (NTVs). Significant differences included that only 1 of 20 NTVs, but 7 of the 14 MTVs, attended the investigatory interview dressed as women. The majority of both groups had commenced partial cross-dressing by age 12, showing no significant difference in this respect; however, 11 (80%) of the MTVs but only half of the NTVs fully cross-dressed by age 15. (Full cross-dressing was defined as wearing underwear, a blouse and skirt or dress, and shoes, but not necessarily a wig, makeup, or accessories.) MTVs fully cross-dressed more frequently than NTVs in the past 2 years, and 12 of the 14 appeared cross-dressed in public, as compared with 9 of the 20 NTVs. When cross-dressed, 9 of the 14 MTVs but only 4 of the 20 NTVs felt like a woman all of the time.

All 34 subjects had experienced heterosexual intercourse, with a nonsignificant tendency for NTVs to experience it earlier and with a greater number of partners. Two (10%) NTVs and 4 (30%) MTVs reported some homosexual experiences. In terms of their Kinsey ratings and penile volume responses to pictures of nude men and women, MTVs showed significantly more homosexual interest than did NTVs. Several subjects in both MTV and NTV groups had fantasies of being escorted by a man when cross-dressed, but not of having sexual contact with him. Typical statements included, "I like being taken out by a man, my chair held out at restaurants, and my cigarette lit, but the thought of sex turns me off," and "I like to imagine I am escorted by a man to a party and that we dance closely, but I would never get into bed with him." There was no difference in the proportion of the two groups who were married or had children. NTVs were of higher socioeconomic status.

To determine the degree to which the 34 transvestites showed the "sissyish" behaviors and poor paternal relationships found more commonly in the childhood of homosexual than heterosexual men (see Chapter 3), they were compared with two control groups: one predominantly heterosexual, made up half of psychiatric and half of orthopedic patients, and the other of subjects seeking treatment for compulsive homosexuality (Buhrich, 1977a; Buhrich & McConaghy, 1978b). The transvestites reported significantly more sissyish behaviors in childhood than the hetero-

sexual group, and significantly fewer than the homosexual group. MTVs reported
more sissyish behaviors than did the NTVs. The transvestite and homosexual groups
reported a similar degree of poor relationships with their fathers.

Freund, Steiner, and Chan (1982) also recognized two groups of transvestites:
those who felt like women only when wearing at least one item of female underwear
and clothing, and those who felt like at women at other times as well. The sexual
identity of the latter group was considered to fluctuate substantially between female
and male, and the authors termed them "borderline transsexuals." These subjects
reported stronger female sexual identity in childhood than did the nuclear transvestite group, which Freund, Steiner, and Chan pointed out confirmed Buhrich and
McConaghy's finding in this respect. This finding of both studies that MTVs had
stronger opposite-sex identity than NTVs from childhood suggests that MTVs but
not NTVs have the potential to develop into transsexuals. MTVs identify as transvestites in early adult life because of their greater heterosexual feelings, compared to
those of subjects who identify at this stage as transsexuals. In middle age, as their
heterosexual interest weakens, their strong opposite-sex identity (present since childhood) influences them to give it full expression.

In the study of Buhrich and McConaghy (1977b), the transvestites who were
termed MTVs because they sought some degree of sex conversion were not older than
NTVs who didn't. This was considered to support the suggestion that transvestites
who develop transsexual wishes differ since childhood from those who do not develop
such wishes. If all transvestites had the potential to develop into transsexuals, it would
be expected that those seeking sex conversion would be older than those not seeking it.
Fagan, Wise, Derogatis, and Schmidt (1988) also found that transvestites who were
unhappy with their biologic sex, compared to those who were not, were more likely to
be bisexual than heterosexual and to have commenced cross-dressing at an earlier age.
There was no difference in the mean current age of the two groups. Fagan et al.
considered their results did not support the concept (J. Meyer, 1974; Stoller, 1971)
that transvestites may become increasingly dissatisfied with their biologic sex.

Partners of Transvestites

G. Brown and Collier interviewed 7 members of a wife-and-girlfriend support
group established by a club for transvestites and transsexuals. All were in a committed exclusive relationship with a transvestite male, 5 being married. Four considered
their partner's transvestism the biggest problem in their relationship. Four of the
partners cross-dressed for sexual activity, but only 1 of the women said she enjoyed
this; 5 did not allow it or tolerated it only because it was necessary for the potency of
her mate. The authors stated that there were overwhelming indicators of low self-
esteem in all of the women. Four showed significant obesity. It was considered that
suffering was an essential ingredient in their relationship.

Brown and Collier considered their findings to be comparable with those of an
earlier study of partners of patient transvestites, in which half of the partners were
patients themselves. Both studies reported mean relationship durations of about 10
years and low incidences of divorce or prior long-term committed relationships.
Brown and Collier pointed out, however, that neither sample may be representative of
the wives of transvestites who do not seek the support of groups. Of the subjects

investigated by Prince and Bentler (1972), 20% reported that their wives were unaware of their cross-dressing; 23% that their wives were completely accepting and
cooperative; 33% that their wives showed a certain amount of permissiveness, with
12% allowing cross-dressing only in the home in her presence and 21% allowing it in
her absence; and 20% that their wives were completely antagonistic. Twenty percent
of the subjects said they liked to be completely cross-dressed during intercourse.

Comparison of Transvestism and Transsexualism in Males

To investigate further the relationship between transvestism and transsexualism
in males, the self-identified members of the transvestite club were compared with 29
nonpsychotic male subjects who consecutively sought sex conversion at a transsexual
clinic (Buhrich & McConaghy, 1977c). As expected, these self-identified transsexual
subjects showed a more intense opposite-sex identity. Twenty-six reported feeling like
a woman all the time, both when cross-dressed and when nude. Thirteen of the 35
transvestite club members felt like a woman all the time when cross-dressed, but only
3 when nude. The transsexual subjects showed a significantly stronger current tendency to cross-dress permanently in public, to fantasize living permanently as wom-
en, to always sit to urinate, to ingest female sex hormones, and to desire a sex change
operation. Most subjects in both groups had commenced cross-dressing before the
age of 9 years, and almost all by the age of 15.

Most transsexuals had never partially cross-dressed, whereas the majority of the
transvestites had done so in adolescence and in the previous 6 months, both these
differences being statistically significant; partial cross-dressing was defined as wearing one or two items of women's clothes. Significantly more transsexuals fully cross-
dressed weekly in adolescence, and 15 had begun to cross-dress permanently by their
early 20s. Currently 18 of the transsexuals were fully cross-dressing permanently, as
compared with 1 of the self-identified transvestites. The latter subject was the only
self-identified transvestite to report no history of sexual arousal to cross-dressing; he
felt like a woman all the time whether cross-dressed or not, and could better be
classified as a transsexual. Twenty-one of the 35 self-identified transvestites and 27 of
the 29 transsexuals had appeared in public dressed as women. The greater role of
grooming behavior in transvestism as compared to transsexualism was indicated by
the fact that 25 of the 35 transvestites took over an hour to cross-dress and apply
makeup, as compared with 10 of the 29 transsexuals. Transsexuals also spent significantly less time examining themselves in the mirror. They were significantly less likely
to be married, to show predominant heterosexual interest, and to have ever experienced sexual arousal to cross-dressing. Transvestite subjects were of higher socioeconomic status. The presence of these significant differences was considered to justify
considering transvestism and transsexualism as separate clinical entities.

Transsexualism

The DSM-III-R diagnostic criteria for transsexualism are persistent discomfort
and sense of inappropriateness about one's assigned sex in a person who has reached

puberty. In addition, there is persistent preoccupation for at least 2 years with getting rid of one's primary and secondary sex characteristics and acquiring the sex characteristics of the other sex. These diagnostic criteria are less restrictive than those advanced by some earlier workers who wished to limit numbers of subjects approved for sex conversion surgery, partly in response to ideological conflict stimulated by the procedure. When it became more readily available in the 1950s, the sudden appearance of a number of men who presented in a distressed state (often threatening self-castration, suicide, or even harm to others if they were not accepted for sex-conversion) polarized clinicians. From the perspective of the proponents of the operation (Benjamin, 1954; Hamburger, Sturup, & Dahl-Iversen, 1953), these subjects were victims of a genetic constitution that resulted in their being women in the bodies of men. Their femininity had been apparent since childhood, and they disliked their male sexual organs. Though attracted to normal men, they were disgusted by homosexual relationships, and their sexual life was largely cerebral and nongenital. Their personalities were essentially those of normal women—though, being unable to live as women, they suffered severe mental stress that could result in secondary neurotic conflict. Clinicians holding this view of transsexuals concluded they could achieve a reasonably contented life only by the operation of sex conversion.

Opponents of the operation regarded transsexuals as suffering from a neurotic condition, largely or entirely psychological in nature. Unlike normal women, they had an emotionally shallow, immature, and distorted concept of what women were like socially, emotionally, sexually, and anatomically. Their histories of their past life were unconsciously reconstructed rather than accurate. The lack of interest in sexual activity they reported was a neurotic aversion; to believe they were women in men's bodies was to accept their formulation. Following sex conversion surgery, they would remain neurotic individuals (Ostow, 1953; Worden & Marsh, 1955).

A major reason preventing resolution of these disparate views was that the clinicians who regarded transsexuals as not primarily neurotic did not diagnosis all subjects seeking sex conversion as transsexual, but only those they regarded as suitable to surgery. As they were aware of the marked opposition of many of their colleagues to the operation, they were understandably under pressure to reject those they thought less likely to show a good response. These were usually subjects with a history of psychiatric treatment, suicidal attempts, or antisocial or criminal activity; those diagnosed as transsexual were therefore the most psychiatrically healthy. One study reported transsexuals to be above average in intelligence and with MMPI scores showing no evidence of major pathology (D. Hunt, Carr, & Hampson, 1981). The finding was based on 22 transsexuals selected from 200 subjects who sought surgery. Lothstein (1980) reported that following establishment of a gender identity clinic, only 14 of over 120 applicants were selected for surgery. Criteria included successful social and work/school adjustment in the adopted gender for at least 1 year, reasonable mental and emotional stability, absence of significant legal problems, and agreement to participate in long-term follow-up studies. Morgan (1978) noted that of the male subjects seeking sex conversion who were unsuited for surgery, 10% had a major mental disorder, and that most of the remainder were sexually ambiguous but had inadequate personalities, or were homophobic bisexuals or homosexuals who could be helped to make a satisfactory adjustment to their sexual orientation.

Additional restrictive diagnostic criteria advanced by Stoller (1971) were that only men who were feminine, not effeminate; who at no stage of their development showed masculine behavior; who were incapable of sexual relations with the opposite sex; and who never showed fetishistic arousal induced by female clothes should be diagnosed as transsexual. Stoller believed such men to invariably prefer masculine "straight" men and to have an almost uncanny ability to detect homosexuals. Their desire for sex conversion had persisted without change from the first few years of their life. Buckman (1974) commented that this restriction of the diagnosis of transsexualism to a very select group of the most severe feminine gender-oriented men represented a marked change of attitude from that previously held by workers in the field. Randell (1971) commented that of 73 transsexuals whom he analyzed in depth, 48% had been married at some time and that it was surprising how many were well-developed males. He suggested that the patient being currently married contraindicated sex conversion surgery, however, as the wife could sue the surgeon for deprivation of conjugal rights. Person and Ovesey (1974) reported of 20 male transsexuals selected for sex conversion that 10 had no significant history of either heterosexuality or homosexuality, and 9 of the 10 showed no evidence of effeminacy in childhood and did not engage in girls' activities or play with girls any more than did normal boys. A further 5 were homosexual transsexuals who were effeminate from early childhood, and 5 were transvestic transsexuals who were masculine in childhood and whose cross-dressing were most often fetishistic.

The tendency of subjects seeking sex conversion to reconstruct their history to maximize their chance of being selected was noted early by Worden and Marsh (1955). Fink commented that as long as the word was out that only classical transsexual histories were welcome, lo and behold, only classical cases appeared (MacKenzie, 1978). Most subjects seeking sex conversion mix in a homosexual culture that accepts their cross-dressing and where they meet other transsexuals, from whom they learn selection criteria. An example of this situation was described in a group of 95 male-to-female transsexuals receiving public assistance in New York, most of whom were black or Puerto Rican (Siegel & Zitrin, 1978). Each had a much larger number of male friends and acquaintances, both black and white who had similar life-styles and aspirations. The 95 were living as women in small cliques in contact with the others throughout the city. Most met in one clinic with a reputation (spread by word of mouth) as a place where they would find a sympathetic and accepting atmosphere—and the possibility of hormonal treatment, group therapy, or referral for surgery—and where everyone seemed to know the inside gossip. Siegel and Zitrin believed there was a spectrum of illusion-sustaining capacities for transsexuals. For many it sufficed to dress in female attire, take a female name, and enact the part. Others were helped by hormonal therapy to sustain the necessary illusion of being a woman. For still others, surgery could be required. For some, even this would not do; repeated surgery and/or suicide often followed.

With the passage of time, more liberal views have developed concerning the need for subjects to meet arbitrary diagnostic criteria of transsexualism to be considered suitable candidates for sex conversion surgery. The major factor determining whether or not they receive it has become the practical test of their ability to live successfully in the role of the opposite sex for a continuous period of time. This was apparent in a discussion in the "Open Forum" (1978) that concluded the Fourth International

Conference on Gender Identity. Fisk commented that "the trial period, be it two years or eighteen months, is phenomenologically sound, and in our experience, it does not matter what the diagnosis really is. . . . In our follow-up there are people who came with a transvestite, or effeminate homosexual, or virile lesbian history, and seem to do as well as those who had a classical transsexual history" (p. 402). While both male and female subjects were undergoing the test of living in the role of the opposite sex, most workers were prepared to prescribe sex hormones for them to aid in altering their appearance toward that of the opposite sex. Some also approved of mastectomy for women whose breast development could not be satisfactorily concealed. Another contributor to the forum discussed the difficulty of attempting to be the patient's total doctor, saying that after 6 years and several hundred patients he felt manipulated and blackmailed. He suggested that where possible, patients should be assessed by a group so that there was no single person who had ultimate responsibility for granting or not granting any kind of treatment.

Subsequently, Standards of Care (1985) were developed and disseminated by the Harry Benjamin International Gender Dysphoria Association that ratified many of the aspects of treatment revealed by the open forum to be commonly practiced. The use of the term *gender dysphoria* for the condition of all subjects who experience discomfort in their biological sex role enabled workers to reserve the term *transsexual* for only some of the diagnostically heterogenous total group of subjects accepted as candidates for sex conversion. The Standards of Care supported a team approach by requiring that the clinical behavioral scientist making the primary recommendation for surgical sex conversion obtain a peer review, in which a colleague would personally examine the applicant on at last one occasion and concur with the decision in writing. Both scientists were to share the moral responsibility with the surgeon who carried out the procedure. In practice, many workers make the decision concerning surgery via a committee that consists of the surgeon as well as behavorial scientists. The Standards of Care further stated that the scientist should have known the patient in a psychotherapeutic relationship for at least 3 months before recommending hormonal sex reassignment and for at least 6 months before recommending surgery. Prior to surgery, the patient should have lived full-time in the social role of the opposite sex for at least 12 months.

Subjects Seeking Sex Conversion

Most clinical studies of subjects seeking sex-conversion diagnosed them all as transsexual, rather than attempting to differentiate transsexual from gender dysphoric subjects. These studies mainly reported all those who sought sex conversion surgery, or those who received it; few investigated those refused the procedure. Most subjects attending clinics seeking sex conversion commenced cross-dressing before puberty; their cross-dressing was usually full rather than partial, and was not accompanied by sexual arousal at puberty; at presentation, up to one-half were cross-dressing permanently; and the majority of the men and almost all women reported sexual attraction to members of their own biological sex (Buhrich & McConaghy, 1977c; Hoenig, Kenna, & Youd, 1970). Two-thirds of women and one-third of men reported relationships of 3 months or longer with members of their biological sex;

one-third of the men reported similar relationships with members of the opposite biological sex (Dixen, Maddever, Van Maasdam, & Edwards, 1984).

Significantly more men than women had married, with one study finding that none of 55 women had done so (Verschoor & Poortinga, 1988). These workers also emphasized the greater stability of the women's same-sex relationships, as Pauly had earlier (1974). Dixen et al. pointed out that when they applied for sex conversion, women were frequently living with a female lover or spouse, whereas men were mainly living alone. Forty percent of their female subjects and 71% of the males had taken hormones, and 1% of the females and 17% of the males had received cosmetic surgery to assist in passing as a member of the opposite sex. In some studies, an occasional woman and up to one-third of the men had engaged in prostitution, both in sex-appropriate clothes and cross-dressed; 24% of the men and 8% of the women had criminal convictions; and 24% of the men and 11% of the women were unemployed (Dixen et al., 1984; Hoenig et al., 1970). Hoenig et al. reported that only 30% of their subjects were free from other psychiatric disorders, and that most were in the lowest socioeconomic class. Eklund, Gooren, and Bezemer (1988) found that almost all female-to-male transsexuals presented before the age of 50, whereas a number of male-to-female transsexuals presented after that age.

J. Meyer, Knorr, and Blumer (1971) reported data obtained by questionnaire from 436 men and 163 women who wrote to their clinic seeking sex conversion. Most were in the lower-middle and lower socioeconomic class. Men were drawn to jobs that were usually considered feminine, which lowered their socioeconomic level. Women were attracted to masculine occupations, but seldom had the education or experience to qualify for positions at higher income and social levels. Twenty-three percent of men and 15% of women had been in trouble with the law, which the authors suggested may have been in part attributable to arrests for impersonation. Forty percent of women but only 12% of men cross-dressed constantly; 30% of men but only 5% of women cross-dressed occasionally. Twenty-four percent of men and 11% of women had taken hormones. Twenty-four percent of men and 32% of women had lived with a member of the same biological sex, and 22% of the men and 11% of the women had been married; few of either sex had done both.

The stability of the relationships of female transsexuals was also noted in those studied following surgery. Kockott and Fahrner (1988) related this to the women, unlike the men, having established the relationships prior to surgery. This was consistent with the findings of Fleming, MacGowan, and Costos (1985) that are discussed subsequently in relation to the life history of female transsexuals. Equivalent information is not available concerning male transsexuals, possibly because they are a less homogenous group and their life-style is insufficiently stable to allow adequate follow-up.

These more recent studies of subjects seeking sex conversion did not report that they showed reduced sexual activity, in contrast to the beliefs of earlier workers (Benjamin, 1954; Hamburger et al., 1953). The earlier workers sought evidence of this reduction in interest from a need to remain confident that subjects receiving sex conversion differed from homosexuals, and from uneasiness that they could be terminating some subjects' heterosexual activity. It is widely accepted that subjects seeking sex conversion modify their history to obtain it. Hence it could be expected that workers who required a history of low sexual interest to approve of sex conversion would be given it by subjects aware of the requirement. An additional factor contributing to the belief of these workers may have been reports of some male subjects taking female sex hormones. These subjects would be likely to experience reduced sexual interest and, if large doses were taken, reduced sexual activity also (see Chapter 2).

It is apparent from these studies that women seeking sex conversion, as compared to men, were more exclusively aware of attraction to members of their biological sex and more likely to establish a relationship based on that attraction; they either cross-dressed permanently or not at all, whereas a percentage of men cross-dressed occasionally; and it was rare for women to present after the age of 50. All these sex differences could result from there being no female equivalent to that form of transsexualism in men associated with a history of fetishistic arousal to cross-dressing.

Male Fetishistic Transsexualism

A number of authors have noted that differences in male subjects seeking sex conversion appear related to three variables—age, sexual orientation, and presence or absence of sexual arousal to cross-dressing in adolescence. J. Meyer (1974) believed that some men seeking sex conversion showed cohesive clinical features sufficient to categorize them as aging transvestites. They sought sex conversion in middle life, invariably gave a history of cross-dressing, and their prior adjustment had been hypermasculine. In Meyer's study of 67 male transvestites there were 10 such subjects, whose mean age was 51 years. They were of relatively high socioeconomic status; 9 had married, and most had children. Homosexual contact had been avoided, but hormone use and attempts to live as women had been common. Meyer suggested that they were not ego-syntonic transvestites, as they did not openly acknowledge and embrace the fetish as a life-style. Bentler (1976) investigated a group of 42 male-to-female transsexuals following sex conversion. Thirteen had been or were married to a woman and reported that they were heterosexual before surgery. Unlike the remainder, they sought surgery in middle age (rather than earlier) and had higher average education, job status, and annual income. They were particularly likely to report sexual arousal with cross-dressing. Rather than follow Meyer in calling these subjects aging transvestites, Bentler termed them "heterosexual transsexuals."

As age and sexual orientation are both dimensional, Buhrich and McConaghy (1978a) investigated the value of classifying male subjects seeking sex conversion in relation to the categorical distinction of the presence or absence of a history of fetishistic arousal. The two groups so formed differed to a statistically significant extent on a number of characteristics, which were considered to justify their separate classification. Those reporting a history of sexual arousal to cross-dressing were termed *fetishistic* and those without this history *classical* transsexuals. Of 29 nonpsychotic subjects who consecutively sought sex conversion, 5 gave a history of fetishistic arousal to cross-dressing. The mean age of the fetishistic group was 40 years, significantly older than the 24 classical transsexuals, whose mean age was 26 years. The fetishistic group were of higher socioeconomic status. Only 4 of the 24 classical transsexuals had experienced heterosexual intercourse and only 2 had married, of whom 1 was separated and 1 divorced. Of the fetishistic group, 4 of the 5 had experienced heterosexual intercourse, and 2 who married were still in the relationship.

Twenty-one of the classical and 3 of the fetishistic transsexuals had experienced homosexual contact to orgasm; 12 of the former, but only 1 of the latter, had this experience at least fortnightly over the previous 6 months. Fetishistic subjects' penile volume responses to pictures of nude men and women were approximately equal; those of the classical transsexuals were significantly greater to the men. In contrast to this evidence of significantly greater age and heterosexual feelings in fetishistic transsexuals, the degree of opposite-sex identity of the two groups of subjects both in adolescence and currently seemed comparable. Four of the fetishistic and 10 of the classical transsexuals fully cross-dressed at least weekly during adolescence, and 3 of the former and 14 of the latter had dressed permanently as women in the preceding 6 months. All but 1 of the fetishistic and 2 of the classical transsexuals felt like a woman all the time.

Freund, Steiner, and Chan (1982) also distinguished transsexuals with and without a fetishistic component, terming them types B and A, respectively. They did not report differences between the two groups other than a categorization as either heterosexual or homosexual. Twenty-two of the 42 fetististic transsexuals they studied were heterosexual, whereas 52 of the 57 nonfetishistic transsexuals were homosexual, the remaining 5 being atypical. Strangely, having classified their transsexual subjects as type B and type A on the basis of the presence or absence of fetishism, they stated that the most useful differentiation of types of cross-gender identity was on the basis of the subjects' heterosexuality versus homosexuality.

In a further study, Buhrich and McConaghy (1979) compared fetishistic transsexuals with 14 marginal transvestites (MTVs) who self-identified as transvestites but expressed a wish for sex conversion. Presumably their wish was not as strong as that of the fetishistic transsexuals, as the latter had acted on their wish by applying to a gender clinic for sex conversion. Also, all the fetishistic transsexuals, but only 6 of the MTVs, were taking hormones, though a further 7 MTVs requested them at interview. Fetishistic transsexuals in comparison to MTVs were significantly more likely to have felt like a woman when nude, to have lived continuously as a woman, and to have experienced sexual interest in men. They showed greater penile volume responses to pictures of nude men than of nude women. The mean age of both groups was about 40 years. Nine of the 14 subjects in the MTV group were married, 2 were widowed, and 1 cohabited with a woman; 2 of the 5 subjects in the fetishistic transsexual group were married.

In opposition to the belief that transvestism could develop into transsexualism (Benjamin, 1966), Buhrich and McConaghy suggested that fetishistic transsexuals— men who experienced sexual arousal to cross-dressing but sought sex conversion usually in middle life—had shown since childhood a stronger female sex identity and homosexual interest as compared to nuclear transvestites, who did not seek sex conversion, and marginal transvestites, who had some wish for it but did not strongly seek it. Presumably factors such as the state of their marriage, the age of their children, and their financial situation would play a role in determining the persistence with which fetishistic transsexuals sought hormones and surgery. Kockott and Fahrner (1987) found that subjects seeking sex conversion who hesitated to accept it when it was offered differed from those who accepted it in being older, more often married, and in a more stable socioeconomic situation. Their current partnerships had existed for significantly longer and were only with subjects of the opposite biological sex.

The classification of transvestites and transsexuals as heterosexual or homosexual used in DSM-III-R accepted a categorical distribution of sexual orientation that prevented recognition of its dimensional relationship with four different groups of cross-gendered men—the groups termed by Buhrich and McConaghy as classical and fetishistic transsexuals and marginal and nuclear transvestites. Classical transsexuals were predominantly homosexual, with no or a minimal heterosexual component. Fetishistic transsexuals and marginal transvestites were bisexual, with the for-

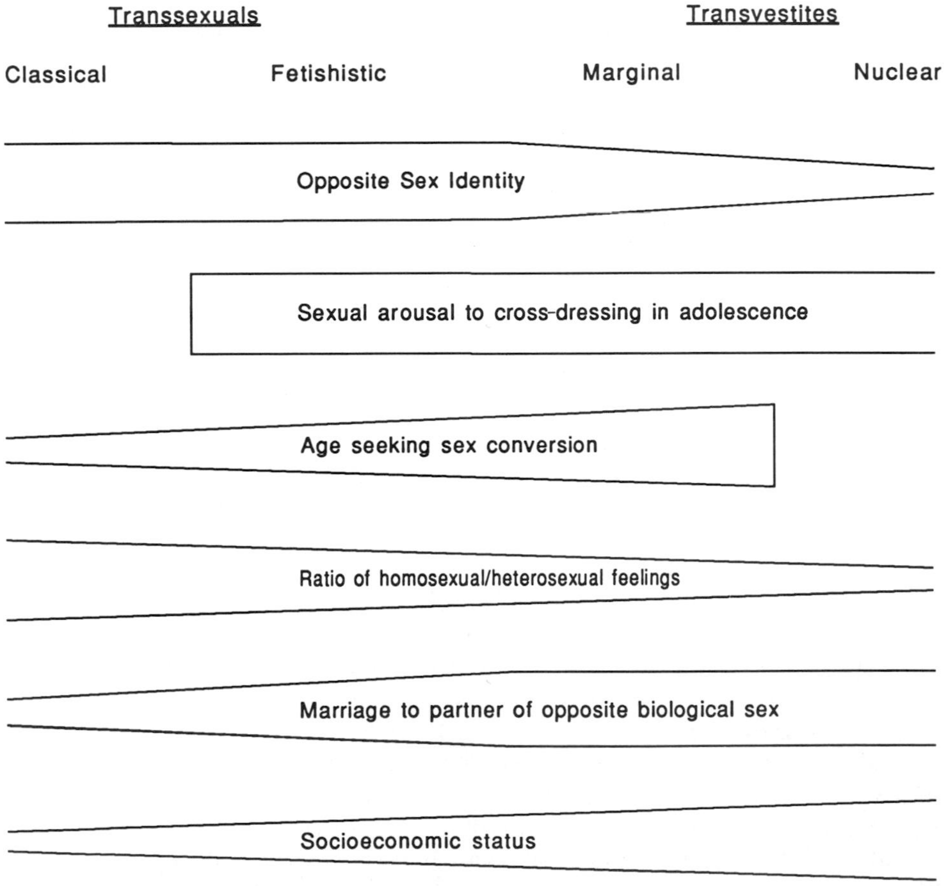

FIG. 4.1. Features of subgroups of men who cross-dress.

mer having a somewhat stronger homosexual component. Classical and fetishistic transsexuals showed equivalent intensity of opposite-sex identity since childhood, the intensity being greater than that of marginal transvestites. Nuclear transvestites were predominantly heterosexual, with only minimal homosexual feelings; they experienced an opposite-sex identity only intermittently and therefore did not desire sex conversion. Differences between subjects in the four groups are summarized in Figure 4.1.

Fetishism in Transsexuals

By separating fetishistic from classical transsexuals, the classification reported maintains an earlier emphasis put on the presence or absence of a history of sexual arousal to cross-dressing in relation to the diagnosis of transsexualism. Such arousal if currently present remains an exclusion criterion in the DSM-III-R classification, though this is not stated in its description of transsexualism but in the discussion of the differential diagnosis of transvestic fetishism. DSM-III-R accepts that transvestic fetishism and transvestism can develop into transsexualism with a wish for sex conversion. Presumably, the belief is that any fetishistic arousal previously present disappears with this development. As discussed above in relation to diagnosis and the Standards of Care recommendations, most workers accept subjects who experience sexual arousal to cross-dressing as suitable for sex conversion, provided they live as members of the opposite sex for an appropriate period. The issue has therefore become largely a semantic one as to whether these subjects should be termed "gender dysphoric" or "transsexual." Blanchard and Clemmensen (1988) considered the existence of subjects who sought sex conversion but also experienced sexual arousal to cross-dressing to require modification of the DSM-III-R criteria for transsexualism to include such arousal.

Ethnic Factors

The possible role of ethnic factors in influencing the syndromes of transsexualism appears worthy of investigation. Tsoi (1990) reported of 200 male transsexuals in Singapore that they could not be differentiated from male homosexuals from their earlier sexual behavior until they started to cross-dress and sought sex conversion. None had ever married or experienced heterosexual intercourse. Tsoi suggested that the availability of sex conversion surgery may have drawn out the Singapore transsexuals earlier and that they had a stronger need for sex conversion, given that homosexuality was not accepted by society there. Tsoi (1988) had earlier reported from Singapore the highest prevalence of transsexualism in the literature; the absence of older bisexual fetishistic transsexuals among his subjects requires explanation. MacFarlane (1984) found that 90% of the transsexual prostitutes she investigated in Wellington, New Zealand, were half- or quarter-caste Maoris, who made up only 9% of the population. Lothstein and Roback (1984) found that black women were grossly underrepresented among applicants for sex conversion to their clinic in Cleveland, Ohio. They considered the few who did apply to be borderline or frankly schizophrenic.

Life History of Female Transsexuals

Pauly (1974) reviewed the literature to that time reporting female transsexuals, commenting that it was much less than that dealing with male subjects. Eighty cases had been described by 39 primary authors. Female transsexuals had a distinct preference for the opposite-sex role from an early age, and 90% had cross-dressed before puberty, 16% consistently and 54% as often as possible. At that stage, many of the girls prided themselves on being the toughest kid in the neighborhood, delighting in outdoing their male competitors. Puberty was traumatic, with the concrete evidence of their femaleness shattering their fantasies of becoming male. They found their developing breasts difficult to conceal, though they attempted to do by using tight binding. They reported a late onset of menarche and described their menstrual periods as scant and irregular.

After puberty they cross-dressed more consistently and obtained employment in positions traditionally held by men, often doing extremely strenuous physical labor. Pauly did not comment concerning the possibility that any female transsexuals experienced sexual arousal to cross-dressing; Blanchard et al. (1987) reported that none of the 72 they studied did. The female transsexuals in the studies reviewed by Pauly had completely adopted a male role by an average age of 19 years, most doing so very convincingly. They developed awareness of sexual attraction to females between the ages of 6 and 22, with a mean of 13.4 years, but homosexual contact was delayed for a further 5 years.

All the cases reported had homosexual experience, though Pauly considered that initial disturbance at awareness of feelings of attraction to women caused some to have a flight into heterosexuality. One-half had experienced intercourse with men, usually only once and without pleasure or satisfaction. Twenty percent married, but invariably divorced. Sixteen percent had children, but did not respond with maternal instincts and a desire to assume the female role and mother children. Homosexuality was ego-alien to them, and though they experimented with a lesbian life-style, they realized it was not for them. Seventy-six percent were involved in ongoing, fairly long-lasting relationships with female partners. Pauly commented that the relationships tended to be more stable than those of female homosexuals. The transsexuals chose sexual partners who were decidedly feminine girls whom they considered to be heterosexual. More than half the transsexuals stimulated the female partner but concealed their own female anatomy, not infrequently deceiving the partners into believing they were males and that their lack of insistence on intercourse was a sign of gentlemanliness; however, 40% allowed the female partner to stimulate their external genitalia.

Though the majority were of lower socioeconomic class, their average IQ was 105. Pauly believed they adopted the opposite-sex role more naturally than did male-to-female transsexuals, who frequently exaggerated it. He also considered them to be better adjusted, freer from paranoid trends, and more realistic in their appraisal of what was possible for them. Though those in the series were frequently given the diagnosis of psychopathic or sociopathic personality disorder, this was usually based on their sexual behavior being considered deviant. Forty-four percent did show acting-out behavior, however, including theft and armed robbery as well as alcoholism. Many reported depression, and 17.5% had attempted suicide, which Pauly considered equivalent to the incidence in male transsexuals. Forty percent had had psychiatric hospitalizations, usually related to depression or suicidal attempts, commonly precipitated by rejection of requests for sex conversion. Pauly stated that suicidal gestures aimed at manipulating physicians into recommending the procedure were less likely in female than male transsexuals.

Fleming et al. (1985) investigated 22 female-to-male transsexuals who had undergone surgery and were living with female spouses for a year or more. The mean length of the relationships was 3.7 years. Seventeen were living as men when they first met their spouses; 8 were in the role of father to one or more children, and 10 planned to include children in their families. All were employed. When the couples were compared to a control group of nontranssexual husbands and their wives matched for age, length of relationship, and education, no differences were found between their scores on the Dyadic Adjustment Scale or their degrees of sexual satisfaction, of sexual problems, and of certainty that they would be together in 10 years. There were also no differences in these variables between the five couples in whom the transsexual had had phalloplasty and the remainder. Eleven of the couples reported that transsexualism was not very or not at all important in their relationships. The remainder reported various problems, including the spouse's family's lack of acceptance, the need to maintain secrecy from families and/or society, and the financial burden of surgery. Spouses of female-to-male transsexuals seem more accepting of their partner's sexual anomalous behavior than do the spouses of transvestites.

PREVALENCE OF TRANSSEXUALISM AND TRANSVESTISM

The observed prevalence of transsexualism has steadily increased since it was first reported. Eklund et al. (1988) cited estimated rates for male-to-female and female-to-male transsexualism of 1 in 100,000 and 400,000, respectively, in the United States in 1968; 1 in 37,000 and 100,000 in Sweden in 1968 and in the United Kingdom in 1974; 1 in 45,000 and 200,000 in the Netherlands in 1980; 1 in 26,000 and 100,000 in the Netherlands in 1983; and 1 in 18,000 and 54,000 in the Netherlands in 1986. Tsoi (1988) reported a prevalence of 1 in 2,900 for male and in 8,300 for female Singapore-born transsexuals. Eklund et al. (1988) reported the recent higher Netherlands estimates and stated that all their subjects had commenced hormone therapy. Eklund et al. pointed out that the ratio of male-to-female as compared to female-to-male transsexuals tended to remain consistent at about 3 to 1.

There was no trend for the age of subjects seeking treatment to be younger in the more recent studies, which Eklund et al. argued would be the case if the true prevalence of transsexualism had risen. They suggested that more transsexuals were seeking sex conversion as a result of the increasingly benevolent social climate concerning the procedure. Tsoi concluded similarly that the high prevalence in Singapore was attributable to the availability of sex conversion surgery. It would seem that a significant number of subjects in the community are potential candidates for sex conversion, so that more seek it as it becomes more available. As discussed earlier, Siegel and Zitrin (1978) reported a large number of men in New York with a spectrum of illusion-sustaining capacities, so that for many it sufficed to dress in female attire, whereas others required hormones and still others surgery. One of the speakers at the Open Forum (1978) commented that most transsexuals never made contact with a gender identity program, but obtained black market hormones.

The prevalence of transvestism is unknown. Most transvestites do not seek medical help, and no community surveys have attempted to assess it. In a question-naire investigation of sexual behaviors by Person et al. (1989), 4% of female and 1% of male university students reported dressing in the clothes of the opposite sex in the previous 3 months. The motivation for the behavior was not reported, but 3% of the men and 2% of the women reported recent sexual fantasies of dressing in clothes of the opposite sex. Fifteen of 138 male medical students, but none of 58 female medical students, reported they had obtained sexual arousal from dressing in the external or underclothes of the opposite sex (McConaghy, 1982). One had done this on seven occasions, and the others on no more than three. It would seem unlikely that marked transvestite behavior is shown by more than 1% of the population.

ETIOLOGY

Sex Identity: Categorical or Dimensional; Learned and Biological Determinants

Once transsexualism was recognized, theories of its etiology stimulated formula-tion of the concept of sex identity. Benjamin (1954) considered transvestism in its transsexual form to fulfill a deep-seated urge that suggested a disharmony of the total sexual sense, a dissociation of physical and mental sexuality. This concept, which raised the possibility that transsexualism was a biologically determined pathological condition not necessarily relevant to normal human development, received little attention. The alternative view of Worden and Marsh (1985) that "the existence of persons who have this distorted subjective perception of their sexual identity offers an opportunity to study the whole problem of how human beings normally get their sense of being a male or a female" (p. 1292) was accepted, and was reinforced by its repetition (Green & Money, 1969). The possibility that studying the development of sexual identity of transsexuals might result in a very distorted concept of the develop-ment of the sexual identity of normal subjects was not considered. Benjamin (1954) had pointed out that the conviction of transsexuals that they were really females with faulty sex organs was profound and passionate. Understandably, it was accepted that the sexual identity of normals was equally profound, a powerful and unified sense that they were either male or female held with the same persistence and intensity as was the opposite-sex identity that drove transsexuals to tolerate the significant diffi-culties of undergoing sex conversion. Research was not considered necessary to establish this categorical concept of normal sex identity.

When the categorical concept of sex identity was unquestioningly accepted in the 1950s and 1960s, the generally held theory of human development was that of psychoanalysis. In this theory, as it evolved in the ideological climate of the United

States, personality development was considered to be entirely learned (i.e., uninfluenced by biological factors) and to be established in the first 5 years of life, very largely by parental relationships. The sexual identity of both normals and transsexuals was considered to be similarly established. This belief had practical significance regarding the treatment of hermaphrodites or pseudohermaphrodites, subjects born with partly male and partly female genitalia, the appearance of which could be sufficiently ambiguous that some were assigned and reared in the sex opposite to their chromosomal sex. Money, Hampson, and Hampson (1955, 1957) opposed attempts to change these subjects' sex of assignment being made after they were 4.5 years old, claiming this would would result in impairment of their adjustment. To justify this claim, they added to the psychoanalytic theory of sex identity a complimentary theory from animal research that attracted attention at the time. Lorenz (1937) found that some species of birds for a defined period of hours shortly after their birth followed a moving object (in the case of his research, himself). This following response could persist into their adult life as an emotional attachment to that object. He proposed that a critical period existed in the development of the nervous system of these birds such that the following response could be learned only during that time span, and if learned then, it was established irreversibly; to use Lorenz's term, it was *imprinted*.

Despite the marked differences in the central nervous systems of birds and mammals, Money et al. (1955, 1957) extrapolated Lorenz's concept of imprinting to human development. They suggested the problems that they believed followed late sex reassignment of hermaphrodites indicated that, in their sexual development and in that of normal subjects, there was a critical period between 18 months and 4.5 years. During that period, the sex identity they were assigned was learned by imprinting. Money et al. (1955) introduced a further term to describe the results of such imprinting: *gender role*, defined as "all those things that a person says or does to disclose himself or herself as having the status of boy or man, girl or woman, respectively. It includes but is not restricted to sexuality in the sense of eroticism" (p. 285). Thus, by this definition, the area of human sexuality established as entirely learned was broadened to include sex identity, sex-linked behaviors identified as masculine or feminine, the sex to which one wished to belong, and the sex of persons to whom one was attracted. The assumption that all these variables were sufficiently closely related to be considered part of one categorical entity (gender role) was not considered to require empirical verification. Freund, Nagler, Langevin, Zajac, and Steiner (1974) developed a scale to measure feminine gender identity in men that provided a combined score of their wishes to be a female, sex-linked behaviors such as preference for housework and girls' games, wearing women's clothes, self-assessed femininity of appearance, identifying with the woman in stories, and at times feeling like a member of the opposite sex.

In an attempt to determine the degree to which the behaviors subsumed in the concept of gender role were associated, their relationship was examined in medical students of the University of New South Wales in two consecutive years. The students anonymously reported the degree to which they showed these behaviors by the questionnaire (McConaghy, 1988b) described in Chapter 3. To assess their sexual orientation, they reported dimensionally their ratio of heterosexual to homosexual feelings. To assess their sex of preference, they rated the frequency with which they wished to be of the opposite sex both between the ages of 6 and 12 years and subsequently. To assess their sexual role, they rated the degree to which they felt they had a component of the opposite sex in their mental makeup, to which they thought other people considered they showed traits of the opposite sex in their behavior, and to which they thought they showed effeminate or butch traits. To assess their sex identity, they rated the degree to which they felt uncertain of their identity as a member of their sex, the strength of their identity as a member of their sex, and the degree to which they felt a member of the opposite sex.

Insufficient numbers of students reported cross-dressing to determine its relationship to the other behaviors. In the total sample of students in both years, the two sex-of-preference items correlated reasonably strongly ($r = 0.6$), as did the three sex-role items ($r = 0.5$ to 0.6). The correlations of the sex-of-preference with the sex-role items were weaker, however, as were the intercorrelations of the three sexual identity items (McConaghy & Armstrong, 1983). These findings suggested that the concept of a categorical gender role that incorporated these behaviors in normals could not be supported.

A further finding emerged when the responses of medical students whose feelings included a current homosexual component were examined separately from the responses of those whose feelings were exclusively heterosexual (McConaghy & Armstrong, 1983). Correlations between the degree to which the subjects reported the various behaviors were markedly stronger in those aware of some homosexual feelings. In regard to the three sexual identity questions, the responses of the exclusively heterosexual group did not intercorrelate to a signifiant extent; those of subjects with a homosexual component did, but in the direction of their showing opposite-sex identity. They reported greater preference to be of the opposite sex, greater opposite-sex-role behavior, and greater opposite-sex identity. That is to say, their opposite-sex identity was markedly stronger and more consistent than was the same-sex identity of the exclusively heterosexual subjects.

Once this was found, it seemed obvious this would be the case—to paraphrase Freud (Chapter 1), it could be accounted for with certainty. Members of a minority group (e.g., blacks as compared with whites, or Jews with non-Jews) can be expected to have a much stronger sense of group identity. Basing concepts of the nature of the sexual identity of the total population on that of minority sexual groups could be misleading. Further evidence that sex identity is not a categorical entity was the finding, discussed earlier, that unlike transsexuals, a number of transvestites feel like a woman when cross-dressed but not when nude (Buhrich & McConaghy, 1977c).

In addition to the lack of evidence for the concept of a unified sex identity as categorical, that supporting its resistance to change was questioned. Hamburg and Lunde (1967) were critical of the findings of Money et al. (1955, 1957) advanced to support the belief that subjects' assigned sex could not be changed after the age of 4.5 years without impairing their adjustment. Hamburg and Lunde agreed that inadequate information was provided to establish how the nature of the subjects' sex roles and adjustment was assessed. Dewhurst and Gordon (1963) noted that some hermaphrodite children behaved as if they belonged to the sex opposite to that in which they had been brought up; they reported a number of such cases whose assigned sex was successfully changed after the age of 4.5 years. Further evidence of this nature was reviewed by Diamond (1965), who advanced data supporting a role for biological determinants in the establishment of sex role and identity. Zuger (1970) pointed out that the sex assigned to hermaphrodites was based on the appearance of their external genitalia, which was determined by biological factors. The possible contribution of these factors would need to be excluded before the sex role successfully adopted by the subjects could be attributed entirely to their learning the sex to which they were assigned.

Money (1970) rejected these criticisms, arguing that early sex assignment was the sole factor determining gender role, as it was equally successful whether or not it conformed with the subjects' biological sex. He had found this to be the case in matched pairs of hermaphrodites of the same genetic and morphological sex, one reared as a boy and one as a girl. As the pairs were not randomly allocated to their assigned sex, however, this quasi-experimental data did not exclude the possibility that biological factors (including genital appearance) were used to determine the sex of assignment. In regard to the reports of apparently successful reassignment of subjects after 4.5 years, this was explained as attributable to their having been reared in an ambiguous sex role prior to the reassignment because of their parents' uncertainty about their sex.

Zuger (1970) pointed out the arbitrary, post hoc nature of this concept, which was advanced without supporting data to preserve the original theory. In rejecting Zuger's criticisms, Money (1970) suggested to the journal editor that rather than publish Zuger's paper, it should be returned for a very radical total revision. Zuger (1970) was able to have the paper accepted, pointing out that the request for such a revision—far beyond the scope of the paper—amounted to stalling it forever. This publication of the evidence of scientific politics in action is rare. Nevertheless, Zuger's criticisms had little effect, possibly because of their suggestion that biological factors could be involved in determining sexual identity, a possibility incompatible with the current ideology. The dogma was maintained that normal subjects developed an unchangeable categorical gender role by learning in the first few years of life (Constantinople, 1979; Gosselin & Wilson, 1980). The alternative proposition, that sex roles and identities of normals (and possibly hermaphrodites and transsexuals) were distributed dimensionally, remains ignored.

On the basis of this theory that sex identity is established by learning and that biological factors are unimportant, Money recommended the reassignment at the age of 17 months of one of a pair of monozygotic male twins whose penis was accidentally ablated. The boy was maintained on female sex hormones; his apparently successful adjustment in childhood was widely reported as a dramatic documentation of the theory (Diamond, 1982). Diamond attempted to investigate the boy's outcome subsequent to puberty and found that there were virtually no research data available concerning this. This suggested the possible suppression of findings that could threaten established beliefs. Diamond commented that it was regrettable that researchers in the United States were dependent on a British Broadcasting Commission investigative journalist team for information concerning a case originally and so prominently reported in the American literature. The evidence available suggested the boy was very poorly adjusted to the female role.

Some workers who accept the theory that sex identity is usually established in childhood by learning have awarded an occasional role to biological factors. Stoller (1968) described the case of an apparently anatomically normal girl raised by unsuspecting parents who wanted a girl. To the bitter dismay of her feminine mother, the child from birth acted as though she was convinced she should be a boy. Stoller commented that all efforts to assign her a feminine gender, so crucial in almost all instances, left the child untouched. Then, at puberty, physical examination revealed she was a male with a penis the size of a clitoris, a bifid scrotum, and cryptorchid testes. Stoller further commented that the child had been right all along, that his gender identity had been male in the face of all of society's pressures to act like a female. He believed there were enough such subjects that one could presume they were not merely coincidences but rather cases in which biological forces became, as they almost never did in normals, the most powerful effect in producing gender identity. Stoller believed this identity usually started to develop from birth as a fundamental sense of belonging to one sex. It could be conceptualized as a core gender identity, produced by the infant-parent relationship, by the child's perception of its external genitalia, and by a biological force that springs from the biologic variables of sex. In Stoller's view, the first two factors were almost always crucial in determining the ultimate gender identity.

Stoller (1968) considered that the core gender identity was established before the age of 5, but that gender identity continued to develop intensively until at least the end of adolescence. This accounted for transvestite men who tried to be very feminine when dressed in female clothes, yet did not truly feel they were females. Their core identity was male, but overlaid by later-developed female elements. Stoller believed that hermaphrodites from the beginning of awareness of their existence may not feel themselves to be members of either sex. Because of their parents' uncertainty as to their "true" sex, they are also uncertain. Stoller saw them as members of a third hermaphrodite gender that was a different core gender identity. They could change sex and change gender role, but not gender identity. The sex of these hermaphrodites could be reassigned successfully after the age of 5 years. If a subject with a well-fixed, unquestioned gender identity is told—and knows the person telling him or her is correct—that he or she is really a member of the opposite sex, however, the effect may be devastating.

Support for a role of biological factors in determining sex identity was advanced from the study of a group of males with an inherited form of hermaphrodism produced by a deficiency of the enzyme 5-alpha-reductase (Imperato-McGinley, Peterson, Gautier, & Sturla, 1979). This resulted in a decreased production of the sex hormone dihydrotesterone during the subjects' intrauterine development with consequently marked ambiguity in the appearance of their external genitalia at birth, leading to some being raised as girls. With the approach of puberty (with its associated increase in production of the sex hormone testosterone), the subjects' voices deepened, and they developed a muscular habitus with substantial growth of the phallus, which previously resembled a clitoris. In most subjects the testes descended into the scrotum, if they had not already done so. There was no breast development. They commenced to have erections and were capable of intercourse with intromission.

Imperato-McGinley et al. were able to investigate 33 such subjects from 23 interrelated families in three rural villagers in the Dominican Republic. Twenty-five were postpubertal, 3 pubertal, and 5 prepubertal. The authors interviewed the affected subjects and, where possible, their parents, siblings, wives, girlfriends, and neighbours. Other men and boys in the villages were interviewed as controls. The interviews were designed to discern any sexual ambiguity in the rearing of the subjects raised as girls and to determine the validity of any change to a male sex, identity, and role. Nineteen of the 33 subjects were considered to have been unambiguously raised as girls. Adequate psychosexual data obtained from 18 of these 19 revealed that 17 had successfully changed to a male sex identity. The 17 began to realize they were different from other girls in the village between 7 and 12 years of age when they did not develop breasts, their bodies began to change in a masculine direction, and masses were noted in the inguinal canal or scrotum. They showed concern over their true sex identity, and a change to a male identity gradually evolved over several years.

A change to a male role occurred in 16 of the 17 subjects during or following puberty, when they were convinced they were men and experienced sexual interest in women. The time of first heterosexual intercourse was 15 to 18 years for subjects raised as girls, 15 to 17 years for those raised as boys, and 14 to 16 years for 20 normal male control villagers. One subject continued to dress as a woman but had the affect and mannerisms of a man, and engaged in sexual activity with village women. The authors did not comment on whether he showed fetishistic arousal to women's clothes, which would have indicated a transvestite adjustment. Fifteen of the remaining 16 were living or had lived with women in common-law relationships.

One subject maintained a female identity and role. At age 16 she "married" a village man who left her after a year. She left the village and lived alone, working as a domestic, and had no further sexual activity with men. She wore false breasts, yet her build and mannerisms were masculine. She denied any attraction to women and desired sex conversion of her genitalia so she could be a normal woman. These findings are compatible with this subject showing predominant homosexual feelings. If the same factors were operating in these subjects to produce homosexual feelings as operate in the normal population, it would be expected that 1 of 18 males would be predominantly homosexual. Imperato-McGinley et al. commented that there were no laws against homosexuality, but there was strong social pressure against it. A predominantly homosexual male reared as a girl could prefer to go on living as a girl rather than change to be identified as a male homosexual. It would be of interest to know if this subject compared to the remainder had shown more "sissyish" as opposed to rough-and-tumble play, discussed in Chapter 3 as characterizing the childhood of homosexual men. This data was not reported.

Imperato-McGinley et al. commented of the earlier reports of matched hermaphrodites whose sex identity remained that of their sex of rearing, contrary to their chromosomal and gonadal sex, that it was not possible to establish the nature of the hormonal milieu to which they were exposed in their intrauterine development. Also, castration and sex hormone therapy were usually given to complement the sex of rearing. The authors concluded that in a laissez-faire environment, when the sex of rearing is contrary to the testosterone-mediated biologic sex, the biologic sex prevails if the normal testosterone-induced activation of puberty is permitted to occur. They further concluded that their findings showed that sex identity is not unalterably fixed in early childhood but is continually evolving, becoming fixed with the events of puberty.

Rubin, Reinisch, and Haskett (1981) suggested that the major methodological problem concerning the conclusions of Imperato-McGinley et al. was establishing that the children had been reared unambiguously as girls; the abnormal appearance of their external genitalia at birth should have made at least their mothers uncertain concerning their sex. Herdt and Davidson (1988) reported 14 subjects with 5-alpha-reductase deficiency in New Guinea. They stated that 5 were wrongly assigned at birth to be reared as girls. All changed to a male role after puberty. Herdt and Davidson believed that the change occurred only under the greatest external public pressure; however, they gave little evidence of this pressure. Three had died, 1 of whom was reported to have shown odd behavior as a child before the condition was discovered: climbing trees and carrying male artifacts, such as a bow and arrows. One of the two still alive suffered ridicule when the condition was discovered following puberty and shifted to a distant town to escape the stigma, but continued to dress and identify as a man there. It would be expected that if the subject's sex identity as a woman was strong, he would have lived as a woman when freed from the stigma. Rosler and Kohn (1983) described a number of subjects with hermaphoroditism attributable to 17-beta-hydroxysteroid dehydrogenase deficiency who were reared as girls but spontaneously adopted a male sex role and identity following puberty. The authors stated that careful inspection of the external genitalia at birth would be required to detect the difference, and all were reared unequivocally as girls.

The lack of resolution concerning the nature and etiology of sex or gender identity is evident in the series of statements concerning it in DSM-III-R. These include that some forms of gender identity disturbance are on a continuum, whereas others may be discrete; that when gender identity is mild, the person is aware that he is a male or that she is a female, but discomfort and a sense of inappropriateness about the assigned sex is experienced; and that disturbance of gender identity is rare. This attempt to accommodate all possible views succeeds in accommodating none. It is not compatible with concepts of categorical gender identity, yet those who believe that sex identity is on a continuum from mild to severe would not accept mild deviations are rare. The prolonged disputes concerning the nature of the sex identities both of normal subjects and those with sexual anomalies, and whether these identities are entirely learned or are influenced by biologically based urges, will require further evidence to be resolved. To support the role of environmental factors, it needs to be established that specific differences occurred in the rearing of the different groups of cross-gendered subjects.

Stoller (1971) considered that transsexualism was produced in men whose mothers encouraged them to be feminine while their fathers remained withdrawn, so that they developed a core opposite-sex identity. Factors responsible for transsexualism in women included the child at birth not appearing feminine or beautiful to the parents, and not being cuddly; the mother being feminine, but removed from the child by emotional illness; and the father being masculine but nonsupportive of the mother in her illness or the daughter in her femininity. The daughter took on the role of succoring husband to the mother and subsequently developed masculine behavior.

In regard to transvestism, Stoller (1972) suggested that the mothers allowed their sons to develop masculinity in the first few years of their life, so that they established a male core identity. Once developed, their masculinity excited revenge in the mother or some other woman, who attacked it by putting female clothes on the subjects. These conclusions were apparently based on psychoanalysis of the reports of a small number of subjects.

Accounts of young men being encouraged against mild initial reluctance to cross-dress are common in transvestite fiction (Buhrich & McConaghy, 1976). In the accounts the men then appear to be beautiful women, and when they are accepted socially as such, they greatly enjoy the experience. Prince and Bentler (1972), in their postal survey of transvestite club members, found no evidence that childhood experiences of wearing female clothes were an etiological factor in their developing the condition. Buhrich and McConaghy (1978b), using self-report, questionnaire, and semantic differential assessment, found no significant differences in the parental relationships during childhood of male transsexuals, transvestites, and homosexuals, indicating that these relationships do not have a specific role in determining the different anomalies. There was a nonsignificant trend for subjects in all three groups compared to normal controls to have experienced less positive feeling towards and involvement with their fathers in childhood. As discussed in Chapter 3 in relation to this finding with homosexual men, it could be attributable to the fathers' response to the greater degree of "sissy" behavior and the lack of interest in sports shown by members of all three groups.

Pomeroy (1967) considered transsexualism a defense against homosexuality in subjects whose strict religious or moral code made it very difficult for them to accept their condition. Homosexuality is associated with some degree of wish to belong to the opposite sex, as well as opposite-sex identity, role, and sex-linked behaviors (Chapter 3). For those exclusive homosexuals who show all these features to a marked extent, acceptance of a transsexual solution could have advantages, particularly if they wish to establish a relationship with a heterosexual man. The advantages could be greater for men of lower socioeconomic class. Farrell and Morrione (1974) reported that of 148 male homosexuals in a large U.S. midwestern city, those belonging to this class were more likely to act in a stereotypic, overtly effeminate way and to see themselves as less accepted by their society. They used feminine nicknames for friends and acquaintances, wore facial makeup, and dressed in women's clothing. Farrell and Morrione considered that lower-class homosexuals were more likely to think of themselves in terms of their sexual behavior first, whereas homosexuals belonging to higher classes thought of themselves more in terms of their occupations or interests. Also, in the lower classes more importance was attached to sex roles, which were stereotypically defined. If transsexualism represents a solution to the conflict of adopting a homosexual role, these findings suggest that homosexuals in lower socioeconomic class would be more likely to adopt it. As discussed earlier, transsexuals predominantly belong to this class. Similar dynamics might contribute to the high prevalence of transsexual prostitution in half- or quarter-caste Maoris in Wellington, New Zealand (MacFarlane, 1984), where Maoris made up only 9% of the population but were more likely to be of lower socioeconomic class. It is possible, however, that unknown additional variables are associated with ethnic status. In studies in the United States and Singapore, discussed previously, ethnic differences were associated with atypical levels of prevalence of transsexualism.

The decision of men who had previously identified as transvestites to seek sex conversion in middle age could result from the biological and social changes that occur at this time. These men tend to have had a stronger desire to be of the opposite sex since childhood and a stronger homosexual component, compared to transvestites who do not seek sex conversion. Changes at middle age that could increase the wish for sex conversion include decreased sexual drive (so that the subjects' heterosexual activity becomes less important), children approaching adulthood (so that pressures to maintain the family are reduced), and midlife crises (producing wishes to explore new avenues of experience).

In the early adulthood of most transvestives, sexual arousal as a motivation for cross-dressing is replaced by a compulsive urge to cross-dress, followed by a feeling of relaxation. This change is consistent with the behavior completion hypothesis of the motivation of compulsive sexual behaviors, discussed in Chapter 8. This hypothesis postulated that these behaviors were initiated by sexual urges in adolescence, but as they became habitual, they were maintained by neurophysiological behavior completion mechanisms (BCMs). The BCM for a behavior produced tension in the subject when he was stimulated to carry out the behavior, but tried not to do so. Completion of the behavior produced relief from tension, a feeling of relaxation.

Biological Factors

From the perspective of the current biological theory of sex-linked behaviors and sexual orientation (Chapter 3), the factor most likely to be involved in determining the differing degrees of opposite-sex identity characterizing transvestism and transsexualism is exposure at some critical stage in intrauterine development to an increased ratio of opposite- to same-sex hormones. For this theory to be valid, some independence must exist between the critical periods that determine the ratio of subjects' heterosexual to homosexual feelings, their sex-linked behaviors, their degree of same- to opposite-sex identity, and their ability to be sexually aroused by crossdressing. This independence is required to explain the facts that of men who are sexually aroused by cross-dressing, nuclear transvestites are predominantly heterosexual, whereas marginal transvestites are bisexual, but more heterosexual than fetishistic transsexual men. Classical transsexual men are almost exclusively homosexual and are not sexually aroused by cross-dressing.

Whether the marked grooming behavior shown by transvestite men is an opposite-sex-linked behavior or is related to fetishistic arousal to cross-dressing requires further investigation. Extremely few if any women appear equivalent to male fetishistic transvestites in that they experience sexual arousal to cross-dressing in adolescence, followed by a strong compulsion to cross-dress in adulthood with minimal sexual arousal. It would seem likely that a biological rather than an environmental cause is required to account for this marked difference. As some men with compulsive transvestism seek sex conversion in middle age, the absence of equivalent transvestite women could account in part for the higher percentage of men who seek sex conversion. A further factor causing more men than women with homosexual feelings to seek sex conversion could be the much stronger relationships of homosexual feelings with opposite-sex-linked behaviors in men as compared with women (see Chapter 3). Men with marked opposite-sex-linked behaviors and wishes to be of the opposite sex could be likely to seek sex conversion, particularly if this would enable them to escape the negative social reaction to these behaviors. Women with homosexual feelings but slight opposite-sex-linked behaviors could be less motivated to seek sex conversion.

Earlier reports of hormonal differences between transsexual and heterosexual men failed to be replicated (Spijkstra, Spinder, & Gooren, 1988). Pauly (1974) stated that there was a high index of suspicion of hormonal or ovarian dysfunction in female transsexuals, in view of their frequent reports of scant or irregular menstrual periods. High 17-ketosteroid levels were found in 10 of 31 cases in whom relevant information was available. Pauly warned that this rate might be spuriously high, however, as only abnormal findings were certain to be reported. Also, some subjects may have been surreptitiously taking exogenous androgens to increase the masculinity of their appearance. Meyer-Bahlburg (1979) concluded from a review of the literature that about a third of homosexual and transsexual women had elevated androgen levels. Futterweit, Weiss, and Fagerstrom (1986) reported a similar finding in the transsexual women they studied, adding that in some it was associated with hirsutism. Eleven of their 40 subjects had definite or probable polycystic ovarian disease, and 2 had amenorrhea. This led the authors to recommend that female transsexuals be investigated endocrinologically before hormonal therapy is commenced.

W. Meyer et al. (1986) found no evidence to support an association between abnormal levels of sex hormones in either 30 female-to-male transsexuals or 60 male-to-female homosexuals they studied. Two of the female-to-male transsexuals had been born with ambiguous genitalia as a result of intrauterine exposure to excess androgen and had been raised as girls. Fourteen of the remainder and 19 of the male-to-female subjects had not previously taken exogenous hormones. The hormone levels of both these groups and the menstrual history of 12 of the female-to-male subjects were normal. Meyer et al. (1981) had previously reported an examination of 9 of these 12 subjects that showed them to have normal physical development. The lack of hirsutism in these female-to-male transsexuals suggests that its presence in the subjects studied by Futterweit et al. could have resulted from self-medication with androgens.

Freund, Steiner, and Chan (1982) reviewed a number of reports of families in which there were at least two transsexuals, suggesting the possibility of familial transmission, either genetic or environmental. Transvestism was reported in two brothers, in a father and son, in a father and three sons (Freund, Steiner, & Chan, 1982) and in a father, a sister, and a brother of three of 70 transvestites (Croughan et al., 1981). Pauly (1974) reported a female transsexual with a chromosome abnormality (XO/XX). An association was found between Klinefelter's syndrome, produced by an XXY genetic constitution, and transvestism or transsexualism, which led to the suggestion that the two conditions were related (Money & Pollitt, 1964). These authors speculated that the XXY genotype may have produced a disposition to defective psychosexual differentiation, and that transvestism not associated with

Klinefelter's syndrome might result from the interaction of another genotype producing this disposition with unknown social and/or physical environmental factors.
Transvestism was not reported, however, by any of the 16 XXY men identified from
4,139 men investigated for the condition (Schiavi, Thielgaard, et al., 1988).

Kolarsky, Freund, Machek, and Polak (1967), in an investigation of 86 male
epileptics, were unable to find a relationship between epilepsy and transvestism. This
had been suggested in earlier studies of small numbers of subjects in which the two
conditions occurred together. Ferrando, McCorvey, Simon, and Stewart (1988) reported transvestism in a 32-year-old man that occurred only on the occasions he
ingested the contents of inhalants containing levo-methamphetamine and other volatile substances. They postulated several biochemical brain mechanisms whereby the
drug could induce transvestism; however, they pointed out that other amphetamine
congeners had been associated with bizarre sexual activities that did not include
transvestism. They did not appear to have considered the possibility that the subject
they reported may have had transvestite impulses that he controlled when not disin-
hibited by the drug.

If prenatal exposure to higher levels of opposite-sex hormones is validated as
contributing to the etiology of heterosexuality/homosexuality (Chapter 3), it may
also prove to be an etiological factor in transvestism and transsexualism. If so, these
conditions might also be by-products of an evolutionarily determined need for a
percentage of subjects in whom sex-linked behaviors are detached to varying extents
from other aspects of sexual behavior.

Treatment

Transvestism

Few transvestites persist with seeking treatment for their condition, though a
number consult psychiatrists at least once at some stage; one-quarter of the subjects
reported by Prince and Bentler (1972), one-third of those interviewed by Buhrich
(1977a), and one-half of those interviewed by Croughan et al. (1981) had done so.
Croughan et al. reported that equal numbers had consulted psychiatrists on their
own decision and in response to pressure from courts, wives, parents, or friends. In
my experience, most transvestites who persist with treatment to cease the behavior
do so to please their female partners. Aversive therapy for this purpose was introduced in the 1960s; Morgenstern, Pearce, and Rees (1965) treated 13 transvestites by
giving them apomorphine so that they experienced nausea and vomiting while they
cross-dressed. Almost all cross-dressed once in the month following treatment, but
none found it produced the pleasure it had previously. At follow-up 8 months to 4
years later, 7 had ceased to cross-dress, though 2 continued to experience strong
urges to do so. The remaining 6 reported reduction in the frequency of cross-dressing, but relapsed in relation to stressful events. A similar response rate was reported
to electric-shock aversive therapy for transvestites (Marks, Gelder, & Bancroft,
1970).

I have found behavioral therapies are markedly less effective in giving transvestites control over the behavior as compared to exhibitionists and voyeurs, suggesting that biological as compared to learned factors play a stronger role in transvestism. My practice is to explore with the subject and his partner the alternative option of their adopting a compromise where he is able to continue the behavior in a form more acceptable to the partner; one possibility is for him to join a club and restrict his cross-dressing to its meetings. Subjects who remain motivated to cease cross-dressing are treated with alternative behavior completion, as discussed in Chapter 8 in relation to the treatment of sex offenders. This frequently needs to be supplemented with temporary androgen reduction by medroxyprogesterone, also discussed there. Prince and Bentler (1972) reported that psychotherapy brought about a temporary cure in only 5% of transvestites who sought treatment, and 53% considered it to have been a waste of time and money. Croughan et al. (1981) reported that treatment, mainly psychotherapy alone, played virtually no role in bringing about periods of abstinence of cross-dressing in the transvestites they investigated.

Transsexualism

Psychological and Social Outcomes of Surgical Sex Conversion

The view of early proponents (Benjamin, 1954; Hamburger et al., 1953) that the desire of transsexuals for sex conversion was irreversible and that its provision by surgery was the only successful treatment remained widely accepted by workers treating these subjects throughout the 1960s and 1970s. A number of uncontrolled studies, recently reviewed by E. Gordon (1991), reported good outcomes in 70% to 90% of subjects, and J. Meyer and Reter (1979) concluded from this literature that obvious psychiatric disturbance, serious postsurgical ambivalence, and gross dyssocial behavior were infrequent complications. As discussed previously, criteria for the diagnosis varied. It was usually required that to receive surgery, subjects must have made a satisfactory adjustment to living as a member of the opposite sex for at least 1 and often 2 years; what constituted a satisfactory adjustment was not clearly defined. It may not have included stable employment, but a lack of significant psychiatric pathology over the period was usually required.

In 1979, a negative quasi-experimental assessment of sex conversion surgery for transsexualism received considerable attention. J. Meyer and Reter (1979) followed up 50 of 100 subjects evaluated for the procedure. They pointed out that their inclusion of a comparison group of unoperated subjects was an important departure from earlier studies. Meyer and Reter was not able to allocate subjects randomly to receive or not receive sex conversion, but compared 11 men and 4 women who received it with the 35 who initially had not. The latter group had not completed the qualifying period of living and working in the desired role while taking opposite-sex hormones for one year; however, 13 men and 1 woman of the 35 subsequently obtained sex conversion, 5 in the program and 9 elsewhere. The group remaining unoperated (16 men and 5 women) were slightly younger and of higher education and socioeconomic status than the other two groups, consistent with the suggestion made earlier that transsexuals of higher socioeconomic class were under less pressure to change their sex. Subjects' outcome was assessed by a composite score in which legal charges, lower work status, cohabitation or marriage with a person of the opposite biological sex, and psychiatric contact were rated negatively.

According to this assessment, no statistically significant differences were found between the three groups, though there was a trend for those subsequently operated upon to have improved less. This trend could have reflected bias in the outcome measure; those obtaining surgery following rejection are likely to have required additional psychiatric contacts to do so. Scoring cohabitation or marriage with a person of the opposite biological sex negatively prejudiced the outcome of subjects with a heterosexual component who may have shown a good adjustment on the other measures. As pointed out earlier, such subjects are likely to be older male-to-female transsexuals with a history of having been sexually aroused to cross-dressing and of marriage, features often leading to their rejection for sex conversion. If such rejection occurred in Meyer and Reter's study, they would have been overrepresented in the subjects obtaining the operation elsewhere. It is possible that if more unbiased outcome criteria had been used, the subjects rejected for surgery who obtained it elsewhere would have shown as good an outcome as those accepted, suggesting that the criteria for rejection required reassessment.

Meyer and Reter put considerable emphasis on the fact that the initially operated-upon group changed little if at all socioeconomically and demonstrated no superiority in jobs or education to the unoperated group. They concluded that sex conversion conferred no objective advantage in terms of social rehabilitation, but accepted that those who received it found it subjectively satisfying. Their emphasis on the need for improvement in socioeconomic status seems surprising, particularly as most subjects were men converting to women, who in general are paid more poorly. Expectation of marked improvement in socioeconomic status is not a usual outcome criterion for psychiatric or surgical treatment of other conditions.

Fleming, Steinman, and Bocknek (1980) trenchantly criticized this outcome study, which they said had been widely cited by professionals and in the popular press as proof that there was no difference in long-term adjustment between transsexuals who received surgical sex correction and those who did not. They pointed out the arbitrary nature of the outcome scale, in that it rated being arrested and cohabiting with a person of the opposite biological sex equally negatively (−1); being admitted to a psychiatric hospital more negatively (−3) than being jailed (−2); and having a job as a plumber and being married to a person of the same biological sex equally positively (+2). Fleming et al. questioned whether cohabiting with a person of the opposite biological sex should be regarded as negative, citing an article approving of a lesbian-feminist orientation in male-to-female transsexuals. In particular, Fleming et al. were critical of the failure of the study to examine the relationship to outcome of postsurgical complications that they believed occurred frequently, as well as its discounting the patients' subjective satisfaction with surgery, Flemming et al. pointed out that patients' feelings were crucial to any understanding of the transsexual phenomenon. They expressed concern that Meyer had not disclaimed the press interpretation of the study as showing that surgery did nothing objective beyond what time and psychotherapy could do.

The influence of Meyer and Reter's negative interpretation of the outcome of sex conversion surgery for transsexualism was indicated by the fact that it contributed to a district court decision that sex conversion surgery was not covered by Georgia's Medicaid program because it was an experimental procedure and no medical consensus existed as to its safety or efficacy (Gordon, 1991). Gordon also stated that Meyer and Reter's study was used as evidence to close the Johns Hopkins surgical program. It would appear to have had less effect on the views of clinicians: A 1986 study found that 52% of physicians believed sex conversion surgery improved the mental health of the subjects, and only 12% considered it definitely harmful. In 1966, 25% of physicians had reported both beliefs. Subsequent to Meyer and Reter's report, a number of studies found significant reduction in neurotic symptoms and improvement in social status of transsexuals following surgery (Gordon, 1991).

Kockott and Fahrner (1987) reported a number of transsexuals who, when offered sex conversion, remained undecided about accepting it. They differed from those with an unchanged wish for surgery in being older, more often married, and in a more stable socioeconomic situation. Also, their current partnerships, although mainly unhappy and not satisfying sexually, had existed for significantly longer and were only with subjects of the opposite biological sex. No details were given of the undecided subjects' sexual arousal to cross-dressing, but their features suggested that they were fetishistic transsexuals. On the basis of their findings, Kockott and Fahrner considered the transsexuals who had not had surgery in the Meyer and Reter study to be equivalent to their undecided group, and hence not comparable with those who received surgery.

Kockott and Fahrner also described transsexuals who, when offered surgery, rejected it. They were also more likely to be in long-standing relationships, and in addition were more satisfied with their jobs at the initial interview, compared to the subjects who continued to desired surgery. The psychosexual adjustment of the three groups as measured by rating scale did not differ significantly. Kockott and Fahrner compared subjects with a continued wish for surgery with those who had received it; the latter were more often well or very well adjusted to their opposite sex role, in which all subjects in both groups were living. They were more often employed, had made fewer suicide attempts, were more satisfied with their sexual experiences, and were better adjusted on the psychosexual rating scale, reporting few difficulties whereas the group still wanting surgery reported marked difficulties. At the time of initial diagnosis, scores of the two groups on the psychosexual rating scale had not differed.

Kuiper and Cohen-Kettenis (1988) pointed out that it was possible to discern a trend in the numerous outcome studies that sex conversion surgery resulted in improvement in patients' subjective well-being, but not necessarily in their actual life situations. They reported this outcome in 105 male-to-female and 36 female-to-male transsexuals, all of whom had started hormone therapy. About two-thirds of both males and females had completed surgery. Sixty-five percent were happy or very happy, the proportion of the four groups not differing in this respect. In many, having a steady partner was a principal factor in their being happy. None ascribed unhappiness to difficulties related to their social, emotional, or physical functioning in the opposite-sex role. Of the four groups, 80% to 100% had no doubt that having surgery was the correct decision; 1 of the subjects who had completed surgery had persistent doubts concerning this, but none about living permanently as a member of the opposite sex. Eighty percent of female-to-male but 50% of male-to-female subjects were satisfied or highly satisfied with the treatment provided. Male-to-female subjects were on average 9 years older, and more often married and with children compared to the female-to-male subjects, thus creating an additional problem for sex reassignment.

No direct relationship was found, however, between these or other variables in relation to outcome. Dissatisfaction was with physical complications, and more especially with lack of adequate psychosocial guidance before, during, or after surgery. Dissatisfied subjects were more likely to have no partner; to receive less acceptance from their direct environment, particularly their families; to have lost social contacts and jobs; and to feel lonelier, contributing to their need for support from care givers. They did not wish more frequently for supplementary surgery. Blanchard, Steiner, Clemmensen, and Dickey (1989) investigated 111 transsexuals who had received sex conversion at least 1 year earlier. None of the 61 homosexual males or the 36 homosexual females consciously regretted surgery, compared to 4 of the 14 heterosexual males, a significant difference. As discussed earlier, more of these heterosexual males could be expected to be older and married. Walinder, Lundstrom, and Thuwe (1978) found age and heterosexual experience to be associated in men with a greater likelihood of regretting sex conversion.

Physical Outcome of Surgical Sex-Conversion

Much less evidence has been provided concerning the physical outcome of sex conversion surgery. Lindemalm, Korlin, and Uddenberg (1986) found only three studies that had followed up a total of 30 male-to-female transsexuals for as long as 3 years following surgery; they reported the outcome of 15 men who had received penile amputation 6 years or more previously. One was abroad, and 1 had committed suicide shortly after vaginoplasty. Vaginal construction had been attempted in 9 of the remaining 13. At follow-up, 3 had atrophic or scarred vaginas, and two had vaginal cavities too small to allow intercourse. The surgical result was judged by the investigators to be fair in the sixth, who reported pain and dryness with intercourse, and as excellent in the remaining 3; however, 1 of the 3 considered it to be virtually a failure. Poor results were attributed by the plastic surgeon to surgical complications or anatomical difficulties in 3, and lack of cooperation (e.g., not performing distension exercises following surgery) in 2. Two of the subjects with poor results, but none of the remainder, expressed some repentance concerning sex conversion. Five subjects had little or no sexual activity with partners before or after surgery. Four were sexually very active after surgery, 3 of whom had been very active and 1 moderately active prior to surgery. Of the 4, 2 were in the group of 3 classified as having an excellent result; 1 had the fair result; and 1 had severe scarring that prevented further attempts to construct a vagina, and reached orgasm by anal intercourse.

Lindemalm et al. commented on the fact that the overall sexual adjustment was often unchanged by surgery and that there were surprisingly small changes in libidinal strength and capacity for orgasm, despite the drastic measures of penile amputation, castration, and estrogen administration. They further commented that

the scanty outcome literature reported similar findings to theirs, that surgical attempts to create a functional vagina resulted in severe complications in about 50% of
biological males. The lack of interest in adequate follow-up of surgery in view of the
poor results reported is disquieting, particularly given the very extensive literature
devoted to the clinical features of transsexualism. Genital sex conversion may have
more symbolic than physical significance for many of the men who undergo it.

Kuiper and Cohen-Kettenis (1988) commented of penoplasty (which 4 of the 25
female-to-male transsexuals who had completed surgery in their study had undergone) that in view of the grave risk of complications and the often disappointing
results, it was unlikely they would continue to provide it. In the Open Forum (1978),
Money had earlier expressed his opposition to penoplasty because of the incredible
surgical complexities of the procedure and the possibility that it would require 10 to
15 surgical admissions.

In addition to the limited data concerning surgical outcome of sex conversion,
little has been published concerning transexuals' requests for additional surgery.
Bentler (1976) stated that the procedure most frequently requested in his study of 42
male-to-female transsexuals was nose alteration. This was requested by 50% of
subjects who stated that they were homosexual prior to surgery, and 20% of those
who stated that they were heterosexual. The former group were also more likely to
request face lifts, skin peeling, larynx shaving, and ear operations. A quarter of both
groups requested breast implants.

Hormone Therapy

W. Meyer et al. (1986) were among the few groups of workers to report the
outcome of hormonal therapy in some detail. Of 60 male-to-female transsexuals who
attended their gender clinic, at their initial visit 41 were taking or had taken some
form of hormonal therapy for between 1.5 and 360 months. Hormones taken included conjugated estrogen, ethinyl estradiol, combinations of birth control pills,
and diethylstilbestrol. The hormone levels, liver function, cholesterol, triglycerides,
and glucose levels of the 19 who had never taken hormones were all normal. Six of
the 19 were never given hormones, 6 were given them at the first visit, and seven
received them 1 to 12 months later. Those given hormones received either conjugated
estrogen (1.25 to 10 mg/day) or ethinyl estradiol (0.05 to 1 mg/day). Therapy was
usually begun at the lowest dose and increased every 3 months until the subjects'
testosterone levels were suppressed into the range considered normal for women.
Patients who at their initial visit were taking one of these hormones in higher doses
than the maximum doses specified had the dose reduced to the maximum. Those
taking other hormones were randomly allocated to take one of the two. Fifteen
subjects were also given an oral progesterone, usually 10 mg/day of medroxyprogesterone, but it was stated to produce no significant effect.

Meyer et al. found that ethinyl estradiol was 75 to 100 times more potent than
conjugated estrogen on the basis of the doses required to lower testosterone to the
adult female range, 0.1 mg of the former and 7.5 to 10 mg of the latter being
necessary. The greater reliability of testosterone suppression was associated with a
greater likelihood of production of liver enzyme abnormalities, with 4 patients show-

ing elevated serum glutamin-pyruvic transaminase and serum glutamic-oxaloacetic transaminase levels on ethinyl estradiol. The levels returned to normal in 3 of the 4 when all were given estrogen instead; they remained elevated in the fourth for 6 months after estrogens were ceased. Meyer et al. stated that the long-term safety ethinyl estradiol as compared to conjugated estrogen could not be determined because of the small number of subjects and the limited period of follow-up. Breast size increased equally with both forms of therapy, but required 2 years to become maximal. It was suggested that surgical breast implants should be postponed for 2 years.

W. Meyer et al. (1986) reported feminization of body habitus was produced, but did not give further details. Neither hormone altered penis length, but estrogens reduced testicular volume. Suppression of spontaneous erections was reported by many subjects, but usually erections occurred during periods of sexual excitement. Similar responses are shown by sex offenders receiving antiandrogens (Chapter 8). Kwan, VanMaasdam, and Davidson (1985) reported that frequency of masturbation was reduced in 5 of 7 transsexuals when they were taking 2.5 to 5 mg/day oral estrogen as compared to placebo. None were having sexual relations with a partner, so the effect on this behavior could not be determined. Goh and Ratnam (1990) warned of the increased likelihood that transsexuals taking estrogens long-term would develop hyperprolactinemia, particularly with estradiol or its conjugates. They recommended that these subjects' prolactin levels be regularly monitored.

Two of the women seeking sex conversion in the study by W. Meyer et al. (1986) were hermaphrodites. Of the remaining 28, 11 at their initial visit were taking or had taken hormones for between 6 and 240 months. Hormones taken included methyl testosterone linquets, intramuscular testosterone proprionate and enanthate, and a testosterone emulsion made for horses. The hormone levels, liver function tests, and cholesterol, triglycerides, and glucose levels of the 17 who had never taken hormones were all normal, as were the menstrual histories of 12 of this group. Three were never given hormones, 5 were given them at the first visit, and 9 received them 2 weeks to 10 months later. All of those taking hormones were asked to cease them and were given intramuscular testosterone cypionate (50 to 200 mg/fortnightly). The dose was increased until menstrual periods stopped or, in the case of castrated patients, until LH and FSH were suppressed into the normal range. Usually 400 mg/month was required; several subjects administered up to 400 mg/weekly against advice.

After hormonal treatment was commenced, menses of the 12 with a normal menstrual history ceased in 4 months, 2 having one period and 6 none. Subjects' serum glutamin-pyruvic transaminase increased statistically but remained within the normal range, and the change was thought not to have clinical significance. Cholesterol and triglycerides increased to above the upper limit of normal, leading the authors to warn of an associated possible risk of coronary heart disease with testosterone therapy that required further study. Doses greater than 200 mg/month produced striking increases in amount and coarseness of hair on the chest, abdomen, and face, though growth of a cosmetically acceptable beard was not predictable. Clitoral growth was rapid and plateaued by 1 year. There was no significant decrease in breast size, in contrast to the finding of the authors' earlier study (W. Meyer et al., 1981). As in that study, Pauly (1974) found that female-to-male transsexuals experienced reduction in breast size when receiving 100 to 200 mg/fortnightly of depo-testosterone. The majority also reported marked improvement in their general emotional state.

Relationship Psychotherapy and Behavior Therapy

The view held by most physicians in the 1960s (Gordon, 1991) that the mental health of transsexuals would not be improved by sex conversion surgery was maintained by some psychiatrists who continued to recommend psychotherapy as the appropriate treatment at least for the majority of subjects seeking sex conversion. Morgan (1978) noted that the man who always thought of himself as a female, who attended interviews dressed and behaving as a totally convincing woman, and who viewed his penis as an abnormal growth was readily accepted for surgery, but made up only 5 of the 100 candidates he saw and still required psychotherapy to prepare him for the realities of the operation and the difficulties of the postoperative period. Much more common was the man whose core gender identity was toward the middle of the male-female continuum.

Morgan was critical of the common procedure of starting these subjects on opposite-sex hormones while they lived and dressed as a member of the opposite sex and received counseling and, in the case of men, electrolysis. He argued that this procedure was not, as was generally assumed, an easily reversible one that gave the subject a trial of the opposite-sex role. In the case of men, the penile atrophy and impotence resulting from female sex hormone administration removed any emotional investment the penis may have had for the patient, and his newly budding breasts were invested as sexual organs, thus increasing what Morgan termed the "transsexual imperative." In fact, as pointed out above, neither penile atrophy or impotence in sexual relationships commonly result.

Morgan suggested that about 10% of transsexual candidates were psychotic and should initially be treated for that condition. Thirty percent were unable to accept their homosexual desires and could be helped through psychotherapy to make a satisfactory homosexual or bisexual adjustment; previously administered hormone therapy greatly complicated this process. Twenty to 25% were sexually ambiguous but also had inadequate personalities. If possible, their wishes for sex conversion should be ignored while they were urged to find a job, return to school, move out of the parental home, or in other ways have their self-esteem increased. To delay administering hormones, the prolonged, painful, and costly procedure of electrolytic removal of facial hair could be commenced, and subsequently a battery of psychological tests carried out. Then the subject should be urged to live, dress, and work as a member of the opposite sex for at least 6 months before hormone therapy was commenced. Morgan noted that the belief that hormone therapy was a harmless screening device had been disseminated in the medical community. He estimated that there were 200 self-diagnosed male-to-female transsexuals in the Philadelphia areas alone who had received estrogen therapy for 1 to 2 years without ever having seen a psychiatrist.

Behavior therapy has also been reported to be an effective alternative to sex conversion. Barlow, Reynolds, and Agras (1973) reported the successful response of a 17-year-old boy who agreed to the treatment, as he was considered too young for sex conversion, which he requested. Aversive therapy to reduce his transsexual fantasy was ineffective. Direct modification of female gender-specific patterns of sitting, walking, and standing was commenced by modeling and videotape feedback, with verbal praise when the patterns changed in the masculine direction. This was successful, but he still felt like and fantasized himself as a girl. Electric-shock aversion and covert sensitization then reduced his awareness of homosexual arousal. At follow-up 6.5 years later, he was continuing a relationship with a girl whom he had been considering marrying 2.5 years previously (Barlow, Abel, & Blanchard, 1979). They had not had intercourse, and it was not stated if he obtained erections when petting with her; however, he believed he was completely sexually reorientated.

Barlow et al. (1979) reported the response of a further 2 transsexuals to similar treatment. Both were college students who had commenced taking female hormones but desisted, having developed doubts that they could behave sufficiently like women to be socially accepted. Following treatment, the first adopted a masculine gender identity all the time, and the second when he wished. Treatment to alter the homosexual orientation of the first subject failed, and the second desired to remain homosexual. Barlow, Abel, and Blanchard (1977) described a reversal of sex identity in a transsexual occurring in 2 hours with exorcism, which presumably demonstrates the role of suggestion and expectancy in this reversal. It was stated that all the components of masculine motor behavior were seemingly acquired in a matter of hours.

As Zucker (1985) pointed out, evidence of the success of psychotherapy or behavior therapy in enabling subjects seeking sex conversion to accept their same-sex identity has been in general poorly documented and based on case reports of one or a few subjects. Lothstein and Levine (1981) reported the results of a research program established in a gender identity clinic to understand better the benefits of psychotherapy and/or surgery with subjects seeking sex conversion. They pointed out that such subjects often refused to discuss anything besides hormones, electrolysis, and surgery, so that psychological methods were difficult to initiate. They did not report how many patients refused them; presumably a number did, as Lothstein (1980) had earlier stated there were over 120 applicants. In the 1981 study, they reported on 50, of whom 70% adjusted to a nonsurgical solution, 20% were still in therapy, and 10% had received sex conversion therapy. The percentage who received sex conversion would appear within the range of that reported by most clinics offering surgery without a program of psychotherapy as an alternative. Zucker (1985) cited Blanchard as concluding that 75% of transsexuals accepted for eventual surgery self-selected against it by not completing the required criteria.

Green in the Open Forum (1978) commented that most patients who seek sex conversion do not want any kind of behavioral modification or "talking" type of intervention that is going to reorient their sex identity. He suggested that those who accepted such approaches were a subgroup apart from the majority of transsexuals. Fisk stated that he offered all patients (including adolescents) in a gender identity program the option of trying behavior modification, but had yet to have a taker. Kuiper and Cohen-Kettenis (1988) stated of their follow-up of transsexuals that they had intended to have two control groups, one of persons who desired treatment but were not considered eligible, and one of persons who after psychotherapy decided to refrain from surgery. All 7 subjects in the first group refused to cooperate, and there were none in the second group. It would seem that the few transsexuals who have been reported to respond to psychotherapy or behavior therapy by abandoning the wish for sex conversion either were atypical or similar to those whom Kockott and Fahrner (1987) classified as "undecided". If so, the reported response of these subjects to psychotherapy would not be relevant to the management of the majority of transsexuals seeking sex-conversion. Following a brief reconsideration stimulated by the report of J. Meyer and Reter (1979), the early belief that the desire of transsexuals for sex conversion is irreversible and that its provision by surgery is the only successful treatment appears to be generally accepted.

Possibly the aspect of transsexualism most in need of explanation is the intense interest shown by sex researchers in all aspects of this condition other than its physical outcome following surgery. Pauly and Edgerton (1986) pointed out that every year since 1970 there have been about 50 articles published on the subject, and every other year more than 100 researchers come together to hear some 40 papers presented to a gender dysphoria symposium. Sixty-two (i.e., 1 in every 7) of the 445 articles published between 1980 and 1990 in the *Archives of Sexual Behavior,* the official journal of the International Academy of Sex Research dealt with transsexualism. When it is considered that the condition is one of the rarest sexual problems, affecting only one in many thousands of individuals, it suggests that cross-gender behavior has a unique fascination. Certainly crudely parodying the opposite sex in cross-dress appears to be one of the first recourses of groups of men, particularly those identified as "macho" (e.g., members of football teams), when they mount a public entertainment.

CHAPTER 5

Sexual Dysfunctions and Difficulties

The various impairments of sexual functioning, the dysfunctions, were divided into four categories in DSM-III-R. *Sexual desire disorders* included hypoactive sexual desire (deficient sexual fantasies and desire for sexual activity) and sexual aversion (extreme aversion to and avoidance of all or almost all genital sexual contact with a partner). *Sexual arousal disorders* included female sexual arousal disorder (partial or complete failure to attain or maintain the genital lubrication-swelling response of sexual excitement until completion of sexual activity, or lack of a subjective sense of sexual excitement and pleasure during sexual activity) and male erectile disorder (either partial or complete failure to attain or maintain erection until completion of sexual activity, or lack of a subjective sense of sexual excitement and pleasure during sexual activity). Failure to attain or maintain erection is the much more common of the male arousal disorders and continues usually to be referred to as impotence. This may be because the term *male erectile disorder* does not make clear which of the two conditions the subject suffers.

The third DSM-III-R category, *orgasm disorders*, includes inhibited female and male orgasm, and premature ejaculation. Inhibited female orgasm is defined as delay or absence of orgasm during sexual activity judged to be adequate in focus, intensity, and duration. Failure to experience orgasm in coitus without manual clitoral stimulation is considered to justify the diagnosis only in women in whom it is judged to represent a psychological inhibition; this judgment might require a trial of treatment. Inhibited male orgasm is delay or absence of orgasm during sexual activity judged to be adequate. It is usually an inability to reach orgasm by ejaculation in the vagina, orgasm being possible with other types of stimulation. Premature ejaculation is ejaculation with minimal sexual stimulation before, upon, or shortly after penetration and before the person wishes it to occur. The fourth dysfunction, *sexual pain disorders* included dyspareunia (genital pain in either males or females before, during, or after sexual intercourse) and vaginismus (involuntary spasm of the musculature of the outer third of the vagina that interferes with coitus). Vaginismus usually prevents penetration of any object larger than a certain size into the vagina, including the subject's finger or a tampon. If intercourse is attempted, vaginismus is commonly accompanied by spasm of the adductor muscles of the thighs, preventing their separation. Vaginismus does not prevent women from experiencing sexual arousal and orgasm with other activities than coitus.

To receive the diagnosis of sexual dysfunction in DSM-III-R, all the conditions are to be persistent or recurrent in the judgment of the clinician, taking into account such factors as the frequency and chronicity of the symptom, the subjective distress it causes, and its effect on other areas of the subject's functioning. The common failure of studies to report how these factors were taken into account when a particular dysfunction was diagnosed means that it is impossible to be certain that the subjects who received that diagnosis in different studies had the same condition. This is particularly the case in regard to the diagnosis of impotence.

SEXUAL PROBLEMS

Studies of both community and clinical populations have revealed that the dysfunctions classified in DSM-III-R are only some—and apparently not the most important—of the problems limiting the enjoyment of sexual activities, at least for middle-class subjects. Frank, Anderson, and Rubenstein (1978) investigated the presence in 100 predominantly white, well-educated, happily married couples of both sexual dysfunctions (the problems of performance) and what they termed "sexual difficulties" (problems related to the emotional tone of sexual relations). The latter included such conditions as the partner choosing an inconvenient time, or not using appropriate foreplay. Frank et al. found sexual difficulties to be not only more prevalent, but also more significant; their presence in the subjects and their spouses correlated more highly with their lack of sexual satisfaction than did the presence of dysfunctions. In the case of men, the correlations between presence of dysfunctions and lack of sexual satisfaction were not statistically significant.

Community studies in Sweden and the United Kingdom, of which the latter specified the subjects were predominantly middle-class (Nettelbladt & Uddenberg, 1979; Reading & Wiest, 1984), also found no association between the presence in men of either premature ejaculation or erectile difficulties and their sexual satisfaction. In the Swedish study, the presence of these dysfunctions in the men did not correlate with the sexual satisfaction of their female partners, either. The authors of the Swedish study commented that the couples' sexual satisfaction was related to their emotional relationship rather than their sexual function. A similar conclusion was drawn by Snyder and Berg (1983a) from a clinical study of couples presenting with lack of sexual satisfaction to a sexual dysfunctions clinic. They found that though dysfunctions were common complaints of both the men and women, none reported by the women correlated with their sexual dissatisfaction, and only failure to ejaculate during intercourse correlated with that of men. Dissatisfaction correlated strongly in both sexes with the partner's lack of response to sexual requests and with the frequency of intercourse being too low.

It would appear sexual dysfunctions are much less important than the emotional aspects of relationships in determining the sexual satisfaction of couples in the community. If replicatory studies confirm that this finding also applies to subjects who seek treatment for dysfunctions, it will explain the commonly reported outcome that they experience increased sexual interest and enjoyment with improvement of the emotional aspects of their relationships, even though the dysfunctions persist.

SEXUAL AND MARITAL DYSFUNCTION

Rust, Golombok, and Collier (1988) discussed the controversy in the literature as to whether sexual and marital dysfunction were related. They pointed out that some scales assessing the two dysfunctions included similar items, possibly producing an artifactual relationship between them. Rust et al. used two scales designed to avoid conceptual overlap to investigate 28 couples attending a sexual and marital clinic. Impotence correlated with a poor marital relationship as perceived by both partners; premature ejaculation, with a poor relationship mainly as perceived by the male. Sexual dysfunctions in the female did not correlate strongly with a poor relationship as perceived by either partner. Sexual dissatisfaction in the male partner correlated very strongly with a poor marital relationship as perceived by both partners; sexual dissatisfaction in the female partner correlated with a poor marital relationship only as perceived by the female. As the authors pointed out, the direction of causality could not be determined, so that it was possible, for example, that sexual dissatisfaction either produced a poor marital relationship or resulted from it. Where the marital relationship was perceived as poor by both men and women, there was less sexual communication; when it was perceived as poor only by men, sexual relations were less frequent.

The results from this small clinical sample indicate that sexual dissatisfaction and dysfunctions in men are related to their and their partners' perception of the marital relationship. Sexual dissatisfaction, but not dysfunctions, in women are related only to their perception of the marital relationship. These findings require replication in larger clinical and nonclinical populations. Brecher (1984) found that 90% of husbands and wives 50 years and over who were having intercourse, and 67% of wives and 71% of husband who were not, reported being happily married. Sexual dysfunctions in husbands are the most common cause for the cessation of intercourse in older couples (see Chapter 2).

INHIBITED ORGASM AND PRETENDING

A number of studies found that not all women consider inhibited orgasm a problem. Many stated they enjoyed intercourse very much, even though they did not reach orgasm (Butler, 1976; Fisher, 1973; M. Hunt, 1974); however, one-third of adolescent girls surveyed by Sorensen (1973) who didn't experience orgasm in sexual relations considered it very important that they did (Chapter 2). Brecher (1984) found that in married couples aged 50 and over, 10% more men and women who experienced orgasm in all or almost all sexual relationships reported being happily married compared to those who did so in half or fewer occasions. The increased likelihood of reaching orgasm could have been a result of the happy marriage, rather than contributing to it; in any case, it was not a major determinant of happy marriages. More than 80% of both men and women who experienced orgasm on half or fewer occasions were also happily married.

Butler (1976) and Steiner (1981) reported that 60% of women stated that they pretended to reach orgasm on some occasions. A similar prevalence was found by Darling and Davidson (1986) in an investigation of 805 professional nurses; 95%

had experienced intercourse, and 58% had pretended to achieve orgasm during it. Of both those who pretended and those who did not, 97% had experienced orgasm; slightly more of those who pretended had experienced orgasm by every form of stimulation, including penetration. The major difference appeared to be in marital status: 82% of widows, 72% of the divorced/separated, 63% of the never married, and 53% of the married had pretended. It is possible that this relationship with marital status reflects the stability of the relationship and hence the degree of the women's concern that it be maintained. As discussed in Chapter 2, older unmarried women have difficulty finding a male partner. Women who wish to maintain a potentially unstable relationship may feel more pressure to pretend to reach orgasm, consistent with their belief (discussed subsequently) that it is important to the male partner that the female partner experiences orgasm in coitus.

Thirty-four percent of those who had pretended felt guilty if they did not experience orgasm, as compared with 21% of those who had not. The most common feeling about pretending, given by 51% of those who had pretended, was "I feel guilty, but it is important I satisfy my partner"; the second, given by 25%, was "I don't like doing it". A number of other differences between the two groups was reported, but most were small, reaching significance only because of the relatively large number of subjects. The authors concluded that many of the women pretended orgasm because they felt trapped, and that therapists should take care not to overemphasize and overvalue the orgasmic experience. They cited with apparent approval Butler's conclusion (1976) that the relatively low frequency with which women experience orgasm during sexual relations needs to be understood as normal behavior, rather than being judged as abnormal by male standards. The authors' ambivalence concerning this issue, however, was reflected by their further statement that women who pretend to reach orgasm were left with congestion of the pelvic blood vessels that could result in backache, irritation, and even chronic vaginal and urinary tract infections.

Steiner (1981) commented that male pretense of orgasm had not been investigated, and found that 36% of male junior-college students reported it. In homosexual relations, most men do not reach orgasm in receptive anal intercourse, and a number report not reaching orgasm by any method in many of their sexual relationships, which they nevertheless enjoy. Women in lesbian relationships appear to attach greater value to hugging and cuddling activities than to genital stimulation resulting in orgasm, as compared to other couples (see Chapter 2).

PREVALENCE OF SEXUAL DYSFUNCTIONS, DIFFICULTIES, AND DISSATISFACTION

Community Studies

The study of Frank et al. (1978) of 100 happily married couples appear to be the only community study to have investigated the prevalence of sexual difficulties and dissatisfaction as well as dysfunctions. Sixty-three percent of the women and 40% of the men reported dysfunctions, and 77% of the women and 50% of the men reported difficulties. Despite the high prevalence of both difficulties and dysfunctions, 85% of both men and women reported that their sexual relations were very or moderately satisfying. In women, the most common dysfunctions were difficulty getting excited (48%) and difficulty reaching orgasm (44%); the most common difficulties were inability to relax (47%), too little foreplay before intercourse (38%), disinterest (35%), partner choosing an inconvenient time (31%), and being turned off (28%). In men, the most common dysfunctions were ejaculating too quickly (36%) and difficulty getting (7%) and maintaining (9%) an erection; the most common difficulties were attraction to persons other than the spouse and too little foreplay before intercourse (21% each), too little tenderness after intercourse (17%), and disinterest and partner choosing an inconvenient time (16% each).

The prevalence of dysfunctions found by Frank et al. were among the highest in over 20 community studies reviewed by Spector and Carey (1990). Unfortunately, few were of representative samples. The reviewers regretted the failure of the National Institute of Mental Health Epidemiologic Catchment Area Program study of the prevalence of psychiatric disorders to provide data concerning the prevalence of specific sexual dysfunctions. That carried out in St. Louis, using Diagnostic Interview Schedules administered by lay interviewers, reported a prevalence of all psychosexual dysfunctions of 24%; this was the second most common diagnosis, after tobacco use disorder. Largely because of a lack of relevant data, Spector and Carey did not report the prevalence of dysfunction in relation to the subjects' age. Age appears to be the most important determinant at least of the major dysfunctions of inhibited female orgasm and male erectile disorders, as demonstrated graphically in Figure 5.1.

In his study of a representative sample of adolescents, Sorensen (1973) found that more than 50% of the girls rarely or never reached orgasm in sexual relationships. This was reported by 25% of women in their first year of marriage, but 11% or less in their 20th year (M. Hunt, 1974, Kinsey et al., 1953). Other studies documenting the increasing percentage of women who experience orgasm in sexual intercourse from adolescence until the mid-40s and its subsequent decline were discussed in Chapter 2.

Of the studies reporting the frequency with which women achieved orgasm in sexual intercourse, only that by Hagstad and Janson (1984) indicated whether orgasm was reached by any form of stimulation or by coitus only. They stated that intercourse could include clitoral stimulation by hand or otherwise. Difficulty in reaching orgasm with masturbation as well as coitus would appear to be prevalent in adolescent girls (see Chapter 2). Less data is available to determine if other female sexual dysfunctions, in addition to inhibited female orgasm, decrease in frequency from adolescence to menopause. Decline in most women's sexual interest appears to commence from the perimenstrual period, but an additional factor of major importance is the presence of a sexually active male partner (Chapter 2). In an investigation of a representative sample of 497 women living with their husbands, hypoactive sexual desire disorder (i.e., absence of sexual desire) was reported by 4% of those aged 38, 3% of those aged 46, 9% of those aged 50, and 21% of those aged 54 (Hallstrom & Samuelsson, 1990). At follow-up 6 years later, the prevalence in the four groups was 0%, 7%, 16%, and 29%, respectively—a significant increase in the

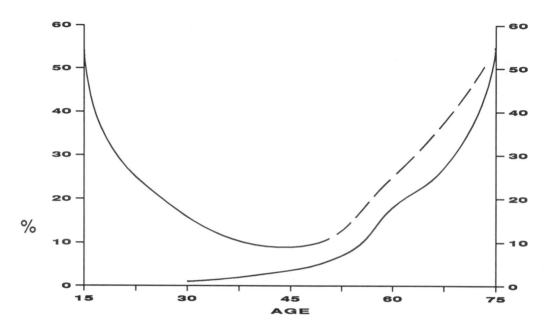

FIG. 5.1. Left-hand graph: percentage of women not experiencing orgasm in sexual relations; right-hand graph: percentage of men totally impotent.

older women. The community studies reviewed by Spector and Carey (1990) reported prevalence of female sexual arousal disorder of 11% to 48%; of hypoactive sexual disorder, 34%; and of dyspareunia, 8% to 23%.

Prevalence rates in community studies of men for complete inability to attain erection, were 1% at age 30, 2% at age 40, 7% at age 50, 18% at age 60, 27% at age 70, 55% at age 75, and 76% at age 80 (Kinsey et al., 1948; Weizman & Hart, 1987); the prevalence of their difficulty in achieving erection without manual stimulation of the penis, experienced with increasing age, does not appear to have been documented. Prevalence rates for premature ejaculation were 36% to 38%; for hypoactive sexual desire disorder, 16%; and for inhibited male orgasm, 1% to 10% (Spector & Carey, 1990). Inhibited male orgasm may range from inhibition on some to all occasions of coitus.

Though 4% of the men studied by Frank et al. (1978) reported difficulty in ejaculating, none reported inability. Difficulty ejaculating was reported by 10% of men in a Swedish (Nettelbladt & Uddenberg, 1979) and 16% of men in a U.K. study (Reading & Weist, 1984). M. Hunt (1974) was critical of the statement by Kinsey et al. (1948) that husbands achieved orgasm in virtually 100% of their occasions of marital coitus, pointing out that the Kinsey study did not obtain detailed data concerning this. In Hunt's study, 15% of men aged under 25 years missed orgasm on at least 25% of occasions. Hunt considered this to be attributable in most cases to erectile failure produced by anxiety, and in some to attempts being made too soon after having reached orgasm previously. Twenty-one percent of the adolescent boys in

Sorensen's study (1973) had masturbated in the previous month without reaching orgasm. No community studies appear to have investigated the prevalence of sexual dysfunctions in homosexual activities.

Lack of Interest in Seeking Help

Only a small percentage of subjects with sexual dysfunctions seek treatment for them. A community sample of 436 women in the United Kingdom (Osborn, Hawton, & Gath, 1988) revealed that 142 reported at least one of four operationally defined dysfunctions: impaired sexual interest (17%), vaginal dryness (17%), infrequency of orgasm (16%), and dyspareunia (8%). Only 32 of the 142 considered that they had a sexual problem, as did a further 10 with no dysfunctions. Of the total of 42 who believed they had a problem, 16 said they desired treatment if it was available; only 1 was receiving it.

Catania, Pollack, McDermott, Qualls, & Cole (1990) investigated a community sample of 458 women and 54 men, of whom more than 80% were recruited at "pleasure parties" in the California Bay Area. (The authors explained that pleasure parties were similar to Tupperware parties, except that the items being sold were sexual in nature.) Forty-three percent reported problems that currently reduced their or their partner's sexual satisfaction; 7.5% of those with problems were having specific therapy for them (4%, marital therapy, 3% psychotherapy; and 0.5% medical sexual therapy). Twenty-six percent had received specific therapy for the problems in the past. Fourteen percent were receiving and 28% had received nonsexual psychotherapy. There was little difference in the amount of specific sexual treatment the subjects who reported the problems were receiving or had received, as compared to the total group. The greatest difference was that 14% of those with the problems, compared to 8% of the total sample, were receiving nonsexual psychotherapy. The authors did not investigate whether this psychotherapy was in part aimed at improving the sexual problems, or indeed if the therapists were aware of them.

Psychotherapists usually do not enquire about sexual problems. If they did they would presumably have to treat them, and in view of their prevalence, would have less time to treat other problems that they—and, hopefully, the patients—consider to be more important. Therapists influenced by psychoanalytic theory do not consider the reality of sexual behavior in itself important, but rather how it is incorporated in the patient's inner fantasy life, which should be the focus of treatment (Malcolm, 1984). Though the presence of problems impairing sexual satisfaction in the subjects studied by Catania et al. (1990) appeared to have little influence on their seeking professional help, most who reported them had sought nonprofessional help for them, mainly from intimates and friends.

Catania et al. pointed out that men and subjects over 50 years of age were underrepresented in their study, but the majority of these subjects also appear not to seek help for sexual problems. Of 1,080 men attending a medical outpatient clinic, 401 on questioning admitted to having erectile dysfunction (Slag et al., 1983); prior to the inquiry, only 6 had been identified as having the dysfunction. The authors commented that the subjects were reluctant to call attention to their dysfunction but were eager to discuss and seek evaluation for it when the physicians broached the topic. In fact only 188, slightly less than half, accepted the offer of evaluation. Their mean age was 59 years; the mean age of those who refused evaluation was 67 years.

Other workers have found older men with sexual dysfunctions to be satisfied with their sexual life (see Chapter 2). Martin (1981) reported that of 188 60- to 79-year-old male volunteers of a Baltimore study of aging, only 10% of the 88 with potency problems had sought medical advice for the condition. He suggested that the majority were uninterested because of low sexual motivation. Buvat, Lemaire, Buvat-Herbaut, Guieu, et al., (1985) found that none of 26 impotent diabetics aged 21 to 55 years reported the dysfunction until they were directly questioned concerning it. Ende, Rockwell, and Glasgow (1984) investigated the 51% of male and 55% of female patients who were found to have sexual problems when they completed a checklist after attending a Boston university medical outpatient clinic. Lack of sexual desire was reported by 27% of women and 13% of men; lack of orgasm by 25% and painful intercourse by 20% of women; and premature ejaculation by 14% and impotence by 12% of men. Forty-three percent of the male and 21% of female patients reported that the doctor had not discussed their sexual functioning. The study was part of an investigation of the effect of training doctors in taking a medical history, of which the doctors were presumably aware. If this was the case, it is likely that more of the doctors discussed the patients' sexual functioning with them than would under usual circumstances.

Subjects Seeking Professional Help

As Spector and Carey (1990) pointed out, the prevalence of dysfunctions in subjects who seek professional help may not reflect the prevalence in the population. Community conceptions that particular disorders can be effectively treated could be expected to lead more subjects with those disorders to present for treatment; LoPiccolo (1978) noted a marked increase in the number of subjects with sexual dysfunctions who sought treatment following the media attention given the publication of *Human Sexual Inadequacy* (Masters & Johnson, 1970). Such conceptions are also likely to influence the type of clinic chosen to provide help. Segraves, Schoenberg, Zarins, Camic, and Knopf (1981) compared impotent men who self-referred to different clinics. Eighty-nine percent of those who attended a sexual dysfunction clinic, as compared with 57% of those who attended a urology clinic, were considered to have psychogenic rather than organic impotence. The authors concluded that the prevalence of causes of impotence reported in different studies will vary depending on the type of clinic where the subjects were identified; however, marked differences have been found in patients attending what appear to be similar clinics. Rates of psychiatric disorder in subjects presenting to sex clinics varied from 14% in 2,367 members of 1,188 couples (Renshaw, 1988) to 34% in male presenters and 50% in female presenters of 200 couples (Catalan, Hawton, & Day, 1990).

In the literature reviewed by Spector and Carey (1990), the prevalences of sexual dysfunctions diagnosed by practitioners mainly paralleled those reported in community studies. In women, prevalence of hypoactive sexual desire, and of sexual arousal and inhibited orgasm disorders were fairly equivalent, and markedly higher than that of dyspareunia. Snyder and Berg (1983a) found about 70% of women patients reported the former three dysfunctions and 20%, dyspareunia. Spector and Casey (1990) suggested, however, that women may interpret pain as a medical symptom and seek help for this from a general practitioner or gynecologist, citing a finding that dyspareunia was a common problem reported to medical practitioners.

Though premature ejaculation is the most common dysfunction found in community studies of men other than the elderly, Spector and Carey found erectile disorder to be the most common complaint in subjects seeking treatment in the 1970s. It was reported by about 40%, whereas 20% reported premature ejaculation. The erectile disorder reported was usually secondary or acquired, with primary or lifelong erectile disorder being infrequent. Inhibited male orgasm was also infrequent, being reported by less than 8% of subjects. Spector and Carey concluded that complaints of hypoactive sexual desire in men increased markedly in the 1980s, reaching more than 50% and outnumbering the percentage of women with this complaint in some studies. This increased prevalence may have reflected lack of representativeness of the few studies available for their review; it was not reported in two recent studies they did not review, which investigated subjects who presented to university sex and marital therapy clinics. Catalan et al. (1990) found that 13 of 113 dysfunctional men suffered impaired sexual interest, compared with 62 with erectile dysfunction and 26 with premature ejaculation. Seventy-two of the 117 dysfunctional women reported impaired sexual interest. Stuart, Hammond, and Pett (1987) stated that they restricted their investigation of inhibited sexual desire to women because of the limited number of men who reported it.

ETIOLOGY

In investigating the etiology of sexual problems, most attention has been given to sexual dysfunctions, though as pointed out earlier, they showed much weaker correlations with men and women's dissatisfaction in heterosexual relations than did the problems related to the emotional tone of their relationships (termed "sexual difficulties" by Frank et al., 1978). The nature of these difficulties—inability to relax, being turned off, too little foreplay before and too little tenderness after intercourse, and the partner choosing an inconvenient time—strongly suggests that poor communication concerning sexual needs is the major factor involved. Correlations were found between poor sexual communication and sexual dissatisfaction (Snyder & Berg, 1983a) and poor marital relationships (Brecher, 1984; Rust et al., 1988).

Organic Causes of Erectile Dysfunction and Male Hypoactive Sexual Desire

In regard to the etiology of male dysfunctions, the most significant change in recent years has been the reversal of the belief that most cases of impotence were attributable to psychological rather than organic factors (LoPiccolo, 1982). Given the lack of adequate community studies of impotence, however, the data are not available to justify either the original belief or its reversal. The original belief that most cases of impotence were caused psychologically was established not by data but by the ideologically determined conviction, strongly held in the United States throughout most of this century (see Chapter 1; McConaghy, 1987b), that behavior was determined entirely by environmental events. The associated refusal to consider that biological factors could be involved led, in regard to impotence, to failure to consider the considerable evidence indicating that they were. The marked increase of prevalence of impotence with age, demonstrated in Figure 5.1, strongly suggested that biological factors associated with aging were etiologically significant.

Frequency of Sexual Activity

Martin (1981) reviewed studies indicating that the frequencies of current sexual activity reported by men in their 40s and older were highly related to the frequencies they reported of their activities in their adolescence and early adulthood. He found this to be the case also in the 60- to 79-year-old men he studied. As experiential factors could be expected to have varied markedly over the subjects' lives, these findings suggest that the frequencies of men's sexual activities throughout their postpubertal lives are largely biologically determined. If this is so, the biological factors involved would seem to be also involved in determining the prevalence of sexual dysfunctions, independent of the important effect of aging. In regard to his elderly subjects' level of sexual activity throughout their lives, Martin found that 75% of the least active, 46% of the moderately active, and 19% of the most active were partially or totally impotent; 21% of the least active, as compared with 8% of the most active, had experienced a long-term problem with premature ejaculation.

Testosterone

The obvious biological factor to be considered as etiological in men's sexual dysfunctions is the major androgen or male sex hormone, testosterone. Almost all testosterone in men is produced by the male gonads or testes. Centuries of experience with removal of the testes (i.e., castration) established that male sexuality, human and animal, was largely dependent on their integrity. Awareness that a chemical they contained was involved has been at least suspected for a hundred years following the report of the physiologist Brown-Sequard of the effect of injections of testicular extract on his own behavior (T. Jones, 1985). Davidson, Kwan, and Greenleaf (1982) emphasized the wonder the clinician experienced in observing the transformation of a hypogonadal male from a eunuchoid state to one of renewed sexuality with administration of testosterone. They pointed out that testosterone appeared to stimulate all the major elements of the hypogonadal man's sexuality—libido, frequency of sexual activity, erectile potency, and ejaculatory capacity. (The term *libido* is usually employed to include such cognitive factors as sexual interest, drive, and pleasure.) In making these observations, Davidson et al. raised an issue that most other researchers have ignored: whether testosterone supports erectile potency directly, or indirectly by maintaining libido and ejaculatory capacity.

As discussed in Chapter 2, a number of studies in the 1980s, unlike some in the 1970s, found relationships between healthy men's sexual interest and their serum levels of testosterone within the normal range. The findings of the 1980s studies, however, are frequently rejected in favor of the negative earlier findings. Schiavi, Thielgaard, et al. (1988) decided there was no convincing evidence that differences in testosterone levels within the normal range were related to sexual behavior in men, though they found this relationship in their investigation of 26 men with chromosomal abnormalities and 52 matched normal controls. The subjects' testosterone levels were negatively related to age at first intercourse, and positively related to number of sexual partners, frequency of extramarital experiences, and unconventional sexual behaviors. Workers who accepted that a relationship did exist were conflicted concerning whether it was significantly stronger for free rather than bound testosterone (see Chapter 2). The relationships found between testosterone levels and sexual behaviors in healthy men in the 1980s studies have also been found in men with sexual problems. Testosterone levels correlated with sexual interest in impotent men (Segraves, Schoenberg, & Ivanoff, 1983), with frequency of intercourse attempts and masturbatory experiences in men with hypoactive sexual desire (Schiavi, Schreiner-Engel, White, & Mandeli, 1988), and with number of ejaculations and frequency of erections in men with hypogonadism (Salminies, Kockott, Pirke, Vogt, & Schill, 1982).

The lack of consistency in the studies investigating relationships between men's sexual activity and their levels of testosterone within the normal range suggest that if the relationship is present, it is weak. The contrary is true of the relationship between men's sexual activity and levels of testosterone that are below normal, or indeed those that remain within normal limits when they are reduced chemically. As discussed above, Davidson et al. (1982) remarked on the dramatic increase in the previously minimal or absent sexual interest of hypogonadal men when they were administered testosterone. In a double-blind study, Davidson, Camargo, and Smith (1979) demonstrated that the increase was not a placebo effect attributable to suggestion or expectancy of improvement. They treated 6 hypogonadal men with pituitary tumors or testicular atrophy, all of whom had serum testosterone levels less than 1.5 ng/ml (the normal range for this assay was 3–10 ng/ml). Following injections of either 100 or 400 mg of testosterone enanthate, 5 of the 6 men showed significant increases in frequency of erections and of coitus and in intensity of orgasms, as compared with their response to placebo injections. The increases were greater following the larger dose. Skakkebaek, Bancroft, Davidson, and Warner (1981) provided further evidence that increase in sexual interest was a result of testosterone administration. Cessation of its administration to 6 hypogonadal men resulted in reduction of their sexual activity and an increase in erectile problems.

Is the Level of Testosterone Required the Same for All Men? It appears that the level of serum testosterone required to maintain normal sexual interest and possibly erectile function varies for individual men, so that in some it may be above what is considered the lower level of the normal range of 3–10 ng/ml. Takefman and Brender (1984) found that of 15 men with erectile dysfunction whose testosterone levels were within normal limits, the 7 who failed to respond to psychological therapy had levels significantly below those of the 8 who showed a successful outcome. Salmimies et al. (1982) found the lower threshold in hypogonadal men to vary between 2 and 4.5 ng/ml; some with levels of above 3 ng/ml showed reduced frequency of erections and ejaculations, which increased in response to administration of testosterone. Reduction in the sexual interest of sex offenders correlated highly with the degree of reduction in their testosterone levels produced by medroxyprogesterone, even though in a number of the subjects the levels remained within the normal range (McConaghy et al., 1988).

These findings suggest that though all men with testosterone levels below 3 ng/ml are hypogonadal and will benefit from testosterone administration, some of those with higher levels who show impaired sexual activity are also hypogonadal. As it is not possible to know what the normal testosterone levels of hypogonadal men are, it is only possible to determine which men are hypogonadal by giving them all a trial of testosterone administration. To establish or refute this possibility would require a prolonged research study involving large subject numbers. A further complication in such research is that some subjects whose sexual dysfunctions are primarily organic develop secondary psychological dysfunctions resulting from conditioning of the anxiety produced by their impaired sexual performance. Their failure to respond to testosterone administration does not mean that their dysfunction was not originally produced by low testosterone.

Testosterone, Erectile Potency, and Sexual Interest. The issue raised by Davidson et al. (1982) as to whether abnormally low levels of testosterone directly reduce only sexual interest or also impair erectile potency remains unresolved. Davidson originally stated that it was not possible to distinguish between changes in libido and potency (Davidson et al., 1979); however, he appeared to abandon this opinion in a study with other colleagues that reported the presence of erectile problems associated with low testosterone levels (Skakkebaek et al., 1981). The erectile problems were considered not to result directly from the low testosterone levels, but to be secondary to the reduced sexual interest consequent on the low levels. It was suggested that the reduced interest could have produced anxiety about successful sexual performance that in turn produced the erectile difficulties. This possibility would seem difficult either to establish or to refute.

Davidson and his colleagues questioned whether reduced testosterone levels directly produced erectile dysfunction in order to account for observations that following castration men have been reported to maintain sexual activity including coitus for many years, and that a small number of castrated and hypogonadal men showed erectile responses to erotic films not significantly different from those of normal controls or from their own responses when given testosterone (Davidson et al., 1982). Davidson suggested that testosterone maintained a pleasurable awareness of sexual thoughts and activity that secondarily stimulated erectile ability. In the absence of this pleasurable awareness, erections could still occur, but only if directly driven by strong visual, tactile, or cognitive stimuli. Castrated men could therefore generate erections to satisfy their partner, but spontaneous erections would tend to be absent. This theory led Davidson to suggest that erections occurring in the absence of adequate levels of testosterone would not be associated with pleasurable genital sensations and that in the absence of these sensations, hypogonadal and castrated men would often perceive their deficient sexual capacities as being problems with erection.

Davidson, Camargo, Smith, and Kwan (1983) investigated a castrated man who maintained satisfying coitus while taking a combination of estrogen and progestin.

When testosterone was substituted in a double-blind trial, he experienced a high frequency of spontaneous erections but loss of sexual interest. This finding suggests that testosterone has direct effects on erectile ability independent of the level of sexual interest, at least in some hypogonadal men. Davidson et al. (1982) doubted that the erections of hypogonadal men could lack rigidity. They questioned the beliefs of Karacan and other workers that full penile circumference increases may be present without sufficient rigidity for penetration, and stated that it was not established that lack of rigidity was a frequent cause of sexual failure. In contradistinction, Slag et al. (1983) reported that nearly half of the impotent men they investigated stated that they developed erections both in relation to sexual stimulation and spontaneously, but that the erections were of inadequate turgidity for coitus. In my experience, this complaint of inadequate rigidity of erections is commonly reported by impotent patients. More information concerning the nature of the erectile ability of castrated men appears required, including its association with pleasurable sensations.

Testosterone and Sexual Interest. Whether or not potency is maintained primarily or secondarily by testosterone, it is incontrovertible that the testosterone level required for normal erections is well below that required to maintain normal sexual interest, at least in younger men. This was demonstrated when the level was reduced by androgen-suppressing chemicals. Intramuscular administration of 150mg of medroxyprogesterone fortnightly reduced treated subjects' serum testosterone levels to an average of 30% of their pretreatment levels, producing in many subjects levels well below the lower range of normal (McConaghy et al., 1988). The effect in 14 of 16 subjects was a lowering of sexual interest without impairing the quality or associated sensations of their erections. The majority of the 14 reported that their frequency and enjoyment of intercourse was unchanged. Two subjects reported difficulty maintaining adequate erections; both had levels lowered to 16% or less of their pretreatment levels.

Testosterone levels of prostate cancer patients were lowered to 5% of pretreatment levels by combined administration of an LHRH agonist and a pure antiandrogen (Rousseau, Dupont, Labrie, & Couture, 1988). Before treatment, 93% of subjects desired and 80% were having intercourse once a week or more. During treatment, only 21% continued to desire this frequency of intercourse, and only 10% achieved it. In all, 38% continued to desire some frequency of intercourse but only 20% continued it, indicating that inability to have intercourse attributable to erectile failure in the presence of sexual interest was the reason in some subjects. This conclusion was supported by the report that prior to treatment, 56% of the subjects reported no difficulty in maintaining erections; following treatment, only 19% reported this. Loss of penile rigidity was reported by 36%. Salmimies et al. (1982) administered testosterone to 15 hypogonadal men. No details of the erectile ability of the subjects were given, but one with a very low testosterone level who reported no ejaculations prior to treatment and had not undergone puberty reported erections with testosterone administration. This finding suggests that in this subject, erections were produced for the first time following testosterone administration and so were testosterone dependent. It is possible that testosterone or other androgens do have a direct action in maintaining erectile ability, but that the level required for this action in most subjects is well below that necessary to maintain normal sexual interest.

Testosterone and Potency. As in most younger men, at least, sexual activity is maintained by their normal level of testosterone through its effect on sexual interest, not potency, only at somewhat lower levels could it be involved in the etiology of impotence. As levels below the normal range have usually been reported to be uncommon in impotent men, most cases of impotence are considered to be attributable to other causes. Schwartz, Kolodny, and Masters (1980) compared 341 sexually dysfunctional men and 199 sexually functional men who accompanied their sexually dysfunctional partners to a clinic for sexual dysfunctions. There was no significant difference in mean serum testosterone levels of the two groups. Post hoc comparison of subgroups with different dysfunctions revealed no differences apart from those with lifelong or primary impotence, who showed significantly lower testosterone levels. T. Jones (1985) suggested that findings of reduced testosterone levels in impotent men could be attributed to failure to allow for the decline in testosterone levels that commonly occurred with aging. As discussed in Chapter 2, there is conflicting evidence concerning whether this decline occurs in healthy elderly men and, if so, whether it could be partially responsible for the reduction in sexual activity that accompanies aging.

In contradistinction to the evidence of Schwartz et al. (1980) that testosterone levels were rarely a significant determinant of impotence, a study claiming the reverse published in the Journal of the American Medical Association (Spark, White, & Connolly, 1980) appeared to be highly influential in reversing the belief that impotence was usually produced by psychological rather than biological factors. The study investigated 105 impotent men, the majority of whom were under 50 years of age. Reduced serum testosterone levels (3.5 ng/ml or below) were found in 34, and other hormonal abnormalities of the hypothalamic-pituitary-gonadal axis in a further 3. Therapy to normalize the levels restored potency in 33 the of the 37. The authors stated that their findings led them to reconsider the concept that impotence was psychogenic in 95% of cases, and to conclude that the role of hormonal abnormalities was substantially greater than was recognized. The impact of their finding was greatly enhanced by the addition of case histories of subjects who had been treated with psychotherapy for some years without investigation of symptoms or signs they showed suggestive of hormonal abnormalities. These included a history of a pituitary tumor; small, soft testes; loss of body hair; and lack of beard growth.

The disparity between the conclusion of Spark et al. that hormonal abnormalities could be expected to be present in a significant number of impotent men, and the finding of Schwartz et al. (1980) that the testosterone levels in men with secondary impotence were normal, could have been attributable to differences in the nature of the subjects they studied. Those investigated by Spark et al. (1980) were referrals to a medical department: 16 of the 37 impotent subjects with hormonal abnormalities had pituitary tumors, 2 had other cerebral tumors; and 12 were noted to have small or soft testes. The high percentage with cerebral tumors suggests that the medical clinic was somewhat specialized to deal with such problems, so that the subjects could have represented a special sample of the total population of impotent men. Subjects in the study of Schwartz et al. (1980) sought treatment at the Masters and Johnson institute and could represent a different but equally nonrepresentative group. The mean age of the subjects studied by Spark et al. was 42 years, and that of those studied by Schwartz et al. was 40 years. The subjects in neither study could be considered representative of the majority of impotent men who are aged over 60 years. As reported earlier, the prevalence of total impotence increases with age, being present in about 2% of men aged 40, 20% of men aged 60, and 55% of men aged 75.

The subjects in the study of Slag et al. (1983), though consisting of men attending a medical clinic, could be regarded as more representative of the total population of impotent men. As stated previously, only 6 of the 1,180 men interviewed in the study had been identified as suffering from impotence, but 401 (34%) reported it on direct questioning. The mean age for both the impotent and nonimpotent subjects was 61 years, so that the percentage who were impotent was reasonably similar to (less than double) what would be expected in a representative sample of the normal population; hypogonadism was found in 19% of those evaluated. Determination of the significance of hormonal factors in the etiology of impotence requires investigation of representative community samples of men with impotence diagnosed according to defined criteria.

Diagnostic Criteria for Impotence. The need for definition of the criteria used to diagnose impotence in research studies was apparent in regard to the conflicting findings of the studies by Spark et al. (1980) and those discussed earlier. All 105 subjects investigated by Spark et al. were described as suffering from impotence. This was attributed in 34 to their reduced testosterone levels, which were around the lower limit of the normal range. Findings discussed earlier indicated that many subjects with testosterone levels somewhat below the normal range reported reduced sexual interest and frequency of spontaneous erections, but not impaired erectile ability; with appropriate physical stimulation, they obtained erections adequate for coitus. Others whose testosterone levels were reduced to markedly below the normal range did report inadequate erections.

It is possible that the nature of the erectile dysfunctions of subjects in all the studies, including that of Spark et al., were similar. Those with reductions in testosterone levels slightly below normal and who showed infrequent but adequate erections (produced by manual stimulation if necessary because of reduced sexual interest) may have been diagnosed as impotent by Spark et al., whereas those with marked reductions in testosterone levels and inadequate erections were considered by Davidson et al. (1982) to be not primarily impotent. Their sexual difficulties were attributed to their markedly reduced or absent sexual interest. Some men who had full erections that were inadequate for coitus as a result of reduced rigidity may not have been diagnosed as impotent by Davidson, in view of his belief that lack of rigidity was not an established cause of sexual failure (Davidson et al., 1982).

To determine if this interpretation was correct (that different diagnostic criteria accounted for the different results reported in these studies), it would be necessary to know the criteria used. When the criteria are reported, degree of rigidity of erections and the method of its determination should be included. Few workers have followed Karacan (1978) in directly assessing the rigidity of subjects' erections, and many may not question the subject concerning this. Nevertheless, lack of rigidity has been attributed significance by most investigators other than Davidson (Rousseau et al., 1988; Slag et al., 1983). No attention appears to have been paid to the possibility that differences in the genital anatomy in addition to the psychological attitude of the partners of impotent men could produce differences in ease of penetration, resulting in some men succeeding in coitus and others not when the degree of rigidity of their erections are the same. If this is established to occur, it would seem worthy of investigation when men's impotence is being assessed.

Testosterone and Hypoactive Sexual Desire. As markedly higher levels of testosterone are required to maintain sexual interest as compared with potency, it could be expected that some men with hypoactive sexual desire without erectile dysfunction would show reduced serum testosterone levels. Schwartz et al. (1980) did not report any subjects with hypoactive sexual desire in their study of 341 nonhypogonadal men who presented to a sex clinic with sexual dysfunctions. O'Carroll and Bancroft (1984) investigated 10 men with low sexual interest not secondary to erectile failure and 10 with erectile difficulties not secondary to loss of sexual interest. All had levels of testosterone within the normal range, but the levels of the group with erectile dysfunction were significantly lower than the levels of those with reduced sexual interest. Schiavi et al. (1988), however, found that the mean nocturnal testosterone levels of 17 physically healthy men with hypoactive sexual desire were significantly lower than those of age-matched nondysfunctional controls. Also, reduction in current sexual interest of 56 impotent men correlated with reduced serum testosterone levels, which in 9 were below the lower limit of the normal range (Segraves et al., 1983).

Apart from this conflict concerning whether reduced testosterone levels are associated with hypoactive sexual desire, other issues await resolution by studies of larger and more representative community samples. These include whether the reduction in testosterone level that occurs with age is restricted to the unhealthy or whether, if found in the healthy, it plays a role in the reduction in sexual interest and increase in impotence both groups show with aging. Also, further support is required for the conclusion of T. Jones (1985) that in the absence of loss of libido or the physical signs of regression of male hair pattern, gynecomastia (increased breast development) or small, soft testes, the testosterone levels in impotent men under the age of 50 years is almost invariably in the normal range.

Prolactin

Seven of the men diagnosed as impotent in the study of Spark et al. (1980) who had low testosterone levels, and 1 with a normal level, showed hyperprolactinemia (HPRL), raised levels of the pituitary hormone prolactin. Other studies also found HPRL to be usually associated with low levels of testosterone, leading to the suggestion that it was the low testosterone levels rather than HPRL that were responsible for the accompanying impotence. Buvat, Lemaire, Buvat-Herbaut, Fourlinnie, et al. (1985), however, argued against this on the basis of earlier findings that the potency of some subjects with HPRL did not return with normalization of their testosterone levels by testosterone administration, but did when their prolactin levels were normalized by bromocriptine.

The findings of their own study supported their conclusion. They treated 10 subjects who showed marked HPRL (above 35 ng/ml) and who made up 1% of the 850 men diagnosed as impotent from 1,053 men consecutively referred for sexual dysfunctions who did not show obvious organic causes (drugs, apparent endocrinopathies, diabetes, neuropathy, and arthritis). Five of the 10 subjects with marked HPRL had testosterone levels within the normal range (3–10 ng/ml), and 6 showed radiologic evidence of a pituitary adenoma. Response of the 10 correlated better with the therapeutically produced reduction of prolactin levels than with the accompanying change in testosterone levels. A further 17 (2%) of the 850 showed mildly raised prolactin levels (20–35 ng/ml). Prolactin levels were normal in the 27 with pure reduced sexual desire.

In regard to the significance of mild HPLT, Buvat, Lemaire, Buvat-Herbaut, Fourlinnie, et al. cited other studies reporting its presence in 2% to 16% of subjects with impotence. None of their subjects with mild HPLT showed testosterone levels below normal or pituitary adenomas, and only 40% showed improved potency following lowering of their prolactin levels to normal. The authors cited a study reporting a 40% response to placebo treatment in impotence and concluded that the mild HPRL in their subjects was not the cause of their impotence but the consequence of the emotional disturbance associated with it.

Thyroid Dysfunction

Two of the 37 impotent patients with hormonal abnormalities reported by Spark et al. (1980) had above-normal testosterone and thyroid hormone levels. The latter levels were consistent with the diagnosis of hyperthyroidism but were not accompanied in either subject by overt signs of the condition, though both had small palpable goiters. When their thyroid function was returned to normal with propylthiouracil, their testosterone levels also fell to within the normal range, and their potency was restored. Spark et al. stated that the increased testosterone levels noted in hyperthyroid patients were not a reflection of increased testosterone production, but an artifact of the increase in production of the protein testosterone-binding globulin that occurs in this disease.

Spark et al. pointed out that hyperthyroidism is not generally considered to cause impotence. They cited a study of 7 consecutive hyperthyroid men (Kidd, Glass, & Vigersky, 1979) in which 4 reported diminution of libido and potency and 1 of libido only. Four of the 5 had serum testosterone levels of over 10 ng/mg. Spark et al. concluded that in impotent patients, elevated serum testosterone levels could be considered a biochemical marker for possible occult hyperthyroidism. In view of the reluctance of most men to report impotence, it could be present in a number of medical conditions without the physician knowing. Impotence was attributed to hyperthyroidism in 1% and to hypothyroidism in 4% of the older medical outpatients evaluated by Slag et al. (1983).

Diabetes

Diabetes, usually accompanied by neurological and vascular complications, was present in 9% of the subjects evaluated by Slag et al. Buvat, Lemaire, Buvat-Herbaut, Guieu, et al. (1985) noted that impotence was present in more than 50% of diabetic men 10 years after onset of the condition and did not result from poor control of the diabetes; that attributable to poor control was temporary and improved when control was attained. Jensen (1981) compared 80 insulin-treated diabetic men with 40 age-matched controls who consecutively attended a general practitioner. Thirty-five of the diabetic men and 5 of the controls reported sexual dysfunctions, mainly erectile dysfunction and reduced libido in the diabetics and premature ejaculation in the controls. Of the complications of diabetes, peripheral neuropathy was found to correlate significantly with the presence of sexual dysfunctions in the diabetic men.

Buvat, Lemaire, Buvat-Herbaut, Fourlinnie, et al. (1985) like Jensen found no hormonal abnormalities to account for persistent diabetic impotence. To determine other possible causes, they investigated 26 potent and 26 impotent diabetics, using Doppler assessment of the penile vascular supply, measurement of motor and sensory conduction velocities of peripheral nerves, urine flow estimation of urinary autonomic and sensory motor nerve status, and bulbocavernous reflex latency evaluation of sensory motor nerves of the penis. Mean scores of both groups showed abnormalities particularly in the penile vascular supply, but only urine flow rate significantly discriminated the two groups. Twenty-four of the 26 impotent diabetics, but only 2 of the 26 who were potent, showed flow rates of less than 18mm per second. The authors commented that the differences were so clear-cut that they wondered if they were specific for a pelvic neuropathic condition or whether they resulted from a psychosomatic mechanism associated with impotence.

To investigate the latter possibility, these workers assessed the urine flow of impotent nondiabetics and found it to be reduced in 43%. They concluded that specific psychological factors might reduce the urine flow in impotent men, but the much higher percentage of the diabetic impotent men who showed reduce flow indicated that many of them suffered from a slight abnormality of the pelvic autonomic system. The authors found that the impotent diabetics also differed significantly from the potent diabetics on psychological assessment, and though they accepted that these differences could be in part attributable to an emotional response to their impotence, they believed the impotent group showed a special psychological frailty. It would seem reasonable, as Jensen (1981) suggested, that psychological and organic predisposing factors interact to produce impotence.

Other Organic Causes of Erectile Dysfunction

It does not appear that any studies have comprehensively evaluated community samples of impotent men to determine the causes of their condition. As discussed earlier, the 401 men who reported impotence on direct questioning (Slag et al., 1983), though they were medical outpatients, would appear to be the most representative group investigated. Of the 188 who agreed to evaluation, 14% were considered to have a psychological cause. Hormonal abnormalities were the most common organic cause; reduced serum testosterone, HPRL, hyper- and hypothyroidism, or diabetes was present in 38%. Another 25% were attributed to effects of wide variety of medications, those most often implicated being diuretics, antihypertensives, and vasodilators. Neurological causes were diagnosed in 7%, urological causes in 6%, and other medical conditions in 4%; no organic cause was found in 7%. Interestingly, Slag et al. found that the prevalence of alcoholism in the impotent men was far lower than in the nonimpotent men but similar to that in the general population. The majority of the men with impotence reported a gradual onset of the condition with continuance of their normal libido. Nearly half of those without diabetes or HPRL were having erections either in relation to sexual stimulation or spontaneously, but in almost all cases, the erections were of inadequate turgidity for coitus.

Slag et al. found that a number of patients who experienced impotence with medications had stopped taking them, but were hesitant to tell their physician why they had and hence were often considered noncompliant. Segraves, Madsen, Carter, and Davis (1985) reviewed the literature reporting associations of pharmacological agents with erectile dysfunction, listing (along with antihypertensive agents) drugs used in psychiatric treatment, including major and minor tranquilizers, monoamine oxidase inhibitors, and tricyclic antidepressants, as well as a long list of other medications and drugs of abuse. They pointed out that the paucity of adequately designed studies in this area made definitive statements about the significance of the associations impossible, but that the number of such reports suggested that male sexual function was highly susceptible to interference from commonly prescribed drugs.

There appears little evidence from surveys of impotent men to support the common clinical observation that alcohol is an important contributing factor (Tsitouras et al., 1982). The finding of Slag et al. (1983), reported above, appeared to support the contrary conclusion. Surveys of men suffering from alcoholism have found prevalences of sexual dysfunctions, mainly impotence or loss of libido, ranging from 8% to 70% (Fahrner, 1987). The significance of the findings is difficult to determine in view of the absence of age-matched healthy controls and the lack of defined diagnostic criteria for impotence. In Fahrner's own study, there was no difference in the incidence of sexual dysfunctions in the 22 subjects who had relapsed and the 58 who were abstinent 9 months following a 4-month inpatient treatment program for alcoholic addiction. Certainly alcoholism could be expected to increase the likelihood of impotence, as it can produce neuropathies, liver damage leading to an increase in estrogens, and testicular damage. Erectile potency appears highly susceptible not only to drugs but to interference from a wide variety of neurological conditions (Mancall, Alonso, & Marlowe, 1985). As discussed previously, the impotence associated with diabetes would appear to be often attributable to the damage to the nervous system produced by the disease.

The absence of any cases of impotence specifically attributed to vascular pathology in the study of Slag et al. (1983) appears inconsistent with the significance attributed to this condition by other workers. Slag et al. did not report their subjects' penile blood pressure index (PBI)—the ratio of their penile to brachial systolic blood pressure—and may not have determined this. Gewertz and Zarins (1985) considered that vascular occlusive disease was too frequently overlooked as a cause of impotence in middle-aged and older patients, and they recommended PBI screening to avoid this. Virag, Bouilly, and Frydman (1985) investigated 440 impotent French men of mean age 47 years for the presence of four factors increasing the risk of arterial disease, diabetes, smoking, hyperlipidemia, and hypertension, in addition to assessing their PBI. Smoking, diabetes, and hyperlipidemia but not hypertension were significantly more common in the impotent men as compared with French men of similar age. Ninety-two percent of the impotent men over 40 years of age had at least one and usually two risk factors.

Virag et al. concluded that much of the increase in impotence with age is associated with arteriosclerotic changes in the arteries and cavernous tissue of the penis. Unless PBI screening is performed following mild exertion by the subject, it may not detect cases of the colorfully named "pelvic steal syndrome" produced by iliac artery pathology. This can result in blood being shunted from the pelvic region to the musculature of the lower extremities when these muscles become active in coital thrusting, producing loss of erection following penetration. Erectile failure at this stage of coitus has been commonly attributed to psychological factors (Segraves, Schoenberg, & Segraves, 1985b).

Wabrek and Burchell (1980) found that two-thirds of men hospitalized for myocardial infarction reported a sexual problem, predominantly impotence, prior to the infarction. Possibly because of the then-current belief that almost all sexual problems were psychologically caused, they considered the infarction to be second-ary to the stress of impotence, rather than that the impotence was attributable to associated vascular disease and medication. In an investigation of 121 impotent male veterans whose mean age was 68 years, Mulligan and Katz (1989) found the coexis-tence of neurological and vascular disorders to be the most frequent cause, being present in 30%; vascular disease alone was responsible for 21%, diabetic neuropathy for 17%, and nondiabetic neuropathy for 10%. In addition to diseases specifically impairing sexual functioning, those associated with pain or that produce debility, anxiety, or depression are likely to significantly reduce sexual interest.

Organic Causes of Premature Ejaculation and Inhibited Male Orgasm

Few studies have reported organic causes for premature ejaculation unaccom-panied by erectile dysfunction or hypoactive sexual desire (Williams, 1984). Williams investigated 25 subjects with premature ejaculation only, all of whom gave a history of previous good control of ejaculation. Two had spinal cord damage, 1 in the sacral region (which responded to treatment with an alphasympathetic blocker) and 1 with paraplegia. Two were secondary to acute bacterial prostatitis: 1 remitted with antibi-otic therapy, and the other needed behavior therapy in addition. The fifth case was associated with evidence of alcoholic peripheral neuropathy and cerebellar dysfunc-tion; as these conditions resolved so did his premature ejaculation.

Strassberg, Mahoney, Schaugaard, and Hale (1990) found 15 premature ejaculators showed significantly shorter latencies to reach orgasm with self-stimula-tion but reported no greater anxiety during the activity compared to 17 non-premature ejaculators. Strassberg et al. cited an earlier study by other workers that found that subjects who experienced premature ejaculation both during intercourse and masturbation did not avoid intercourse, unlike those who experienced pre-mature ejaculation only during intercourse. The latter group showed some degree of erectile disturbance and experienced anxiety feelings with intercourse. On the basis of these findings, Strassberg et al. suggested that at least some premature ejaculators had a physiologically based hypersensitivity to sexual stimulation. They were unable to support the hypothesis, which they attributed to Kaplan, that premature ejaculators were less able than controls to evaluate accurately their level of physiolog-ical sexual arousal.

Difficulty or inability to reach orgasm and/or to ejaculate are not infrequent results of medications, commonly those that in other men produce erectile difficulties, and of neurological disorders (Munjack & Kanno, 1979). In their study of 1,053 men with sexual dysfunctions without obvious cause, Buvat, Lemaire, Buvat-Herbaut, Fourlinnie, et al. (1985a) found mildly raised prolactin levels in 13 (10%) of 124 men with premature ejaculation. They did not report the subjects' response to lowering the levels to normal. Though prolactin levels were normal in the 51 subjects with anejaculation without orgasm, the authors pointed out that individual cases of HPRL had been reported with anejaculation that had responded to reduction of the HPRL with bromocriptine.

Organic Causes of Female Sexual Dysfunctions

Sex Hormones

As discussed in Chapter 2, the nature and significance of the influence of hormonal factors on the sexual interest and activity of women remains unestablished, and psychological variables (particularly the presence and nature of a relationship with a male partner) appear to be the major determinants. In women, unlike men, the marked increase in hormone levels that occurs with puberty is not immediately accompanied by increase in sexual interest and regular achievement of orgasm. The significant hormonal fluctuations that occur throughout the menstrual cycle have not been demonstrated to be accompanied by consistent fluctuations in sexual behaviors. The effects of removal of women's ovaries, oophorectomy, were so much less apparent than those of testicular castration that Kinsey et al. (1953) considered them negligible. Subsequently there has been general agreement that the menopausal symptoms, including hot flashes and atrophic vaginitis, that follow oophorectomy are accompanied by reduced sexual interest and activity. As discussed in Chapter 2, however, it is not established whether the reduction in sexual interest and activity is primary, caused by direct effects of hormones on the central nervous system, or secondary to the hot flashes and atrophic vaginitis.

Conflict also persists concerning the nature of hormonal therapy required to reverse the loss of sexual interest in women following oophorectomy. Dennerstein and Burrows (1982) found that estrogen administration alone produced significant reversal compared with placebo, whereas Sherwin and colleagues (Sherwin & Gelfand, 1987; Sherwin et al., 1985) found it did not. Dennerstein and Burrows's result was supported by Dow, Hart, and Forrest (1983). Unlike Sherwin et al., Dow et al. found that estrogen alone was as effective as the combination of androgen and estrogen. Both therapies produced significant improvement in psychological, somatic, and vasomotor symptoms, including hot flashes, as well as in sexual interest and responsiveness. In the studies by Sherwin et al. in which the combination produced positive effects, it was associated with above-normal levels of androgen, resulting in the longer term in mild hirsuitism in about one-fifth of the women treated.

As discussed in Chapter 2, the increased sexual interest following androgen administration may be secondary to abnormally high androgen levels producing hypertrophy and increased sensitivity of the clitoris. Adamopoulos, Kampyli, Georgiacodis, Kapolla, and Abrahamian-Michalakis (1988) pointed out that the generally accepted concept that androgen was a—or the—libido hormone in women was based on early uncontrolled reports that female cancer patients experienced no change in sexuality following oophorectomy but a severe decline after adrenalectomy, with its associated loss of the androgens produced by the adrenal glands. The effects of the marked physical and psychological effects of this major surgical procedure would need to be excluded before the decline could be attributed to its hormonal effects (Donovan, 1985).

It has not been possible to explore the effect of chemical hormone reduction on the level of sexual interest in women to the extent this has been possible in men. A significant number of male sex offenders are treated by hormone reduction (Chapter 8). My experience with the few women who sought this treatment, following failure to respond to psychological therapy for distressing levels of compulsive masturbation, was that they showed no response to chemical reduction of their androgen levels. These women showed marked personality disturbance, however, unlike most men who responded well to testosterone reduction. Adamopoulos et al. (1988) investigated another group of women in whom there was a role for chemically induced androgen reduction. These were women with hirsuitism who had high androgen levels; they also required addition of estrogen to maintain menstruation, thus confounding the effect of the androgen reduction.

Adamopoulos et al. compared the sexual activity of 38 women who received the combined treatment with that of a control group of age-matched nonhirsute women. Prior to treatment, the hirsute women with partners reported a higher rate of masturbation and a lower rate of coitus compared to controls, but the frequencies of the combined activities of the two groups were no different. After 6 months of chemical reduction of the treated subjects' total and free testosterone levels with resultant reduction of their hirsuitism, there was no reduction in their total sexual outlets; however, their frequency of coitus rose and of masturbation fell. The major rise in frequency of coitus was between 2 and 6 months following commencement of treatment. Adamopoulos et al. argued that this alteration in type of sexual outlet was unlikely to be caused by the endocrine changes, as these had occurred prior to 2 months, and attributed it to psychosocial factors such as improved self-image or attractiveness.

Most of the women in the study of Adamopoulos et al. suffered from polycystic ovary syndrome. A further study of women with high levels of testosterone as a result of this condition also found no evidence that they showed increased libido. Fifty women with the syndrome reported normal levels of sexual activity before and following wedge resection of their ovaries (Raboch, Kobilkova, Raboch, & Starka, 1985). Following the operation their testosterone levels were in the normal range, though higher in those with lower rates of experiencing orgasm in coitus. An earlier study of 11 women with the syndrome (Gorzynski & Katz, 1977) reported that 8 almost invariably initiated sex, in contrast to 1 of 16 controls. The authors stated that a sense of uncontrollable sexual urge may be a symptom of the condition; however, they reported that there was no significant difference in the capacity of the two groups of women to experience sexual arousal in response to specific stimuli. It would appear that this and other earlier reports of marked increases of libido in women with high levels of androgen (as a result of either excess production or administration) need further replication in carefully controlled studies. Although some women taking oral contraceptives report reduced libido and ability to orgasm, other state that their sexual interest and enjoyment is increased; there appears to be no agreement among researchers as to whether these effects are induced hormonally or psychologically.

The markedly conflicting findings concerning the nature and degree of direct influences of hormones on the sexual interest and activity of women as compared with that of men suggest that in women, their influences are much weaker, and hence psychological and social factors are more important. The lack of evidence of involvement of sex hormones in the common sexual dysfunctions of premenopausal women is consistent with this conclusion.

Other Organic Factors

The role of organic factors other than genital and pelvic pathology appear to have been investigated much less in women than in men. Vaginal lesions, dermatitis, or infections are likely to be associated with dyspareunia on penetration, and inflammation or disease of the pelvic organs with pain on deep penile thrusting. The effects of neurological and vascular disease and of medications and drugs of abuse on the sexuality of women are much more poorly documented than their effects on that of men. Clinically it is found that many women taking drugs used in psychiatric treatment, including major and minor tranquilizers, monoamine oxidase inhibitors, and tricyclic antidepressants, will on inquiry report reduced libido or ability to reach orgasm. A double-blind study of two such drugs, phenelzine and imipramine, found them to produce a high incidence of impairment of sexual function in depressed patients compared with placebo, through the incidence was higher in men than in women (Harrison, Rabkin, & Ehrhardt, 1986).

In contrast to the high rates of sexual dysfunction reported in clinical studies of alcoholic women, a national survey of 917 women found that the relationship between sexual dysfunctions and drinking were weak. Moderate drinking was associated with lower rates of several dysfunctions than lighter or heavier drinking or abstinence (Klassen & Wilsnack, 1986). Jensen (1981) found no significant difference in the percentage of insulin-treated diabetic women (27.5%) who reported sexual dysfunctions compared to age-matched controls (25%) who consecutively attended a general practitioner. Peripheral neuropathy was more prevalent in the diabetic women with than in those without dysfunctions. As in men, diseases associated with pain or that result in debility, anxiety, or depression will significantly impair women's sexual interest.

Psychological Causes of Sexual Dysfunction

Learning to Relinquish Control in Women

The gradual increase from the age of 15 to middle age in the ability of women to reach orgasm in sexual relationships, demonstrated graphically in Figure 5.1, suggests learning is strongly involved. This possibility is supported by consideration of the differing demands placed on girls and boys in their sociosexual development. Mead (1950) pointed out that adolescent girls are expected to restrict the limits of sexual relationships, and boys to extend them. This must result in girls attempting to limit their sexual arousal in physical relationships, as well as experiencing anxiety if it increases. When they no longer need to restrain their arousal, they have to learn to relinquish the control they have regularly practiced, and to lose their anxiety at becoming aroused. Women who consistently experienced orgasm during coitus, as compared to those who did not, were found to be more likely to report inability to control their thinking or movements as they approached orgasm (Bridges, Critelli, & Loos, 1985). They also obtained higher scores on a hypnotic susceptibility scale. This was considered to reflect a greater ability to suspend effortful, controlled cognitive processes.

This concept that women need to learn to relinquish control to experience orgasms with coitus is consistent with the behaviors men have been encouraged to adopt in their sexual relationships. Mead (1950) commented approvingly that happy sexual relationships in France and Samoa are based on the man's taking pride and pleasure in arousing the female. In M. Hunt's U.S. survey (1974) of sexual behavior in the 1970s, women emphasized the role of men in helping them to learn to become aroused: "A man . . . taught me how to move my body, how to feel my own rhythms"; "I talked it over a lot with two of them [her lovers], hoping to work it out and become a better and more exciting woman"; "A man . . . got me to read several books on peak experiences and joy . . . to blow my mind", (pp. 164, 165). The men emphasized the importance of arousing their partner: "She let me know what it was that I did that got to her"; "You try to create something in your partner"; "I began to learn . . . how to make a woman rise up higher and higher"; "I really work at getting the girl so hot", (pp. 162, 163).

Darling and Davidson (1986) found that opinions of clinicians differed concerning the prevalent practice of men asking their partner immediately after intercourse if she had experienced an orgasm. They pointed out that the women may believe the men were seeking confirmation of their own skill as lovers, in which case the women could feel under pressure to pretend orgasms in future. M. Hunt (1974) reported this reaction in some of the women in his survey, one of whom commented that "men seem to be so hung up about making the woman have an orgasm—so I often fake it, and go ape, and tell them they were fantastic" (p. 164). Hunt suggested that some men who failed in attempts to reach orgasm shortly after having done so could pretend they were successful. If this is correct, it suggests that both men and women fake orgasm to satisfy male expectations.

The apparent importance of the role of men in helping women learn to become sexually aroused might seem at variance with Morokoff's statement (1978) that she found little evidence to support a relationship between male sexual technique and female orgasm. It could be, however, that having learned to reach orgasm, women are no longer dependent on the technique of the male. Also, the type of learning suggested by the statements of the women in Hunt's survey do not appear to involve physical techniques so much as psychological factors. This is compatible with the failure of evidence to support the commonly held belief that inadequate genital stimulation in sexual relationships is an important determinant of women's inability to reach orgasm. Terman (1938) found that duration of intercourse did not differ greatly between married women who usually and who rarely experienced orgasm.

Butler (1976) misinterpreted Gebhard's (1966) findings from his study of married women, concluding that they showed a strong positive relationship between the women's ability to attain orgasm and length of intromission. In fact, there were no meaningful differences in the percentage of women obtaining orgasm with durations of intromission of 1 to 2, 2 to 4, 4 to 7, or 8 to 11 minutes. There was a trend for fewer women to experience orgasm with durations of less than 1 minute in contrast to more than 12 minutes, but even if this was not a chance finding, it may not have indicated a causal relationship. Women who reach orgasm after prolonged coitus would presumably encourage their partners to regularly prolong it; women who rarely or never reach orgasm despite prolonged stimulation would be less likely to do so. This explanation could also account for the positive relationship found by Gebhard between duration of foreplay and ability to attain coital orgasm.

Huey, Kline-Graber, and Graber (1981) found no differences among durations of foreplay or intromission reported by 153 women who did not experience orgasm with coitus or other sexual activities, 114 women who reached orgasm with other sexual activities apart from coitus, and 24 women who experienced orgasm with coitus and usually with other sexual activities. All the women had sought treatment at a sexual therapy clinic. Consistent with the concept that orgasmically inadequate women are those who fear losing control, and that it is not the male's sexual technique as such, but his encouraging the woman to let her feelings of sexual arousal take over, that enables her to learn to reach orgasm, Morokoff (1978) believed that in our culture sexual arousal and orgasm in women are associated with a letting go or loosening.

Supporting the role of learning in women's achieving the ability to experience orgasm in sexual relationships, Morokoff cited a number of studies finding that this ability was strongly developed in societies in which women were expected to possess it, and weakly developed or absent in those in which they were not. Female orgasm was reported to be unknown on Inis Beag, an island off the coast of Ireland where the cultural expectation was that women received no pleasure from sexual activity. Premarital coitus did not occur there, and sexual activity within marriage was extremely circumscribed. In contrast, on the Polynesian island of Mangaia, as far as could be determined all women reached orgasm. There it was believed that women must be taught to have orgasms, a task formerly allotted to older women but more recently carried out by the young girls' initial lovers. Sexual activity began at puberty and premarital coitus was expected with different partners.

Mead (1950) reported a similar contrast between two primitive Pacific societies: the Mundugumor, in which women were expected to derive the same satisfaction from sex as men, and the Arapesh, in which female orgasm was unrecognized, unreported, and had no name. Culturally determined changes concerning female sexuality were considered the likely explanation for the higher frequency of orgasm in women in the United States born later in the present century (M. Hunt, 1974; Kinsey et al., 1953), and for the disappearance in Hunt's later study of the association between orgasmic responsiveness and higher socioeconomic class found by Kinsey et al. Mead (1950) concluded that the human female's capacity for orgasm was to be viewed much more as a potentiality that may or may not be developed by a given culture, or in a specific life history of an individual than as an inherent part of her full humanity.

Parental Relationships: Personality Factors in Women

Psychoanalytic theory emphasized the importance of children's parental relationships in the first few years of their lives in determining their later behavior, including their sexual behavior. Terman (1938, 1951) found little support for the theory in his studies of factors determining married women's ability to attain orgasm in sexual activity. Degree of attachment to or conflict with mother or father, the resemblance of husband to father, childhood happiness, type of childhood discipline, and amount of punishment were all unrelated. A premarital attitude of disgust toward sex was also unrelated, but quality of sex instruction showed a positive relationship in both studies. Morokoff (1978) cited the study of Fisher (1973) as not finding this relationship. It also found no relationship with parental attitudes of permissiveness or repressiveness concerning sex or nudity, or with the subject's openness in displaying affection, reaction to the onset of menstruation, or attitude toward her mother. Heiman, Gladue, Roberts, and LoPiccolo (1986) found overall quality of home life, parental attitudes and openness about sex, early religious attitudes, parental strictness, and family abuse did not enter a discriminant analysis that distinguished sexually dysfunctional from functional women. No personality traits have consistently been found to be associated with reduced sexual responsiveness in women. Degree of femininity, aggressiveness, passivity, guilt, impulsiveness, and narcissism were all unrelated (Fisher, 1973), as were neurotic illness (Winokur, Guze, & Pfeiffer, 1959) and neuroticism (Cooper, 1969).

Learning in Men

Much less attention has been given the possible role of cultural and personality factors in determining men's ability to become sexually aroused and to climax. In addition to the need discussed for men to learn how to arouse women sexually, some men also appear to need to learn to enjoy coitus, or at least to overcome inhibitions limiting enjoyment. As discussed in Chapter 2, Schofield (1968) found that fewer than half the boys and one-third of the girls in a representative sample of English teenagers said they liked their first experience of intercourse. When followed-up 7 years later, the majority had continued to have intercourse and only 5% did not enjoy it (Schofield, 1973). Men who report inability to reach orgasm in the presence of a partner appear to suffer the same fear or embarrassment at loss of emotional control as do women with the same disorder, and seem to respond to similar treatment.

Conditioned Anxiety Concerning Sexual Activity

The psychodynamic view that sexual dysfunctions resulted from unconscious fears of castration established in the first 5 years of the child's parental relationships was significantly modified by Wolpe (1958), enabling him to develop the now gener-

ally accepted direct cognitive-behavioral treatment of these conditions. In the ,
of his conceptualization of all neurotic conditions as persistent unadaptive bel
learned by conditioning, Wolpe suggested that anxiety could be conditioned to
sexual activity by experiences that occurred at any stage of life, not merely the first 5
years. These experiences could include cognitions obtained from simple misinforma-
tion or from the development of complex mistaken attitudes toward society, other
people, or the patient himself or herself. They could include beliefs that masturbation
weakens the body and the mind, that sexual activity is sinful and will be punished by
hellfire, or that sexual behaviors are painful or aggressive (the last beliefs resulting
from overhearing or observing the sexual activities of parents or others). A single
episode of impotence or of premature ejaculation caused by fatigue, illness, or indul-
gence in alcohol could lead to anxiety about future sexual performance, particularly
in subjects whose ability to perform sexually is important to them.

When anxiety occurs in association with sexual activity, it is linked to it by
conditioning and so will recur when sexual activity is subsequently considered or
initiated, even though the experiences may have been forgotten or the beliefs abandoned that originally produced it. This conditioned anxiety could partially or totally
inhibit the subject's sexual responsiveness, resulting in sexual arousal disorders. Inadequate sexual arousal could secondarily result in hypoactive sexual desire or sexual
aversions. Fear of loss of control could lead to inhibition of orgasm, and fear that
sexual activity will be painful or will result in an undesired pregnancy or an agoniz-
ing labor could lead to vaginismus. Anxiety is associated with heightened activity of
the sympathetic nervous system, which is primarily involved in ejaculation in the
male. Anxiety could therefore lead to premature ejaculation, which would then be
maintained by a fear of its recurrence.

Clinicians have generally accepted the concept that anxiety is responsible for
sexual dysfunctions, though pointing out that other negative emotional responses
can also play a role: "Fear or anxiety is the major etiologic factor in all of the sexual
dysfunctions, but anger at the partner is also a highly prevalent cause for the loss of
sexual interest" (Kaplan, 1979, p. 90). In contrast, a number of experimental studies
found that anxiety did not consistently impair sexual arousal (Hale & Strassberg,
1990). These authors pointed out that the anxiety was produced by injections of
epinephrine, exposure to anxiety-provoking material (e.g., films of fatal car accidents), or threat of electric shock, and the fact that fear of sexual activity itself was
not examined may have been responsible for the negative findings. In a study of 54
healthy men aged 21 to 45 years, Hale and Strassberg investigated the effect on their
sexual arousal of two forms of anxiety: threat of a painful but not harmful electric
shock, and threat of sexual inadequacy. The men had no history of sexual dysfunctions. Their sexual arousal was assessed by their penile circumference responses to
videos of sexual activity by heterosexual couples. Though as discussed in Chapter 1,
penile circumference assessment is markedly less sensitive than penile volume assessment in detecting sexual arousal using mildly arousing stimuli, it is capable of
discrimination when strong stimuli of couples engaged in intercourse are used.

The threat of sexual inadequacy was produced by showing the subjects bogus,
unusually low tracings of their penile responses during a baseline assessment, and
informing them that low tracings were associated with increased risk of developing
sexual problems. Hale and Strassberg found that both forms of anxiety reduced the

subjects' sexual arousal. They suggested their finding that threat of shock reduced sexual arousal, in contrast to its failure to do so in an earlier study of 12 college students, could have been attributable to the older age and larger size of their sample, and the fact that the 12 students were exposed to a sample of the electric shock prior to assessing the effect of the threat of its administration; the experience of sampling it may have reduced the threat. Hale and Strassberg concluded that their study provided empirical support for the concept that anxiety about sexual performance was a factor in erectile dysfunctions in men. They commented that if the sexually functional men in their study were sufficiently concerned by the possibility that their sexual performance was subnormal, the effect of such cognitions could be expected to be much greater in men with reasons for concern, such as an episode of erectile failure following heavy alcohol intake. If replicated, Hale and Strassberg's findings provide evidence that anxiety need not be directly associated with sexual activity to impair performance.

As stated earlier, Strassberg et al. (1990) found that premature ejaculators reached orgasm by masturbation significantly more rapidly than did controls, though they did not report greater anxiety. Strassberg et al. concluded that premature ejaculation was not necessarily caused by anxiety and could result from a physiologically based hypersensitivity to sexual stimulation. They cited a study by other workers, however, that found two groups of premature ejaculators, one who ejaculated prematurely both with masturbation and coitus, and one who did so only with coitus. The latter group showed some degree of erectile disturbance and experienced anxiety with intercourse.

Masturbation, Foreplay, and Orgasm in Women

Evidence does not appear to support the beliefs that the nature of foreplay activities or masturbatory experiences improve women's ability to reach orgasm in coitus. Kelly, Strassberg, and Kircher (1990) investigated 24 orgasmic women whose mean age was 30 years and 10 anorgasmic women whose mean age was 23 years. All reported moderate to high levels of sexual activity and interest. The anorgasmic women achieved orgasm on at most 5% and the orgasmic women on at least 70% of occasions of intercourse, or of oral or manual genital stimulation by their partner. Kelly et al. found the anorgasmic women did not experience a more limited range of sexual experiences, including those involving more direct clitoral stimulation. They pointed out that a number of theorists and clinicians had considered clitoral stimulation essential for many women to become sufficiently aroused to achieve orgasm.

Leff and Israel (1983) investigated the masturbatory behavior of 117 middle-class women aged 20 to 65, of whom 75% were married. Sixty-nine used direct masturbation, defined as digital manipulation of the clitoris or use of a vibrator in the genital area. Twenty-five used indirect masturbation, stimulation of an area adjacent to the clitoris, by rubbing the thighs together, rocking backwards and forwards while seated, rubbing against an object, pressing on the pubic area, or vaginal insertion of an object other than a vibrator. Thirteen were nonmasturbators. Seventeen percent of the 94 masturbators had used the same style from their initial masturbation. There were no differences in the three groups in the frequency with which they reached orgasm during, compared with or before, or after intercourse with their partners' assistance. To obtain orgasm in coitus, nonmasturbators used manual or other stimulation of the clitoris by themselves or their partners significantly less frequently than did both groups of women who masturbated. As discussed in Chapter 2, Lightfoot-Klein (1989) questioned the acceptance in Western sexological literature that the clitoris must be stimulated to produce orgasm, reporting that it was experienced by the majority of Sudanese women who had undergone excision of the clitoris.

Communication

Kelly et al. (1990) asked orgasmic and anorgasmic women to rate the difficulty of communicating with their partner about a range of sexual activities of heterosexual couples they were shown on video. The anorgasmic as compared to the orgasmic women anticipated significantly greater discomfort regarding communications about sexual activities involving direct clitoral stimulation. They also showed less sexual knowledge, more sexual guilt, and more negative attitudes toward masturbation. Kelly et al. considered that whether the discomfort about communication was a cause or a result of the anorgasmia, their finding highlighted the importance of communication in sexual interactions. The orgasmic women in the study of Kelly et al. were 7 years older than the nonorgasmic women. Though statistical techniques were used in an attempt to control for the age difference, in view of the strong association in women between age and ability to achieve orgasm, a replicatory study in orgasmic and nonorgasmic women of the same age would seem desirable. If the findings are replicated, they may not establish the importance of communication as directly involved in determining sexual functioning. As the investigation was a quasi experiment, the possibility would need to be excluded that ability to communicate about clitoral stimulation is associated with other variables that are the actual cause (e.g., ability to accept becoming sexually aroused).

Multifactorial Etiology

The findings reported indicate that the etiology of sexual dysfunction is multifactorial. Factors involved appear to include fear of loss of emotional control, of inability to perform adequately, and of the consequences of sexual activity; inability to communicate sexual needs; and negative feelings toward the partner. These psychological factors appear to interact with cultural factors that establish sexual expectations and demands, and with biological variables that influence innate sexual interest and arousability. The nature of the sexual technique currently used may not be of major importance, provided that in the case of women, those previously inhibited about expressing their sexual excitement have learned to overcome this.

DIAGNOSIS

Diagnostic Criteria

A problem with diagnosis that preoccupies academics is that of reliability, the degree to which diagnoses made by different clinicians identify the same patients

(Chapter 1). Though the issue is of little practical concern to clinicians in their management of their own patients, it is of importance for studies that report findings concerning patients diagnosed as having particular sexual dysfunctions. DSM-III-R (APA, 1987) left it to the clinician to take into account the frequency and chronicity of the symptom, the subjective distress it caused, and its effect on other areas of the subject's functioning. Reference was made earlier to the difficulty this produced in relation to the diagnosis of impotence employed in different studies. DSM-III-R does not provide a specific term for the condition; male erectile disorder can mean either impotence or lack of a subjective sense of excitement or pleasure during sexual activity.

The main criterion currently employed for the diagnosis of impotence would appear to be the patient's report that he has a problem attaining or maintaining an erection adequate for coitus. The nature of the impairment, the percentage of all attempts at intercourse on which it occurs, and the frequency of the attempts may not be investigated. Depending on their degree of concern about performance, one man will succeed in coital penetration, whereas another will not attempt it, though both show the same degree of reduction in penile rigidity. The nature of their relationship with their partners could be a major factor determining the degree of their concern. As mentioned earlier, the possible role of the partner's genital anatomy does not appear to have been investigated. If it is demonstrated that it influences ease of penetration, this influence could become crucial when a degree of erectile impairment develops. Some men never discuss with their partners the fact that they are having erectile difficulties and attempt intercourse only when they are confident of their potency. This can be during the night, when they wake with an erection and then proceed to awaken their wives and immediately initiate coitus.

The criteria used for the diagnosis of hypoactive or inhibited sexual desire seem even more arbitrary. Stuart et al. (1987) classified 59 of 90 married women who presented to a sex and marital therapy clinic as having inhibited sexual desire on the basis that they reported at least three of nine criteria of low sexual interest. The 59, compared to those not so diagnosed, had engaged in premarital intercourse significantly more often and showed no difference in frequency or duration of intercourse or duration of foreplay. The frequency of intercourse of 13 men regarded as showing inhibited desire was half that of men reporting a healthy sex life; however, their mean age was greater (43.6 years vs. 37.4 years), and their frequency of masturbation was 20% higher (Nutter & Condron, 1985). In diagnosing hypoactive or inhibited sexual desire, it would seem appropriate that the frequency and degree of enjoyment of sexual activity are taken into account in addition to the complaint of reduced interest. This could help exclude the possibility that a number of women and men are diagnosed as suffering from hypoactive sexual desire when the reason they report reduced desire is that they are dissatisfied with their sexual relationship. Nutter and Condron suggested that their subjects may have lacked sexual interest in their partners. At times, men present as suffering from premature ejaculation when they cannot prolong ejaculation for 10 minutes or more following intromission, and their partner takes longer than this to reach a climax. There appears to be no concept of retarded orgasm in women equivalent to that of retarded ejaculation.

Assessment of Organic Factors

The exclusion of organic causes or determination of their significance when they are found to be present is of most importance in regard to male sexual dysfunctions, particularly impotence. It may be apparent from the history that the cause of a dysfunction is psychological, for example, if it occurs in relationships with one partner and not others; or, with impotence, if adequate erections can be maintained in nonstressful situations such as masturbation, and the pelvic steal syndrome is excluded. Segraves, Segraves, and Schoenberg (1987) reported that many centers nevertheless routinely screen all patients who complain of erectile difficulties with the expensive techniques discussed subsequently, NPT assessment, and Doppler determination of penile blood flow, as well as complete hormone investigation. Segraves et al. found that a history of early morning or masturbatory erections adequate for coitus differentiated subjects with psychogenic from those with organic impotence. Slag et al. (1983) reported an investigation of 188 impotent men, of mean age 59 years, by intensive psychological and medical examination and hormonal screening. The presence of normal erections in situations other than with their usual partners characterized the 14% of men diagnosed as having psychogenic impotence.

If it is clear from the history that the dysfunction is psychogenic, some psychotherapists do not carry out a physical examination, believing that it could have a negative effect on the therapeutic relationship. All dysfunctions that are not clearly psychogenic require that a medical history be taken and a physical examination performed to evaluate use of medication and alcohol, tobacco, or other drugs of dependence and to exclude relevant physical illnesses, including diabetes. Negative findings with this assessment are usually considered adequate grounds to initiate a trial of psychological therapy in men with premature ejaculation and in those complaining of impotence in sexual activity with their partner who have normal sexual desire and erections adequate for coitus in other situations. If they report reduced sexual desire, they require hormonal screening. Dyspareunia or other indications of genital and pelvic pathology in men or women require gynecological or urological examination.

Investigation of Organic Factors in Impotence

A number of specialized investigations have been introduced to exclude or determine the significance of organic factors in impotence. When impotence is not clearly psychogenically caused, it appears to be fairly general practice to exclude diabetes and determine subjects' testosterone, LH, FSH, prolactin, and thyroid hormone levels. Jones (1985), however, noted that in the absence of loss of libido or the physical signs of regression of male hair pattern, gynecomastia (increased breast development), or small, soft testes, the testosterone levels in impotent men under the age of 50 years were almost invariably in the normal range. When these investigations reveal no abnormality, most workers continue to place considerable value on nocturnal penile tumescence assessment, the investigation of the subject's erections during sleep.

CHAPTER 5

Nocturnal Penile Tumescence. Karacan (1978) advanced the belief that if men with erectile dysfunction show erections during dream sleep (nocturnal penile tumescence, or NPT) similar to those of normal men, their dysfunction is attributable to a psychological rather than organic cause. He recommended that dysfunctional men undergo NPT assessment by continuous recording of their penile circumference, the procedure being conducted in a sleep laboratory on 3 consecutive nights. On the third night, those who showed erections were awakened for them to assess its fullness and to have the rigidity determined by the pressure necessary to produce buckling. Wasserman et al. (1980) pointed out that the basic assumption that NPT can distinguish psychogenic from organic impotence had never been demonstrated when the two conditions were diagnosed by criteria independent of the NPT measurements. They also pointed out the lack of agreed criteria for assessment of NPT as to whether it should be based on the frequency and/or duration of full erections only or all erections, and whether the criteria should be modified for patients of different ages.

Wasserman et al. stressed the necessity for including direct observation if NPT assessment was undertaken, reporting a subject whose nocturnal erection was revealed by observation to be inadequate for intercourse when it would have been considered adequate by penile circumference assessment. Investigations revealed the man to have hyperprolactinemia; when it was corrected, his potency returned, and he showed adequate NPT as assessed by observation. Karacan (1978) found that 20% of the patients he studied had impaired NPT but no demonstrable organic cause for their impotence. Though he believed these patients may have had defects not detectable by available techniques, Wasserman et al. (1980) felt that psychogenic factors could be responsible. They reviewed a number of studies that demonstrated that psychogenic factors could impair NPT. The erections of normal men were diminished during the first night of assessment, presumably because of anxiety associated with the novel situation, and also during dreams with a manifest content of aggression, anxiety, or other negative affect. Absence of nocturnal erections were found in a number of men with impotence diagnosed on clinical grounds as psychogenic, and in elderly men who reported having erections adequate for intercourse.

Schiavi et al. (1984) investigated 12 sexually functional and 17 impotent healthy men aged 23 to 36 years. Their NPT was assessed over 3 to 6 nights, and penile rigidity of erections determined. Five of the 17 were considered to suffer from primary impotence as they had never been able to achieve intercourse, though they obtained full erections with masturbation and had adequate sexual desire. The remaining 12 developed impotence secondarily; 3 were unable to achieve full erections by any means, and 3 had reduced sexual desire. NPT parameters of the secondary impotence group did not differ from those of the controls, whereas those of the primary impotence group were significantly reduced. One of the latter showed no episodes of full tumescence over 5 nights, yet after psychotherapy he was able to have intercourse and remained potent 12 months following termination of treatment. The authors concluded that psychological factors could depress NPT in some subjects.

This conclusion was supported by Thase, Reynolds, and Jennings (1988), who compared the NPT assessed over 3 nights with rigidity determined by buckling pressure assessment on the third night in 34 depressed men, 14 nondepressed men with organic impotence, and 28 healthy controls. Forty percent of the depressed men showed reduction of duration of NPT (corrected for diminished sleep time) by more than one standard deviation from that of the controls, and in the same range as that of the organically impotent men. Thirty-eight percent of the depressed men showed diminished erectile rigidity.

Men with reduced testosterone levels caused by hypogonadism or estrogen administration showed normal erectile response to sexual films and fantasy, but impaired NPT (Kwan et al., 1985). This finding suggests that the physiological mechanism responsible for NPT is not identical with that responsible for erections produced by sexual arousal. If so, this would explain why normal NPTs are found in some subjects with organically caused impotence, and abnormal NPTs in some with psychogenic impotence.

In their recent critical evaluation of NPT assessment, Meisler and Carey (1990) considered a conservative appraisal to be that it may misdiagnose as many as 20% of the subjects investigated. Nevertheless, it appears that NPT assessment of erectile dysfunction will continue to be widely used in assessment of erectile dysfunction, commonly in modified form, over fewer than three nights and without determination of penile rigidity.

Penile Brachial Index. The technique most commonly employed in assessing vascular pathology in impotent men is determination of the penile brachial index (PBI), the ratio of the blood pressure in the penile arteries (measured by Doppler ultrasound probe) and the conventionally measured blood pressure in the brachial artery in the arm. It is generally stated that arterial insufficiency is very likely to be the cause of the impotence of subjects with a PBI of less than 0.6, but that a higher ratio does not exclude the possibility, though a PBI of over 0.9 should indicate sufficient perfusion to maintain erection (Gewertz & Zarins, 1985). Metz and Bengtsson (1981) provided data supporting these conclusions from a study of healthy men and men with peripheral arteriosclerotic disease, half of whom were impotent. More than 90% of those with PBIs of 0.6 or less were impotent, and all the healthy controls had PBIs above this ratio. The authors emphasized that PBIs above 0.6 did not exclude vascular disease as a cause of impotence. They suggested that in this situation, other methods for determining the adequacy of the penile blood supply be employed. These methods include arteriography, outlining the blood supply by the injection of chemicals opaque to X-rays.

Saypol, Peterson, Howards, and Yazel (1983) questioned the reliance of clinicians on NPT and PBI assessment in impotence, arguing that many patients could be evaluated adequately by a psychiatrist and a urologist without these expensive tests. They compared the two forms of evaluation in 33 consecutive patients with impotence and found close agreement between the diagnoses of the psychiatrist and urologist, reached by clinical examination alone, and the diagnoses reached on the results of the patients' fasting blood sugar and testosterone levels and their PBI and NPT assessments. They suggested that expensive tests be reserved for patients regarding whom the psychiatrist and urologist disagree or cannot determine the diagnosis.

Pharmacologic Assessment. Krysiewicz and Mellinger (1989) recommended as practical and cost-effective a procedure for evaluation of impotence that frequently enabled NPT assessment to be eliminated. If no organic cause was apparent from the history and physical examination of the patient, pharmacologic assessment was carried out. A chemical vasodilator, such as papaverine, was injected into one of the corpora cavernosa of the patient's penis. Papaverine relaxes the smooth muscle of the vessels supplying blood to the penis, bypassing neurogenic factors to mimic the hemodynamic changes of normal erection. If the patient developed a full erection following the injection, severe vascular insufficiency could be excluded and psychogenic, neurogenic, hormonal, or mild vascular disease implicated as the cause of the impotence. On rare occasions, a less than full erection could occur as a result of the high level of autonomic activity in highly anxious subjects; Krysiewicz and Mellinger had not established what dose of alpha-blocker medication should be administered with the papaverine to prevent this.

Apart from this rare occurrence, a less than full erection following the injection indicated severe vascular insufficiency, but did not distinguish arterial from venous incompetence as the cause. To establish this, these workers mapped the vasculature of the penis by sound waves (duplex sonography), first with the penis flaccid and then following intracavernous administration of papaverine. If this procedure showed the penile arteries to be distensible, and the peak blood flow was subnormal, they recommended arteriography to establish the presence of obstructive lesions in the arteries supplying blood to the penile arteries. Such lesions could be amenable to treatment. If the penile arteries were not distensible, the authors believed the expensive and uncomfortable procedure of penile arteriography should not be carried out merely to confirm the diagnosis, but only in subjects likely to respond well to vascular reconstruction. They should also have the penile venous system evaluated, as it was estimated that between 50% and 70% of subjects have both arterial and venous disease. Evaluation of the penile venous system was the only definitive procedure for diagnosis of corpora cavernosal venous leaks. It involved inserting two needles, one in one cavernosal body to record intracavernosal pressure, one in the other body to infuse first papaverine and then saline. If a leak was detected, opaque contrast material was infused for its visual demonstration by radiography.

Neurological Assessment. If an organic cause is still suspected after medical, endocrine, and vascular factors have been excluded, neurological investigation has been recommended (Freund & Blanchard, 1981). In my experience, this has only been required when obvious neurological signs or symptoms were present. The techniques developed to investigate impairment of nerve transmission, however, such as the latency of bulbocavernous reflex and the latency and form of cerebral potentials evoked by stimulation of the glans penis and the peroneal nerve (Ertekin, Akyurekli, Gurses, & Turgut, 1985) may be demonstrated to be of value.

Segraves, Schoenberg, and Segraves (1985) found that in approximately 15% of men with a history and NPT assessment suggestive of an organic problem, multidisciplinary evaluation will fail to show any disease process.

Assessment and Treatment of Psychogenic Factors Causing Sexual Dysfunctions

In assessing and treating psychogenic factors responsible for or significantly contributing to the maintenance of sexual dysfunctions, it is necessary to decide if they result mainly from the subjects' personalities, their relationship with their partners, or specifically sexual concerns. This should be apparent from interviewing the subjects alone and then with their partners. As discussed in Chapter 1, the presence of personality problems can usually be determined from the nature of the relationship the subject consciously or unconsciously attempts to establish with the therapist, in combination with their history of behaviors at school, at work, and in their social and sexual relationships. This information, assessed in light of the behavior the subject shows toward his or her partners when they are interviewed together, usually allows the quality of the relationship to be assessed. In general, if there is evidence of marked personality disorder in the subject or if it is obvious in the interview that the relationships with the partner are overtly hostile, many sex therapists refer the subject for alternative treatments. A great variety of treatments of personalities and emotional relationships are available, most adopting a psychodynamic or depth psychology orientation, but some have been developed from cognitive-behavioral theory. The majority of patients presenting with sex dysfunctions, however, are suitable for treatment aimed directly at that problem.

The concept advanced by Wolpe (1958) that the major psychological factor responsible for sex dysfunctions was anxiety concerning sexual activity has become the basis for the direct therapy of these conditions employed by most clinicians, whether or not they label it a cognitive-behavioral approach. Using this model the therapist, when interviewing the subjects, investigates their attitudes toward sexual activity. If it is not one of acceptance, experiences are sought that could explain this. Misconceptions or incorrect interpretations of such experiences that have led the subjects to believe such activities are harmful or evil are cognitively corrected. Any beliefs of a religious nature that are not appropriate to challenge are discussed to determine what sexual behaviors are acceptable to the subjects. Concerns about past failures of sexual performance are explored, with reassurance concerning the normality of occasional failures.

Education will be needed if the subjects are unaware of the basic facts of sexual activity and the anatomy of the sexual organs. With older patients, the woman's menopausal status and the man's possible need for manual stimulation to attain erection will require discussion. A number of men whose wives do not touch their penis in sexual activities cease coitus when this condition develops, rather than discuss the situation with their wives and incorporate manual penile stimulation into their foreplay. My experience has led me to the conclusion, also reached by Marshall and Barbaree (1990b) from their program to enhance the enjoyment of heterosexual activities of sex offenders, that extensive detailing of the anatomical or physiological aspects of sexual functioning is unnecessary. They believed it could result in attention being focused on the objective and physical aspects of sex rather than crucially important interpersonal features.

Desensitization

Systematic Desensitization

To treat the anxiety conditioned to sexual activity that persisted following the correction of faulty cognitions, Wolpe (1958) recommended desensitization. This could be carried out by a procedure he developed, termed *systematic desensitization in imagination*. In its initial form, the patients were first trained to relax in several sessions during which they progressively tensed and relaxed different muscle groups. When it was considered that they had mastered the ability to relax, the therapist determined the patient's individual hierarchy of anxiety-provoking situations, from those that produced the least to those that produced the most anxiety. The patient was then instructed to relax and to visualize the anxiety-provoking situation lowest on the hierarchy. The state of relaxation was considered to inhibit reciprocally the low level of anxiety produced, so that the subject soon ceased to experience any anxiety while visualizing the situation and was asked to signal when this occurred. He or she then was instructed to visualize the next situation. Treatment progressed in this way until the patient was able to visualize the highest item on the hierarchy without anxiety.

The treatment relied on the phenomenon of generalization identified by Pavlov (1927). Pavlov found that when a dog developed a conditioned response to a stimulus (Chapter 1), it showed a similar, though weaker, response to a related stimulus. For example, if the dog was regularly presented with a tone of 1,000 cycles that was followed by food that caused it to salivate, it would develop the conditioned response of salivating to the tone. When it had developed this response, it would also salivate if it was presented with a tone of 990 cycles, producing slightly less saliva than to the original tone. A tone of 980 cycles would produce a still lesser amount of saliva. Pavlov termed the process *generalization,* and that of the reduction in its intensity the more the new stimulus departed from the original stimulus, the *gradient* of generalization.

Systematic desensitization relied on the reduction of anxiety produced to the lowest item generalizing to the next item on the hierarchy, so that the amount of anxiety that item produced would be reduced when the subject initially visualized it. This reduced level of anxiety would rapidly be inhibited by the state of relaxation as the subjects continued to visualize the item. This inhibition would generalize to the next item on the hierarchy, so the subject could then visualize it with less anxiety, and so could proceed through the hierarchy. Generalization also enabled the reduction in anxiety to the visualized situations to extend to the real situations. Where possible, as the subjects experienced minimal anxiety to the visualized situations in imagination, they were given homework assignments in which they were encouraged to enter and remain in the real situations.

In treating patients with psychogenic sexual dysfunctions with systematic desensitization, hierarchies were developed in relation to sexual situations that patients were able to identify as making them anxious. Some patients with hypoactive sexual desire report they do not experience any feelings, including anxiety, in sexual situations. To treat these subjects, it is assumed that they have repressed awareness of the anxiety. They are exposed to a hierarchy of situations in which they visualize being sexually aroused, from the initiation of sexual activity by stroking, cuddling, and kissing through to reaching orgasm in coitus.

Modifications of Systematic Desensitization

For men with impotence, Wolpe appeared to believe desensitization in reality could be more effective, as he instructed them to cuddle naked with their partners but not to attempt penetration, even if they obtained adequate erections, until he gave them permission to do so. Anxiety concerning their ability to perform adequately was therefore no longer activated in these sexual situations, and the component that was conditioned to past threatening situations was gradually inhibited by the continued exposure to this nonthreatening situation. The subjects' sexual arousal, once it was no longer blocked by anxiety, commenced to result in adequate erections. When this was occurring sufficiently regularly to establish the men's confidence, they were instructed to attempt coitus. Wolpe pointed out that subjects frequently commenced coitus prior to his giving permission.

The use of systematic desensitization for sexual dysfunctions was adopted in the 1960s by clinicians in the United Kingdom, Australia, and presumably South Africa, where Wolpe initially worked. Like many of these clinicians, I found the procedure could be significantly modified and still produce what appeared to be equally effective results. The major modification I introduced was marked curtailment of the length of the training in relaxation. As stated above, with systematic desensitization, patients were trained over several hours in a progressive muscular relaxation procedure (Wolpe, 1958). I use the procedure outlined in Chapter 8 in relation to alternative behavior completion. It is carried out within 5 minutes, with the therapist conveying complete conviction that the patient will be relaxed at its termination. It is extremely rare for patients not to signal they are. This apparent conviction that they are relaxed appears to be all that is necessary for systematic desensitization to be effective.

Resistance to Desensitization Therapy in the United States: Masters and Johnson

In the United States, unlike the many countries where desensitization for emotional and sexual disorders was rapidly accepted in the 1960s, the treatment was largely ignored. It would seem likely that its political associations (attributable to its derivation from Pavlovian theory developed in the USSR) was less a factor than its ideological foreignness. Psychiatrists and many clinical psychologists in the United States were at that time committed to a psychoanalytic approach. The then-small number of psychologist-behavior therapists were equally committed to an operant conditioning or social learning approach. Both approaches rejected the significance of neurophysiology. Concepts of relaxation producing reciprocal inhibition of anxiety were outside the cognitive awareness of these therapists. Very few mainstream therapists adopted Wolpe's approach, and little attention was given to those who did.

Chapman (1968) published a report in the *Journal of the American Osteopathic Association* of the treatment of 74 women who failed to enjoy sexual relations and/or achieve orgasm, by what he termed an expanded concept of Wolpe's reciprocal inhibition. To avoid fears of performance, they were instructed not to engage in sexual intercourse until instructed, but their partner was to pet, fondle, and in all ways arouse them without any threat of coitus. These sessions lasted 3 to 8 weeks and were combined with weekly interviews in which Chapman monitored compliance, and provided information and cognitive correction with the goal of establishing healthy sexual values for the couples. He reported an improvement rate of 80% overall and of 94% for the 48 subjects he was able to follow up for 5 years.

LoPiccolo (1978) pointed out the consequence of the neglect by most main-stream U.S. therapists in the 1960s of the direct approach to treating sex dysfunctions. In 1970, Masters and Johnson published *Human Sexual Inadequacy,* reporting results of their treatment program also based on desensitization, though not relating it to the work of Wolpe. Though the results they claimed were in the same range as those reported by Chapman, as Zilbergeld and Evans (1980) documented, the enthusiastic reviews the book received in major newspapers praised the program as a breakthrough in the treatment of human sexual inadequacy, some accepting Masters and Johnson's suggestion that such inadequacy could be substantially eliminated in 10 years. This media attention gained for the program the attention of a wide public, bypassing mainstream therapists and academic critics. The resulting demand for sex therapy led to its being provided by a large number of minimally qualified or untrained persons.

Current Desensitization Therapy

The program developed by Masters and Johnson involved the subjects and their partners being seen both individually and jointly by a male and a female therapist, at times working individually and at times jointly. The majority of subjects treated came from elsewhere in the United States to St. Louis to receive the treatment, which was carried out in daily sessions for 2 or 3 weeks. In addition, the couples were given nightly homework assignments.

Treatment of Couples. Most therapists do not follow the format of the Masters and Johnson approach precisely, as the majority of patients are unwilling or unable to give up 2 or 3 weeks for treatment and can do homework assignments of an hour's duration a few times weekly at most. Also, many sex therapists, finding their results satisfactory, continue to work individually rather than involve a cotherapist of the opposite sex. They see the couple weekly or less frequently. In these interviews the cognitive phase of Wolpe's approach is initiated, so that the couple are provided with appropriate information and their faulty cognitions corrected. They are then given instructions concerning their homework activities, and their performance of these are monitored in the following treatment session. They are asked to organize their activities so that they can put aside two or more periods of an hour's duration weekly when they are relaxed and will not be disturbed. This often takes a good deal of negotiation, dealing with issues of how interruptions from children, as well as house and external work demands, are to be managed.

For some patients the instructions appropriate for the homework sessions follow the procedures of Masters and Johnson, which elaborated Wolpe's injunction not to attempt intercourse into two phases. In the initial phase, the couple are instructed that in the sessions one is to be passive and the other active for half the period, and then they are to change roles. The active partner is to stimulate the passive partner sensously by massaging, stroking, or kissing how and where he or she is told by the passive partner, except that their genitals and, in the case of female subjects, their breasts are not to be touched. The aim is that they enjoy the sensuous experience without attempting to become sexually aroused. This procedure, termed "sensate focusing" by Masters and Johnson, enables the couple to have a physical relationship confident that coitus will not occur and free from any pressure to perform sexually. The subjects' anxieties conditioned to physical relations from past fears that coitus will be unpleasant or painful, or that their sexual performance will be inadequate, will begin to be extinguished. Also, in the passive role they learn to communicate verbally about what they enjoy in foreplay activities, and in the active role they gain experience in how to carry out the activities their partner enjoys.

When subjects in this initial phase report that they are communicating effectively, are enjoying the sensous experiences carried out by their partner, and are comfortable and relaxed, they are instructed to proceed to the second phase. In this they include stimulation of the genitals and breasts of the partner when he or she is in the passive role, but still do not attempt intercourse. If they feel it is appropriate they can reach orgasm by other means, such as manual or oral stimulation, at the end of the session. Men and women who are unable to ejaculate or to reach orgasm in physical relations are instructed to attempt to do so during the session. They are told that it may take an hour or more of masturbatory stimulation for them to reach orgasm initially, and that they will need to experiment to find the type of stimulation that most arouses them. Some women find direct stimulation of the clitoris unpleasant and need to be stimulated near it. Some men may require very vigorous stimulation. Some subjects, more commonly women, do not wish to stimulate their genitals themselves, and it may be adequate if their partner does so. Others prefer to masturbate on their own in separate sessions.

Occasionally women who cannot touch their own or their partner's genitals in this phase benefit from the addition of individual sessions of desensitization to this activity in imagination. If anorgasmic men or women do not respond to prolonged stimulation when with their partner or alone, they are encouraged to use an electric vibrator. If fear of loss of control or embarrassment at behaving emotionally is considered to be a factor preventing subjects reaching orgasm with their partners when they can do so alone, role-playing loss of emotional control and reaching orgasm in the presence of their partners can overcome this. LoPiccolo (1990) found that the use of "orgasm triggers" can aid women who report being unable to reach orgasm, although they become highly aroused. Orgasm triggers are behaviors that occur involuntarily during orgasm, which if performed voluntarily can initiate orgasm. The ones described were holding the breath, bearing down with the pelvic muscles, pointing the toes and tensing the leg and thigh muscles, throwing the head back, and thrusting the pelvis.

The partners of women with vaginismus are instructed to commence digital vaginal dilation when the women are sexually aroused. Initially they use one finger and in later sessions, provided the women remained relaxed, two and then three. The woman may feel less anxious if she initiates vaginal dilation with her own finger, or if graded vaginal dilators are employed at first. Subjects with hypoactive sexual desire who do not report experiencing sexual arousal in the second stage are recommended to use erotic videos and books and sexual fantasy in addition. Some people with hypoactive desire seem to have reduced ability to enjoy any sensuous experiences. They should be encouraged to incorporate appropriate ones into their recreational life, expanding this if necessary. These can include such physical activities as walking, sun-baking, and swimming, or emotional ones, such as going to rock or classical concerts or art galleries.

The partners of men with premature ejaculation are instructed to sit between the men's legs, facing them, and to masturbate them. The men are told to monitor their arousal and, when they feel they are about to ejaculate, to tell their partners, who then cease stimulation until told the sensation has disappeared. They then recommence masturbation. Subsidence of erection may occur temporarily. The subject becomes aware that he can prolong erection prior to ejaculation, thus reducing his anxiety that he will ejaculate prematurely. This "stop-start" procedure was recommended for premature ejaculation by Semans (1956), but apparently attracted little attention at the time. Semans believed that ejaculation occurred more rapidly when the penis was wet, and as the subject became able to prolong erection with the technique, he advised use of a lubricant with masturbation. When the subject could prolong erection indefinitely when masturbated with his penis lubricated, Semans suggested that the moist surface of the vagina would no longer produce premature ejaculation. He reported case histories of 8 subjects who showed a successful response. Semans also recommended masturbation as a treatment of coital anorgasmia in women.

Like Semans, Masters and Johnson (1970) also advised the use of masturbation for premature ejaculation. When ejaculation was imminent, however, they recommended not temporary cessation, but use of the "penile squeeze." The partners were told to place their first fingers on the subject's glans penis, the second fingers just below it, and their thumbs under it, so they could firmly but not painfully squeeze the glans. This inhibited ejaculation and usually resulted in some loss of erection. Masturbation was then recommenced as with the stop-start procedure.

When in the second phase of the homework activities the subjects are adequately aroused and report no anxiety at the thought of having coitus, they are instructed to initiate this in a third phase. Couples in whom the receptive partner in vaginal or anal intercourse presented with negative feelings toward the activity, or in whom the active male had premature ejaculation, are told to initiate it with the active male lying on his back. Penetration then occurs by the partner squatting or kneeling over him and sitting on his erect penis. In this way the partner with some remaining anxiety concerning being penetrated is able to feel in control. The partner of the premature ejaculator who feels he is about to ejaculate can, when informed, cease stimulation by raising herself or himself off the penis and using the penile squeeze if necessary. Men with inability to ejaculate into the vagina or rectum can masturbate to the point of ejaculation and then penetrate. Usually when they have ejaculated into the vagina or rectum on one or a few occasions, their inhibition is overcome.

LoPiccolo (1990) reported the use of nocturnal penile erections in three men with lifelong erectile failure in all situations who had failed to respond to desensitization. Their wives were instructed to remain in another room while their husbands went to sleep. After an hour or two she was to check every 15 minutes until she observed he had an erection. She then gently stroked his penis until he woke to the unique experience of having an erection during sexual activity with his wife. LoPiccolo said this enabled the wife to accomplish vaginal intromission, while her husband was awakening, to consummate the marriage after 7 years. He did not report the long-term outcome of the procedure.

Treatment of Subjects without Partners. The use of desensitization to actual sexual experiences in treating sex dysfunctions requires that the subjects have cooperative partners. If they seek treatment when they are without partners, some may be prepared to accept working through the program with a surrogate therapist. In my experience, many men but few women are prepared to do so. Fortunately, women appear less likely than men to require a partner to respond successfully. This may reflect the greater performance demands on male sexuality in that it requires that the man maintain an erection; women appear able to complete coitus successfully in the absence of any response. Sexual anxieties of subjects without partners can be treated by education, cognitive correction, and systematic desensitization in imagination. Where appropriate, use of erotic literature and videos and directed masturbation in homework sessions is advised (McConaghy, 1985). In my experience, good results are obtained with these procedures in women who present with hypoactive sexual desire, sexual aversion, and anorgasmia, and with men who report inability to reach orgasm in the presence of a partner. Men with impotence and premature ejaculation respond less well.

Group treatment by two male cotherapists was used with men without partners who were impotent in sexual relationships but not with masturbation (Lobitz & Baker, 1979). Education and cognitive correction of faulty attitudes concerning women's expectations was followed by training in muscular relaxation and then desensitization to a hierarchy of sexual situations of increasing intimacy, up to coitus. The subjects were given homework assignments of masturbating to full erection, letting the erection subside, and repeating the procedure. They also practiced the stop-start penile squeeze techniques, as most had anxieties about premature ejaculation. In one session, three female therapists joined the group for the men to role-play communicating self-disclosure of their sexual problem and suggesting that coitus not take place in their initial sexual activities. Dekker, Dronkers, and Staffeleu (1985) found that treatment outcome in male-only groups was improved when training in dating skills and communication techniques was emphasized. In their treatment of male-only groups by rational emotive therapy, masturbation exercises, and social skills training, however, no effect was found in the subjects without partners. The authors considered that the subjects may have improved, but as they had no new sexual experiences, they completed their posttreatment assessments on the basis of their pretreatment experiences.

Flowcharts in Figures 5.2 and 5.3 summarize the assessment and direct desensitization treatment of women and men with the common sexual dysfunctions.

OUTCOME OF TREATMENT OF PSYCHOGENIC SEXUAL DYSFUNCTIONS

Methodological Considerations

In attempting to evaluate whether a treatment is effective, it is usually recommended that the outcome of the subjects receiving it is compared with that of subjects

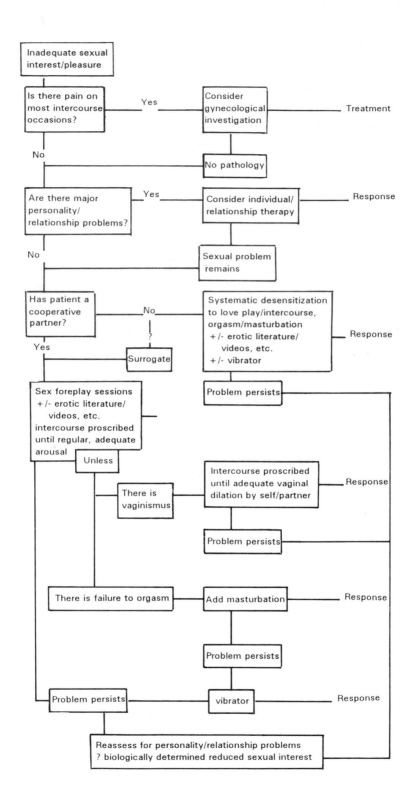

FIG. 5.2. Management of sexual dysfunction in women.

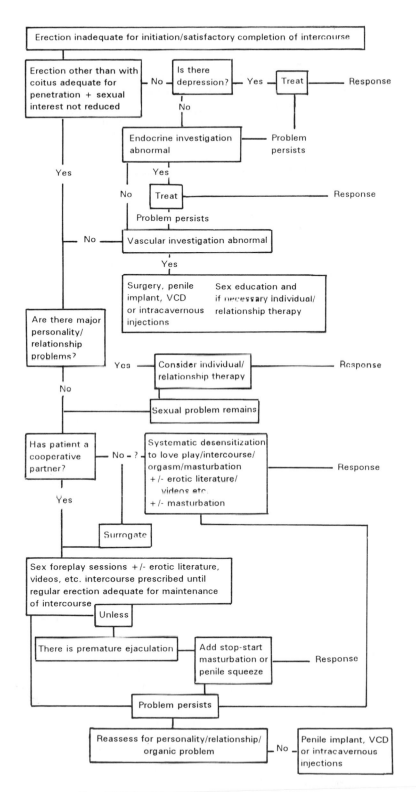

FIG. 5.3. Management of sexual dysfunction in men.

who do not (Marshall & Barbaree, 1990b; Steketee & Foa, 1987). To control for possible differences in the two groups apart from those attributable to the treatment, the subjects need to be randomly allocated to the treatment or nontreatment groups, for the reasons discussed in Chapter 1. Though this design is widely accepted, it is of dubious value. The only appropriate method to establish that a treatment has a specific effect is to compare it with a placebo procedure, that is, one accepted to have no specific treatment effect. It is essential that the subjects receiving the active treatment and those receiving the placebo both believe to the same extent that the treatment they are receiving is likely to be effective. Otherwise the expectancy of improvement of the two groups will differ, and this, of course, could affect the outcome.

Expectancy of improvement is generally accepted to contribute significantly to the results of psychological treatments. Untreated controls have no expectancy of improvement. In the evaluation of drug therapy it is possible to prepare dummy tablets identical in appearance to the active drug, so that neither patients or investigators know which patients are receiving the drug and which the placebo. It is much more difficult to design a psychological procedure that will be ineffective, yet appear to the patients to be as effective as the active treatment. For example in a study of Milan, Kilmann, and Boland (1988), the researchers decided on follow-up that the procedure introduced as a placebo was an effective treatment.

In evaluative studies using untreated controls, for ethical if not humanitarian reasons, it is usually necessary that the subjects denied treatment eventually receive it. They are informed they will be given treatment, but only after a waiting period during which their outcome without treatment will be evaluated. While waiting to receive treatment, many subjects who sought it are unlikely to make efforts to improve. Any who do may minimize or not report the improvement, fearing it would jeopardize their being given treatment later. If the delay in their receiving treatment is significant and they know other patients are receiving treatment immediately, some may feel resentment and anger. This could result in deterioration of their condition. In contrast, subjects given a placebo therapy that they believe is effective are likely to make efforts to improve. The possible negative consequences of being denied treatment could result in untreated controls showing an inferior response to that of patients allocated to immediate treatment, even if the treatment had no specific effect.

The most powerful evidence indicating the inappropriateness of untreated subjects as controls is the consistent finding of meta-analyses of treatment outcome studies. These have shown that the responses of untreated subjects are markedly inferior to those of subjects who received placebo therapies (McConaghy, 1990a). Unless it is possible to design a placebo therapy that subjects consider as likely to be effective as the active therapy when they are informed one could be a placebo, I consider the only useful evaluative studies to be those comparing treatments believed to be effective. These studies provide the information of value to clinicians. Clinicians do not deny patients treatment, but use the one they consider most effective.

Spontaneous Improvement

Little information is available concerning the spontaneous improvement rate of untreated sexual dysfunctions. It would be of some value in determining the usefulness of treatment, though subjects with a dysfunction who have not sought treatment cannot be considered equivalent to those with the same dysfunction who did. The wish to change in itself is likely to be of considerable significance in motivating the subject to improve. The reduction without treatment in women's inability to reach coitus in sexual activity that occurs from their early to middle adulthood was discussed earlier. It may be inappropriate to consider this inability a dysfunction in most of the women experiencing it; however, researchers who treat it as a dysfunction need to be aware of its marked degree of spontaneous recovery. This was ignored by Milan et al. (1988) in their investigation of women with orgasmic dysfunction 2 to 6 years after they and their partners had become randomly allocated to active treatment or a series of didactic lectures. The lectures were originally incorporated to act as a placebo. When the patients who had received the active treatment were found to show no greater improvement in orgasmic frequency than did those who received the lectures, it was decided that the latter group had not improved spontaneously, but that the lectures were an effective treatment. It was also possible that the improvement in orgasmic frequency in the women in all groups would have occurred without treatment. At follow-up their frequency of intercourse was below pretreatment levels—another likely spontaneous change, because it occurs with aging (see Chapter 2).

Hallstrom and Samuelsson (1990) followed up a representative sample of married women aged 38 to 56 after 6 years. At the original interview 36 (7%) of the 497 reported absence of sexual desire. Half regained desire without treatment over the following six years, 70% to a weak and 30% to a moderate extent.

Uncontrolled Outcome Studies

The most widely cited of the uncontrolled outcome studies of treatment for sexual dysfunctions would appear to be that of Masters and Johnson (1970). They reported a failure rate of about 29%, one of the best in the literature. The report has been severely criticized, at greatest length by Zilbergeld and Evans (1980). The subjects treated needed to give 2 to 3 weeks to the treatment, and in 90% of cases to travel to St. Louis for it, so it is likely they were much more highly motivated than subjects treated in most studies. In addition, couples were rejected who were considered to be not really interested in reversing their basic dynamics, which Zilbergeld and Evans pointed out may have screened out subjects in disturbed relationships, who would be less likely to respond. There was no mention of patients who dropped out of therapy, and it was not reported whether patients asked to leave therapy were counted as failures.

The fact that Masters and Johnson reported the number of failures rather than successes was interpreted by most readers, apparently incorrectly, as meaning that the remainder responded completely. The definition of failure used, however, was failure to initiate reversal of the basic symptomatology. Zilbergeld and Evans considered that in the case of an anorgasmic woman, this could mean that she felt less guilty about sex, became less performance oriented during sex, enjoyed sex more, had an orgasm with masturbation, or had an orgasm in intercourse. Criteria for failure with male dysfunction were also imprecise, as were those employed in a 5-year follow-up.

In the follow-up, only 7% of those who were not treatment failures had relapsed, but it was not made clear what percentage of the total sample treated were available for the follow-up evaluation; Zilbergeld and Evans believed it to be 29% of the total sample treated. They pointed out that other studies have not found such a low relapse rate, citing one of 54% in subjects treated by two psychiatrists trained by Masters and Johnson.

When results comparable to those of Masters and Johnson have been reported by other therapists, they have usually been open to some similar criticism. LoPiccolo and Stock (1986) treated 150 women for orgasmic dysfunction with a behavioral desensitization program including directed masturbation. Following treatment, 95% were able to reach orgasm with self-masturbation, 85% with genital stimulation from their partner, and 40% with penile-vaginal intercourse. No information was provided as to whether any patients dropped out of therapy.

Reported dropout rates vary remarkably. Catalan et al. (1990) offered sex therapy to 110 and marital therapy to 23 of 200 couples referred for assessment to a sexual dysfunction clinic. Despite the careful selection of patients for treatment, almost half of the 70% offered sex therapy who accepted it dropped out. Renshaw (1988) found that of 1,225 couples who attended a medical school sex clinic over 15 years, only 49 (4%) did not complete a 7-week program. She reported an 80% reversal of symptoms in the completers, but details of the reversal were not given. Forty percent of 140 couples assessed by Hawton, Catalan, Martin, and Fagg (1986) as suitable for treatment did not complete it; the treatment averaged 15 weekly sessions. Seventy-six percent of all the couples were followed up 1 to 6 years later, including 61% of those who had completed treatment. At termination of treatment, the therapists' ratings of the subjects' responses were that the problem was totally resolved in 36 (26%), was resolved with some difficulties persisting in 45 (32%), improved in 25 (18%), showed no change in 31 (22%), and was worse in 3 (2%). At follow-up, recurrence or continuing difficulty with the presenting problem was reported by 64 (75%) of the 86 couples whose relationship was still intact. This had caused little or no concern to 22 (34%), and only 11 had sought further help. Nine couples (10%) reported that a new sexual problem had developed. Slightly more than 50% of both the men and women reported they were very or moderately happy with their sexual relationship. Significant improvement in the couples' general relationship had been found at termination of therapy and was still present at follow-up.

Comparison Studies

Studies comparing treatments with placebo or nontreatment tend to report less impressive responses than those that are uncontrolled. This was true of the long-term follow-up study mentioned earlier by Milan et al. (1988) that treated anorgasmic women, employing a placebo procedure later considered an effective therapy. At posttreatment and follow-up, the mean response of the subjects was that they reached orgasm on fewer than 50% of occasions of coitus. Munjack et al. (1976) also investigated anorgasmic women; 22 most of whom were happily married, were randomly allocated either to immediate or delayed treatment with an education, communication, and desensitization program. Following treatment, one-third of the treated women were orgasmic on at least 50% of sexual relations, whereas there was no change in the untreated group. As pointed out earlier, untreated groups cannot be regarded as a satisfactory comparison group.

Kuriansky, Sharpe, and O'Connor (1982), using a behavioral desensitization program derived from that of LoPiccolo, reported equivalent responses in treated and untreated anorgasmic women. Of the 19 who completed treatment, at termination 68% experienced orgasm with masturbation, and 37% with a partner; at 2 year follow-up comparable figures were 21% and 47%. Four women were accepted for treatment, but did not start or dropped out. When interviewed 2 years later, 3 of the 4 were experiencing orgasm with a partner. Given the small numbers, the authors pointed out it was difficult to draw conclusions. Their results with treatment were much less impressive than those reported in the uncontrolled study of LoPiccolo and Stock (1986): As stated above, following treatment 95% of their subjects were able to reach orgasm with masturbation, and 85% with genital stimulation from their partners. No adequate placebo controlled studies or studies comparing recommended treatments appear to have been carried out in recent years.

Response of Different Dysfunctions

Hypoactive sexual desire disorder is generally considered to be the dysfunction most resistant to therapy. The only exception appears to be the report of Renshaw (1988), which found an 80% reversal of symptoms in over 1,000 couples, of whom 442 of the women and 250 of the men showed no interest in sex. Hawton et al. (1986), in their 1- to 6-year follow-up, found that though 70% of women with impaired sexual interest reported its resolution at termination of therapy, more than half had relapsed. As pointed out earlier, Hallstrom and Samuelsson (1990) found a spontaneous remission 6 years later in half of the women of their community sample who reported absence of sexual desire. Only 1 of the 50 male presenters in the study of Hawton et al. reported reduced interest. De Amicis et al. (1985) found regression to be worse than pretherapy levels at 3-year follow-up in both men and women treated at a sexual dysfunctions clinic for sexual desire disorder, and Kaplan (1977) reported limited success in women with this condition.

There is inadequate but suggestive evidence that retardation and particularly absence of ejaculation may also respond poorly to treatment (Munjack & Kanno, 1979). The good response at termination of treatment among men with premature ejaculation and with erectile dysfunction was maintained at follow-up only by the latter group (De Amicis et al., 1985). In the study by Hawton et al. (1986), the problem remained resolved in 60% of men with erectile dysfunction but only 25% of those with premature ejaculation. De Amicis et al. (1985) found that the good immediate response of women with anorgasmia persisted at 3-year follow-up. Vaginismus has also been consistently found to respond well to treatment. Success, usually defined as ability to have coitus, was the immediate outcome in 80% of cases in 37 studies reviewed by van de Weil, Jasper, Schultz, and Gal (1990). Persistence of response was found at 1- to 6-year follow-up in 18 of 20 female patients (Hawton et al. 1986).

Patient Characteristics

A number of studies have examined the characteristics of patients with sex dysfunctions in regard to their acceptance of and response to treatment. Predictably, a hostile relationship with the partner has been consistently found to predict a poor response (Snyder & Berg, 1983b; Takefman & Brender, 1984). Segraves et al. (1981) found marked differences between 46 men with erectile dysfunction who self-referred to a sexual dysfunction clinic and 47 referred from a urology department. Twenty-seven percent of the former and 56% of the latter declined the offer of behavioral sex therapy. Of those who accepted treatment, all the self-referred patients completed six or more sessions; 57% of the urology-referred men dropped out before six sessions. Segraves et al. found a marked lack in urology-referred as compared to self-referred patients of willingness to accept a possible role of psychological factors in their dysfunction. They commented that the current models of behavioral sex therapy were developed on a highly sophisticated self-referred population.

Catalan et al. (1990) found that couples who dropped out as compared to those who completed sex therapy had shown less initial motivations for treatment and more marked relationship and marital problems, and the presenting person had shown greater anxiety. Hawton et al. (1986) found a history of psychiatric disorder, particularly in the female partner, to be the major pretreatment predictor of poor outcome at 1- to 5-year follow-up. Couples who rated themselves before treatment as able to communicate anger showed a better response. The authors considered that communication of anger reflected the couples' general ability to communicate with each other.

Treatment Format and Components

In their review of the significance of the format of psychological treatments for sex dysfunctions, Libman, Fichten, and Brender (1985) found that whether they were administered by therapists to individuals, couples or groups, or as bibliotherapy, (i.e., by the subject's use of self-help treatment books, combined with minimal therapist contact), they appeared equally effective. LoPiccolo and Stock (1986) subsequently reported use of a self-treatment book and film for women to become orgasmic, combined with limited therapist contact, to be as effective as a complete program of therapist-administered sex therapy. Bibliotherapy alone was found to be ineffective (Libman et al., 1985), leading Rosen (1987) to criticize the commercialization of psychotherapy involved in the publication and recommendation for use without therapist supervision of self-help treatment books for sex dysfunctions. Libman et al. (1985) found no empirical support for the frequently expressed beliefs that cotherapists are more effective than single therapists or that the gender of the therapists affects treatment outcome.

Review of studies comparing different components of sex therapy revealed that in the treatment of orgasmic dysfunction in women, directed masturbation for primary anorgasmia was more effective than sensate focusing combined with supportive psychotherapy, and there were few differences between sensate focusing, systematic desensitization, and communication training (Fichten, Libman, & Brender, 1983).

Response Despite Persistence of Dysfunctions

Consistent with the low correlations between the presence of dysfunctions and sexual satisfaction discussed earlier, a common finding of outcome studies has been that despite minimal improvement of the specific dysfunction with which they presented, many subjects reported increased sexual interest and enjoyment following psychological treatment (Adkins & Jehu, 1985; De Amicis et al., 1985; Hawton et al., 1986). These changes presumably resulted from the marked improvement in many couples' general relationships that Hawton et al. pointed out was found by many workers to follow the treatment of sex problems. Hawton et al. considered this improvement to be a consequence of the improved communication between the couples that was also frequently reported to follow treatment.

These consistent findings that following psychological therapy for sexual dysfunctions, there were greater gains in sexual satisfaction and emotional relationships than in improvement in the dysfunctions led LoPiccolo, Heiman, Hogan, and Roberts (1985) to conclude that this therapy is more effective in changing the way people think and feel about their sexual life than in totally eliminating the presenting complaint. The findings emphasized that a good sexual relationship involves more than just an erect penis or an orgasm; that patients should be encouraged to enjoy the sexual process rather than to strive for results. Though this conclusion would seem true of subjects who seek and persist in psychological treatment for sexual dysfunctions, it may not apply to those who seek physical treatment—and who, if referred for psychological treatment, as Segraves et al. (1981) demonstrated in the study referred to above, are unlikely to persist with it.

TREATMENT OF ORGANIC FACTORS CAUSING SEXUAL DYSFUNCTIONS

As with psychogenic sexual dysfunctions, little information is available concerning the long-term outcome of organic dysfunctions not treated with sexual therapy. Fifty female and 51 male diabetics consented to be studied 6 years after an initial assessment (Jensen, 1986). Six of the 8 women and 8 of the 14 men who had sexual dysfunctions at that assessment had recovered 6 years later. Eight of the 14 women and men who recovered had a new partner; 4 of the remainder attributed the recovery to improvement in their emotional and social security. Five of the 14 had objective signs of peripheral and autonomic neuropathy at both interviews.

In regard to the treatment of organic factors producing or complicating sex dysfunctions, when genital or pelvic pathology is present, referral to a gynecologist or urologist is usually indicated. The use of hormones in menopausal women was discussed in Chapter 2.

Testosterone Administration

Most workers appear to agree that men with hypoactive sexual desire or impotence whose testosterone levels are below the lower limit of the normal range (3 ng/ml) should be given a trial of testosterone administration. If correction of their testosterone levels does not significantly improve their dysfunction, a trial of desensitization treatment should be instituted. Though their dysfunctions may have originally been attributable to inadequate testosterone, they could have developed secondary psychological reactions as a result of anxiety being conditioned to sexual activity in their past experiences of failure of performance. T. Jones (1985) concluded, presumably on the basis of clinical experience, that testosterone administration did not reliably improve the coital performance of men with low testosterone in the later decades of life. In fact, there is no consistent evidence of its effectiveness in men of any age group when their testosterone levels are not markedly below the lower limit of the normal range. LoPiccolo (1990) and Schwartz et al. (1980) concluded that it was generally agreed that the use of testosterone administration for sexual dysfunctions in men with normal levels of testosterone is without value.

Two complicating factors, however, could have contributed to these negative findings. As discussed earlier, levels above the lower level of normal range could be abnormally low for some men with dysfunctions but not others; as the normal levels of these men are not known, the two groups cannot be distinguished. Only the former group of men would respond to testosterone administration, and not all of them, as some would have developed secondary psychological causes. In view of the finding of Salmimies et al. (1982) that testosterone administration increased the frequency of erections and ejaculations in some men with pretreatment serum testosterone levels of up to 4.5 ng/ml, it would seem reasonable to use this level as a cut off point below which to give men with sexual dysfunctions, particularly reduced sexual interest, a trial of testosterone administration.

Physical Treatments for Organically Determined Impotence

Few men with impotence of organic etiology are found to be suitable for vascular surgery. This aims to improve the blood flow in the penile arteries or to correct venous leaks, but the results have so far often been unsatisfactory. Currently, one of three procedures are employed to enable men with impotence of organic etiology to obtain adequate erections. Discussion of these procedures in men with sexual dysfunctions obviously of psychological origin who attended expecting a nonpsychological cure has, in my experience, encouraged a number to accept cognitive-behavioral approaches. This also has occurred with some men with organic dysfunctions. When they realized the nature of the alternative procedures, they accepted a behavioral approach on the basis that it might enable them and their partners to enjoy sexual activity even if they did not develop full and rigid erections.

Penile Prostheses

The physical procedure with the longest history of use is implantation of a prosthesis in the penis. It can be a semirigid rod made of soft plastic that increases penile rigidity but not its size, or a device that can be inflated by the subject using a pump placed in the scrotum (Steege, Stout, & Carson, 1986). Steege et al. reviewed studies investigating patient satisfaction with penile implants. Of 90 private patients who received Small-Carrion semirigid prostheses 1 year or more previously, 80%

reported they were completely or somewhat satisfied, and 20% were rather or completely dissatisfied. Sixty percent rated their sexual relationships as improved and had increased their modal frequency of intercourse from once to 2 or 3 times weekly. One-quarter had some physical or social discomfort associated with the constant erection produced. Ninety-five percent of 245 men who received the Scott inflatable penile prostheses were reported by Scott, Byrd, & Karacan (1979) as able to use it to their satisfaction. In another study, 20% of men who received this prosthesis were dissatisfied because of mechanical problems, discomfort, and loss of sensation. Though 75% were very or fairly satisfied, only 30% described the erections produced as the same as natural erections.

Of 60 men who received Small-Carrion implants, 31 allowed their female partners to be interviewed. Fewer than half the women were totally satisfied with the results of the operation. Their complaints included dyspareunia, the partner's hypersexuality, and the decreased postoperative size and rigidity of his penis. Fifty percent of partners of men who received the operation privately reported total satisfaction, compared to 33% partners of men who received it at Veterans Administration (VA) hospitals. Sixty percent of partners of those treated privately and 20% of those treated by the VA had preoperative consultations with the surgeons; it was suggested that this participation by the partner in the decision-making process may have produced the more favorable response.

Steege et al., in their own survey of 52 respondents (of 85 men surveyed) who had received penile prostheses 7 to 26 months earlier, found that on a scale of 1 to 10, they rated their sexual satisfaction at 8.3 before their impotence, at 2.4 while it was present, and at 5.9 after surgery. There was no significant differences between the responses of those who had received semirigid and inflatable prostheses. Approximately one-half reported a change, almost always a decrease, in ejaculatory sensations. Even so, 90% considered that they would have the surgery again given the choices they felt they had at the time of the procedure. Schover (1989) was critical of reports of good outcomes following penile implants, arguing that there was considerable potential for distorted recall of presurgical sexual functions; that the measures of satisfaction employed in these reports, such as questions about whether the men would undergo surgery now, were usually those most responsive to cognitive dissonance; and that the clinicians who took part in reported studies generally worked in an academic setting and tended to be more sophisticated (and not only in regard to their surgical skills) in comparison to colleagues whose results were not investigated and were likely to be less satisfactory. The last criticism could be directed at outcome studies of most therapies, including cognitive-behavioral therapy.

Vasodilators and Vacuum Constriction Devices

The effects of the other two physical procedures for producing erections are not irreversible. They are carried out by the subjects following training. With one, they inject chemical vasodilators into one of the corpora cavernosa of the penis; with the other, they use a vacuum pump to evacuate air from an acrylic tube placed over the penis and pressed against the body to produce an airtight seal. The erection produced using this apparatus, termed a *vacuum constriction device* (VCD), is maintained by

an elastic band that has loops attached to aid its later removal. The band is trans-
ferred from the base of the acrylic tube to the base of the penis, and the tube is
removed.

Szasz, Stevenson, Lee, and Sanders (1987) reported a double-blind comparison
of intracavernosal injection of saline alone and saline and chemical vasodilators. Four
of 11 impotent men obtained full erections, and a further 5 erections sufficient for
intercourse, 3 hours after injection of papaverine and phentolamine and penile mas-
sage by themselves or a partner. None obtained erections after injections of saline
alone combined with the same stimulation. In an uncontrolled study, Zorgniotti and
Lefleur (1985) reported that intracavernous injection of the same chemical vasodilators combined with sexual stimulation produced adequate erections for coitus
in 59 of 62 men with diagnosed vascular impotence who had a sex partner. Eighteen
accepted the offer of training in self-injection and were able to have regular coitus,
achieving adequate erections within 4 to 10 minutes. All had rejected penile implants
and were unsuitable for penile microsurgical revascularization because of age or
disease. In a brief review of the literature concerning the procedure, Althof et al.
(1987) found prolonged painful erections, or priapism, had been reported in 4% to
16% of subjects using it; however, it was considered that this could usually be
avoided by gradually increasing the dose of chemicals to the appropriate amount.
Penile plaques, nodules, or fibrosis had been found to occur at the injection sight, but
the data published indicated that this was rare.

Althof et al. reported on the first 82 patients admitted to their program. Forty-
three, whose mean age was 57.9 years, were organically impotent; 28, whose mean
age was 58.4 years, had mixed ctiology; and 11, whose mean age was 46.8 years, had
psychogenic impotence. Fifty-two were in stable relationships. Men with psychogenic impotence received the treatment only if they failed to respond to a 6-month
trial of individual, marital, or sex therapy. Injections produced satisfactory erections
in 50 of the 52 subjects who progressed through the program's trial dose phase.
Periodic bruising occurred at the injection sight in 26%, and plaquelike nodules were
noted in 21%, but the latter did not cause penile bending or pain and did not require
termination of the treatment.

Twenty-nine subjects had completed 3 months of self-injections, doing so on an
average of 4.8 times a month. Seventy percent of the injections produced erections
sufficient for coitus. Compared with the pretreatment condition, frequency of intercourse increased, frequency of masturbation decreased, and satisfaction after sexual
activity increased. Their partners also reported greater frequency of intercourse,
greater arousal during intercourse, and greater satisfaction after sexual activity. The
couples were also reported to engage in regular noncoital sexual activity without
using the injection and to be less focused on intercourse. The 35% dropout rate
indicated that intracavernous self-injection is not the treatment of choice for all
impotent patients. Siraj, Bomanji, and Akhtar (1990) reported that prostaglandin E_1
produced a better erectile response than did papaverine.

Cooper (1987) reported on the use of the vacuum constriction device (VCD) in 5
diabetic and 4 healthy men with impotence of several years' duration. All were aged
over 40 and had failed to respond to other therapies, including cognitive-behavioral

desensitization. The men with no apparent organic disease could develop adequate erections with masturbation. Use of the VCD was initially supervised, and all subjects were able to develop erections within 7 to 20 min., although 3 had difficulty learning to maintain an airtight seal, which was essential for success. Two non-diabetic subjects complained of mild pain and mild numbness, but all 9 were willing to use the VCD in coitus, and they and their partners were given no further advice or treatment. When assessed 6 months later, the subjects had used the VCD from 3 to 28 times, with 5 using it 20 or more times and only 1 less than 10 times. Two complained of severe pain in the glans and 1 of these, who had used the VCD 3 times, did not intend to use it again. Three more were uncertain that they would continue to use it, apparently in part because of the negative feelings of their partners. The remaining 5 believed they would use it when they had strong sexual needs.

Sexual Counseling

Whichever physical procedure is being considered for the treatment of impotence, it would seem necessary to assess the couple's relationship and determine that they have a reasonable possibility of benefiting from the procedure. It would appear that the subject's partner is frequently not interviewed, possibly at times because it is not considered necessary, but often because the subject refuses consent. The advisability of providing a penile prosthesis to men in relationships without preliminary investigation of the partner's attitude could seem questionable, but less so in regard to intracavernous injection or VCD treatment in view of the reversibility of their effects. The latter could be used on a trial basis to establish the couple's ability to recommence coitus using a procedure that either or both may consider unnatural or unesthetic. Such a trial might be useful in determining the likelihood of couples maintaining a sexual life following penile implants, particularly in subjects whose partner is not available for interview. Anecdotal reports are frequent of men who requested and received penile implants, though they were in relationships that the most superficial assessment would have established were unsatisfactory. Some of the men in such relationships were reported to have believed that once they could maintain an erection, problems in the relationship would vanish. Schover (1989) cited a finding that interviews with the wife as part of the evaluation for penile implant surgery altered the sexual dysfunction diagnosis in 18% of the subjects, and changed the recommended treatment in 40%.

Schover suggested that candidates for penile prostheses would benefit from three or four sessions of brief sexual counseling. Recommended areas to be dealt with included sex education with emphasis on the effects of aging, attitude change from a performance orientation, resumption of sex in couples who had discontinued it, the use of sensate focusing, discussion of any physical disabilities present in the candidate, and brief marital counseling. Schover also recommended brief assessments at 3 and 6 months following surgery. He believed a similar counseling approach was indicated in men using intracavernous injections; this would, of course, also apply to those using VCDs.

Sexual counseling is likely to be of value to the majority of subjects with chronic medical problems and disabilities. Few, though, receive it. Tuttle, Cook, and Fitch (1964) found that two-thirds of men recovering from myocardial infarction received no advice, and in the remainder, it was vague and nonspecific advice. They concluded that without specific advice, the patients markedly reduced their sexual activity because of fear of further heart attacks and sudden death. Counseling of subjects with sexual dysfunctions to improve their physical fitness, and if appropriate to reduce their weight and intake of alcohol and tobacco, is generally recommended. The increase in sexual interest and activity found in men who improved their fitness by an exercise program and reduced smoking (J. White, Case, McWhirter, & Mattison, 1990) supports this recommendation. The strong association between sexual activity and good health found in the elderly (Chapter 2) provides further support.

Who Should Counsel?

Many psychiatrists and psychologists would consider that a member of their profession should conduct sexual counseling. In regard to the assessment of men and their partners for physical treatments of impotence, Blake, McCartney, Fried, and Fehrenbaker (1983) reported a successful outcome in subjects screened by the surgeon who performed the penile implants. Factors taken into account included the subject's apparent emotional stability, absence of depression, positive reinforcement from the partner (when present), absence of hostility toward the surgeon, degree of motivation for the procedure, and presence of reasonable expectations regarding its outcome. Twenty-two subjects who received penile implants after this screening, and their spouses when available, were examined by a psychiatrist. Only 1, who did not engage in coitus after surgery, was considered to reveal evidence of poor psychological adjustment to the procedure.

On a scale from 1 to 10, both patients and spouses rated the prosthetic erections between 4 and 10, with means of 6.4 and 6.3, respectively. More than half the couples regained their preimpotence frequency of intercourse; in general, older patients did not. All but 1 would recommend the operation to others. The report did not make clear if some subjects who received implants did not agree to be interviewed. The authors concluded that the surgeon can effectively choose implant candidates who will be satisfied with the procedure. This study conformed to Schover's evaluation (1989) of outcome studies of penile implants, in that the surgeon involved worked in an academic setting. As noted, Schover argued that these clinicians tended to be more sophisticated than many of their colleagues.

No doubt there are a number of workers treating sexual problems and dysfunctions who possess all the relevant knowledge of human behavior, gynecology, urology, and endocrinology to do so effectively. It is likely, however, that there are some who do not. In opposition to the somewhat politically motivated view of professionals that members of their discipline should continue to treat these conditions individually, the time has probably come when close liaison or, preferably, a team approach would be more effective. This might have the further advantage of reducing the number of patients who drop out of treatment in the initial stages. Some patients with sexual dysfunctions come determined to find a physical solution, just as others seek a psychological one. A team whose individual members are seen as providing these different approaches is likely to be acceptable to more subjects than a single person identified as providing only one. There should be no economic reason for professional competition: Surveys reveal that a distressingly large percentage of the population report limited enjoyment or cessation of sexual activities as a result of problems for which few seek help, though the problems are responsive to treatments currently available.

Chapter 6

Child-Adult Sexual Activity
Child Sexual Abuse

Possibly the most dramatic of the many changes that have occurred in the last two decades in beliefs concerning human sexual behavior have been those related to child-adult sexual activity. In contrast to the earlier acceptance that incest occurred in about one in a million families (Ferracuti, 1972; Weinberg, 1955), a 1972 survey found that 14% of 982 males and 9% of 1,044 females in 24 U.S. cities reported involvement in incest, if this included sexual acts such as light petting between family members (M. Hunt, 1974). The prevalence was higher in the subjects younger than 35 years. Hunt reported that many over 35 years failed to answer the question, however, so that the true prevalence in that age group may have been underestimated. Nevertheless, he believed there had been an increase in prevalence in the younger subjects of from 25% to 50%, which he attributed to sexual liberation ideology.

In retrospect, the absence of influence of feminist politics on Hunt's analysis of this data is striking. Males and females were regarded as equal participants in incestuous sexual activities, and most of the activities were considered only marginally deviant because most commonly they were between cousins, went no further than light petting, occurred before the age of 12 years, and ended within the same year. Hunt considered it reasonable to assume that most of the experiences consisted of childish sex play, so that the incestuous activities he estimated had increased in prevalence were far less momentous than they seemed at first glance. His comment that with the exception of brother-sister contacts, incestuous acts within the nuclear family remained extremely rare seems a somewhat unreasonable interpretation of his finding that 0.5% of the women reported sexual contacts with their fathers, and 0.6% with uncles. About 3.5% of both sexes reported contact with a sibling.

The lack of abhorrence shown toward evidence of incest and child-adult sexual activity in Hunt's report, published in 1974, presumably reflected current attitudes. In a questionnaire investigation of a representative sample of U.S. adolescents, 25% of boys and 13% of girls aged 13 to 19 considered false the following statement: "A parent and a child having sex with each other is something that I would consider abnormal or unnatural, even if both of them wanted to do it" (Sorensen, 1973, p. 401). Comparable percentages had the same attitude toward a brother and sister having sex together. Fifty-six percent of boys and 35% of girls aged 16 to 19 years did not believe there should be laws against having sex with a girl under the age of 16.

Fewer than 5% of adults involved as children in sexual experiences with adults believed the experience had a severe negative impact on their lives (Gagnon, 1965; Landis, 1956). Children were described as initiating and maintaining the sexual relationship with the abuser, and at times as making false accusations (Bender & Blau, 1937; Weiss, Rogers, Darwin, & Dutton, 1955). Plummer (1981) cited several workers in the 1960s and 1970s as agreeing with Schultz that most of the sexually assaulted children, where no violence was employed, were engaged in affection-seeking behavior and did not perceive the effect as traumatic. Of the 30 studies on the effects of childhood sexual experiences reviewed by Constantine (1981), 20 reported some subjects without ill effects, 13 concluded that there was essentially no harm for the majority of subjects, and 6 identified some subjects for whom the experience was positive or beneficial.

The contrast with current attitudes and beliefs is of major sociological interest. In the 1980s, sexual activity of children with postpubertal subjects 5 years or more older was defined as sexual abuse, and a specialty of victimology developed with its terminology of victim or survivor and perpetrator or offender generally accepted. This specialty adopted a medical model, so that the sexual behaviors were proscribed not on ethical, moral, or legal grounds, but because they were considered commonly to produce long-term psychological harm to the victim. This abandonment of ethical and legal judgments had the unfortunate result that objections to the sexual activities of children with subjects some years older required evidence that such activities, irrespective of their nature, commonly produce long-term harm. An inevitable consequence has been a marked reluctance to subject the evidence produced to the critical methodological analysis necessary to determine its validity. The few workers who have attempted this were not infrequently labeled skeptics, allowing their analyses to be rejected without further discussion (Finkelhor & Browne, 1988; Walker, 1988). They risk being considered not opposed to—or even covert supporters of—sexual activity of children with older subjects. In other areas of scientific knowledge, skepticism is considered essential to establish the validity of findings.

The change in attitude toward child sexual abuse appeared to have encountered some initial resistance. Sgroi (1975) commented that the professional who was sufficiently concerned and knowledgeable about the issue to be consistently alert to the possibility that sexual molestation may have occurred often produced a response of incredulity or frank hostility from colleagues. Nevertheless, she found that reporting of suspected abuse was increasing rapidly following strengthening of statutes making it mandatory and the establishment of telephone hotlines. Sgroi considered it unconscionable that any member of the helping profession would violate the law, as well as withhold potential help from the child victim, by failing to report suspected sexual abuse; however, a survey at that time indicated that 90% of incest cases were not being reported (Weeks, 1976).

Weeks suggested that the way adults handled the child and the situation after a sexual assault was probably the single most important factor in determining the effect of the event on the child, suggesting that she believed mandatory reporting may not always be in the child's best interest. Gibbens, Soothill, and Way (1978) quoted an earlier comment that the victims of physically incestuous relations with fathers often seemed far less seriously disturbed psychologically than would be supposed possible, and by contrast, that a highly emotional situation between father and daughter without physical relations could be extremely disruptive. On the basis of interviews with 109 Californian subjects who had incestuous relationships, C. Symonds, Mendoza, and Harrell (1981) concluded that "sexual relations with siblings or other close relatives can provide a satisfactory method for children to satisfy their initial sexual curiosity. Contact between parents and children can sometimes offer the child a well-rounded introduction to sexual functioning in a secure and nonthreatening environment" (p. 161). They decided the abhorrence of contact with kin is strictly a social prohibition that has little to do with practice.

Finkelhor (1981), though stressing that a significant number of sibling incestuous experiences had an exploitive character, reported that positive and/or peer-oriented sibling sexual experiences had lasting, apparently healthy effects on some of the female partners' sexual outlooks. Where boys were concerned, some workers challenged the distinction between assailant and victim, considering that it did not fully represent the true facts. Advancing this view, Ingram (1979) stated that children could be seductive toward adults, participate fully in and enjoy sexual acts with them, and suffer greatly when the acts were discovered and there was a family scene followed by police investigation and court proceedings. He concluded that counseling should replace prosecution except where there is violence or sadism or some other reason for intervention by the law. Plummer (1979) argued that the children's problems could be compounded by police and court action and quoted evidence that only 5% of victims had damaged adult lives, and that the damage could have diverse origins.

PREVALENCE OF CHILD-ADULT SEXUAL ACTIVITY

During the 1980s, questioning of the harmful effects of child-adult sexual activities ceased as the number of cases reported in the United States escalated dramatically from 60,000 in 1974 to 2.5 million in 1989 ("Social Worker," 1990). LaBarbera, Martin, and Dozier (1980) reported that child psychiatrists in the United States who responded to a survey all viewed father-daughter incest as moderately to extremely harmful to the daughters, though the greater the psychiatrists' clinical experience with such incest, the less psychologically injurious they considered it. An extensive literature documented both the prevalence of sexual activities with adults reported by women and their association with subsequent psychological maladjustment.

Probably the most widely quoted estimate of the prevalence of such experiences was that provided by Russell (1986) from a 1978 study of 50% of a probability sample of 930 adult women in San Francisco. Russell defined incestuous abuse as any sexual contact or attempted contact with a relative 5 years or more older that began when the woman was less than 18 years of age. The experience was defined as abuse whether or not she considered it to be neutral or positive. Unwanted nonforceful kissing was abusive; exhibitionism and verbal propositions without some gesture were not. Experience with a relative less than 5 years older was abusive if the woman was not the initiator, and if she reported long-term effects or some distress at the time or retrospectively. Extrafamilial abuse was defined more narrowly to include unwanted sexual experiences ranging from unwanted petting (touching or attempted touching of breasts or genitals) to rape before the victim was aged 14 years, and attempted or completed forcible rape between 14 and 17 years. For girls of this age, unwanted petting and intercourse in dating situations were not defined as abusive.

Russell (1986) found that 38% of the women reported at least one experience of incestuous or extrafamilial abuse before the age of 18, 16% with a relative and 31% with a nonrelative. Corresponding figures for such experiences before the age of 14 were 28%, 12%, and 20%, respectively. Using a broader definition of abuse incorporating the noncontact experiences some of her subjects reported, at least 54% had experienced sexual abuse before age 18 and 48% before age 14. Of the perpetrators, 11% were total strangers, 29% were relatives, and 60% were known but unrelated to the victims. The perpetrating relatives were mainly uncles (25%), biological (14%) or nonbiological fathers (10%), male first cousins (16%), and brothers (13%). Seventeen percent of women reared by a stepfather were sexually abused by him before the age of 14, compared with 2% of those reared by a biological father. For stepfathers who were with the victim for shorter periods of time, the risk may have been substantially higher (Russell, 1984). Cross-generational incest was likely to occur over an extended period, which Russell attributed to the power and authority involved; brothers and first cousins were more likely to use physical force. Five percent of incest perpetrators were female. Perpetrating nonrelatives were mainly acquaintances or family friends. Only 2% of the intrafamilial and 6% of the extrafamilial experiences of child sexual abuse were reported to the police.

Russell (1988) considered her findings to be most comparable with those of a questionnaire survey of the prevalence of child sexual abuse reported by 796 undergraduates of six New England colleges and universities, carried out by Finkelhor (1979). In his study, abuse included intercourse, oral-genital contacts, fondling, and being exhibited to by a person at least 5 years older. Seventeen percent of women reported such abuse by age 12, and 6% between ages 13 and 16—19% in all, correcting for those with multiple experiences. Russell (1986) contrasted the low percentage of cross-generational incest (14%) in Finkelhor's study with the 60% that she found. In Finkelhor's study, 39% of perpetrators of incest with women were brothers; uncles made up 9%, and fathers and stepfathers 4%. Russell considered the higher prevalence of such more taboo experiences of father-daughter and other cross-generational abuse found in her study to be attributable in part to the subjects being more likely to disclose these experiences when the information was collected by the method she employed of face-to-face interviews by women trained to encourage such disclosure. She commented of the training "that it would have been foolish to send *supposedly* unbiased interviewers into the field without first educating them about the issues involved" (p. 21). Finkelhor (1984) pointed out that in Russell's study, 14 separate questions were asked about situations where child abuse may have occurred, and that it was likely that "all this probing turned up experiences that are either not remembered or not seen as relevant when more general screening questions are asked" (p. 81).

The belief of Russell and Finkelhor that the method of obtaining the data from the women investigated influenced the prevalence of childhood sexual experiences with older subjects reported was supported empirically by Wyatt and Peters (1986a, b). They attempted to determine the reasons for the much lower prevalence of childhood sexual abuse found by Finkelhor as compared with Russell and with Wyatt in her Los Angeles study (1985). Wyatt and Peters concluded that the definition of childhood sexual abuse accounted for only a portion of the discrepancy in the prevalences reported. The major factor was the method of collecting the data: Face-to-face interviews in which multiple probing questions were asked about specific types of abusive sexual behaviors by interviewers given special training in ideologically correct attitudes were associated with much higher prevalence rates. Variations in the age of the subjects may have had an effect, but use of random sampling techniques, the area of the United States in which the study was conducted, and the educational level and ethnic composition of the subjects did not appear to be influential.

Like Russell, Wyatt (1985) investigated women's experiences in face-to-face interview by workers said to be selected for their sensitivity to the issue of sexual assault and then given 65 hours of training that included information about rape and incestuous abuse. Her Los Angeles study found the highest prevalence as yet to appear in the literature, with 62% of women reported having experienced sexual abuse prior to the age of 18 (Wyatt, 1985). It would be of sociological interest to investigate whether the current absence of questioning of possible bias by interrogators trained to detect child abuse was paralleled by absence of questioning of the possible bias of interrogators trained to detect witchcraft in the seventeenth and eighteenth centuries. Finkelhor (1984), like Wyatt and Peters (1986b), recommended that probing by interviewers trained in a particular ideology be used in future research of child sexual abuse. This methodology does not appear to have been used as yet to determine the prevalence of sexual abuse of males.

Wyatt and Peters's conclusion that failure to employ this interrogatory method was associated with markedly lower prevalence rates was supported by recent surveys. Siegel, Sorenson, Golding, Burnman, and Stein (1987), as part of the Los Angeles Epidemiologic Catchment Area Project, interviewed 1,645 women, of whom about one-quarter were Hispanic and the remainder largely non-Hispanic whites. The women were asked once if anyone had tried to pressure or force them to have sexual contact. Seven percent reported such experiences before the age of 16 years. In opposition to another of Wyatt and Peters's conclusions, though, the subjects' ethnic background was influential; non-Hispanic white women under 40 years of age reported a prevalence of 15%. In relation to the lower prevalence of abuse found in their study as compared to those of Russell and Wyatt, Siegel et al. suggested that prompting of respondents and the younger age of the subjects contributed to the higher rates of other studies. Prepubertal experiences with postpubertal partners not obtained by force or pressure were not classified as abusive in their study, another difference that would have reduced the prevalence found. The assailants' relationships to the victims were comparable to that found by Russell: Strangers comprised 22%, acquaintances 56%, and relatives 23% (of whom 13% were parents). Continued assault was more likely to be carried out by a relative, and 93% of the assailants were male.

Increase in Prevalence

Russell (1986) found that 8% of women in their 60s, 12% in their 50s, 22.5% in their 40s, 24% in their 30s, and 17.7% in their 20s reported incestuous abuse. She considered the reports to reflect the actual prevalence of abuse, rejecting the possibility that older women were less willing to regard or report incidents as abusive on the questionable basis that the youngest group of women reported less abuse than the two cohorts in their 30s and 40s. Russell concluded that the prevalence of childhood sexual abuse had quadrupled from the early 1900s to 1973, most of the increase in incestuous abuse until age 18 occurring after 1937, and in extrafamilial abuse until age 14 after 1960. In contradistinction, Wyatt and Peters (1986b), to reconcile the results of their Los Angeles survey with those of Russell, concluded that the prevalence of child sexual abuse may have been higher in the post– than the pre–World War II era, but had not increased appreciably in the last 30 years.

Russell attributed the rise in prevalence of child abuse that she believed she had detected over the recent period to such factors as increased access to child pornography; the all-sex-is-OK philosophy of the sexual revolution; a backlash against sexual equality by men terrified of dealing with adult women as equals and turning to children; an increase in the number of stepfamilies (as children are at much greater risk of abuse from stepfathers than biological fathers); and, finally, lack of treatment of male victims of child abuse resulting in many becoming perpetrators. Russell suggested that child sexual abuse was likely to grow geometrically on the basis of this last causative factor alone, possibly doubling in each generation. This conclusion seemed at variance with her finding of a reduced prevalence of childhood abuse in her youngest cohort, those in their 20s—the age by which incidents of most abuse of victims had occurred.

Also, it would appear to lack a historical perspective. DeMause (1974), in his review of the evolution of childhood, concluded that the further back in history one went, the lower the level of child care was, and the more likely children were to be killed, abandoned, beaten, terrorized, and sexually abused. Sexual activity with children, particularly girls, was considered normal for many centuries (particularly in the East), and a marriage age for girls of 12 years was accepted in England until 1929 (Bender & Blau, 1937). If DeMause is correct, a reduction in the prevalence of sexual abuse has occurred over the centuries despite the absence of treatment for victims. Also despite its absence, the prevalence of sexual abuse remained relatively unchanged from 1909 to 1940 according to the data provided by Russell, at variance with her conclusion that it should have grown geometrically. Finkelhor (1984) believed it was not possible to establish whether the prevalence of child sexual abuse had altered in the present as compared with previous centuries. Nevertheless, Russell's conclusion required that attention be given to the sexual abuse of males, a somewhat ignored issue. In the recent *Handbook on Sexual Abuse of Children* (Walker, 1988), child sexual abuse almost invariably meant abuse of female children.

Prevalence in Males

Finkelhor's study (1979) was one of the earliest of the rare surveys that investigated the prevalence of abuse in male as well as female children. Finkelhor (1985) pointed out that the initiation of attention to sexual abuse by the women's movement coalesced around the incest model, which was less relevant to abuse of boys. The resultant neglect of boys as victims was compounded by two presumptions that he considered to be poorly supported by evidence—that boys often initiated and, in any case, were less negatively affected by sexual contact with older persons. Nine percent of the male undergraduates in Finkelhor's study reported being sexually abused by an older person by age 16, about half the rate for women. In 91% the experience was initiated by the older person, who in 33% of cases was a family member. The boys, like the girls, were mainly abused by older men.

Fritz, Stoll, and Wagner (1981), in another questionnaire investigation of college students, found that 4.8% of men (as compared to 7.7% of women) reported experiencing at least one sexual encounter with a postadolescent individual before they reached puberty. Unlike the Finkelhor study, physical contact of an overtly sexual nature was required, which along with the lower age limit would account at least in part for the reduced prevalence. A further difference was that a majority (60%) of the men reported that the molester was a woman. As in Finkelhor's study, the molesters of the men were less likely to be family members, and the men were much less likely than women to have talked about the molestation to family members. Positive coercion by reward, rather than negative coercion by threat of attack, was much more likely to have been experienced by male as compared to female victims.

To obtain an estimate of the prevalence of sexual abuse of boys under 13 years of age by partners 5 or more years older, Finkelhor (1985) reviewed the small number of studies then available, none of which were national samples, and only a few of which were random samples. He found a marked consistency, with between 2.5% and 5% of males reporting abuse. Finkelhor suggested that the fact that few male victims were reported in clinical studies of sexually abused children was evidence of the reduced likelihood of male victims being identified by helping agencies. That boys were both more likely than girls to be abused outside the home, and less likely to report the abuse, contributed to this situation. Finkelhor attributed the reluctance of boys as compared to girls to report abuse to fear of the stigma of homosexuality and the possible loss of the greater freedom and independence they were given as compared to girls. Subsequent to the studies reviewed by Finkelhor, a U.S. national survey reported that 27% of women and 16% of men were molested in childhood (Finkelhor & Lewis, 1988); the Los Angeles Epidemiologic Catchment Area Project (Siegel et al., 1987) found that 3.8% of the total sample of 1,480 men and 6.5% of those who were non-Hispanic whites under 40 years of age reported being pressed or forced into sexual contacts, and a national survey of 2,000 adults in Canada found that 22% of women and 9% of men had experienced serious and unwanted sexual abuse before the age of 18 (Carver, Stalker, Stewart, & Abraham, 1989).

In contrast to these figures from community surveys in which half as many male as female children were sexually abused, a national incidence study that collected data on all cases known to professionals in the United States (Alter-Reid, Gibbs, Lachenmeyer, Sigal, & Massoth, 1986) found 83% of victims to be female. Alter-Reid et al. quoted similar findings from an equivalent United Kingdom study. Also, the annual national statistics on sexually abused children provided by the U.S. child protection system consistently report male cases to be 20% or less compared to female cases (Faller, 1989). Faller reported 373 cases of sexual abuse referred to

Michigan child protection agencies between 1979 and 1986; 28% were male, the highest percentage reported in noncommunity studies.

FEATURES OF CHILD SEXUAL ABUSE

In regard to the incidence of intrafamilial versus extrafamilial abuse, 23% of boys and 14% of girls in nationally reported child protection cases were sexually abused by nonfamily members (Faller, 1989). Faller's study reported comparable figures, with 37% of boys and 11% of girls suffering extrafamilial abuse. Faller pointed out that the incidence of extrafamilial abuse is higher in both males and females investigated in community surveys. In Finkelhor's 1979 and 1984 studies, 83% and 77% of boys and 56% and 66% of girls, respectively, were abused by nonfamily members.

In regard to the age of the victims when sexually abused, in Faller's study (1989) of reported abuse, the mean age at the onset was 6.3 years in boys and 5.5 years in girls. In a study of 566 sexually abused children seen at a sexual assault crisis center of an inner-city hospital, the age of the male victims showed one modal peak at age 7, whereas the female distribution showed modal peaks at ages 6 and 15 with a sharp decrease in reported cases between 6 and 11 (Alter-Reid et al., 1986). Faller (1989) commented on the inconsistency in the literature concerning whether the mean age at onset of abuse was higher in boys or girls. Victims in community surveys tended to be older, the mean age of those at first assault in the Los Angeles area project (Siegel et al., 1987) being 9.5 years. For the victims of continued assault, however, it was 8.5 years, the assaults ending at a mean age of 13.1 years. The higher age of the victims and the increased prevalence of extrafamilial abuse in cases reported retrospectively in community studies, as compared with those reported at the time of occurrence, suggest that extrafamilial abuse is more prevalent in older children and is less likely to be reported.

Little information is provided by most studies as to the socioeconomic status of victims of sexual abuse. Alter-Reid et al. (1986) stated they would present data concerning this when it was available, but presented none. Russell (1986) stated that unlike earlier surveys, her study found incest victims to be more likely to have come from families with higher incomes and slightly better education. She did not consider the possibility that when questioned by ideologically correct interrogators, educated women might remember more abusive experiences. She found no relationship with the fathers' level of education or occupation. In Finkelhor's questionnaire study (1980) of students, 33% of girls from families with incomes of less than $10,000 reported being sexually victimized, compared to 19% of the total sample. In cases of confirmed abuse reported to a national clearinghouse, the income of families of sexually abused children fell in the lower end of the socioeconomic spectrum, but was somewhat higher than for all forms of child abuse cases. This data was heavily biased toward abuse committed by parents and other caretakers, and 87% of the victims were girls (Finkelhor, 1983). In Faller's study (1989), 46% of male victims' families were middle-class, and 54% were working-class; 20.5% of female victims' families were middle-class and 79.5% working-class, the difference being statistically significant. Faller attributed the difference to the fact that a higher percentage of girls were abused within the family.

In regard to the sex of the offenders, as the predominance of males is high, this information is commonly not reported. In surveys of adolescents and adults retrospectively reporting childhood abuse, women were the abusers of female children in 4% (Russell, 1983), 5% (Fromuth, 1986), 10% (Fritz et al., 1981), and 19% (Finkelhor, 1985) of cases; they were the abusers of male children in 17% (Finkelhor, 1985), 40% (Johnson & Shrier, 1987), 50% (Risin & Koss, 1987), 60% (Fritz et al., 1981), and 75% (Fromuth & Burkhart, 1989) of cases. As at least twice as many girls are abused as boys, it is possible, as Russell (1986) believed, that women may abuse more girls than boys. An investigation of sexually abused children referred to a project on child abuse and neglect found that of girl victims, 81% were molested by males, 1% by females, and 28% by both males and females; of boy victims, 63% were molested by males, 8% by females, and 29% by both males and females (Faller, 1989). It is possible that with the recent increase in reporting of child abuse of males, the percentage of women revealed to be involved has also increased. Krug (1989) reported 8 cases of sexual abuse of male children by their mothers, and suggested that it may not be as rare as commonly believed. Feldman, Mallouh, and Lewis (1986) found that 5 of 15 condemned murderers had been sexually abused as children, 2 by their mothers. Cavanagh Johnson (1989) investigated 13 girls treated in a program for perpetrators: Their child victims had a mean age of 4 years and were mainly members of their family, and twice as many victims were boys as girls.

To assess the likelihood of familial sexual abuse, Finkelhor (1980) developed a Sex Abuse Risk Factor Checklist for women victims: stepfather, ever lived without mother, not close to mother, mother never finished high school, sex-punitive mother, no physical affection from father, income under $10,000, and two friends or less in childhood. In children with none of the factors sex abuse was virtually absent. Its likelihood increased as more of these factors were present, with two-thirds of those girls with five factors present being abused.

NATURE OF CHILD SEXUAL ABUSE

The major research studies of the prevalence of child abuse classified acts as abusive that ranged from exposure and forced kissing to anal and vaginal penetration. As all child-adult sexual activities tended to be regarded as equally harmful, little information was usually provided concerning the frequency of the various acts. Herman (1985) reported that abuse of daughters usually began when the child was between the ages of 6 and 12, the initial contact being fondling and gradually proceeding to masturbation and oral-genital activities. Vaginal intercourse was not usually attempted at least until the child reached puberty. Physical violence was rare, the authority of the parent being sufficient to gain compliance. The sexual contact was repeated for years, secrecy being ensured by threats of family breakup or expulsion of the child, so that the abuse ended only when the child found the resources to escape. In Russell's study (1986) of San Francisco women, in almost half the cases of abuse by stepfathers and a quarter of those by biological fathers, the abuse was in the category classified as very serious, which included activities ranging from forced penile-vaginal penetration to nonforceful attempted fellatio, cunnilingus, analingus, and anal intercourse. The most serious experience reported by male students from an approximately representative national sample who were molested before 14 years of age was exhibitionism in one-third; fondling in one-third; and attempted or successful penetration in one-third (Risin & Koss, 1987).

Gomes-Schwartz, Horowitz, and Sauzier (1985) investigated 112 children attending a family-crisis program for sexually abused children. The most serious sexual acts they had experienced were vaginal or anal intercourse in 18%, oral-genital contact or penetration by a foreign object in 38%, and fondling in 23%. Younger children were abused for a shorter time and were less likely to have experienced intercourse. The threat or use of force was not mentioned. Freund, Heasman, and Roper (1982) pointed out the enormous discrepancy in reported incidences of the use of force in sexual abuse of children, ranging from 0% to 58%; they attributed the discrepancy to the different samples of victims studied. None of the 18,000 persons interviewed by the Kinsey group claimed to have been sadistically victimized as a child (Quinsey, 1986). Berliner (1985) pointed out the common absence of physical evidence in reported cases of child abuse. Frude (1985) and Finkelhor and Lewis (1988) suggested that most child sexual abuse did not involve violent attack on children but the use of authority or misrepresentation.

THE FAMILY IN FATHER-CHILD INCEST

In their review, Alter-Reid et al. (1986) found only one study of family pathology related to child sexual abuse. Mrazek, Lynch, and Bentovim (1983) reported its presence in 56% of families of victims they studied. In 34%, the pathology consisted of poor marital relationships; in 25%, emotional problems in the child; in 14%, parental mental illness; in 13%, unemployment; in 10%, alcoholism; in 10%, previous parental criminality; in 9%, sexual abuse of other siblings; and in 6%, physical abuse of a child. Cammaert (1988) commented that the literature prior to this decade concerning the family in father-child incest was based on clinical impressions and tended to treat the wife of an incestuous husband as a facilitator, if not the primary cause, of the incest. She was seen as failing to make sex gratifying for her husband, reversing roles with her daughter by deliberately working outside the home, or collusively providing opportunities for incest to occur and then turning a blind eye. Cammaert pointed out that little research had investigated incestuous families to substantiate these beliefs. The few studies she found indicated these families were experiencing stress caused by larger than average family size, high family discord, wife battering, and mental health problems. Though problems existed in the marital sex relationship, the father was usually able to command sex from his wife. Cammaert also reviewed a number of studies investigating the personality of the nonoffending mothers that found them to show less self-esteem, passivity, depression, and alcoholism. She considered that these findings provided little support for the strongly pejorative clinical descriptions of the women and that the negative aspects of their personality reported could be the result of living in an atmosphere of male violence.

De Jong (1988) investigated the mothers of 103 children following their evaluation at a sexual assault center for Philadelphia County. He reported that 31% of the mothers were nonsupportive of the child, believing the abuse complaint to be a lie or attributable to misunderstanding, or that the abuse was primarily the child's fault. Mothers were more likely to be nonsupportive in cases of abuse by fathers or by mothers' paramours, as compared with cases of abuse by other perpetrators. Nonsupportive mothers felt frustrated that the police and protective services were doing too much, whereas supportive mothers complained they were doing too little.

The concept of mother-daughter role reversal was upheld in a study (Herman, 1981) that found that 45% of 40 women victims of incest had been pressed into service as "little mothers" by the age of 10. In 55% of these families, the mother was ill, disabled, or absent for a period of time during which the father did not assume the maternal role, which fell to the oldest daughter. Fifty-eight percent of the victimized daughters never told their mothers of the incest, though they gave vague and indirect indications of distress. Longing for their mothers to rescue them, they felt betrayed and disappointed at their mothers' failure to recognize the nature of the problem. Of the mothers who knew, most were unable or unwilling to defend their daughters. Herman commented that most of these mothers saw no option other than submission to their husbands. They conveyed to their daughters the belief that a woman is defenseless against a man, that marriage must be preserved at all costs, and that a wife's duty is to serve and endure. Like other workers (Browne & Finkelhor, 1986), Herman found that more victims were hostile to their mothers than to the offending fathers.

The tendency of incestuous families to accept a pathological exaggeration of the patriarchal norms of society, noted by Herman, was also emphasized by Asher (1988). She discussed the societal implications of child sexual abuse, arguing that it contributed to the perpetuation of a society in which men dominated in terms of political and economic power and of the control they exerted over women's bodies. Such a society contributed to the sexual victimization of women and children, and the victimization created women who simultaneously feared, overvalued, overidealized, and were dependent upon men because of their immense power. Asher reviewed evidence supporting the conclusion that the typical family in which incest occurred was male dominated and authoritarian. She suggested that the girls growing up in such families became passive, dependent, and lacking in coping skills, and that the boys learned to devalue women at an early age and began to experience power over them, so that the dynamics of such families were transmitted intergenerationally.

LONG-TERM EFFECTS OF CHILD SEXUAL ABUSE

Finkelhor and Browne (1988) concluded that though the belief of clinicians that sexual abuse in childhood can have serious long-term effects was based on less than rigorous studies, it was confirmed by subsequent nonclinical studies. They quoted three random sample community surveys and five studies investigating college students that found that women in the general population with a history of child sexual abuse had identifiable mental health problems compared to nonvictims. They pointed out that the findings of these studies challenged the objection that the problems found in clinical studies were simply a function of the clinical setting. They did not confront the major methodological problem with the community studies that, presumably because of the current political atmosphere, has been virtually ignored. This is that the studies were quasi-experimental.

Quasi-Experimental Evidence of the Effects of Child Sexual Abuse

As discussed in Chapter 1, in quasi as opposed to true experiments, subjects are not randomly allocated to the experimental and comparison condition, usually because it is not possible to do so—one cannot randomly allocate half of a sample of children to sexual abuse and the other half not. Random allocation of subjects controls for any differences between the two groups other than exposure to the experimental or the comparison condition. Without random allocation, it is not possible to attribute differences found between sexually abused and control subjects to the effect of the abuse without first excluding all other possible causes. The first step to exclude such possible other causes is to match the abused and the control subjects on all other variables that could possibly be considered to affect the outcome measured.

This matching procedure would not seem possible with child sexual abuse. The psychological abuse, parental neglect, or family disorganization that commonly accompany sexual abuse (Finkelhor, 1984) are virtually impossible to match in the control group; failures of matching have been frequently reported (Conte & Berliner, 1988; Jackson, Calhoun, Amick, Maddever, & Habif, 1990). A number of factors other than sexual abuse could contribute significantly to subsequently found pathology. Weeks (1976) suggested that how the report of the abuse was handled by the surrounding adults was a determinant of its consequences. In relation to abuse by a biological relative, a genetically transmitted personality factor may have caused him or her to offend and, independently, produced the pathology in the victim. Acceptance by therapists of the belief that childhood sexual abuse is invariably traumatic could result in their treating subjects reporting abuse with more than usual concern. From a behavioral perspective, this would reinforce and so increase illness behavior in the vulnerable subject, producing an apparent association between reported abuse and psychiatric symptoms. Personality vulnerabilities of the victims could result in their victimization, after which the vulnerability could be attributed to the abuse.

In the current political climate, one factor possibly contributing to the relationship between reported child sexual abuse and later pathology can be suggested only at the risk of being considered an abuser. This is that some psychologically disturbed subjects could be more likely than the nonabused to interpret incidents in childhood as sexually abusive. In any other context, it would be considered poor clinical judgment to accept automatically the statements of subjects with borderline personality disorders, in view of their tendency to distort reality and their marked needs for attention (Chapter 1). Yet their frequent statements that they were incestuously abused as children are the basis for the commonly accepted belief that such abuse is a major etiological factor in borderline personality disorder (Mrazek &

Mrazek, 1981). Armsworth (1989) investigated 30 female psychotherapy patients who reported experiencing incest in childhood or adolescence. She stated that in some instances, they had no memory of the incest until they talked to the third or fourth professional from whom they sought help. She found that 23% of these women reported sexual involvement with a therapist, and an additional 23% reported that a therapist exploited and victimized them in other ways; one way was by not believing their reports of incest. Armsworth appears to demand that such statements be unquestioningly accepted. In view of her finding that 46% of incest victims reported abuse by therapists, particular caution would appear advisable in the treatment of these patients.

From a methodological point of view, the factors are almost endless that need to be excluded before it can be accepted that child sexual abuse in itself is responsible for the psychological symptoms found retrospectively in subjects who report such abuse. Prospective studies that followed up a cohort of subjects from early childhood into adolescence and adulthood could provide more convincing evidence. They would allow investigation of the relationship between observed changes in the subjects' mental health or behavior and the time of occurrence of any reported abuse. Though studies following up children have been carried out, they do not appear to have investigated this relationship (Burnam et al., 1988). In the meantime, an appropriate control to include in retrospective studies of the long-term effects of child sexual abuse would be to record the presence of other stressful experiences, sexual and nonsexual, in the subjects' histories. These would include victimization by exhibitionism, obscene telephone calls, and unwanted exposure to pornography, as well as by stressful social, educational, and work experiences. This information would enable the possibility to be excluded that childhood sexual abuse is one of a number of nonspecific stresses to which vulnerable people are inevitably exposed and that are therefore found associated with their later demonstrated pathology. Multivariate analysis could establish whether the sexual abuse of itself was associated with additional long-term effects. It would seem that for most child and adolescent health workers, sexual abuse has replaced maternal deprivation as the major childhood experience producing long-term psychological problems. Maternal deprivation held that position in the 1960s and 1970s, on the basis of equally methodologically unsatisfactory but politically powerful evidence (McConaghy, 1979).

Finkelhor (1984) emphasized the need for great caution in interpreting quasi-experimental data in relation to his finding that students who as boys were sexually victimized by older men were over four times more likely to be currently engaged in homosexual activity than were nonvictims:

> It must be emphasized that these data show a "correlation" between sexual victimization and later "homosexual" behavior, but this is by no means saying that the former causes the latter. . . . Much theorizing has taken place about the "causes" of homosexuality that has harmed homosexuals and their public image. . . . In short, these kind of findings cannot and should not be used to increase our culture's already intense fear of homosexuals. (p. 196)

He did not caution against interpreting the equivalent relationship between sexual abuse of girls and their subsequent pathology as evidence that the abuse caused the pathology. It would seem the requirements for interpreting research findings vary in rigor depending on the social and political consequences of the interpretation.

Nature of Symptoms Associated with Abuse

Whether or not a causal relationship is involved, the evidence is substantial that reported child abuse is associated with some degree of emotional disturbance in later life in the majority of female subjects investigated in clinical studies. It is uncertain how representative these subjects are of victims of sexual abuse in the total population.

Community Studies

Studies of community samples have produced inconsistent results. Tsai, Feldman-Summers and Edgar (1979) investigated adult female victims of childhood sexual abuse recruited by a media request that offered therapy, but emphasized that the project was open to women who considered themselves well adjusted and not in need of therapy. Molested women not seeking therapy did not differ from matched nonmolested controls on MMPI personality profiles or in current sexual activities and satisfaction. Molested women seeking therapy showed elevated Psychopathic Deviate and Schizophrenia scale scores on the MMPI and reported reduced sexual satisfaction. Compared to subjects not seeking treatment, they reported a higher frequency, longer duration, and later age of cessation of molestation and stronger negative feelings to the experience. Finkelhor (1984) pointed out the molested subjects in this study could not be considered representative of those in the total population, a criticism that could be made of all clinical and many community samples. Fritz et al. (1981) investigated 952 college students by questionnaire; 10% of men and 24% of women molested as children reported current sexual problems. The prevalence of the problems in the unmolested students was not reported. As discussed in Chapter 5, depending on how sexual problems are defined, they can be reported by more than half of the normal population.

Finkelhor (1984) found that both female and male students who reported childhood sexual abuse had lower levels of sexual self-esteem than the nonabused students. Fromuth was unable to replicate this finding. She used an anonymous self-report questionnaire modified from that used by Finkelhor to investigate 383 female college students (Fromuth, 1986) and 582 male university students (Fromuth & Burkhart, 1989); 22% of the women and 14% of the men reported at least one abusive experience. No relationship was found in either women or men between childhood abuse and scores on the Beck Depression Inventory, Rosenberg Self-Esteem Scale, Locus of Control Scale, a self-rated adjustment scale, or the Finkelhor Sexual Self-Esteem scale. Low scores on the Parental Support Scale were correlated with childhood sexual abuse in women but not in men. There was some evidence that the sexually abused women experienced a wider range of sexual activity and were more sexually active than the nonabused. This has also been reported of women victims of postpubertal sexual assault (Chapter 7). The women sexually abused in childhood were no more likely than the nonabused to experience sexual problems.

In contrast to the findings of Finkelhor (1984) and Johnson and Shrier (1987), Fromuth and Burkhart (1989) found sexually abused men were no more likely than the nonabused to report a homosexual experience occurring after the age of 12.

Fromuth (1986) found that sexually abused women were more likely to report this. In Fromuth and Burkhart's study, somewhat less than half the men were from a midwestern university, and the remainder from a southeastern university. Abused men from the midwestern sample showed a higher frequency of noncoital sexual behavior, reported more difficulty in achieving and maintaining erection, and obtained scores more indicative of pathology on the Hopkins Symptom Checklist. Abused men in the southeastern sample were more likely to report problems with premature ejaculation. The authors suggested that in the southeastern United States, sexual relations between a boy and an adult, particularly a woman, might be viewed less negatively and so be less likely to produce later maladjustment. A very large number of statistical relationships were investigated in the study, most of which were insignificant. No adjustment of probability levels was made to correct for the numbers of relationships tested, so that the few significant differences found may have been chance false-positive (type I) errors (see Chapter 1).

Clinical Studies

Finkelhor and Browne (1988) pointed out the nature of the disturbances found in clinical studies of adult women who reported childhood sexual abuse appeared not to be specific. Asher (1988) also reached this conclusion in her review and commented on attempts to define a postabuse syndrome that not all incest victims will fit one pattern of symptom presentation, and that the victim's account of abuse should not be discounted because she presents with symptoms not commonly associated with childhood sexual abuse. Such a presentation would be rare, in the light of Asher's earlier statement concerning the "myriad of symptoms that have been mentioned as long-term effects of childhood sexual abuse" (p. 10). Lists of reported consequences of child sexual abuse found in women seeking treatment included depression, self-destructive behavior, anxiety and tension, anger and hostility, poor self-esteem, feelings of isolation and stigma, fear of and difficulty in trusting others (especially men), homosexuality, promiscuity, physical and sexual revictimization, marital and relationship problems, sexual difficulties, sleep disturbances (including nightmares), eating disorders, drug and alcohol abuse, multiple and borderline personality disorders, schizophrenia, and murder (Asher, 1988; Browne & Finkelhor, 1986; Finkelhor & Browne, 1988; Mrazek & Mrazek, 1981; R. Palmer, 1990).

As more than 50% of women and 20% of men have been found to be victims of child sexual abuse, depending on the criteria used, a similar percentage of subjects with any psychiatric condition or emotional problem would give a history of child abuse if there was no relationship between the abuse and the condition or problem. So the first stage of demonstrating that a causal relationship exists between abuse and the subsequently detected pathology is to establish that subjects who reported being sexually abused as children showed a higher prevalence of the pathology than did subjects who were not abused. Strangely, Finkelhor and Browne (1988) stated that this had been done for only a few of the pathological conditions attributed to child sexual abuse, but they went on to quote a large number of comparison studies confirming that almost all the conditions were more common in clinical studies of victims of child abuse as compared to nonvictimized controls.

Browne and Finkelhor (1986) considered vulnerability to revictimization later in life one of the most alarming long-term effects. A number of studies found victims to experience higher rates of subsequent rape, and two studies found them to be more liable to abuse from husbands. Browne and Finkelhor did point out a noncausal explanation for the association, though considering it unlikely: that subjects who report child sexual abuse feel more comfortable reporting other forms of abuse. Scientific skeptics could advance other explanations, including that subjects who interpret childhood experiences as abusive are more likely to interpret adult experiences as assaultive. Though commenting without explanation that this was not the best comparison, Finkelhor and Browne (1988) quoted a finding that 24% of a sample of mothers from families in which there was physical abuse reported incest experiences in their childhood, compared to only 3% of a sample of mothers recruited from community organizations. Certainly the prevalence of incest reported by the community sample was very low compared to that of other community samples.

Few clinical studies of adolescent and adult male victims of childhood sexual abuse other than incarcerated offenders have been reported. Briere, Evans, Runtz, and Wall (1988) investigated adult subjects presenting to a crisis counseling program, selecting 20 men and 20 women who gave a history of childhood sexual abuse and 20 men and 20 women who did not. Though the women were more extensively abused to a later age than the men, both reported an equally high likelihood (55%) of previous suicide attempts, as opposed to a 20% and 25% likelihood, respectively, for nonabused men and women. Both abused groups showed equally raised scores for dissociation, anxiety, depression, and sleep disturbance on a trauma symptom checklist, compared to the nonabused groups.

Twenty-five male adolescents who reported childhood sexual abuse were compared by Johnson and Shrier (1987) with age-matched controls. Twenty-eight percent of those molested by women and 57% of those molested by men identified as homosexual or bisexual, as compared with 8% of controls; 21% and 28% of the two molested groups reported sexual dysfunctions, respectively, compared to 4% of controls. Fifty-four percent of those molested by females and 50% of those molested by males experienced the abuse as having a strong or devastating effect on their lives at the time of the study several years later. Petrovich and Templer (1984) found that 59% of 83 incarcerated male rapists had been heterosexually molested as children, one-quarter by two or more women. Eighty percent of the cases involved sexual intercourse. The authors pointed out that this contrasted with the preponderance of more innocuous acts, such as fondling and looking, reported in most investigations of male child molestation. Finkelhor and Browne (1988) reviewed the many studies that advanced evidence that sexually victimized children later become abusers. They believed the major weakness of the studies to be that most investigated male incarcerated convicts. They did not reveal why they considered it a weakness; perhaps it was because such men may falsely report having been sexually abused as children in the hope of being treated more leniently (Freund, Watson, & Dickey, 1990).

Browne and Finkelhor (1986; Finkelhor & Browne, 1988) concluded that it was difficult to establish the severity of the risk of child sexual abuse being followed by significant long-term effects. They accepted that when tests developed to assess the adjustment of members of the normal population were used to investigate victims of child sexual abuse, most showed up as normal or only slightly impaired. Browne and Finkelhor considered such standardized tests to be not sensitive to more subtle forms of discomfort and difficulty, and Asher (1988) pointed out that they might not be measuring the symptoms or behaviors directly related to the abuse experience.

Nature of Abuse

Browne and Finkelhor (1986; Finkelhor & Browne, 1988) reviewed clinical studies investigating the effects of various kinds of abuse, commenting that only a few had enough cases and were sufficiently methodologically sophisticated to examine this issue. Probably their most surprising conclusion was that findings conflicted concerning the relative severity of symptoms following incestuous as compared with nonincestuous abuse. This contrasts markedly with the frequently stated view that incest involves a particular breach of trust. Russell (1986) termed father-daughter incest the supreme betrayal; in her study, 54% of the victims of such abuse reported being extremely upset by it, compared to 25% of victims of all other forms of incest. She also found, however, that female victims of brother-sister incest were less likely to marry. In the studies reviewed by Browne and Finkelhor, duration of abuse, age at which it occurred, and abuse involving intercourse (compared to other types of genital touching) were also found not to be consistently related to severity of long-term symptoms. In regard to the degree of force employed, Browne and Finkelhor (1986) stated that they were inclined to give credence to the studies that showed force to be a major traumagenic influence, despite the fact that a number of studies did not find an association. Though few studies examined the effect of the age and sex of the offenders, those that did found that their being male and older were associated with the experience being considered more traumatic. The general clinical impression that children who felt compelled to keep the abuse secret suffered greater subsequent psychic distress was not supported by research studies.

IMMEDIATE AND SHORT-TERM EFFECTS OF CHILD SEXUAL ABUSE

Asher (1988) reviewed the literature concerning the observed immediate effects of child sexual abuse. This, of course, can only investigate children who come to the attention of mental health professionals, and therefore could include more victims with serious immediate effects. This would not be the case if Frude (1985) is correct in considering that chance factors play a major role in determining which few of the large number of cases of abuse are detected. He pointed out that incest may be revealed during regular casework if there is social worker involvement with the family, during investigation of truancy, or in medical examination. As many victims of child abuse are too young to verbalize information concerning their abuse, Asher argued that it was imperative that professionals be aware of the signs and symptoms of child sexual abuse, many of which are typical of other emotional disorders of childhood. She considered that these included in the preschool child sudden weight loss or gain, abdominal pain, vomiting, and urinary tract infections, and that more clearly indicative signs were perineal bruising and tears, pharyngeal infections, and venereal disease. Behavioral symptoms she listed included sleep disturbance, nightmares, compulsive masturbation, precocious sex play, loss of toilet training, finger sucking, and clinging. These latter behaviors are generally interpreted as the result of fear and anxiety concerning being punished, rejected by the family, or not believed if they reveal the abuse. Asher pointed out that attribution of the symptoms to sexual abuse was based on clinical impression. She believed that a history of physical abuse should raise the question of sexual abuse either in the child or siblings; Finkelhor (1984) concluded that they were closely related only when mothers were the abusers. Cantwell (1981) pointed out that sexually abused children are often seductive, having been taught that sexual behavior is what is expected, and that such seductiveness can result in major problems in relationships with peers and adults.

One hundred and twelve victims of childhood sexual abuse that had occurred or been revealed in the previous 6 months obtained scores on the Louisville Behavior Checklist between those of healthy children and children receiving psychiatric services (Gomes-Schwartz et al., 1985). Only 17% of the preschool but 40% of the school-aged children met the criteria for clinically significant pathology; however, 27% of the preschool and 36% of the school-aged children scored above clinical and general population norms on sexual behaviors, which included open masturbation, excessive sexual curiosity, and frequent exposure of the genitals. School-aged children commonly showed anger or destructive behaviors, but only 16% reported the somatic symptoms of headaches, vomiting, and abdominal pain commonly found in clinical studies. Tong, Oates, and McDowell (1987) investigated 49 sexually abused children at a mean interval of 2.6 years after victimization. The children's scores on the Piers-Harris Self-Concept Scale and the Youth Self-Report of competence and behavior problems were significantly lower than controls, but were not in the clinical range. Subjects' self-ratings correlated poorly with those of the nonoffending parents and teachers. Low self-esteem and problematic behaviors were more apparent in girls than in boys.

Sexually abused older children and boys were more likely to show externalizing reactions, such as aggression and delinquency, and younger children and girls internalizing reactions, such as depression, anxiety, and somatic concerns (Friedrich, Urzuiza, & Beilke, 1986). An association between incestuous abuse and running away from home and delinquency was reported in several studies of girl victims (Browne & Finkelhor, 1986). Consistent with the finding of no greater severity of long-term effects following not revealing sexual abuse, children who did not reveal that they were abused, at least not immediately, showed fewer symptoms (Finkelhor & Browne, 1988).

Conte and Berliner (1988) reported an investigation of 369 sexually abused children, three-quarters of whom were girls. They were assessed at or near the time of disclosure of their victimization by their social workers using a symptom checklist, and by the nonoffending parent using a child behavior profile. The behavior profile was also completed by a sample of parents of nonabused children to provide a comparison group. Factor analysis of the behavior profile revealed eight factors: poor self-esteem, aggression, fear, conscientiousness, difficulty in concentration, withdrawal, acting out, and anxiety to please. Differences between abused and nonabused children on all factors were statistically significant. Conte and Berliner, however, pointed out that the differences could not be taken as evidence of the effects of the abuse, as the two groups differed on a number of demographic and other variables. Correlation of social workers' scores and the behavior profile factors was low to very low. Twenty-one percent of the sexually abused children showed none of the symptoms thought to be behavioral indicators of child sexual abuse, such as behavioral regression, somatic complaints, and fearfulness.

Conte and Berliner suggested that not all children react in the same way and cautioned against undue reliance being placed on children's behavior to determine if they have experienced sexual abuse. They found substantial disagreement in studies attempting to identify factors to account for the different reactions of victims of sexual abuse. In their study, both passive submission and resistance to abuse were associated with reduced impact of the abuse. Children tended to report one or the other approach, and Conte and Berliner suggested that the approach used could reflect the child's general coping strategy in life (i.e., active efforts to control events versus general acceptance of events); hence, either could be a healthy strategy for a particular child. They also argued that evidence did not support the traditional assumption of many health professionals concerning the attributions victims make concerning responsibility for the abuse. They suggested that blaming oneself in an uncontrollable situation could be the only means of maintaining a sense of control and therefore could also be a healthy strategy associated with a less serious impact.

Another source of information of the immediate effects of child sexual abuse are the victims' retrospective reports in adulthood. One-third of the abused women in Russell's study reported being extremely upset; 20%, very upset; 27%, somewhat upset; 12%, not very upset; and 9%, not upset at all (Russell, 1986). In Finkelhor's study (1979) of students, 66% of girls and 38% of boys rated the experience as negative, boys being more likely than girls to cite interest and pleasure as reactions. The male students in the study by Fritz et al. (1981) also reported less negative immediate reactions to childhood sexual abuse, most feeling they were neutral or even positive about the experience; the female students assigned it a negative or harmful quality. Sixty percent of the sexually abused male university students in the study of Fromuth and Burkhart (1989) reported a response of interest or pleasure, 28% one of surprise, and only 12% fear or shock. Older women constituted 75% of the perpetrators in this study. Condy, Templer, Brown, and Veaco (1987) reported the immediate response recalled by male prisoners and college students to a childhood sexual experience with a woman 5 or more years older. Many stated that they found it good if it was nonincestuous and no force was used.

Finkelhor (1985) suggested the positive immediate response reported retrospectively by a high percentage of male victims might be a false attribution, produced by the need to maintain the male ethics of self-reliance and the portraying of youthful sexuality in adventuresome terms. He pointed out that when long-term effects (as measured by impact on sexual self-esteem in his study) were considered, boys seemed as much or more affected than girls. As discussed earlier, however, Fromuth (1986; Fromuth & Burkhart, 1989) was unable to replicate this finding of reduced sexual self-esteem in either male or female students abused as children. In contrast to the experience of childhood sexual abuse being recalled as positive by most of the nonclinical male subjects in these studies, most adolescent male patients investigated by Johnson and Shrier (1987) recalled the experience negatively. Seventy-three percent of victims of adult women and 64% of victims of men recalled the immediate impact as strong or devastating.

Nelson (1986) reported the evaluation of incest by 46 women and 54 men who responded to newspaper requests for subjects who had had incest experience, whether good or bad. Only one case had been reported to the police. Forty-three subjects reported positive experiences. These subjects were more likely than the remainder to be older at the time of the experience, male, the older of the two partners, and to have a consenting partner. Fifty-eight of the 87 subjects who had opinions regarding incest laws thought they should be changed to allow consensual incest.

ASSESSMENT AND IMMEDIATE MANAGEMENT OF REPORTED CHILD ABUSE

Mandatory Reporting

Reporting of suspected child abuse is now mandatory in all 50 U.S. states. Nevertheless, Finkelhor (1984) found that only 86 of 327 workers in Boston child abuse agencies had reported their last case to the mandated authority. When allowance was made for those cases already reported by someone else or where the victim was not a child, 36% of cases were not reported that should have been. The belief that reporting was not always advantageous would appear to have persisted. Kalichman, Craig, and Follingstad (1988), relying on reported responses to vignettes, concluded that clinicians' tendency to report depended on their level of certainty that abuse was occurring. Finkelhor pointed out that criminal action was taken five times more often in cases of reported sexual than of physical abuse, and foster care placement occurred in 17% of sexual as compared to 12% of physical abuse cases. He considered this an excessive response to the emotional outrage that sexual abuse provoked. Vitulano, Lewis, Doran, Nordhaus, and Adnopoz (1986) found that supportive and protective services were much more likely to be provided for cases of sexual as compared to physical abuse reported to the Connecticut Child Protective Services.

Though some workers have argued powerfully in favor of mandatory reporting (Sgroi, 1975) others have claimed that it can discourage victims (Frude, 1985) and abusers from seeking treatment or revealing such abuse in individual or group therapy (S. Smith & Meyer, 1984; Wald, 1982). The Child Abuse Prevention Service in Sydney has overcome the latter problem by allowing offenders to seek and receive treatment without revealing their surnames or addresses. Smith and Meyer (1984) suggested that there be a qualified immunity from prosecution for abuse conducted prior to seeking therapy, though pointing out practical difficulties that would need to be solved. These included making therapy available to the relatively large number of families of low socioeconomic status in which abuse plays a role and who cannot afford psychotherapy. Weinstock and Weinstock (1988) considered the mandatory reporting of long-past child abuse, for the sole purpose of punishing the perpetrator when no child was in danger, to be a serious and unprecedented erosion of confidentiality. If information given by a perpetrator in a clinical interview may be provided to others, he or she should be informed that the confidentiality commonly expected in such interviews does not apply. Professionals who do not report suspected abuse must recognize the necessity for examination of the child involved, and, if relevant, their siblings if there is any possibility of psychological or physical harm or infection. Sgroi (1978) provided an account of a comprehensive procedure for examination of the abused child.

Assessment

Cantwell (1981) considered the destructive consequences of sexual abuse to be so great that the possibility of such abuse should be routinely investigated in all medical history taking. She stressed that all children old enough to be verbal should be asked about their bodies, possibly separately from the accompanying parent and that the subsequent physical examination must include inspection of the perineum. Spencer and Nicholson (1988) provided a detailed guide for individual interviews with the sexually abused child, the nonperpetrator spouse, and the perpetrator.

Videotaping Playroom Interviews

Walker (1988) described the technique she used of videotaping playroom interviews of the child, which can be observed by attorneys and the perpetrator from behind one-way mirrors. She believed many more abusers would accept responsibility for their sexual misconduct if given the opportunity to see and hear the child's descriptions in such videos. She also pointed out, however, that legal battles between experts are not uncommon regarding the interpretation of such data. Yates (1987) discussed modifications of court procedure to make the process less traumatic for the child. He discussed one case where the treating psychiatrist served as the court examiner and recommended the procedure, though pointing out that its constitutionality needed to be tested.

Anatomically Detailed Dolls

The use of anatomically detailed dolls in interviewing children to determine if they have been sexually abused was discussed by Walker (1988). She pointed out the lack of empirical data that sexually abused children use the dolls differently from children who have not been abused. Goodman and Helgeson (1988) reported that in two studies, the use of anatomically detailed dolls to help children describe what has happened enabled observers blind to children's abuse history to discriminate groups of allegedly abused from allegedly nonabused children. Though some allegedly nonabused children were incorrectly identified as abused, Goodman and Helgeson pointed out that they may have been victims of undetected abuse, an hypothesis impossible to disprove. Everson and Boat (1990) found, in a large and demographically diverse sample of 2- to 5-year-olds, that higher rates of explicit doll play were associated with being older, poor, black, and somewhat with being male; more than 20% of some subgroups displayed such behavior. Realmuto, Jensen, and Wescoe (1990) reported the use of anatomically detailed dolls in interviews in which the assessor followed a standardized protocol but was blind as to whether the children were sexually abused. Sixty-six percent of abused and 33% of nonabused children were incorrectly categorized (in all, 47% of the total group). The authors recommended caution when decisions were based on a single instrument.

Drawing Human Figures

Hibbard and Hartman (1990) were unable to replicate an earlier report that sexually abused children showed a significantly increased frequency of incorporating genitals when requested to draw human figures, which would justify the use of such drawings as indicators of possible sexual abuse. Hibbard and Hartman also found no significant differences in the number of other indicators of emotional disturbance in the drawings of the two groups.

Anal Changes

McCann, Voris, Simon, and Wells (1989) emphasized the need for normative data in view of the significance being attached to findings of anal changes in the diagnosis of child sexual abuse. They investigated the incidence of such changes in 267 prepubertal children screened to attempt to exclude any possible cases of sexual abuse. Perianal erythema was found in 40%; increased anal pigmentation in 30%; venous congestion in 7% initially, 52% at the midpoint, and 73% at the end of the examination; anal skin tags, folds, and scars in 11%; and anal sphincter dilation in 50%. Sixty percent of those who showed sphincter dilation also showed intermittent opening and closing of the sphincter. In only one child was the dilation greater than 20 mm, and the authors discussed the possibility that he may have been sexually abused. J. Adams, Ahmad, and Phillips (1988) also reported that anal gaping up to 15 mm in the knee-chest position was seen in many children who denied rectal penetration. They chose a limit of 20 mm after 30 seconds as the conservative definition of gaping.

Hobbs and Wynne (1989) emphasized the importance of routine anal examination in identifying child sexual abuse in suspected cases, considering the findings of paramount importance with preverbal children when the diagnosis had to rest on evidence other than the statement of the child. They described the anal findings in 243 girls and 94 boys in whom a diagnosis of probable or confirmed sexual abuse was made, apparently at times largely on the basis of the anal findings. Perianal erythema was found in 30%, venous congestion in 10%, and scars and tags in 6%. They considered anal dilation the most dramatic sign found in sexually abused children, finding it present in 18% of their cases and in 42% of those with anal signs, but in only 4% of total referrals for possible abuse. They suggested that dilation of over 5 mm without the passage of wind did not occur in normal children. They pointed out that their experience differed from the widely held view that most sexual abuse involved touching and fondling, leading over a long seduction period to intercourse in the preadolescent or adolescent period; they believed that 83% of boys and 29% of girls (40% of girls aged 0 to 5 years) in their own study had suffered anal abuse. Hobbs and Wynne did not consider the possibility that this much higher incidence of anal abuse than that generally reported indicated a lack of validity of the anal signs as evidence of abuse. They used a left lateral position to examine the anus, whereas McCann et al. (1989) used a knee-chest position. Nevertheless, in the absence of normative data for the method employed by Hobbs and Wynne, the fact that the anal signs used in their study to diagnose child abuse were present in a high percentage of nonabused children in the study of McCann et al. is disquieting.

Vaginal Examination

Cantwell (1983) reported that routine vaginal examination resulted in a doubling of the identification of cases of sexual abuse in girls under 13 years of age referred to a crisis care unit in Denver, Colorado. She considered it to be urgent that health professionals dealing with prepubescent girls include such examination as a standard procedure to detect those in need of protection. Sgroi (1975) had earlier emphasized that legal measures must be introduced to enforce such basic minimum standards of medical services. Cantwell (1983) believed that girls showing vaginal diameters larger than 4 mm in the horizontal plane were possible sexual abuse victims. J. Adams et al. (1988) pointed out that normative data for hymenal diameter in nonabused children were still needed. They investigated 116 girls referred for sexual abuse examinations, but did not report the data separately for girls who were not victims of digital or penile vaginal penetration. It appeared, however, that a significant percentage showed horizontal vaginal diameters larger than 4 mm.

Ability of the Child to Provide Accurate Evidence

A major issue in the evaluation of reports of child sexual abuse is the ability of the child to provide accurate evidence. Goodman and Helgeson (1988) argued that there was no evidence that children frequently fantasized sexual attacks or that they could be led by parents or others to report such events falsely. They reviewed the evidence from laboratory studies of children's memory and concluded that, though children as eyewitnesses often retained and reported less than did adults, their errors tended to be ones of omission rather than commission, and that children as young as 5 years of age could answer objective questions about simple concrete events as well as could adults. Four-year-old children who watched a videotaped event or experienced a medical procedure all correctly resisted such incorrect suggestions as "He took your clothes off, didn't he?" Three-year-olds made about 33% of false affirmations to this and similar leading questions. Goodman and Helgeson pointed out that leading questions may be necessary in child sexual abuse cases to break a frightened or embarrassed victim's silence, and that parents may have to question the child over relatively long periods of time before abuse is revealed. Defense attorneys would argue that the child has been "brainwashed" into falsely believing the event had occurred. Goodman and Helgeson considered the most ambiguous cases to be those involving custody disputes, where the complaining parent's method of obtaining the child's report was likely to come under scrutiny. They did not appear to believe, however, that the child could be influenced to provide a false report in this situation. The evidence they cited from laboratory studies did not address this problem, as the children in these studies had no motivation for lying.

Yates (1987) discussed a case of a 5-year-old girl who was influenced incorrectly to remember incidents of sexual abuse. Benedik and Schetky (1987) reported one of a 7-year-old boy coerced by his mother to give a false report. They commented that some clinicians adhere to the myth that children never lie, despite the fact that they may be parents of normal children who "fib," and stated that they had been told repeatedly by children that authorities did not allow them to go the bathroom or eat until they agreed to "tell what really happened." Walker (1988) pointed out that though many professionals find it difficult to believe, it is possible to use brainwashing techniques on young children so that they will falsely report being abused. J. Kaplan (1990) believed that children's desires to please others (including parents, therapists, or lawyers) and their capacity for fantasy could result in their making invalid statements. He quoted cases of children of 6 years of age or less who, under the prodding of their mothers or lawyers, told fantasized stories of sexual abuse by fathers or stepfathers and in many instances had come to believe they were true. Referring to the devastating effects of mass hysteria on the evidence of children in the Salem witch trials, Kaplan concluded that several variables, including the child's makeup, the environmental pressures he or she perceives, and the uniqueness of the given situation, will all have an input in determining whether or not the child will lie. To be able to predict if a child will tell the truth in a given situation is usually not possible.

Though some professionals believe children will not falsely report being abused, they all accept that children will falsely report not being abused. Summit (1983) stated that "whatever a child says about sexual abuse, she is likely to reverse it" (p. 188). Herman (1985) discussed how she dealt with such denial in her relation to crisis intervention with incest cases. Burgess, Groth, and McCausland (1981) and Wild and Wynne (1986) argued that some children in sex initiation rings falsely denied or retracted statements of sexual involvement. Outside the area of child sexual abuse there is general acceptance of evidence that children frequently lie, though conflict as to whether they do so more frequently than adults (Stouthamer-Loeber, 1986).

TREATMENT

Play therapies appear to be the treatments used most commonly with younger children subjected to sexual abuse. Walker and Bolkovatz (1988) reviewed different forms. They included in the goals of therapy assisting the child to heal from the experience, preventing or reversing the development of shame and stigma, supporting the development of emotional intimacy, providing a trust experience, and enabling the child to regain personal power. Gomes-Schwartz et al. (1985) considered that with young children who exhibit little manifest distress, repetitive probing into the details of the abuse should be avoided, and that treatment should be focused on developing the child's understanding of when an adult's approach is inappropriate.

There appear to be no studies comparing the outcome of different forms of individual therapy to determine their relative efficacy.

Furness (1983) discussed the three types of intervention employed in cases of incestuous abuse of older girls, the form of child abuse most commonly treated. Primary police intervention was by definition punitive, resolving the issue by removing the father from the family. Finkelhor (1983) reported that criminal action was taken in almost half the cases when the initial report was to the police, and in one-quarter of cases receiving primary social service intervention, the second type of intervention Furness discussed. Furness claimed that social services act like "better parents" and set themselves against the parents to protect the child. He considered this intervention to threaten the child with removal from the family. Such removal was easily interpreted by the remaining family members as the expulsion of the core of moral evil. The child felt punished and blamed and was prevented from resolving the confusion stemming from the incest, which could only be done in a family context. The third intervention, the primary therapeutic approach, aims to change the family relationships and the underlying dynamics that led to and maintained the incest. It used temporary separation of family members to assist the therapeutic aim. Furness suggested that it might initially appear that the father and daughter were most in need of treatment, but as the intervention proceeded, the mother often became central to the therapy. Finkelhor (1983) reported that criminal action was taken in only 4% of cases of child sexual abuse reported to private agencies.

Herman (1985) considered crisis intervention to be the appropriate model for treatment of revealed father-daughter incest, with its associated threat of disruption of the family. She found that the father, faced with possible loss of his wife and family, social stigmatization, and criminal sanctions, usually reacted with denial. The mother, faced with social stigmatization and the possibility of raising her family alone, may after initially supporting the daughter rally to her husband's side unless she receives rapid and effective support. The daughter may find herself shamed, punished, and still unprotected from continued sexual abuse. Suicide and runaway attempts are particularly common at this time. Herman warned against regarding incest as merely a symptom of family dysfunction, stressing that its criminal and addictive nature must be recognized. Rather than a traditional individual or family therapy model in which the rule of confidentiality is observed, she argued that effective crisis intervention required an active, directive, and even coercive approach, with cooperation between the therapist and agencies of the state in the belief that no therapist can treat incest alone.

Herman recommended that the initial focus of crisis intervention should be on stopping the sexual abuse and establishing a safe environment for the family. Reporting to the mandated authorities should be done promptly. The therapist must assume that the child's complaint of sexual abuse is valid, and should not be confused by initial denial on the part of parents. If safety cannot be guaranteed at home, it is much preferable to have the father leave during the crisis period. The child should be praised for her courage in revealing the incest secret and told that many children retract their initial complaints under pressure, but that she will not be abandoned should this happen in her case. If the parents separate, the mother will need help with issues of practical survival in addition to emotional support. In the postcrisis period, Herman found the incestuous family so fragmented that family therapy was not possible and group therapy for mothers, fathers, and child victims was far more promising. Individual therapy may also be necessary. Herman pointed out the lack of well-documented treatment outcome studies.

Giarretto (1978, 1981) developed a Child Sexual Abuse Treatment Program (CSATP) from a humanistic psychology perspective. Like Herman, he decided that conjoint family therapy was not suited to incestuous families immediately following disclosure and recommended individual counseling for mother, father, and daughter, succeeded by mother-daughter, then marital and father-daughter, and finally group counseling. Average length of treatment was 9 months. Parents United/Daughters United program self-help groups were incorporated, and the authority of the criminal justice system was considered essential (Giarretto, Giarretto & Sgroi, 1978). Encouragement of self-awareness was also an important feature. In the course of the treatment, the father was induced to admit he was totally responsible for his incestuous advances to his daughter. The mother would generally admit that she was party to the incestuous situation and contributed to the underlying causes. She and, as soon as possible, the father were to tell the daughter firmly that she was the victim of poor parenting. In time, the daughter would confide that she was not entirely a helpless victim and be gently encouraged to explore this self-revelation. The goal of the program is to reconstitute and resocialize the incestuous family whenever possible, returning the perpetrator and/or victim to the home when clinically warranted. In an independent evaluation of the program, Kroth (1979) reported this occurred in about three cases out of four.

Kroth found a recidivism rate of 0.6% followed the CSATP, compared with an average of 2% reported by other programs. Reliance on the validity of the recidivism rate must be tempered by the disquieting finding that at entry to the CSATP only 18% of perpetrators and spouses believed that if future abuse occurred they might conceal it; following the CSATP, 40% did (Kroth, 1979). Kroth suggested this could have reflected their unhappiness with the criminal justice system rather than with the program. The mean age of the victims treated was between 12 and 13 years, well above the mean age of victims in population samples (Russell, 1983). The incestuous sexual assaults of children revealed in community surveys tend to end as the victims approach 13 years of age (Siegel et al., 1987). This finding suggests that the abuse of children treated in the CSATP would in many cases have ceased for other reasons than the treatment.

In his evaluation, Kroth (1979) compared an intake sample of victims with those near termination. He did not report how many dropped out of treatment; if there were any, they may have shown a poorer response than those who remained. Nearly half the victims at intake displayed nervous or psychosomatic symptoms. Ninety four percent of those near termination were symptom free and showed significant improvement in their relations with their father, but only a trend toward improvement in relations with their mother. Three percent showed substance abuse, 3% promiscuity, 6% involvement with authorities, and 1% ran away. Kroth suggested that these low figures provided evidence of the lack of deterioration that would have been expected from the literature. The data on the victims was provided by adults, and Kroth believed its accuracy could be questionable. Long-term effects on the victims were not reported.

Friedman (1988) discussed a family systems approach in which incestuous families were treated from the beginning as a system or unit, the procedure Herman and Giarretto considered inferior to initial separate treatment of family members. No comparison data exist to support the superiority of either method. Kitchur and Bell (1989) reviewed studies reporting group therapy for sexually abused children and adolescents, finding that they did not provide sufficient outcome data to aid practitioners in selecting the most efficacious techniques or models. In particular, no standardized outcome measures were employed. Kitchur and Bell reported a study employing two standardized measures to evaluate a 16-week therapy group with seven 11- or 12-year-old girls. The psychometric data allowed no definite conclusion about treatment effectiveness, and the authors suggested that as the girls' pretreatment means on one measure—the Piers-Harris Self-Concept Scale—were within normal limits, it may not be an effective instrument for evaluating outcome.

A nationwide survey of 553 child sexual abuse programs (Keller, Cicchinelli, & Gardner, 1989) found that though over 88% focused on the victim, the majority took a family-oriented approach; only 15% focused on the child and 6% on the adult victim exclusively. Sixty-seven percent focused on the nonoffending spouse as well as the victim; half of the 67% also included the perpetrator. Incest cases were most often emphasized. More than half indicated restrictions of client participation. Apart from residential and procedural restrictions, these were based on the victim's age, sex, and ability to function normally, and on the nonoffending parent's willingness to support and protect the victim. Ability to pay for treatment was not mentioned, but clients' fees accounted for 13% of the funding. Offenders were excluded for reasons reported in Chapter 8. A second national survey of intrafamilial sexual abuse treatment centers also found that the most frequently treated persons were the sexually abused children and the nonoffending spouses (Cammaert, 1988). Nonoffending spouses spent twice as much time in therapy as did perpetrators, consistent with Furness's conclusion (1983) that as the intervention proceeded, the mother often became central to the therapy. Cammaert argued that therapists of nonoffending mothers should aim to empower the women by emphasizing their strengths that enabled them and their children to survive within the father-dominated family.

Conte and Berliner (1988) emphasized the importance of attempts to identify sources of variation in the effects of child sexual abuse, in order to determine a more rational way of distributing services to abused children. They believed this distribution was often determined by which child had the most assertive worker and perhaps by class, race, economic factors, or professional bias about the problem, giving as one example that incest victims were more likely to receive treatment. Conte and Berliner suggested that in a more rational system, victims with a number of risk factors known to be associated with more serious effects, or those whose current functioning indicated a severe effect, would be identified so that they could receive the more intensive (and hence more expensive and less available) interventions.

The most disappointing aspect of treatment of sexual abuse is the lack of methodologically adequate evaluative studies. Cohn and Daro (1987) discussed four studies, representing a $4 million federal investment, that evaluated 89 different demonstration programs treating 3,253 abusive families at the cost of $40 million. Sexual abuse made up less than 25% of the abuse. Though outcomes of different programs were compared, subjects were not randomly allocated to the different programs, making the comparison of dubious value. One-third or more of parents maltreated their children while in treatment, and more than one-half were judged likely to mistreat their children following termination; the response in cases of sexual abuse was considered better than that in cases of physical abuse. Cohn and Daro concluded that putting all resources into intervention after the abuse did not make sense.

PREVENTION

A number of programs have been developed aimed at preventing child sexual abuse. These include school programs to reduce children's fear of saying no to a family member or friend, and to increase their awareness of what constitutes appropriate and inappropriate touching. Brassard, Tyler, and Kehle (1983) recommended that the latter issue be included in accompanying parent education programs. Films and video presentations are available with such programs or for presentation on public television, where resistance by management to presenting sensitive material may occur. A recent campaign on Australian television stressed "stranger danger" without referring to the high risk of sexual abuse from family members.

Conte and Berliner (1988), in relation to their finding that both passive submission or resistance by children to sexual abuse served to reduce the impact of the abuse, suggested that either could be a healthy strategy, depending on the child. They pointed out that their finding did not necessarily support the aspect of popular programs teaching children to escape, resist, or avoid abuse. Asher (1988) argued that prevention programs in which children as young as 3 are taught what to do when approached by strangers, with the aim of empowering them, may instill fear of men and further reinforce the concept of men as powerful, as well as implicitly convey that children are in part responsible for their own victimization. No attempt appears to have been made to direct programs to normal heterosexual men to educate them that a number have a significant potential to be sexually aroused by female children of which they are not aware (Chapter 8). Without this awareness, they can impulsively express this arousal if they are unexpectedly exposed to a situation in which the arousal is provoked.

Given the difference of opinion among professionals concerning what constitutes effective prevention strategies, it is unfortunate that little appears to have been done to evaluate different programs comparatively in terms of their effectiveness in reducing sexual abuse. Taking the easier option, studies have predictably demonstrated that school programs increase student knowledge concerning the information included in the programs (Brassard, Tyler, & Kehle, 1983).

APOLOGIA FOR SCIENTIFIC SKEPTICISM

The data reviewed in this chapter do not make it possible to reject the null hypothesis that child-adult sexual activities do not have significant effects other than the immediate physical and emotional trauma of the experiences. It is possible that for some experiences, the immediate trauma is markedly less than that produced by the reaction of the child's family and community. In community studies, adult subjects reporting childhood sexual experiences with adults have not shown marked pathology, and it has not been excluded that the pathology was attributable to other factors than the experiences themselves. Such factors could include concomitants, such as family pathology and the community reaction, as well as vulnerability of the victim to the many life stresses encountered additional to the experiences. Clinical studies of subjects who seek therapy find that those who report having been sexually abused as children show more pathology than those who do not. This could be caused by patients with more severe pathology, such as borderline personality disorder, remembering or interpreting experiences as abusive that those with less pathology would not remember or interpret in this way. Such experiences would be more likely to be elicited by therapists trained to expect the patient to have been sexually abused.

Questioning whether adult-child sexual experiences of themselves have long-term effects should be seen as a necessary part of the scientific process, not as associated with attempts to weaken the opposition to child sexual abuse. This opposition should be based on other grounds than dubious evidence of such effects. If it is found that the abuse does not of itself have significant long-term effects, this could have the beneficial effect of reducing the alarmed reaction of the victims' families and the community, and the victims' resultant conviction that they have been tainted for life. The major aim of those labeled scientific skeptics, however, is to separate the need for appropriate methodology in establishing scientific findings from opposition to child-adult sexual activities. The labeling of these activities as child sexual abuse is a political act, based on the belief that these activities constitute an exploitation of the child. However willing some victims may be claimed to be, they lack awareness of the complex significance attributed to sexuality by the society in which they live. They are therefore not able to make an informed choice concerning their involvement.

It is on the grounds of this infringement of the human rights of the child that their sexual abuse should be opposed. Such opposition does not require evidence that the abuse has long-term harmful effects. If this is considered necessary, it should be equally necessary to examine the long-term effects of the fear of sexuality that has motivated some of the opposition to child-adult sexual activities. It has been argued that the ambivalence in the United States concerning sexuality is responsible for its teenagers' poor contraceptive practices and their resulting high level of unwanted pregnancies and need for abortions, compared to those in the other countries of the developed world (Chapter 2). The rejection of homosexual adolescents by their families has been considered responsible for many becoming prostitutes (Chapter 3). Repression of sexuality is accepted to be one factor producing sexual dysfunctions (Chapter 5). More specific to the issue of child-adult sexual activities, media evidence has been advanced of the harm done to families in several countries by accusations of incest from professionals who lacked objectivity because of their conviction that child sexual abuse has devastating long-term effects. Researchers in all areas of sexuality need to acknowledge the influence of political pressures, and seek to determine and maintain the appropriate methodology that will enable the findings of their endeavors to remain unbiased by it.

CHAPTER 7

Sexual Coercion and Assault

Primary credit for recognition of the importance of sexual coercion and assault in the United States must be given to the feminist politics of the 1960s stimulating the establishment of consciousness-raising groups and "speak-outs" against rape. Burgess (1985) pointed out that at that time almost all jurisdictions defined rape as "illicit carnal knowledge of a woman, forcibly and against her will," with "carnal knowledge" customarily interpreted as vaginal penetration by the penis. One of the first achievements of the antirape movement was the introduction of the Michigan Criminal Sexual Code, which broadened the criteria of assaultive sexual acts, extended protection to separated spouses and males, eliminated requirements of resistance, and restricted use of the victim's sexual history. By 1976, 49 other states were revising or had revised their rape statutes. The U.S. federal government established the National Center for the Prevention and Control of Rape, broadening the definition to include criminal sexual assaults, heterosexual or homosexual, that involved the use or threat of force and the coercion or bribery of children. Some clinical researchers have further broadened the concept to include more subtle forms of sexual pressuring from persons in positions of power relative to the victim.

Despite the change in legal definition, the community's and even many victims' conception of rape appears to remain that of sexual assault involving penetration of a woman by a stranger, reflecting the type commonly reported to the authorities and in the media. A study of sexual coercion of university students found that only half the women forced to have intercourse against their will regarded the experience as rape (Koss & Oros, 1982). The possibility that some men were the victims of sexual aggression was not investigated. The estimated prevalence of rape and sexual assault will therefore vary considerably depending on the degree of coercion classified as assaultive by the victim or the investigator.

NATURE AND PREVALENCE OF RAPE

Blitz and Confidence Rape

A study comparing cases of rape reported to police with those not reported found that the more the features of rape were those of what was termed a classic case, the more likely it was to be reported (Holmstrom, 1985). In classic cases, the assailants broke into the victims' homes, attacked them in their automobiles, or abducted them from public places; the assailants were strangers or acquaintances rather than friends or relatives; and the assailants threatened the victims with weapons or seriously injured them. Rapes of women reported to police in London from 1978 to 1986 (Keating, Higgs, Willott, & Stedman, 1990) were of this nature. All were carried out by adult males, mainly strangers. Nearly half took place indoors, where victims were more likely to be bound and blindfolded. One-third occurred out of doors, and one-sixth in vehicles; in one-third, weapons were carried. One-fifth were carried out by two or more men. Oral intercourse occurred in one-sixth and anal intercourse in one-twelfth of the offenses.

As such cases are markedly less frequent than marital or date rapes, the term *classic case* could have the unfortunate effect of maintaining the stereotype that such rapes are typical rather than atypical. The terms *blitz rape* and *confidence rape*, introduced by Burgess and Holmstrom (1980), would seem more appropriate. Bowie, Silverman, Kalick, and Edbril (1990) pointed out that though the classification by Burgess and Holmstrom was based on a study of fewer than 100 female rape victims seen in an inner-city hospital emergency room setting during the course of 1 year, their own study of 1,000 consecutive rape victims seen at a Boston rape crisis intervention program over a 10-year period demonstrated the same two predominant types of rape. Blitz rapes are sudden surprise attacks by an unknown assailant. Confidence rapes involve some nonviolent interaction between the rapist and the victim before the attacker's intention to commit rape emerges. Incidents could be classified as blitz rapes in 60% of cases and confidence rapes in 36% (Silverman, Kalick, Bowie, & Edbril, 1988).

Bowie et al. found that victims who reported blitz as compared to confidence rape were more likely to be or have been married, to have completed a higher level of education, to be working in a professional or managerial position, and to have been living alone at the time of the rape. Blitz rapes generally occurred in settings the victims assumed to be secure, with significantly more occurring in the victim's home. Blitz rape victims were more likely to have experienced actual threats to their lives and were twice as likely as confidence rape victims to have seen a weapon or had the presence of one implied by the assailant. Blitz victims resisted their assailants less frequently than confidence victims and attempted to flee the situation only half as often.

Confidence rape victims were three times more likely than blitz victims to have consumed alcohol or other drugs, to have spent some time with the assailant in a public or private place, or to have been in transit with him prior to the assault. The rape was more likely to have taken place in the rapist's home or automobile. Confidence victims reported feeling more anger during the incident and were more likely to have offered resistance, particularly attempts to flee. They waited significantly longer before seeking medical attention or help from the crisis program. Confidence rape assailants were more likely to be of the same race as their victim, to have known the victim's name and/or address, to have consumed alcohol or other drugs before committing the rape, and to have prolonged the incident beyond 5 hours.

Some confidence rape victims, particularly victims of date rapes, were unclear that the assault or forced sexual encounter to which they were subjected constituted rape. In a questionnaire investigation of women university students (Koss, 1985) 13% of women reported experiencing oral, anal, or vaginal intercourse against their will by force or threat of force, but only just over half acknowledged it as rape. Of those who did, 8% reported it to the police, and 48% did not discuss it with anyone. Sixty percent, and all of those who had the experience but did not acknowledge it was rape, knew the assailant; 30% of those who acknowledged the rape and 76% of those who didn't were romantically involved with him. Mean age of the acknowledged victims at the time of the assault was 18.9 years, and of the unacknowledged victims, 17.3 years. The prevalence of rape of women university students appears not to have increased over the past 30 years. Kanin and Parcell (1977) repeated a 1957 study and found that as in the earlier study, about half the female students reported having experienced sexual coercion in the previous year, one-quarter having been forced to have intercourse.

Groth and Burgess (1977) investigated 92 adult women victims of rape, treated at the Boston City Hospital, for whom there were complete data on the presence or absence of sperm. The authors found that it was present in only 32 cases; they commented that the statistic was even more impressive when it was noted that sperm was present in only half the women raped by more than one man. Though the classification of blitz and confidence rape was developed from the study of these victims, the relationship of presence of sperm to the two forms of rape was not reported. It would be expected that it would have been absent more often in cases of blitz rape. Groth and Burgess considered the finding to be evidence of sexual dysfunction in sexually assaultive men (see Chapter 8). They emphasized that absence of sperm did not mean that rape had not taken place.

Rape of Males

In most studies of rape, it is taken for granted that only women are victims. As Finkelhor (1985) pointed out, concern about sexual assault originated in the women's movement of the 1960s and quickly coalesced around the model of father-daughter incest. Hence, little attention was initially given to the rarer situations where boys and men were the victims. Groth and Burgess (1980) combined data from offender and victim samples to describe 22 cases of male rape. Average age of the victim was 17.5 years. Groth and Burgess concluded male subjects were at greater risk when engaged in solitary pursuits; in two-thirds of cases, they were hitchhiking or engaged in out-of-doors activity. Most were intimidated by threat of physical harm or were suddenly hit or overpowered. Three were entrapped by the offender getting them drunk. The concepts of blitz and confidence rapes would seem equally applicable to rapes of men as of women. The majority were sexually penetrated, and in half the cases the offenders attempted to make the victims ejaculate, in 7 cases performing fellatio on them. Half the offenders were known to the victims.

Societal beliefs that men should be able to defend themselves, concern that their masculinity would be suspect, and embarrassment concerning the act of reporting made male victims reluctant to report sexual assault. Rapes they reported resulted in more physical trauma than those reported by women (Kaufman, DiVasto, Jackson, Voorhees, & Christy, 1980). These workers found an increase of from 0% to 10%

from 1975 to 1978 in the percentage of male as compared to female victims of male sexual assault presenting to a sexual assault team in New Mexico. Five of the 14 males were over 18 years of age. Seven males and 23 of the 100 female victims had been attacked by more than one assailant. Eight male and 12 female victims were attacked on multiple occasions. Nine male victims were beaten, 5 severely, so that they suffered more physical trauma than the 11 female victims who were beaten. All 14 male victims were sodomized, and 9 were forced to commit fellatio. Five did not report their sexual assault during their initial contact with emergency department staff, preferring to seek treatment solely for their nongenital trauma. The authors speculated that a far smaller proportion of male as compared to female victims report their assault. More may be prepared to do so, though, as community attitudes change in response to feminist political activity.

A recent study investigated 100 male victims in London who had sought help from a volunteer-run service, "Survivors," after being sexually assaulted (Hillman, O'Mara, Taylor-Robinson, & Harris, 1990). Their mean age was 14.5 years at the time of the assault and 25.3 years at presentation so that most were reporting past assaults. Of 37 for whom the information was available, before the assault 38% considered themselves heterosexual, 51% homosexual, and 11% bisexual. This finding suggests that predominantly homosexual compared to heterosexual adolescent males are either more vulnerable to sexual assault or more willing to reveal it. The former possibility was supported by the report of McConaghy and Zamir (1992c) that male students aware of homosexual feelings were more likely to have been sexually coerced than those who were not.

In the study by Hillman et al. (1990), 72 of the 100 victims knew their assailant, who in 28 cases was a family member. The perceived sexual orientation of the assailant was heterosexual in 72%, homosexual in 16%, and bisexual in 12% of the 69 cases where this information was available. Seventy-five victims had been assaulted on more than one occasion, 43 reported multiple assailants, and 15 reported women assailants (in 12 cases in combination with men). Assaults occurred most commonly in the home of the victim or assailant. Receptive anal intercourse was reported by 75% of the victims, receptive oral intercourse by 59%, insertive oral intercourse by 43%, masturbation by the assailant by 55%, and forced vaginal intercourse by 10%. In 88 cases the assailant ejaculated, as did 53 of the victims. Fifty-one victims felt their life had been endangered. Thirty-three suffered skin or mucosal damage, which the authors considered similar to the percentage reported in other studies of male victims and greater than that reported in studies of female victims. Seventeen sought medical help; 12 of the 17 revealed the sexual assault to the medical staff. Police were involved in 12 cases, but in only 2 did the victims feel they were helpful. Assailants were taken to court in 5 cases, but only 2 were successfully prosecuted.

National Statistics of Rape Prevalence

Burgess (1985) summarized prevalence figures for rape in national statistics. Though those reported in the FBI national crime statistics doubled from 1971 to 1981 to reach 34.4 of every 100,000 women, they remained less than one-hundredth of the prevalence revealed in community surveys. No male victims were included. The National Crime Survey, which attempts by a continuing survey of representative households to identify cases not disclosed to law enforcement agencies, reported rates that were 10 times higher, yet still substantially below those of community surveys. The marked increase in the number of reported rapes continued in the 1980s, particularly in urban areas (Hochbaum, 1987).

The age group of both women and men most commonly victimized was that aged 15–24 years, according to the National Crime Survey rates in 1979. In terms of cases per 1,000, the prevalence in women was 2.5 for the group aged 12 to 15, 5.7 for those 15 to 19, 4.7 for those 20 to 24, 2.1 for those 25 to 34, 1 for those 35 to 49, and 0.1 for those 50 and over; prevalence for men was 0.2, 0.7, 0.5, 0.4, and 0.1 per 1,000 subjects for the age groups 12 to 15, 15 to 19, 20 to 24, 25 to 34, and 35 to 64 years, respectively (Burgess, 1985). Abramson and Hayashi (1984) compared the prevalence of reported rapes in various countries, stating that in the United States it was 34.5 per 100,000 population; in England, 10.1; in West Germany, 10.7; in France, 3.2; and in Japan, 2.4.

Sexual Assault in Adolescence

In relation to the prevalence of sexual assaults in adolescents, the most representative study appears to be that of Ageton (1983). Yearly from 1978 to 1980, subjects were interviewed who self-identified as victims or perpetrators of sexual assault, which was defined as all forced sexual behavior involving contact with the sexual parts of the body, the "force" varying from verbal pressure to physical beatings. They were selected from 73% of a national probability sample of 2,360 subjects, who were aged 11 to 17 years at the beginning of the study. Ageton did not report the number of male victims or of homosexual assaults, stating they were not typical and could result in misleading conclusions.

Generalizing conservatively from her findings, Ageton concluded that in each year from 1978 to 1980, 5% to 7% (i.e., 700,000 to 1 million) teenage females were sexually assaulted in the United States. In Sorensen's earlier study (1973) of a national probability sample of U.S. adolescents, 4% of nonvirgin girls aged 13 to 15 years reported that the first boy with whom they had intercourse was someone who raped them. Sexual assaults that involved physical violence and/or the use of a weapon were experienced by approximately 1% of the adolescent girls in Ageton's study. She calculated this to be twice the prevalence of all forcible rapes and attempted rapes reported in the National Crime Survey, and 20 times that reported in the Uniform Crimes Report. The Uniform Crimes Report provides annual statistics on crime in the United States as measured by arrests and offenses that come to the attention of law-enforcement agencies.

The victims in Ageton's study reported that the offenders were mainly boyfriends or dates in their age range; fewer than 20% were unknown to them. Victims considered time of day, location, and the offender being sexually excited and/or drunk to be major factors in precipitating the assault. Half the assaults occurred in the offender's home or an automobile, and one-quarter in the victim's home. The most common pressure reported by victims was verbal, but in each of the 3 years, 27% to 40%

experienced some pushing, slapping, and mild roughness. The majority were successful in deterring the assault. There were no significant race or social class differences in the total sample of victims, though urban girls were more vulnerable. Those who reported violent sexual assaults were typically black, lower-class urban adolescents. Victims of rape reported in the National Crime Survey were also more likely to be lower-class urban adolescents, consistent with the evidence that violent sexual assault is more commonly reported. In Ageton's study, one-third of victims of assault in 1 year experienced at least one further assault in the same year, and their risk of being assaulted in the next year was three to four times that for all female adolescents.

Comparison of victims and nonvictims suggested that involvement in a wide variety of delinquent behaviors and with delinquent peers might account for the victims' initial and continuing vulnerability. Data obtained 2 years prior to the commencement of Ageton's study showed the victims and controls to be substantially different in terms of exposure to delinquent peers, relations with family, and attitudes toward deviance. Ageton pointed out that if one is behaviorally and attitudinally delinquent, conventional protestations with regard to requests for sexual intercourse may fall on deaf ears. This would not explain her finding, however, that girls who showed equivalent delinquency and exposure to delinquent peers were as likely to be physically as sexually assaulted. A more likely explanation would be that both forms of assault characterize the behavior of delinquent males toward their female associates.

Only 5% of the assaults recorded in Ageton's study were reported to the police. These were mainly blitz rapes, that is, those carried out by unknown or multiple assailants and involving threats or employment of violence. Completed assaults made up more than half of reported assaults, but 20% of unreported assaults. Consistent with the features of confidence rapes discussed earlier, Ageton suggested that attempted nonviolent assaults by dates or boyfriends may not be defined by the victims as legitimate sexual assaults for purposes of reporting to officials. One-third of the victims assaulted by their romantic partners reported no change in the relationship. Approximately 60% of those whose husband or boyfriend was not the offender informed their partner of the assault, the majority reporting that their subsequent relationship was closer and more affectionate. More than two-thirds of the victims told their friends, but more than three-quarters did not inform their parents, presumably accounting in part for the reduced prevalence of rape reported in the National Crime Survey data. Few victims sought professional assistance.

As Burgess (1985) pointed out, these research findings reflect the peer orientation common among adolescents and their typical reluctance to communicate with adults, including therapists. Most adolescents may expect and wish to avoid the negative reactions the majority of parents show if they are informed of the assault (discussed subsequently). Victims' reactions to date rapes had not changed from those reported by Kanin (1959). The majority of university freshman he investigated who reported sexual aggression from a partner did not terminate the relationship. Few of the total assaulted informed their parents.

It is of interest that no episodes of incestuous abuse were reported in Ageton's study (1983), in which subjects were asked whether in the last year they had been sexually attacked or raped or whether an attempt had been made to do so. This would appear to mean that adolescent girls do not consider that the incestuous relationships they experienced involved the use of force, including verbal pressure. In the light of the data discussed in Chapter 6, a significant percentage must have experienced incestuous abuse. Four percent of the women studied by Russell (1986) reported experiencing initiation of incestuous abuse between the ages of 14 and 18 years, in addition to the 12% with whom it was initiated earlier. Ageton's failure to discuss the issue of incestuous abuse suggests that researchers as well as victims may not regard such abuse as sexual assault. Consistent with this view, Johnson and Shrier (1987) reported of male adolescents attending a medical outpatient service that none under the age of 15 years reported being sexually assaulted prior to puberty. A clinical study of adolescent rape (Mann, 1981) also failed to mention incestuous abuse.

Mann, unlike Ageton, did report assaults of males as well as females, stating that of 122 adolescent victims attending a sex abuse treatment center in Honolulu, 14% of those 12 to 14 years old and 8% of those 15 to 17 were male. All the offenders were male; two-thirds were known to the victim, and one-third to their parents. Vaginal, anal, or oral intercourse occurred in 88% of cases, and force in the form of verbal threats, physical overpowering, or weapons was employed in 80%. Incestuous and nonincestuous abuse was investigated in a study of 34 female and 6 male adolescents who attended a child sexual abuse clinic in Perth, Australia (Gardner & Cabral, 1990). All 17 whose abuse had continued for longer than a month, but only 4 of 23 whose abuse had been of shorter duration, were incest victims. In the other 19, the offenders were mainly peers or strangers. About half the nonincest victims were more akin to a "street kid" or delinquent population and presented reluctantly to the clinic as a result of intervention by acquaintances or police. Their affect was considered inappropriate in that they seemed undisturbed by the sexual incident.

The large number of episodes of sexual coercion of adolescent males by females revealed in retrospective surveys of adults are not reported to authorities, nor do they directly lead subjects to seek treatment.

Community Surveys of Sexual Assaults

The prevalence of reported rape in five community surveys of adult women reviewed by Sorenson, Stein, Siegel, Golding, and Burnam (1987) varied from 5% to 24%. The highest figure was obtained in Russell's San Francisco study (1986), which used the narrowest definition of rape (forced intercourse or intercourse obtained by physical threat or completed when the woman was unable to consent). Her study also reported the highest rate for attempted rape, 44%. Russell's data were obtained by trained interviewers using multiple probing questions, the method that produced markedly higher prevalence rates of child sexual abuse, compared to the use of questionnaires or interviewers asking only one question (see Chapter 6).

Russell would presumably reject Ageton's comment (1983) that, regarding adolescent victims of sexual assault, she believed there was a natural tendency for those who feel victimized to justify themselves by maximizing their description of the assault. Most rapes in the surveys reviewed by Sorenson et al. (1987) occurred to victims when they were younger than 20. In a subsequent community study, 1,157 adult women were interviewed 1 year after their participation in the NIMH North

Carolina Epidemiologic Catchment Area (ECA) program (Winfield, George, Swartz, & Blazer, 1990). Sexual assault was defined as a situation where someone pressured them against their will into forced contact with the sexual parts of their body or the offender's body. Seven percent of those 44 years of age or younger reported having experienced assault, compared with 3% of those between 45 and 64 years of age. Prevalence was higher in urban than rural residents, and in respondents with at least some college education. Sex of the offender was not reported.

An earlier ECA study investigated male as well as female victims of assault as a supplement to the Los Angeles project (Sorenson et al., 1987). The subjects were 1,480 men and 1,645 women, mainly Hispanics and non-Hispanic whites. Sexual assault was any pressured or forced touching of the victim's or offender's sexual parts, or sexual intercourse. Thirteen percent of women reported having been sexually assaulted in adulthood, and 16% in their lifetime; comparable percentages for men were 7% and 9%. Sexual assaults were reported more often by white non-Hispanics and by younger subjects and those with some college education. Age of the victim at the time of first assault was 5 or younger in 6%, between 6 and 10 in 13%, between 11 and 15 in 19%, between 16 and 20 in 34%, between 21 and 25 in 15%, and 26 or older in 12%. Modal age of the victim at the time of assault was 18 years. One-third reported one assault, and two-thirds two or more. The most recent assault involved a male assailant in 75% of cases, who acted alone in 90% of cases, and was acquainted with but not related to the victim in 77% of cases. In 26% of cases the assailant was a spouse or lover, more being spouses in the case of women and lovers in the case of men. Verbal pressure was used with 62% of the male and 27% of the female victims, and harm or threat of harm in 37% of female and 9% of male victims. Eighty-three percent of the victims tried to resist, and the outcome was some form of intercourse in 50% of women and 39% of men.

Higher prevalences of sexual assault were reported to female as compared to male interviewers by both men and women. For non-Hispanic white women interviewed by women, prevalence rates of lifetime and adult sexual assault were 27% and 22%, respectively. Within this group, more than 30% of those above the median education level reported a sexual assault. The sex of the victims of the 25% of female assailants was not reported, and the fact not discussed that the percentage was at variance with the previous literature, which has taken for granted that sexual assailants of adults were male. In reviewing explanations why younger and more educated subjects report higher rates of sexual assault, Sorenson et al. did not consider the possibility these subjects were more prepared to recognize excessive pressure for sexual activity as assaultive. A higher rate of sexual assault was also reported by younger women in the North Carolina ECA study (Winfield et al., 1990). Women differ in their concept of what constitutes sexual assault; among college women who had experiences that legally qualified as rape, only 27% conceptualized themselves as rape victims (Koss & Dinero, 1989; Koss & Oros, 1982).

Sexist and Nonsexist Questionnaires

Koss and Oros developed the Sexual Experiences Survey to investigate the concept that rape represented an extreme behavior that was on a continuum with normal male behavior within the culture. Two continua were investigated in their questionnaire: Men were asked to report the forms of pressure, including threat of or use of force, that they had employed to obtain sexual activities from women. Women were asked to report the forms of pressure of which they were the victims. McConaghy and Zamir (1992b) modified the questionnaire to investigate the possibility that continua also existed on which women were the aggressors and men the victims.

Fourteen percent of female and 13% of male Sydney medical students reported experiences in which their partner was so aroused they could not stop them, even though they did not want sexual intercourse. In Koss and Oros's study (1982), 33% of Kent State University women students reported this experience. Eleven percent of the Sydney men and 6% of the women reported they were so aroused they could not stop, though their partner did not want intercourse. Twenty-three percent of the Kent State men reported this experience. Two percent of the Sydney men and women and the Kent State men reported they used force to attempt to obtain sexual intercourse. Two percent of Sydney women, as compared to 6% of Kent State women, reported having been raped. No Sydney men reported having raped or been raped. The Kent State men were not asked this question; 3% reported having sexual intercourse with a woman when she did not want to, because they used some degree of physical force.

These data support the dimensional concept of sexual aggression. It could be expected that subjects' level of consciousness concerning rape would determine at what point in the continuum they would label as sexual assault the behavior they had experienced as aggressor or victim. Christopher (1988) found that the most common pressure reported by women victims was persistent physical attempts, which were not classified as the use of physical force. In a second study of Sydney medical students, 14% of the women and 20% of the men reported they had made constant physical attempts to have sexual activity with a member of the opposite sex; 1% of the women reported they had made constant physical attempts with a woman (McConaghy & Zamir, 1992c).

Struckman-Johnson (1988) also concluded that both men and women engage in a continuum of sexually exploitive behaviors ranging from verbal pressure to use of physical force and restraint. She found that 16% of male as compared to 22% of female university students reported at least one episode in which they were forced to engage in sexual intercourse on a date. Most men were coerced by psychological pressure and most women by force, but 28% of men were coerced by both. In a study of psychology students, more men (63%) than women (46%) reported experiencing unwanted sexual intercourse (Muehlenhard & Cook, 1988). Many of the men's reasons for engaging in unwanted intercourse related to sex-role expectations (e.g., fearing to appear homosexual, unmasculine, inexperienced, or shy).

Marital Rape

Attention has only recently been directed to marital rape. As it is excluded from most sexual assault statutes, victims are often unable to report it. The few who go to authorities do so for being beaten (Holmstrom, 1985). Yllo and Finkelhor (1985) pointed out that this means that a marriage license is in effect a license to rape. They believed marital rape to be the least recognized form of rape, and its victims the most silenced. The exclusion of marital rape from statutes supports the feminist concept that criminalization of rape was not designed to protect women as women but as male property.

Studies of marital rape have tended to use the narrowest definition of sexual assault. Yllo and Finkelhor (1985), though recognizing the existence of forms of nonphysical coercion, limited their research to the frequency of husbands using force or the threat of force to obtain sexual activities, not exclusively vaginal intercourse. They pointed out that Russell's definition (1982) remained fairly close to legal definitions, requiring forced vaginal, oral, anal, or digital penetration. Yllo and Finkelhor considered that because of reluctance or forgetting on the part of some women, marital rape was experienced by more than the 10% and 14% of married women, respectively, who reported it in their survey of Boston women and in Russell's survey of San Francisco women. They concluded that this made sexual assault by husbands the most common form of sexual assault. In Russell's study, more than twice as many women had been raped by a husband as had been raped by a stranger.

Kilpatrick, Best, Saunders, and Veronen (1988) investigated 391 women who participated in a study of lifetime victimization by sexual assault, physical assault, or robbery. Of the 91 who reported being raped, assailants were husbands in 24%, dates in 17%, and strangers in 21% of cases. In Yllo and Finkelhor's study (1985), since the age of 16, 10% of women had been sexually assaulted by a husband, but only 3% by a stranger. In the ECA community survey of Sorenson et al. (1987), which used a broader definition of sexual assault than the use of force or threat of force, 13% of adult assaults of women were carried out by spouses, and 13% by lovers; 22% were carried out by strangers, and 48% by acquaintances. This study also found 6% of sexual assaults of men to be carried out by spouses and 18% by lovers—forms of assault as yet little investigated. Though pointing out the particular vulnerability of battered wives to marital rape, Yllo and Finkelhor (1985) found that wife rape occurred separately from battering in a sizable minority.

The Handicapped: Sexual Torture

Other groups whose vulnerability to sexual abuse has been insufficiently emphasized are the handicapped (Rinear, 1985) and the mentally retarded (Tharinger, Horton, & Millea, 1990). These workers pointed out the failure to provide adequate protection and services for the special needs of these groups. Also the significance of sexual aspects of torture are being recognized. Two hundred and eighty-three victims, mainly from Europe, Turkey, and Latin America, were questioned about methods of torture (Lunde & Ortmann, 1990). Eighty percent of the women and 56% of the men had experienced sexual torture, ranging from physical sexual assaults and violence against the sex organs to mental assaults including forced nakedness and witnessing others being sexually tortured.

EFFECTS OF SEXUAL ASSAULT

Immediate Effects

Studies of the immediate effect of sexual assault are limited to those where the assault is reported, and hence are mainly of blitz rapes. Burgess and Holmstrom

(1974) studied 92 women, aged 17 to 73 years, admitted to an emergency department with the complaint of rape. Similarities in their symptoms justified identification of a clinical entity Burgess and Holmstrom termed *rape trauma syndrome,* characterized by an acute or disruptive phase followed by a long-term reorganization process. Burgess and Holmstrom (1985) subsequently reported that subjects in the acute phase showed all four cardinal features required for the DSM-III diagnosis of posttraumatic stress disorder. Their symptoms had a temporal and presumably causal relationship to a stressor beyond usual human experience. The victim reexperienced the trauma, most frequently by recurrent and intrusive imagery, in daytime experiences, dreams, and nightmares. Numbing of responsiveness occurred, the victim complaining of being in a state of shock or feeling that the assault was not real and losing the ability to emotionally respond normally. Finally, they showed at least two of a list of symptoms not present prior to the event: hyperalertness, sleep disturbance, guilt, impairment of memory and concentration, avoidance of situations reminiscent of the trauma, and symptoms related to the trauma. In relation to rape, the latter symptoms could include sexual dysfunctions.

In addition to these features of posttraumatic stress disorder following sexual assault, Burgess and Holmstrom (1985) described two additional features. One they termed *compounded reactions,* which included depression, psychosis, psychosomatic disorders, suicidal behavior, and drug use. The second was a *delayed response* to a much earlier unresolved sexual trauma that was not reported. Following the acute phase, which could last days or weeks, a second phase of long-term reorganization occurred in which the victim had the task of restoring order to and control over her or his life-style. This phase could last months or years.

Nadelson, Notman, Zackson, and Gornick (1982) concluded from a review of studies of recently assaulted female victims that for months following the assault, nearly every aspect of their lives were affected, including functioning at school, work, or in the home. Behavioral symptoms reported included sleep disturbance, nightmares, and eating disorders; somatic symptoms included headache, nausea, and exhaustion; and emotional and cognitive responses included fears, generalized anxiety, difficulties in concentration, intrusive thoughts about the assault, irritability, anger, self-blame, and guilt. Victims moved their residences or sharply curtailed their activities.

Bowie et al. (1990) contrasted victims of blitz and confidence rape. They found the immediate concerns of blitz rape victims to center around their sense of safety—fearing the rapist might return—and dismay at having failed to ward him off. Chief concerns of confidence rape victims were guilt and self-blame; if they sought help, it was usually after a significant delay. Most rapes reported by the national probability sample of adolescents studied by Ageton (1983) were confidence rapes. In the week following the assault, 50% of the victims reported feeling anger, depression, embarrassment, and guilt; and 20%, fear of the offender's return, of other men and of being alone. These percentages halved during the following 6 months, and Ageton concluded that the typical assault, a date rape, did not generate many negative reactions that persisted for 6 months. Reactions to the assault were not differentiated by race, age, social class, number of offenders, relationship to the offender, or the amount of force experienced. Only the completion of the assault had a significant influence, being associated with more negative reactions in the following year.

The absence of marked negative reactions persisting for 6 months following sexual assault of adolescents was also reported by Gomes-Schwartz et al. (1985). They investigated 14 to 18-year-old subjects presenting to a family-crisis program for sexually abused children in whom the abuse had occurred or been revealed in the preceding 6 months. The majority of cases were of incestuous abuse, in contrast to the study of Ageton (1983), in which subjects of this form of abuse apparently did not report it. Gomes-Schwartz et al. (1985) compared victimized subjects with adolescents in psychiatric treatment, using the Louisville Behavior Checklist E-3 as a measure of emotional distress. On 10 of the 13 scales, sexually abused adolescents showed less pathology than those in treatment. Few exhibited severe pathology on most scales, using the criterion proposed by the author of the checklist.

Asher (1988) concluded that child victims of sexual abuse approaching adolescence, compared to younger victims, showed more antisocial behaviors (e.g., petty crime, drug use, promiscuity, and prostitution) often associated with running away from home. Gomes-Schwartz et al. (1985) suggested that the adolescents evaluated in their study fell predominantly into the anxious, inhibited category. They hypothesized that their failure to find significant pathology in teenage victims of sexual abuse could be attributable to those who were more severely disturbed running away or being placed in welfare institutions. Only the less severely disturbed would turn to a family-crisis program for help and hence be included in their study.

In contrast to the findings of the studies by Ageton and Gomes-Schwartz et al., which investigated community samples or used standardized outcome measures, studies of adolescents seeking treatment and investigated clinically found severe effects following sexual assault. Asher (1988) concluded that depression and suicidal attempts were more common in adolescent victims and pointed out that the adolescent girl was at risk of becoming pregnant, either by an incest perpetrator or another male. Herman (1985) commented of incestuous abuse that as it continued from childhood into adolescence, the distress of girl victims often increased. The father might have initiated attempts at intercourse, with the possible risk of pregnancy. Also, he frequently responded to the daughter's increased social involvement, normal at this stage of life, with jealousy verging upon paranoia. Runaway or suicide attempts, indiscriminate sexual activity, and early pregnancy were frequent reactions. As the older daughter became more resistant, the father could turn his attentions sequentially to younger daughters.

Long-Term Effects

Ageton (1983) was able to assess reactions of adolescent girls to sexual assault for up to 3 years in a subsample of victims. After the marked decline noted in the first year, 2 to 3 years later a number of subjects reported depression and fear of men and of being alone. These reactions were not related to features of the assault, and Ageton concluded that factors such as support from significant others, history of traumatic events, and personality traits may be more instrumental in affecting long-term reactions. She also suggested that these late-reported reactions might have been artifacts of the repeated interview situation. Certainly if they were not and many victims of attempted assault by dates or boyfriends experience fear of men and of being alone 2 to 3 years later, these symptoms should be very common in adolescent girls, in view of the prevalence of this type of assault by dates or boyfriends. Ageton considered that it could be regarded as almost a standard feature of dating.

Nadelson et al. (1982) pointed out that though earlier follow-up studies carried out at 1 year indicated that rape victims had recovered from the acute trauma by this time, two recent studies reported contradictory findings. One that followed up 213 victims found that at 1 year, at least one-third still experienced rape-related adjustment problems, including decreased social activities and worsened sexual relations with their partners. In the other, half the women felt that it took years to recover. Nadelson et al. interviewed 41 of 130 women who had attended a rape crisis program 1 to 2½ years earlier. Sixty-one percent felt restricted and would go out only with friends, 51% reported sexual difficulties, and 49% noted fears of being alone.

In regard to individual symptoms following sexual assault, psychosexual dysfunctions were those most commonly reported in clinical studies. A number of these studies found the victims' satisfaction with sexual behaviors with their partner was significantly reduced, particularly behaviors forced on the victim during the assault, though not all studies reported that the frequency of the behaviors was reduced (Foley, 1985). Sexual dysfunctions reported included vaginismus, dyspareunia, and difficulties with arousal and orgasm. Dysfunctions could persist for years following the assault. In a community study, Koss (1985) investigated female university students who had intercourse with dates against their will by force or threat of force. Those who acknowledged this as rape reported more liberal sexual values and a larger number of sexual partners. Koss considered this consistent with the hypothesis that sexual victimization altered sexual standards and behavior. Students who did not acknowledge the experience as rape showed no difference in sexual behavior from the less victimized group of women.

Effects of Sexual Assaults on Men

Few clinical studies have reported the effects of sexual assault on men. In their study of 14 male and 100 female victims, Kaufman et al. (1980) reported that 11 of the male victims of assault studied showed a controlled response of a calm, composed, or subdued affect, rather than an expressive style of crying, sobbing, smiling, or restlessness. They contrasted this with Burgess and Holmstrom's report (1974) that the responses of female victims were more or less equally divided between the two styles. Kaufman et al. were able to follow-up 6 subjects, of whom 1 became delusional, 1 exhibited severe denial, and 1 (a child) ran away from home. The authors believed male victims might experience major, hidden trauma. Other clinical studies reported effects similar to those of sexual assault of women. Groth and Burgess (1980) concluded that male victims of men often experienced rape as life threatening. They subsequently reported disturbances of sleep and appetite, thinking about it a lot, and having a fear of men. Victims were especially concerned when the offender had attempted or succeeded in getting them to ejaculate. Psychosexual disorders were reported to follow sexual assault both in this study, in which offenders were male, and the study of Sarrel and Masters (1982), in which men were assaulted by women. Of the male and female victims of sexual torture investigated by Lunde and Ortmann (1990), 40% reported sexual difficulties, compared to 19% of victims of nonsexual torture. The prevalence of the difficulties were not associated with age or gender.

Preexisting Pathology in Assault Victims

Burnam et al. (1988) questioned the significance of clinical studies of victims of sexual assault, pointing out that the findings were of limited generalizability because subjects attending clinics were not representative of victims of sexual assault, the majority of whom did not seek professional help. Those who did could have higher rates of psychopathology. Burnam et al. reported additional findings from the ECA Los Angeles community study discussed earlier (Sorenson et al., 1987). Subjects received psychiatric diagnoses made by lay interviewers using the NIMH Diagnostic Interview Schedule (Robins et al., 1981); as discussed in chapter 1, diagnoses made in this way can differ markedly from those made by psychiatrists. Subject who reported having been sexually assaulted, compared with matched controls, showed significantly higher prevalences of major depression, alcohol and drug abuse or dependence, antisocial personality, and phobia prior to their first assault. Risk ratios for onset of disorders following the assault were 2 to 4 times higher for major depression, alcohol and drug abuse or dependence, phobia, panic disorder and obsessive-compulsive disorder.

Burnam et al. (1988) found that major depression, alcohol abuse or dependence, panic disorder, and obsessive-compulsive disorder were more likely to develop in assaulted subjects in the year following the assault as compared with controls, suggesting that the assault contributed directly to the disorder. Data were not available to investigate the prevalence of sexual dysfunctions in assaulted subjects. Burnam et al. found that the impact of assault on mental health did not differ significantly between men and women, except that men were more likely to develop later alcohol abuse or dependence.

Effects of Marital and Partner Rape

In their discussion of the effects of marital rape, Yllo and Finkelhor (1985) considered that, contrary to common opinion, it could leave a woman feeling much more powerless and isolated than if she were raped by a stranger. They pointed out that a woman raped by her husband has to continue to live with her rapist, not just a frightening memory of a stranger's attack. Of 92 wives of violent men, those raped by their husbands (41% of the sample) experienced more severe nonsexual violence and had more negative reactions overall. When the severity of nonsexual violence was controlled, marital rape was significantly related to low self-esteem, negative attitudes toward men, not wanting sexual relations, and withholding sex. Another study found that battered women who had also been raped were more likely to call the police. Only 36% of these women reported positive consequences of the call; 16% felt the blame was placed on them, and 12% experienced retaliation from their husbands. In Russell's study (1982), increased negative feelings and behavior toward men in general were reported by 37% of the victims of marital rape. Fifty-two percent of women raped by husbands and 52% raped by a relative reported a great effect on their lives, as compared with 39% raped by a stranger, 25% by an acquaintance, and 22% by a friend, date, or lover. Kilpatrick et al. (1988) found that women sexually assaulted by husbands and dating partners were more likely to sustain physical injury than those assaulted by strangers. Victims of date rape were more likely to fear injury or threat to their lives than the other two groups. More victims of rape than nonvictims met diagnostic criteria for major depressive episode, social phobia, and sexual dysfunctions as assessed by a modification of the Diagnostic Interview Schedule. Prevalence of the disorders did not differ in subjects raped by husbands or dates as compared with strangers.

Relationship with Features of Assault

Norris and Feldman-Summers (1981) investigated relationships between features of rape and its impact in 129 subjects who had reported the offense to police and/or sexual assault centers and 50 who had not. Impact was assessed by changes in psychosomatic symptoms, sexual behavior, and reclusiveness. Reporting of the offense was unrelated to outcome. Severity of the assault significantly predicted an increase in psychosomatic symptoms; the presence of understanding men in their social network predicted increased frequency of going alone to movies and concerts; and the presence of understanding women predicted increased frequency of going alone to bars. None of the factors assessed predicted increased sexual difficulties.

Becker, Skinner, Abel, and Treacy (1982) investigated 83 female victims of rape and/or incestuous assaults. Thirty-six reported no sexual problems, and 47 at least one problem related to the assault. Incest victims compared to rape victims showed higher rates of primary and secondary anorgasmia. More women subjected to assaults with minimal verbal and marked physical coercion did not report dysfunctions, compared to the remainder. Victims of such assaults experienced less guilt, as they labeled the attack as clearly offender initiated. Penetration, compared with feeling of the body, was much more likely to be followed by sexual problems.

In a later study, Becker et al. (1984) investigated 178 female survivors of rape and/or incestuous assaults and 50 controls, using the Beck Depression Inventory (BDI) to assess their level of depression. Assault victims showed significantly higher scores on the BDI, but there was no significant difference between those subjected to incest as compared to rape. Presence of a weapon was significantly associated with higher BDI scores. Other assault characteristics, including known versus unknown assailant, number of assailants, level of aggression, whether penetration occurred, and whether the assault was reported, failed to show any association. The authors suggested that sexual assault may be such a traumatic experience in itself that specific aspects are insignificant.

Ellis (1983), in a review of additional studies that investigated the relationship between severity of the victims' reactions and circumstances of the rape, came to a similar conclusion. She found no consistent relationships with any features of the rape, including the degree of force and whether a weapon was used. Characteristics of the victim were associated with slower recovery; these included prior victimization, economic stress, lack of social support, a history of prior psychiatric or physical

health problems, and suicidal ideation or attempts. As stated previously, Ageton
(1983) also found in her community study of adolescent girls that symptoms reported by some victims 2 or 3 years after the assault were not related to features of the
assault; personality traits and a history of traumatic events were important determinants.

Ellis (1983) considered these findings to be consistent with a crisis-theory model
of response to rape. The outcome of a crisis is not solely determined by antecedent
factors such as the nature of the stress; the victim's previous experience and personality or character structure load the dice in favor of a positive or negative outcome.
This belief of Ellis could explain the inconsistency among studies, some of which
found that the majority of rape victims recovered fairly rapidly and others that a
significant number showed slow and minimal recovery. The later studies could have
investigated more subjects with vulnerable personalities.

Physical Harm

Little information has been provided in the literature concerning the degree of
physical harm inflicted during sexual assaults, possibly because excessive force is
used only in a minority of cases (APA, 1987; Palmer, 1988). Palmer found that 15%
to 20% of victims of rape reported to the police required hospital treatment for
physical injuries, and that severe, lasting physical injuries were rare. As discussed
previously, reported rape constitutes only a small percentage of total sexual assaults
and could be expected to include most cases where significant physical injury was
inflicted. Quinsey and Upfold (1985) investigated 95 completed rapes and 41 attempts made by 72 men referred to a maximum security psychiatric institution; 69
victims were not injured, 8 were treated in clinics and released, 7 were hospitalized
overnight, and 2 were killed. Less than 1 rapist in 500 is convicted (Swift, 1985), and
those who are injured their victims more severely (Ageton, 1983; Herman, 1990).
The incidence of sex murders is minute in comparison to that of sexual assaults
(Revitch, 1980). The few sex murders that do occur usually receive national or
international media attention. Sex murders are discussed in more detail in relation to
the perpetrators in Chapter 8.

Effect on Relatives and Partners

In contrast to the relatively benign effect of sexual assault on the victims' relationship with husbands and boyfriends reported in the national probability sample of
adolescent girls by Ageton (1983), a clinical study of a small number of subjects cited
by Foley (1985) reported that 50% to 80% of women raped suffered loss of their
boyfriends or husbands as a result. In regard to male partners' initial reactions, most
studies reported that the primary concern of the majority was for the victim's well-
being (Miller, Williams, & Bernstein, 1982). Moss, Frank, and Anderson (1990)
found that the psychological functioning of married and single victims did not differ
in the first 4 weeks following rape. For the married women, lack of support by the
partner, particularly if unexpected, was significantly related to poor functioning.

The emotional impact of rape of adolescents who sought treatment was rated by health professionals as more severe on the parents than the victims; 71% of parents were assessed as showing a severe response, compared with 37% of victims (Mann, 1981). No parents showed a mild response, as compared to 20% of victims. The major concern reported by 65% of victims was fear for life or bodily harm, a concern shared by only 50% of parents, almost exclusively those whose children had been physically injured. The next concerns of victims were feelings of shame, self-blame, and guilt. Forty percent of parents blamed their child directly for the rape, especially if there were preceding intrafamilial problems. Anger at the assailant was expressed by 45% of victims and 69% of parents. Two-thirds of parents, but only 21% of victims, believed the assault would cause future sexual anxieties or problems. Victims expressed marked concern regarding their peers' reactions to them, and 80% expressed a wish not to be treated differently but to be considered "normal like everybody else." Eighty percent of the victims complained about increase communication problems with their parents after the rape.

Similar findings were reported in relation to 44 victims of exhibitionists, most of whom were adolescents at the time of the offense (Gittleson, Eacott, & Mehta, 1978). Forty reported the offense, in 32 cases to their families. In 28 cases those told were upset, compared to 25 of the victims who were upset. In 17 cases, the degree of upset of those told was greater than that of the victims, and in 14 it was more traumatic to the victim than the offense.

Causal Relationship of Assault to Long-Term Effects

Though the quasi-experimental evidence is convincing that subjects reporting sexual assault show more psychological symptoms than do nonvictims, establishing the degree to which the assault in itself was responsible for the symptoms present some time following the assault is of considerable methodological difficulty. Studies such as those of Ageton (1983) and Burnam et al. (1988) found that assaulted subjects differed from the nonassaulted prior to the assault; hence preexisting differences could account for some apparent long-term effects. Subjects also differ as to whether they label the same sexual experience an assault. Some of those who do may have always had more emotional problems, thus producing a noncausal association between sexual assault and psychopathology.

As Burnam et al. pointed out, what are now needed are prospective studies of probability samples of children that investigate their psychological health at regular intervals until they reach adulthood and that also record the occurrence of sexually assaultive episodes, as well as life stresses and any other possibly traumatic experiences. Though it is likely that many sexually assaultive episodes would not be reported at the time, it would appear from studies of the sexual behavior of adolescents (discussed in Chapters 2 and 3) that most episodes would be reported by the subjects when they reached adulthood. If sexual abuse and assault commonly produce long-term mental impairment, and their reported prevalence in up to 60% of U.S. women (Chapter 6) is correct, the mental health of women should be markedly inferior to that of men.

COPING STRATEGIES FOLLOWING SEXUAL ASSAULT

Burt and Katz (1988) reviewed studies of women's reports of the strategies they used to cope with the distress following sexual assault. Those reported most frequently were explanation (aimed at understanding why the rape happened), minimization (viewing what happened as better than other other possible scenarios), suppression (avoiding thinking about the rape), and dramatization (extensive expression of feelings about or discussion of the rape). Women who used one or more of these strategies to reduce anxiety, who adopted action-oriented behaviors such as changing residence or traveling, and who had positive self-esteem recovered faster. Decreased activity (e.g., staying at home and withdrawing from people), substance abuse, prior victimization, chronic economic stress, and lack of social supports were associated with slower recovery.

FEMINIST AND SOCIOLOGICAL MODELS OF RAPE

One consequence of the role of the women's movement in increasing public awareness of sexual assault has been widespread acceptance of the feminist perspective that rape is a political act by men to "keep women in their place." Rape is seen as normative male behavior, and rapists as conforming to a socially encouraged perception of male sex-role expectations. Rape laws are considered to protect women not directly but as men's property in transactions in which sex is treated as an exchange of goods. This view can be advanced more convincingly if its proponents minimize the evidence discussed that men are the victims of one-third of sexually coercive acts, and a significant percentage of women carry them out: "The findings that most victims are female and that the vast majority of offenders are male have been reproduced in every major study" (Herman, 1990, p. 177).

It could be that the sexually coercive acts of women are ignored because they rarely involve the use of physical force. Nonforceful coercion by men, however, was included in most estimates of the prevalence of sexually assaultive behaviors (Koss & Oros, 1982; Russell, 1986) employed to support the feminist view. Minimization of the evidence of sexual coercion by women is not limited to the feminist view but characterizes the related sociological theories that attempt to account for sexual coercion and assault. In their review of this literature, Stermac, Segal, and Gillis (1990) referred almost exclusively to studies which, like that of Koss and Oros (1982), investigated women only as victims and men only as perpetrators. Stermac et al. however did refer to two studies that found that men were the victims in one-quarter to one-third of reported incidents of sexual harassment within work settings. They did not report the sex of the perpetrators.

A recent example of research whose methodology was biased toward supporting feminist ideology investigated men's violation of their partners' lack of consent (Margolin, Moran, & Miller, 1989). The violation investigated was that of a man kissing a woman on a date when she indicated explicitly that she did not want to be kissed.

Like the study of Koss and Oros (1982), data were collected only for women as victims and men as perpetrators. Feminist theorists were cited to support the belief that violation of consent in kissing was strong enough to generalize to more extreme forms of sexual assault. In Russell's frequently cited study (1986) of sexual abuse of women, unwanted nonforceful kissing was one form of abuse. The study by Margolin et al. (1989) found that both male and female psychology students considered the man's violation to be less unacceptable in long-term dating and marriage, and the men found it less unacceptable than the women. The women found the woman's right to say no more acceptable than did the men. The findings were considered to demonstrate acceptance of the concept that men have increased rights of sexual access and women less rights to refuse them, the longer the duration of the couple's relationship and the more formal their commitment.

Subsequently, Margolin (1990) published a study that investigated the acceptability of both men and women to violate their opposite-sex partner's lack of consent to kissing when out on a date. Men and women university students considered it to be more acceptable for a woman than a man to deny consent; women were neutral and men slightly approving of a woman violating the man's consent. The results of the first study were discussed in terms of the man's sexual rights over the woman. Violation of their consent was treated as on a continuum of violence and disregard for women. In contrast, the results of the second study were reported as revealing that a disproportionately large number of subjects did not find a sexually diffident male very sympathetic. Unlike the man's forced kissing in the first study, there was no reference to the woman's forced kissing being a sexual violation on a continuum of violence and disregard for men. The man who rejected being kissed was referred to as withholding consent rather than expressing his right to say no. The fact that the findings were not in agreement with the hypothesis of the earlier study (that men were more committed than women to maintaining male dominance and female passivity) was not pointed out. The first study was published in the journal *Violence and Victims*, and the second in the *Archives of Sexual Behavior*.

Regarding rape as an act of social control led many feminists to argue that it is not sexually motivated and indicates nothing about male sexuality (Palmer, 1988). Darke (1990) used this belief to account for the failure of penile circumference assessment to distinguish rapists from nonrapists (discussed in Chapter 8). Herman (1990) considered that in early feminist consciousness-raising, it was necessary to define rape as an aggressive rather than a sexual act to challenge the widespread belief the victims derived pleasure from being assaulted. She implied that now this belief had been successfully challenged, it should be recognized that sexual assault not only asserts male dominance and intimidates women, it also provides the aggressor with sexual pleasure.

Palmer (1988) investigated the empirical as opposed to the political support for the belief that rape was not sexually motivated. He considered it to receive its most influential endorsement from Groth's concepts of power and anger rape (see Chapter 8). Palmer critically examined and rejected 12 reasons advanced to support the belief; however, he did not mention what appears to be the most powerful argument against it, the evidence that sex offenders—including the sexually assaultive—respond to chemical reduction of their level of testosterone (Chapter 8). Furthermore, the reduction produced in the intensity of their deviant impulses correlated strongly with the reduction in their hormone levels (McConaghy et al., 1988).

Failure to subject the relevant data to adequate critical analysis is further evidenced in the common use of the term *rape myths* for a set of beliefs that are accepting of rape. Items in a scale of rape-myth acceptance developed by Burt (1980) included "a woman who goes to the home or apartment of a man on their first date implies she is willing to have sex"; "in the majority of rapes, the victim is promiscuous or has a bad reputation"; and "many women have an unconscious wish to be raped, and may then unconsciously set up a situation in which they are likely to be attacked." Burt reported an investigation of 598 Minnesota subjects 18 years and over, in which agreement with rape myths in both men and women correlated with acceptance of interpersonal violence, of sex-role stereotyping, and of the belief that sexual interactions between men and women were adversarial.

Acceptance of all four sets of beliefs were more frequently reported by older and less educated subjects. As pointed out in Chapter 2, however, they continue to be held by a significant percentage of adolescents. Burt concluded that only by promoting the idea of sex as a mutually undertaken, freely chosen, fully conscious interaction rather than a battlefield can society create an atmosphere free of the threat of rape. While agreeing totally with the desirability of this change, one could question whether labeling rape-supportive beliefs as myths is the most effective way of promoting it. A set of rape myths could equally easily be created that would caricature the more extreme feminist view of rape: "There is no difference between women who are raped and those who are not"; "men and women are equally likely to initiate sexual intercourse"; "women who express initial reluctance to the initiation of intercourse never enjoy it"; and "all men are potential rapists."

Though rape-accepting beliefs must be challenged, if in people's experience there is even a small element of truth in them, to label them myths is to encourage skepticism. This small element of truth in rape myths must be accepted and dealt with. How is society to be changed so that, for example (as discussed in Chapter 2), adolescent boys no longer feel under pressure to initiate sexual activity and girls, that they must limit it? Or how are men to be convinced that women should not be coerced into sexual activity when they report the experience of coercing some women who then appeared to enjoy the experience? Muehlenhard and Cook (1988) found that both male and female students who had experienced unwanted sexual activity tended to believe that women's resistance to sex is often merely token, done so that women can have sex without appearing promiscuous. Fifteen percent of female and 12% of male medical students at the University of New South Wales reported the experience of being initially coerced into, but then enjoying sexual activity (McConaghy & Zamir, 1992c). Ten percent of heterosexual couples who initially rejected their partner's sexual approach changed their mind because they got turned on (Byers & Heinlien, 1989).

That some people respond to a degree of coercion for sexual activity with initial rejection, followed by arousal leading to enjoyment, has to be acknowledged and dealt with by ideologies that oppose coercion in all its forms. Labeling such behaviors as rape myths puts pressure on researchers not to investigate or report them, and on journal reviewers to reject the submissions for publication of those who do. The term is now so established that it would seem impossible to change; however, it is to be hoped that it does not become a general practice to label as myths behaviors that are difficult for ideologies to accommodate. Theory that departs from reality reduces its ability to understand and change reality.

Burgess (1985) reviewed evidence of the rape-supportive nature of sex-role learning, traditional dating patterns, and adherence to rape myths, finding that females associate femininity with softness, nonassertiveness, and dependence on men, but also with the setting of limits in sexual situations. Males are conditioned to be strong, powerful, and aggressive and to view women's resistance to sexual overtures as face-saving gestures. In Sorensen's national probability sample (1973) of adolescents aged 13 to 19 years, 26% of boys and 25% of girls agreed with the statement that "if a girl has led a boy on, it's all right for the boy to force her to have sex." A survey of adolescents at the end of the 1970s revealed similar attitudes (Burgess, 1985). As stated above, the belief that women's rejection of sexual advances is only token continues to find acceptance even by some women (Muehlenhard & Cook, 1988). Bart (1979) questioned why many women hold conventional ideologies about rape, stating that women jurors were never considered especially sympathetic to rape victims. She suggested that it was difficult for women to live with the knowledge that all women are vulnerable and that they are frequently raped by men they know. If they believe that only bad women are raped and only crazy men who are strangers rape, they can feel safe.

Ageton (1983) and Koss and Dinero (1989) were unable to support the aspect of the male political dominance theory that holds that women who subscribe to traditional notions of femininity and accept common myths about rape are vulnerable to rape. These women were considered to act passively toward men, to expect men to be dominant and forceful, and to be slow to realize that an interaction was progressing toward rape. In their community studies, neither Ageton nor Koss and Dinero found an association between the subjects' gender-role attitudes and rape-supportive beliefs and their likelihood of being sexually victimized.

Anthropological evidence was advanced that rape is common in cultures characterized by patrilocality (the marital pattern requiring couples to reside with the groom's family), worship of a sole male creative deity, glorification of war, a high level of feuding, raiding of other groups for wives, interpersonal violence, an ideology of male toughness, women holding little political or economic power, segregation of the sexes, and care of children being an inferior occupation (Herman, 1990; Stermac, Segal, & Gillis, 1990). Marshall and Barbaree (1990a) agreed with the authors that these features characterized U.S. culture and related this to the evidence that the rate of reported rape was higher in the United States than in other Western societies.

As discussed previously, reported rape is a poor index of the actual incidence of rape. More evidence is needed from community studies of its incidence, using identical methodologies. Questionnaire surveys of Australian and U.S. students indicated that the rate of sexual coercion and rape of women by men was higher among the U.S. students (McConaghy & Zamir, 1992b, c). The number of men reporting a likelihood that they would carry out sexual coercion and rape if they could do so without risk of discovery was comparable in the surveys. If reported likelihood to carry out assault is a meaningful entity, this would suggest that Australian students felt there was a greater possibility of disclosure or punishment if they actually carried it out. In a study of different cultures, Otterbein (1979) found a correlation of $r = -0.68$ between severity of punishment and frequency of rape.

Pornography

Herman (1990) commented that the most articulate expression of the sociocultural characteristics of a male-dominated society could be found in literature that enjoys a predominantly male mass audience, such as pornography, and in the works of lionized literary figures. The possible influence of pornography in causing rape has been expressed most emphatically by feminist authors. Wheller (1985) quoted from this literature that pornography is violence against women that masquerades as sexuality; that it is the undiluted essence of antifemale propaganda; that male power is the raison d'etre of pornography, and degradation of the female the means of achieving this power; and that there are remarkable similarities in the way it feels to be violently raped as an adult, incestuously abused as a child, or sexually harassed on the job and the way it feels to view pornography.

Wheller commented that feminist analyses had not sharply differentiated child pornography from pornography in general, but it was seen as linked to it in that women were identified with children as helpless and submissive, with childlike women such as Marilyn Monroe being seen as ideals. She considered child pornography and pornography in general to be backlashes to the women's movement, accounting for the coterminous rise of women's liberation and of brutal adult and child pornography and of child prostitution. She provided no evidence of the rise of child prostitution, perhaps accepting the view of Barry, which she cited, that feminist research on porn is "busy work" and that such research should not get sidetracked on false issues such as freedom of speech and research to provide what feminists already know (i.e., that porn is harmful to women) through their commonsense experience. Pornography may influence the nature of men's sexual demands of women. Ten percent of the San Francisco women interviewed by specially trained interrogators (see Chapter 6) answered affirmatively the question, "Have you ever been upset by anyone trying to get you to do what they'd seen in pornographic pictures, movies, or books?" Two percent were victims of sexual assault arising out of the situation (Russell, 1986).

Murrin and Laws (1990), in their review of the literature investigating the possible influence of pornography in causing rape, paid little attention to what was perhaps its major methodological problem, the use of reported rape statistics as the measure of prevalence of rape. Any relationship found between measures of availability or use of pornography and the prevalence of reported rape must take into account the factors determining the reporting of rape. For example, more liberal attitudes toward pornography could be associated with a higher level of consciousness concerning what constitutes rape and, hence, a greater willingness to report it. Since 1970 there has been a marked increase in the use of pornography and in the number of reported rapes in the United States; however, the prevalence of sexual assaults in a community survey of comparable populations showed no evidence of having increased (Kanin & Parcell, 1977). Kutchinsky (1991) pointed out that though from

1964 to 1984 most crimes increased in frequency, there was no increase in rates of rape compared to those of nonsexual violent offenses, either in the United States, Denmark, Sweden, or West Germany. In all four countries the availability of various forms of pictorial pornography, including violent/dominant varieties, increased from extreme scarcity to relative abundance. He somewhat overconfidently commented that the finding seemed sufficient to discard the hypothesis that pornography caused rape.

In their review, Murrin and Laws (1990) cited one study that took into account four population characteristics stated to have been shown to be highly correlated with rape statistics: percentage living in urban areas, percentage who were black, percentage living below the poverty level, and per capita males aged 18 to 24 years. Having controlled for these characteristics, the study found 83% of the variance in rape rate to be accounted for by six factors: consumption of eight soft-core magazines, indices of sexual inequality, economic inequality, social disorganization, level of urbanization, and unemployment. Murrin and Laws pointed out that further analyses of the same data set were not consistent with the hypothesis that the relationship with use of pornography was causal. Although the circulation of soft-core pornography magazines was related to rape rate, so was that of such outdoor magazines as *Field and Stream*. Circulation of a hard-core pornography magazine was not; nor were other indices of exposure to hard-core pornography, such as number of adult theatres or bookshops.

Murrin and Laws suggested that a variable that could produce a relationship between increased use of pornography and rape rapes was the presence of a "hypermasculine" culture, characterized by social values supporting male domination and use of women as sexual objects. When this was statistically controlled in the data concerning the populations investigated, the relationship between rape rates and sex magazine circulation became insignificant. This would not exclude the possibility that sex magazines contributed to the maintenance of a hypermasculine culture.

Female Pornography

No studies appear to have examined the possible effects of what have been labeled "Mills and Boon" novels written for women in maintaining a hypermasculine culture. Coles and Shamp (1984) cited a report that such novels had 20 million loyal readers. They summarized their contents as a struggle for emotional and physical dominance between an initially innocent nubile teenager and a sensual older man with the man's inevitable triumph, from initial rape to eventual domesticity. During the course of the struggle the characters experienced improbable adventures, most of which involved explicit descriptions of sexual scenes, often including bondage and rape. This content seems at variance with that popular in Australia, in which the age gap of heroine and hero is not great and sexual scenes are not explicit. Coles and Shamp found that women who read these novels (as compared to nonreaders) fantasized significantly more during intercourse, and they concluded that the novels were a form of soft-core pornography that women read for sexual stimulation.

In view of the importance of romantic rather than specific sexual feelings in womens' physical relationships as compared to men's (Chapter 2), it would be expected that pornography for women would be more relationship oriented and less genital than pornography for men. In sociological theory, these novels provide scripts that encourage their women readers to respond sexually to roles of male domination and female submission, attitudes that in the male political dominance theory of rape are believed to encourage their victimization. It would seem that the feminist opposition to heterosexual pornography viewed by men should also be directed to "Mills and Boon" novels and stories read by women, as well as their equivalent in literature regarded as belonging to high culture (e.g., the novels *Jane Eyre* and *Wuthering Heights*) and indeed much art of the romantic movement, all of which similarly advance aggressive males and subservient women as sexual role models.

Feminist/sociological analyses have paid little attention to the extensive pornography produced for male homosexuals, in which men are at times treated as coercively as are women in the pornography produced for heterosexual men. The monograph *Pornography and Sexual Aggression* (Malamuth & Donnerstein, 1984) gave little attention to child pornography and none to homosexual pornography. Wheller (1985) commented, "What remains constant from one example to another [of pornography] is the view of females as dehumanized sexual objects to be used by men" (p. 376). To support her view that pornography is one of the important mechanisms for the social control of women by men, she cited a long description of a woman bound in a painful way. She did not discuss the political significance of similar male-bondage pornography. If the latter is also a mechanism for social control, one would expect it to be found oppressive by the homosexual men at whom it is directed.

PSYCHIATRIC-PSYCHOPATHOLOGICAL MODEL OF RAPE

Bart (1979) and Scully and Marolla (1985) contrasted feminist and sociological perspectives of rape with the earlier psychiatric-psychopathological model in which rapists were regarded as driven by irresistible sexual impulses, as psychologically disordered, or as acting under the influence of alcohol, and in which victims were considered to in part have precipitated the offense. They considered rape to be in this way removed from the realm of the everyday or normal world. Scully and Marolla argued against the beliefs accepted in the psychiatric-psychopathological view on the basis that in one study of rapes reported to authorities, 71% of the offenses were premeditated and so could not be impulsive. As discussed earlier, however, reported rapes are not representative of the much larger number that are not reported. It is these unreported rapes that provide the basis for the belief (which Scully and Marolla accepted) that rape is an extension of normal male sexual behavior. Also, many patients report impulses to carry out such apparently premeditated behaviors as gambling and shoplifting, yet it is accepted that these impulses can be irresistible, and they are classified in DSM-III-R as disorders of impulse control. Following treatment, subjects gain control of these (McConaghy, 1988c; McConaghy & Blaszczynski, 1988) and of sexually assaultive behaviors (Chapter 8), indicating that they previously were uncontrollable. Evidence that men's personality characteristics and their use of alcohol and other drugs influence their likelihood of carrying out sexually assaultive behaviors is reviewed in Chapter 8.

Victim Vulnerability

The belief that characteristics of victims may influence the likelihood of their being assaulted was supported by the studies of Ageton (1983) and Burnam et al. (1988), which demonstrated that some victims, particularly those subjected to repeated assault, differed from nonvictims prior to the assault. Koss and Dinero (1989) investigated a representative sample of 2,723 college women in a study they considered to provide a strict test of the hypothesis that some women are vulnerable to rape. A background of childhood sexual abuse, liberal sexual attitudes, alcohol use, and sexual activity with more partners characterized 10% of the women whose risk of rape was 37%, as compared with 14% for the remaining 90%. This risk profile predicted 25% of rape victims. Too few respondents had delinquent associations to investigate the significance of this variable, which was found by Ageton (1983) to predict victimization. Duncan (1990) reported that lesbian and gay students were two to three times as likely to report having sex against their will as their heterosexual colleagues. The current ratio of homosexual as compared to heterosexual feelings of male but not female medical students correlated significantly with their reporting having been sexually coerced, both by men ($r = 0.5$) and by women ($r = 0.24$; (McConaghy & Zamir, 1992c).

Frank, Turner, Stewart, Jacob, and West (1981) investigated an earlier report that one-third of adult rape victims had a history of prior psychiatric treatment; they found a similar percentage in the female victims they studied. More than 14% had been hospitalized for such treatment. Also, 20% had a past history of alcohol abuse. The authors cautioned that their sample, who had made contact with a rape crisis center, might be biased toward subjects who were psychologically needy. Such a bias, however, was not present in the representative subjects of the ECA community study reported by Burnam et al. (1988). This study also found significantly higher prevalences of major depression, alcohol and drug abuse or dependence, antisocial personality, and phobias in victims prior to their assault as compared with matched controls. This evidence that some subjects are vulnerable to assault, of course, in no way implies they were responsible for the assault, nor provides any justification for it. As there is evidence to support both the sociological and psychiatric-psychological models of sexual assault, it would seem that, as they are not incompatible, some integration of the two will ultimately be accepted.

TREATMENT

Burgess and Holmstrom (1985) recommended immediate crisis intervention when rape is disclosed. The aim was to return the victim to her or his previous level of functioning as rapidly as possible; they believed that the speed with which the victim was treated following the rape was crucial in improving the prognosis. Hochbaum (1987) suggested that the skills required of the therapist in the immediate care of the victim could be divided into four categories: recognition and management of emotional trauma, assessment and treatment of physical injuries, prevention of venereal disease and pregnancy, and appropriate collection of evidence. Hochbaum provided guidelines for these procedures.

Symonds (1980) emphasized the importance of avoiding "the second wound"—the failure to support or the rejection of the victim by her family, friends, community, agencies, and society in general. If she seeks help at a busy hospital emergency department, she could be prioritized behind other patients with life-threatening ill-nesses or injuries, resulting in delay that aggravates the emotional trauma she has already experienced. Legal and technical aspects involved in evaluation of sexual assault and subsequent testimony concerning it could cause physicians and nurses to erect a psychological barrier against the victim. To overcome these problems, it may be necessary to educate and screen all personnel who have contact with rape victims and to establish a specialized admission service. Hochbaum (1987) pointed out that in almost three-quarters of rapes reported in Michigan in 1982, no evidence was forwarded to the police crime laboratory. He related this to the suggestion that physicians were uncomfortable in the role of evidence collectors and provided a simple form, developed by the police department in cooperation with physicians, to encourage physicians to carry out this duty. Help with advocacy services and mobili-zation of the victim's support system were recommended by Burgess and Holmstrom (1985).

McCombie and Arons (1980) hypothesized that the therapeutic task with rape crisis counseling was to provide sufficient containment of powerful affects within the counseling relationship to enable the client to remember, reexperience, understand, and come to terms with the assault. They found staff stress to be prevalent in rape counseling, and the rape counselor to be confronted with both her own personal vulnerability to danger and her own masochistic and sadistic feelings, particularly if she was of similar age and background and identified with the victim. They felt that the issue of the rape fantasies women commonly experience (Chapter 8) should be dealt with to eliminate possible shame and guilt concerning these. The difference between such fantasies, which are sexually arousing, and the actual experience of rape needed to be emphasized; otherwise the victim could experience the rape as a punishment for her fantasies and the counselor could find herself confused in her reaction to the victim's account of the rape, feeling both titillated and repelled. This might lead the counselor to avoid seeking information about the rape, or to express either her censored masochistic fantasies by disgust or fear or her sadistic feelings in an outburst of anger.

McCombie and Arons stated that counselors commonly remark on their wishes to "kill that bastard" or to castrate or torture him. They suggested that the counselor should be able to accept the role of a nonjudgmental, noncontrolling interviewer who identifies and supports the victim's ego strengths and does not encourage regression. The victim needs to begin to acknowledge and comprehend the impact of the rape and give herself permission for a time of healing without harsh self-criticism or unrealistic expectations. She can then move to an active and mastery-oriented posi-tion.

Burgess and Holmstrom (1985) followed treatment of the acute phase of post-traumatic stress disorder with rape work to treat this second phase of long-term reorganization, in which the victim has the task of restoring order to and control over her or his life-style. They considered this phase could last months or years. Additional help could be needed for what they termed compounded reactions, which included depression, psychosis, psychosomatic disorders, suicidal behavior and drug use. Rape work aided the victim in regaining a sense of safety and reestablishing mutually satisfying partner relationships in a world where rape remained a reality for all women. Burgess and Holmstrom considered that traditional psychotherapy could encourage the victim to internalize the blame and adopt a self-critical attitude. In their review of the literature concerning treatment of the posttraumatic stress disorder of rape victims, however, Steketee and Foa (1987) found that some workers recommended treatment by dynamic psychotherapy as a final component of crisis intervention.

Steketee and Foa reviewed programs treating sexual assault victims with combined or multimodal cognitive-behavioral approaches. A stress-inoculation training program began with an educational phase, in which it was explained that anxiety had become conditioned to stimuli associated with the rape experience. This was followed by a number of anxiety reduction techniques, including relaxation, modeling, and thought-stopping. A 4- to 6-hour Brief Behavioral Intervention Program was designed for use immediately after rape. The victim was encouraged to recall the rape events in imagery and to experience and express emotional reactions to it; feelings of guilt and responsibility for the rape were reduced by discussion of societal expectations and rape myths. Coping skills, such as self-assertion, relaxation, thought stopping, and methods for resuming normal activities, were then taught.

Interest has recently been shown in an eye-movement desensitization procedure for posttraumatic stress disorder (Shapiro, 1989). Subject were instructed to visualize the traumatic scene and to rehearse a statement concerning their negative feelings associated with the scene while they followed the therapist's finger with their eyes. The therapist then moved her finger rapidly back and forth across their line of vision. A single session of the treatment was reported to desensitize traumatic memories successfully and to alter dramatically the cognitive assessments of the situations in 22 subjects, some of whom were victims of rape and childhood molestation.

In the treatment of adolescent rape, Mann (1981) found that crisis workers spent more time counseling and calming the parents than the adolescents. They relied mostly on the parents' information about the victims' reactions and thus often did not appreciate the victims' feelings of guilt and self-blame and their worries about bodily, mental, and moral integrity. Instead the therapists tended, like the parents, to express anger toward the perpetrator and to be more concerned about future sexuality, pregnancy, and venereal disease. They found the parents to be more supportive of the victim than the victim did; only if parents were overtly hostile were parent-child communication problems perceived. Mann argued that this resulted in teenagers perceiving therapists as unsupportive and therefore refusing counseling. He recommended that the specific rape concerns of victims and parents be identified in separate interviews; that because adolescents do not freely communicate their worries, active inquiry be carried out using a checklist of important areas; and that if victims' and parents' concerns differ, parents should be helped to accept and support their children's concerns. Professionals treating adolescent rape victims, Mann suggested, should receive specialized training in regard to the differences in the rape stresses experienced by adolescents.

Miller et al. (1982) reported significant improvement in both marital and sexual adjustment following conjoint marital cotherapy in 18 couples in whom the female partner had been raped. Fourteen reported sexual difficulties, and the majority had avoided sexual relations since the rape. Though improvement was not maintained at 6 months follow-up, the authors regretted that the large majority of rape victims did not seek or obtain relationship counseling. Rodkin, Hunt, and Cowan (1982) found that a men's support group enabled the significant others of rape victims to understand and support the victims better. Treatment of revealed father-daughter incest by crisis intervention (Herman, 1985) or a humanistic approach (Giarretto, 1978, 1981) was discussed in relation to child sexual abuse (Chapter 6).

Evaluation

Herman (1985) pointed out the lack of well-documented outcome studies evaluating response to treatment of sexual assault. Steketee and Foa (1987) approved of the increased number of assessment measures used in these studies, without commenting on the effect on treatment efficacy, cost, or patient compliance (Chapter 1). They suggested that no-treatment controls should be included, again without discussing the methodological or ethical problems involved in their use. Few subjects with significant levels of pathology would seem likely to give informed consent to participating in a no-treatment control study, and those who do are unlikely to be representative of the population of sexual assault victims seeking treatment. In any case, no-treatment controls provide little information of value. In virtually all meta-analyses of psychotherapy outcome studies, patients who received placebo therapy showed marked improvement when compared to no-treatment controls. Unlike subjects receiving active or placebo therapies, no-treatment controls are unlikely to make efforts to improve while awaiting treatment and may experience negative feelings from being denied the immediate treatment they sought (McConaghy, 1990a).

More useful information would be provided by studies comparing different treatments claimed to be effective. One treatment worth evaluating in such a comparison study would be a self-defense program, in view of the many positive changes reported to follow this (Ozer & Bandura, 1990). Some doubt of the value of standard treatment in sexual assault centers was cast by the findings of Norris and Feldman-Summers (1981). Follow-up of assault victims who reported to both police and a sexual assault center, as compared to those who reported to police alone or who did not report the assault, revealed no difference in outcome measures, which included indices of psychosomatic effects, decreased sexual activity and satisfaction, and reclusiveness. It is possible, however, that the victims who reported the assault were more severely traumatized and, without treatment, could have had a worse outcome than those who did not seek help.

The largest outcome research project evaluating treatment of sexual assault reported so far is the series of studies comparing systematic desensitization and cognitive-behavioral therapy (Frank et al., 1988). With systematic desensitization, subjects were trained to relax and then, while relaxed, to imagine themselves in situations of which they were fearful and that they had avoided. Initially, they imagined scenes that provoked minimal anxiety. Cognitive therapy aimed to help subjects identify and test the reality of distorted and dysfunctional beliefs. Subjects completed a weekly activity schedule in which they recorded daily activities and the amount of mastery and pleasure they experienced from the activities. They were given graded task assignments to reach difficult goals, such as going out alone, and were trained to detect automatic negative thoughts provoked by the assigned activities.

In the major study, 138 subjects who attended centers for violent crime or rape volunteered to accept therapy. They were randomly allocated to one or the other of the two forms of treatment. Subjects were classified as immediate treatment seekers if the rape had occurred days or weeks previously, and late treatment seekers if it had occurred several months previously. They completed a battery of assessment measures before and following treatment. In the 60% of subjects who remained in the study, there were no significant differences in response to the two treatments, which produced marked improvement in both immediate- and late-treatment subjects. Frank et al. discussed their results in relation to the number of studies showing that rape victims improve markedly within 3 months of the assault without treatment. They pointed out that this was not true of their late-treatment subjects, who prior to treatment showed at least as much pathology as the immediate-treatment group. They considered the fact that equivalent improvement followed treatment of both immediate- and late-treatment groups to support the conclusion that the improvement was attributable to the treatment.

TREATMENT OF ADULTS SEXUALLY ABUSED IN CHILDHOOD

Accompanying the general acceptance that sexual abuse in childhood can result in significantly impaired mental health in adulthood, there is also acceptance that the impairment requires specific treatment. In this respect, the experience of incest appears to have attracted more attention than extrafamilial abuse. Courtois and Sprei (1988) commented that retrospective incest therapy draws heavily on the feminist perspective, which stresses belief in and support of the survivor and her experience. They argued that the therapy stance should be nurturing and reality based rather than abstinent and aloof, and that the therapist must be active in view of the denial, shame, stigma, and repression many survivors experience. They anticipated that with survivors who suffered the most serious repercussions, the therapist could assume the therapy would take years and stated that the patients were likely to be discouraged or enraged by the length of treatment. They believed the countertransference of the therapist could lead to such problems as avoiding discussion of or showing voyeuristic interest in the incest experience, treating the patient as overly fragile, making special efforts to accommodate her, expressing rage about the experience prematurely or too intensively; or sexualizing the relationship due to a rescuing fantasy, possibly rationalized this as a "corrective emotional experience".

Therapists treating incest victims need to take into account the possible legal implications of Armsworth's statement (1989), discussed in Chapter 6, that failure to believe a report of incest is a form of abuse of the patient, and that 46% of incest victims are abused by their therapists. My clinical experience with patients previously treated by some therapists as victims of child sexual abuse is that the therapists' unquestioning acceptance or encouragement of the report that abuse had occurred was a form of abuse. I believe it led patients with personality disorders to adopt the role of perpetual victim and maintained their inability to work or relate to others effectively, a situation that was extremely difficult if not impossible to reverse.

Courtois and Sprei (1988) recommended an eclectic approach incorporating gestalt, psychodrama, psychodynamic, cognitive, behavioral, social learning, trans-actional analytic, and humanistic strategies along with bibliotherapy. They suggested that a group modality would benefit some patients but would be unsuitable for others. Carver et al. (1989) would appear to agree. Of 95 women who accepted referral to a group for adult survivors of childhood sexual abuse, 16 were judged inappropriate, and 11 decided the group was not for them. Reasons subjects were considered inappropriate included obvious thought disorder, current drug or alcohol abuse, or severe individual psychopathology marked by extreme egocentricity, inter-personal paranoia, or a severe lack of connectedness to affect. Perpetrators of the abuse were mainly family members, most of whom were fathers. Forty percent of the women had a history of psychiatric hospitalization, 63% had previous therapy, and 47% were currently in therapy.

The group in the Carver et al. study was structured to provide some sense of security and to make it possible for each participant to begin talking about the sexual abuse from the onset. Disclosure of painful memories and feelings were aided by films, art therapy, and childhood photographs. Of 57 women who commenced thera-py, 15 dropped out. Those who were employed, were not currently in therapy, and had never been hospitalized were less likely to drop out. The 20 subjects who completed questionnaires before and following treatment showed significant im-provement on all but the paranoia scale of the Symptom Check List 90, but not on self-esteem as measured by the Texas Social Behavior Inventory or on the Zung Self-Rating Depression Scale.

Behavioral (Rychtarik, Silverman, Van Landingham, & Prue, 1984a) and cog-nitive-behavioral (McCarthy, 1986) approaches have also been used to treat adult survivors of childhood sexual abuse. McCarthy felt that one of the most powerful interventions in the latter approach was confrontation of the perpetrator, and he discussed the preparation of the victim for this. Kilpatrick and Best (1984) criticized the behavioral approach, suggesting that an exclusive focus on anxiety was short-sighted and that destructive irrational cognitions could persist. Rychtarik et al. (1984b) rejected this view, arguing that treating feelings of anxiety and irrational cognitions as independent created a false dichotomy. Such controversies, based on theoretical considerations and lacking any empirical data to aid their resolution, indicate the need for controlled comparisons of the various treatments being used with adults reporting childhood abuse.

PREVENTION OF SEXUAL ASSAULT

Swift (1985) pointed out that primary prevention of sexual assault is an idea that has not been tested, and that conventional attempts to prevent rape focused on advising women to restrict such activities as going alone into parks or out at night. A possibly more reasonable approach of this nature was the provision of a safety van service by a student federation to provide transport for female students living off campus, with the aim of reducing their exposure to sexual assault. Its introduction was reported to have increased the evening use of study-related facilities; no evidence was provided of its influence on the incidence of sexual assault (Baylis & Myers, 1990). Swift criticized the lack of efforts directed to reducing men's likelihood of sexually coercing women, apart from treatment after they have offended.

Herman (1990) argued that sex education for all children should be a valuable aspect of primary prevention, but that the existing sexual education establishment could not be relied upon to appropriately provide this in view of its male-oriented, libertarian position. She recommended a program that combined full presentation of accurate information, respect for individual privacy and choice, and an articulated vision of socially responsive conduct. Issues of power and exploitation would be addressed explicitly. Boys and young men might be considered a priority for preventive work, and organized male groups that foster traditional sexual attitudes targeted, including athletic teams, college fraternities, and the military. Primary prevention work with groups at high risk for victimization could be expected to result in early disclosure of sexual assaults that have already occurred, with the possibility of immediate treatment of offenders and hence prevention of further assaults by them.

Herman hypothesized that vigorous enforcement of existing criminal laws prohibiting sexual assault might be expected to have some preventative effect, given that both compulsive and opportunistic offenders were keenly sensitive to external controls. This view is supported by the cross-cultural study, cited earlier, that found a correlation between severity of punishment and frequency of rape of -0.68 (Otterbein, 1979). Herman recommended prosecution as particularly important where traditional cultural standards legitimate and condone sexual assault, for example, in marital or date rape or the rape of prostitutes. In these situations, prosecution would serve an educational function. Swift (1985) pointed out that research had confirmed that punishment reduced crime only in relation to its certainty and that 90 percent of cases of rape are unreported. She reported that in 1,000 cases, only 2 convictions resulted. Like Herman, she believed that rigorous enforcement of legal sanctions against rape would signal strong public sentiment that rape is unacceptable and thus influence behavioral norms. Legislation codifying women's equality and rights in educational, economic, political, and social areas would, by empowering women, be part of a primary prevention strategy.

Herman (1990) considered another requirement for primary prevention of sexual violence to be engagement with the organized sex industry, including its nominally criminal component in prostitution, child sex rings, and child and hard-core pornography, as well as its legitimate component in soft-core pornography and men's magazines. She decided from the experience of the temperance movement that abolition of the industry in its entirety must await completion of a feminist revolution. A short-term strategy would be regulation of material dealing with sexual violence; when pornographers and advertisers employed this material, direct action and boycott strategies had proved effective against them.

Individual Strategies

In regard to techniques for reducing the individual woman's likelihood of being raped, Swift (1985) pointed out the consistent evidence of the efficacy of resistant behaviors, such as fleeing, screaming, and kicking as compared with crying, pleading, or doing nothing. A study of 13 adult women, all of whom had both been raped and avoided rape, found that completed rapes were more likely when the victim had a previous sexual relationship with the attacker, when she used only talking or pleading as a strategy, when force was threatened, when the assault took place in the victim's home, and when the victim's primary concern was with not being injured or killed (Bart, 1981). Rapes were more likely to be avoided when the assault took place outside, when the victim used multiple strategies, when the assailant was a stranger, and when the woman's primary concern was with avoiding rape.

Similar conclusions were reached by Quinsey and Upfold (1985) from detailed descriptions of the 145 attempted and completed rapes reported by rapists in a maximum-security psychiatric institution. They concluded that screaming or yelling was a good strategy and not associated with subsequent injury. Physical resistance was only effective in outside locations; however, they pointed out that commonly the physical resistance was grappling, which must penalize the weaker opponent. In the three cases when striking the assailant was used, it was successful. No victims kicked, kneed, used eye gouges, or weapons of convenience. Though physical resistance was associated with victim injury, the authors suggested that the finding could be misleading, as some victims may have resisted as a consequence of injury.

A further study by Bart and O'Brien (1984) investigated women in the Chicago area who had been sexually attacked. Forty-three were raped, and 51 successfully avoided rape. The women who avoided rape were taller and heavier, played football or another contact sport often in childhood, engaged in sports regularly, were more often unmarried and living alone, and were attacked between midnight and 5 a.m. The most effective strategy was fleeing from the rapist. More than 80% of women who tried this avoided being raped, as did almost 70% of women who fought their attacker. The modal strategy for women who avoided rape was a combination of screaming/yelling and physical resistance. Bart and O'Brien concluded that by fighting back, a woman significantly increased her chances of rape avoidance and somewhat increased her chance of rough treatment; however, not resisting was no guarantee of humane treatment. Women who used physical strategies were less depressed following the event, even if they had been unsuccessful in avoiding rape. Use of cognitive verbal tactics such as reasoning, verbally refusing, threatening, and conning—though frequently advised—did not differentiate raped women from those who avoided rape, and were considered ineffective when used alone.

These findings support the value of training women in physical resistance, a rape prevention strategy currently sponsored widely by feminist groups and police departments. Ozer and Bandura (1990) investigated 43 women enrolled in a five-session self-defense program, 38% of whom had been assaulted physically, and 27% sexually. Following completion of the program they were significantly more active in social, recreational, and community activities, an improvement maintained at 6 months follow-up. Of the hundreds of women who completed the program, 40 subsequently experienced attempted sexual assaults, of whom 38 escaped rape. Thirty stunned and disabled the assailants, and 8 frightened them off with counterstrikes. The 2 women raped did not fight back, as the assailants were armed.

Swift (1985) considered that the strategy of teaching women techniques to avoid rape may not reduce its prevalence. There was evidence that assailants abandoned attacks on resistant women and sought locales and victims offering minimum resistance and threat of detection. Such victims could include the very young, the physically or mentally disabled, or the elderly. Haseltine and Miltenberger (1990) reported the successful training of 8 adults with mild mental retardation in self-protection skills needed to discriminate and respond safely to abduction and sexual abuse situations.

WHY RAPE IS RARELY REPORTED AND PROSECUTED

As stated above, Swift (1985) concluded that 90% of cases of rape were unreported, and that of 1,000 cases, only 2 convictions resulted. Though little empirical research has investigated the reasons why rape is rarely reported, the reluctance of victims to do so is understandable in the light of much of the data discussed in this chapter. Some victims of confidence rapes report feeling partly to blame for the rape. If they were drinking with the rapist, they might believe this will be regarded as evidence of complicity. Girls with a history of delinquency are likely to be distrustful of the institutions where help is available. In the literature dealing with the treatment of rape victims, the need for specialized treatment centers with trained personnel was frequently stressed. In their absence, the distressed victim may encounter marked delay in receiving attention. The attention may be provided in a negative manner; professionals were noted to be reluctant to collect evidence for legal purposes.

The vigor with which criminals are apprehended ultimately depends on the attitude of police. Their enthusiasm in bringing to justice offenders against property or perpetrators of nondomestic physical violence is widely acknowledged in film and television. Their negative attitude toward rape victims, however, is frequently reported in anecdotal accounts (P. Murphy, 1980). Murphy also pointed out that victims may not call the police because of fear of the rapist; fear of the reaction of a husband, boyfriend, or parent; or the desire to avoid further ordeal in the police and court process. He considered a major factor in this ordeal to be the long delay from the time the suspect was arrested until he went for trial, often more than a year later. Many victims found that this prevented their resuming their normal lives. This may in part account for the finding of one jurisdiction that whereas 19 of 20 offenders charged with minor sexual crimes were tried, only 1 of 9 serious crimes (all of alleged rape) came to trial; in 5, the victim refused to testify (Beck, Borenstein, & Dreyfus, 1986). The first stage of identifying the factors preventing the reporting of rape is well advanced. The marked change in public attitudes and institutional procedures necessary to correct them and ultimately to prevent or at least minimize the incidence of rape has barely begun.

CHAPTER 8

Sexual Deviations
Paraphilias and Sex Offenses

Paraphilias is the term employed in DSM-III-R (APA, 1987) for the conditions cate-gorized in other classifications as sexual deviations. DSM-III-R describes paraphilias as characterized by arousal in response to sexual objects or situations that are not part of normative arousal-activity patterns, and that in varying degrees may interfere with the capacity for reciprocal, affectionate sexual activity. It then contradicts itself by pointing out that the imagery in paraphilic fantasy is frequently the stimulus for sexual excitement in people without a paraphilia, thus accepting—correctly, in my opinion—that arousal to the objects and situations that excite paraphiliacs can be part of normative patterns. The DSM-III-R description further states that the term *paraphilia* is preferred to that of *sexual deviation* used in other classifications, as *paraphilia* correctly emphasizes that the deviation (*para*) lies in that to which the person is attracted (*philia*). It then contradicts itself again by stating that the diag-nosis of paraphilia is only made if the person has acted on the urges or is markedly distressed by them. This must mean that the same "philia" may or may not justify the diagnosis, depending on whether or not it distresses the subject. The term *sexual deviation*, unlike *paraphilia*, is descriptive and implies nothing about etiology. As early as 1929, Pavlov pointed out the advantage scientifically of terms that do not imply a hypothesis. Many workers are currently suggesting that sexual attraction ("philia") is not involved in a number if not all sexual deviations.

Perhaps the time is not far distant when sex researchers will accept that the introduction of terms such as *sexual deviations* and *paraphilias* was a political act to sustain the concept that sexual activities that were currently socially unacceptable were pathological. The terms represent attempts to find, within a medical-biological model of sexual behavior that excluded sociological factors, properties these ac-tivities shared that distinguished them from acceptable sexual activities. This is most evident in regard to sexual activities between adults and children or adolescents. As discussed in Chapter 2, these remain accepted in some areas of the developing world, as they were in advanced civilizations in the past. When they occur in Western societies today they are regarded with abhorrence and are considered evidence of pathology in the adults involved, whereas they remain of anthropological interest and uncriticized in societies regarded as primitive.

Masturbation, now established as statistically the most normal of sexual activities for the majority of adolescent and elderly males in Western societies, was in the past considered an abnormal sexual deviation that resulted in major physical and mental health problems; with virtually no discussion, it has ceased to be regarded as pathological. The decision to no longer classify homosexuality as a sexual disorder was made overtly with total awareness of its sociopolitical significance. It was accepted that there was no evidence homosexuality was necessarily associated with psychiatric pathology, and that its classification as a disorder was contributing to the maintenance of the social and legal discrimination against homosexuality. A similar argument could be advanced in regard to other sexual practices currently classified as paraphilias, including fetishism, sadomasochism, and transvestism. Meanwhile, as discussed in Chapter 3, the marked effeminacy that is a precursor in boys of adult homosexuality remains classified as a disorder of gender identity.

A sizable minority (or possibly the majority) of the normal population experience fantasies of involvement in some sexual activities regarded as deviant; it is likely that a similar number of adolescent males carry them out. Acknowledgement of these facts and their subsequent acceptance by the community may encourage a shift in meaning of the term *sexual deviation*. Deviant behaviors would then be regarded nonjudgmentally as sexual behaviors that deviate from those that directly express the biological purpose of sexual activity: heterosexual arousal leading to noncoerced coitus. It then could be left to other agencies to determine the social and legal attitudes to the various deviant practices. For those proscribed legally, the term currently in use, *sexual offenses,* is appropriate. Of course, sexuality researchers should and will continue political activity to influence these social and legal attitudes whenever they individually consider that the attitudes conflict with their beliefs concerning individual freedom as well as its appropriate limitations. Where these beliefs have been incorporated into classifications of sexual behavior, however, it would seem necessary to attempt to identify and eliminate this. The resulting classifications would continue to move toward the scientific ideal of being free from politically motivated influences and based solely on the relevant empirical descriptive data.

Not all deviant behaviors classified as paraphilias in DSM-III-R are sex offenses. Some that are not sex offenses however, can lead to them. Subjects with fetishes for particular clothes may enter private property seeking them. Also, some sex offenses— in particular, most sexual assaults and the sexual activity of adult men with postpubertal boys—are not classified as paraphilias. This has resulted in somewhat independent classifications being developed of paraphilias and of sex offenses. DSM-III-R provides criteria for most of the paraphilias commonly encountered clinically.

DSM-III-R CLASSIFICATION OF PARAPHILIAS: SEXUAL DEVIATIONS

Exhibitionism

The DSM-III-R criterion for exhibitionism is that over a 6-month period, the person either has acted on or is markedly distressed by recurrent urges or fantasies involving the exposure of one's genitals to an unsuspecting stranger. Exhibitionists are typically postpubertal males who obtain high levels of excitement from exposing their penis to one or a few females, most commonly strangers at or just past puberty. Though in adolescence the excitement would appear to be sexual, by the time exhibitionists come to attention in adulthood many do not consider that it is. Rather, as Smukler and Schiebel (1975) pointed out, they report experiencing a state of expectation-excitement and a paniclike feeling prior to exhibiting, and the act is followed by a feeling of transient relief. This is rapidly followed by feelings of shame and guilt. Many report they do not have an erection when exposing; a number, however, masturbate during or after the exposure. As discussed in relation to adult transvestites, many of whom also report no sexual arousal to their deviant behavior (Chapter 4), it is likely that some sexual arousal is present but is masked by general arousal developed as the behavior becomes increasingly under the control of behavior completion mechanisms (discussed subsequently).

Exhibitionism usually commences in adolescence, when the subject may report he was somewhat shy with girls and was slower to begin dating than his peers. A number report at this stage experiencing sexual excitement following an episode of accidental exposure. While undressing, they may have become aware they were being observed by a female neighbor, or a female relative may have walked unexpectedly into the room. This situation might be repeated intentionally on a number of occasions, following which the adolescent is motivated to expose himself in other situations. Subjects are rarely charged with exhibitionism until they reach adulthood, suggesting that women victims are reluctant to report the behavior when the offender is an adolescent. Occasionally exhibitionism occurs for the first time in elderly men, many of whom do not show evidence of dementia, but are usually without sex partners or have ceased sexual relationships because of impotence.

Exposure is usually carried out in secluded locations—parks, beaches, quiet streets, shop alcoves, public transport, or from an automobile. In the subjects who come to clinical attention, exhibitionism has a strong compulsive quality. Offenders can be legally charged repeatedly despite their strongly stated desire to cease the behavior. Its compulsiveness is particularly evident in those subjects who exhibit from automobiles, as they are aware of the virtual certainty their behavior will be reported, yet they still cannot cease it. Many exhibitionists report they repeat the offense several times a day for weeks on end, particularly in the summer months, when they are aroused by the greater exposure of women's bodies. Exhibitionists in my experience do not report any consistent motive for the behavior, apart from the feeling of compulsion. Langevin and Lang (1987) reached a similar conclusion.

Freund (1990) pointed out that homosexual men frequently expose their penis to strangers in washrooms or parks as an invitation to sexual interaction. Freund considered that they were mostly men who lived as heterosexuals, were often married, and wanted to remain anonymous; however, these may simply be features of the men with this behavior who seek treatment. Literature by homosexual writers describing homosexual life-styles indicate that many subjects who identify as homosexual also seek casual relationships in this way (Lahr, 1986). Freund did not regard this behavior as exhibitionism, but considered true exhibitionism to appear less rarely in homosexual pedophiles. Kinsey et al. (1948) reported that the most specific erotic activities of children involved genital exhibitionism and genital contacts with other children.

Exhibitionism has been reported extremely infrequently in women, when it usually appeared to be motivated by attention seeking rather than excitement (Blair & Lanyon, 1981; O'Connor, 1987). Grob (1985), however, reported a case of a woman who exposed her breasts to truck drivers while she drove her automobile beside them. If they responded favorably she exposed her genital area, experiencing marked sexual excitement and occasionally orgasm. On an average weekend she drove 600 miles repeating the behavior, which also recurred at brief periods throughout psychoanalytic therapy. Her exhibitionism would seem to have been as compulsive and persistent as that of men.

Exhibitionism probably is the most common of the sexual deviations; 30% to 50% of women report being victims (DiVasto et al., 1984; Zverina, Lachman, Pondelickova, & Vanek, 1987). Gittleson, Eacott, and Mehta (1978) interviewed 100 nurses whose mean age was 33 years. Forty-four stated they had been victims of exposure on 67 occasions. Their mean age at the time of the exposure was 16.1 years, and 27 (40%) of the occasions had occurred prior to menarche. In 10 cases, (15%) the victim knew the offender. Exhibitionism was reported to account for about a third of convictions for sexual offenses in England, Germany, the United States, Canada, and Hong King (Rooth, 1973). Rooth hypothesized from the frequency with which it was discussed in the medical literature that it was much less common in France or Italy. In correspondence with doctors, mainly psychiatrists, in other countries, he was informed that exhibitionism was rare in South America and in Middle Eastern, African, and most Asian countries, including Japan. It was apparently more common in Chinese populations, as it was well recognized in Taiwan and in Hong Kong.

More exhibitionists seek treatment than other deviants and sex offenders. They made up 21 of the 45 subjects consecutively seeking treatment in two studies (McConaghy et al., 1985, 1988). The majority reported they were happily married, and most of the remainder were having satisfactory heterosexual relationships, consistent with the findings of Smukler and Schiebel (1975) and Langevin and Lang (1987). Smukler and Schiebel commented of the personality of exhibitionists that their data did not support any definitive character type or evidence of severe pathology; apart from the exhibitionism, they appeared relatively normal. Of the 21 in the two studies by McConaghy et al. (1985, 1988), 10 reported additional offenses or charges—mainly heterosexual pedophilia, reflecting the tendency of exhibitionists, found by Gittleson et al. (1978), to choose victims around the age of puberty. One reported voyeurism, and another sexual assault. Langevin and Lang (1987) also found an association of exhibitionism with pedophilic behavior but not with sexual assault. Freund and Blanchard (1986) reported that about half the exhibitionists they investigated reported other paraphilias, mainly voyeurism.

Voyeurism

The DSM-III-R criterion for voyeurism is that over a 6-month period, the person has acted on or is markedly distressed by recurrent urges or fantasies involving the act of observing an unsuspecting person who is naked, in the process of disrobing, or engaged in sexual activity. Gebhard, Gagnon, Pomeroy, and Christenson (1965) used the term *peepers* for males who for sexual gratification looked without consent into a private area or room with the hope of seeing partially or completely nude women. Commonly, peepers spend hours walking or driving through a neighborhood at night seeking lighted bedrooms or bathrooms in motels, blocks of units, or houses in the hope of observing a woman undressing. To do so commonly involves them entering private property, thus putting them at risk of arrest. They may return regularly to situations where they have been successful in the past, increasing their likelihood of being caught. The behavior appears to be as driven as exhibitionism, and the subjects report the same feelings of anxious excitement in relation to the act, at times associated with intense autonomic arousal (high heart rate and intense sweating).

Freund and Blanchard (1986) pointed out that not uncommonly, exhibitionists report occasional episodes of voyeurism, and three-quarters of the voyeurs they studied had also exposed. Peeping into private property and observing a vulnerable woman or valuable possessions may tempt the peeper into sexual assault or theft; Langevin and Lang (1987) reported an association between these conditions. While indulging in voyeurism, the subject frequently masturbates. Compared with peeping voyeurs, those with the rarely reported form of observing couples having intercourse in parked automobiles are much less likely to be apprehended and charged. The latter form may be at least as common. One of my patients, who sought treatment after being pursued in a car chase by an irate naked victim, informed me that he regularly attended a number of areas such as "lovers' lanes," where he was usually successful in satisfying his voyeuristic urges. He said there were always several other voyeurs in the areas.

Langevin and Lang (1987) cited Money as stating that few if any voyeurs are homosexual. Some homosexuals, however, seek treatment to cease compulsively spending considerable amounts of time in public lavatories observing others involved in homosexual activities. This would not be classified as voyeurism if it is required that those observed be nonconsenting. This requirement would also exclude troilism (the observation of consenting subjects, in some definitions a sexual partner, in heterosexual sexual activity). Coprophilia (an affinity for feces and urine) is in its most common form the observation of subjects urinating or defecating. Smith (1976), in his comprehensive review of voyeurism, considered its inclusion questionable, however, possibly because of the other forms it may take. Some subjects with coprophilia appear to frequent lavatories to hear rather than observe the excretory activities of women, and the urge of some homosexual men to be urinated upon has been referred to in recent gay literature. The latter behavior is regarded as a form of masochism in DSM-III-R.

Freund (1990) considered an auditory analogue of voyeurism to be the listening (by telephone and for a fee) to tapes of women describing their feelings during masturbation and intercourse. As some subjects continue this behavior despite complaints from their wives concerning the resulting high telephone bills, it would appear that it can become compulsive. Langevin and Lang (1987) included in their definition of voyeurism the public watching of strip shows or censored erotica. This inclusion of a common and widely socially accepted behavior perhaps has heralded the development of the nonjudgmental concept of sexual deviations. A 1974 study cited by Murrin and Laws (1990) reported that 29% of normal subjects reported a desire to own pornography, and one-half of these did. Fifty-eight percent of male and 37% of female university students reported watching or reading pornographic material in the preceding 3 months (Person, Terestman, Myers, Goldberg, & Salvadori, 1989).

Peeping appears to be exclusively carried out by men. Smith (1976) referred to a case report of a woman being an eager observer in a troilistic act. Substantially fewer voyeurs than exhibitionists come to clinical attention, perhaps in part because they are less likely to be detected. Like exhibitionists, they commonly report that they were somewhat shy and slower than peers to commence dating, and that their paraphilia usually began in adolescence, at times after their being excited in a typical situation; they may have accidentally observed a woman undressing or a couple having intercourse. By the time they present for treatment, they are usually married or in satisfactory sexual relationships. In personality they appear within the range of subjects of equivalent age and socioeconomic status.

Pedophilia

The DSM-III-R criteria for pedophilia are that over a 6-month period the person has acted upon or been markedly distressed by recurrent urges or fantasies involving sexual activity with a prepubertal child or children, and that the person is at least 16 years old and at least 5 years older than the child or children. Strangely, the homosexual attraction of adults to immediately postpubertal boys, termed *hebephilia* (Freund, Heasman, & Roper, 1982), is not included among the paraphilias in the DSM-III-R. Both attractions are commonly exclusive and resistant to treatment. To act on them is both illegal and socially condemned, so that they are major problems for their subjects and for society. Pedophilia and hebephilia are usually recognized only when the behavior comes to the attention of authorities or when it is reported retrospectively by the victims. From 10% to 50% of women and 5% to 16% of men retrospectively report having had sexual activity with an adult in their childhood (see Chapter 6); the variation in prevalence in part resulted from the way the activity was defined and the information elicited. The percentage of perpetrators who were male varied from 81% (Finkelhor, 1985) to 96% (Russell, 1983) for molestation of female children, and from 25% (Fromuth & Burkhart, 1989) to 83% (Finkelhor, 1985) for molestation of male children. As at least twice as many girls are abused as boys, it is possible, as Russell (1986) believed, that women abuse more girls than boys.

Little information is available concerning the percentage of a representative normal population who have carried out pedophilic acts. As there are on average one to two female victims of a pedophile, if it is accepted that 90% of pedophiles are male, that 30% of women are their victims, and that there are about four times as many adults as children in the population, about 5% of men and 0.5% of women would molest girls. Herman (1990) cited Finkelhor and Lewis as finding that between 4% and 17% of men in a nationwide random-sample survey acknowledged having molested a child, the sex of whom was not specified. About 15% of male and 2% of female university students in the United States and Australia reported some likelihood of having sexual activity with a prepubertal child if they could do so without risk (Malamuth, 1989b; McConaghy & Zamir, 1992b).

Female Pedophiles

As discussed in Chapter 6, the majority of men in nonclinical samples who were prepubertally molested by postpubertal women reported that the molestation did not involve the use of force, and they recalled their immediate response to the experience as positive. Evidence indicated that it was not followed by significant psychopathology in the victims' adulthood. Only in the case of girl victims have most investigators of child sexual abuse followed Russell (1986) in regarding sexual acts by older perpetrators as abusive whether or not the victims considered their reactions to be neutral or positive. These facts presumably account for the little attention given women molesters of children. Understandably, therefore, women are seldom charged with pedophilia and may not be conceptualized as pedophiles either by themselves or their victims. Wilson and Cox (1983) commented of a self-help pedophile club they investigated that though membership was theoretically open to women, hardly any had joined.

Unlike males, female pedophiles rarely present for treatment if they have not been charged with offenses. I have found that some women while being treated as inpatients reported pedophilic behaviors, usually to other staff members than their primary therapist. These women showed marked features of borderline personality disorder. The pedophilic behaviors they reported involved significant physical violence, so that it was highly likely the infant or child victims would have needed medical attention. Nevertheless, I was unable to confirm that the offenses had taken place. The patients had not been charged with the offenses, and they either reported inability to remember the details necessary or refused permission for the people to be contacted who could be expected to know of the offenses, claiming the thought of such contact was too traumatic for them to tolerate. The reports of the offenses were made in a manner suggestive of an expectation that they would horrify the staff informed and thus result in the patients receiving special attention. This was likely to occur unless appropriate management was immediately instituted to prevent splitting of the staff into those who rejected and those who sympathized with these patients. The information available concerning postpubertal women detected or convicted in relation to sexual activities with prepubertal children is discussed in relation to sex offenders.

Heterosexual and Homosexual Male Pedophiles

Homosexual male pedophiles commonly report molesting many hundreds of victims; heterosexual male pedophiles molest only a few. As about half as many men as women report childhood victimization, there must be many more male offenders of female than of male children. The two types of offenders differ markedly. Groth and Birnbaum (1978) investigated 175 men convicted of pedophilia. Most homosexual pedophiles were single and had been exclusively attracted to male children since puberty. The victims were usually strangers or casual acquaintances; their mean age was 10 years. Almost all homosexual pedophiles (and hebephiles) who consulted me gave similar histories. They commonly sought victims in pinball parlors or other situations where young people congregated. Typically they were usually of average intelligence or above, yet were totally disinterested in social as well as sexual relations with adults. Possibly to avoid detection, the offense was rarely repeated with the same victim unless they were able to form an emotional relationship with a boy, which many wished to do. Most gave a history of stable employment. Their offenses usually commenced in adolescence.

The majority of convicted heterosexual pedophiles investigated by Groth and Birnbaum (1978) were predominantly attracted to adult women and were married. They had rarely shown evidence of pedophilic interest in adolescence and may have been sexually deprived at the time of the offense. Their victims were related or well-known to them and had a mean age of 8 years. Other workers found heterosexual as compared to homosexual pedophiles to be more likely to be heavy drinkers, to be of lower socioeconomic class, to have had little schooling, to have committed other criminal offenses, and to have repeated the offense with the same child on many occasions (Lukianowicz, 1972; Swanson, 1968). The association with lower socio-economic class may not be entirely attributable to offenses in such subjects being more likely to be reported to authorities. Of the college undergraduates investigated by Finkelhor (1980), 33% of girls from lower-income families (compared to 19% of the total sample) reported childhood sexual abuse. Gordon (1989) considered that biological fathers would have greater commitment to the father role than would stepfathers, so that when biological fathers sexually abused daughters it would be in a family environment characterized by relatively high levels of personal, social, and economic stress. Using data from 17 states, drawn from the 1983 National Study on Child Neglect and Reporting, he found, consistent with his expectation, that biological fathers compared to stepfathers showed significantly higher levels of drug and/or alcohol abuse, marital problems, and insufficient income.

The marked differences between homosexual and heterosexual pedophiles are summarized in Table 8.1. They appear to be recognized by pedophiles themselves. Wilson and Cox (1983) requested members of a pedophile self-help club to complete questionnaires anonymously. Of the 75 who complied, 68 reported an exclusive homosexual and 2 an exclusive heterosexual preference. Though the authors noted the absence of women, they did not attach any significance to the fact that the club was made up almost exclusively of homosexual pedophiles. Heterosexual pedophiles are likely to have social and sexual relations with adult peers; they would have less need of a support group than homosexual pedophiles, who lack both and also have few age-appropriate interests. Homosexual pedophiles appear to be less guilty about their deviant urges and behaviors than heterosexual pedophiles. They may therefore be more willing to identify themselves by joining a club.

In my experience, heterosexual pedophiles who do not show evidence of anti-social behavior, below-average intelligence, or low moral and ethical standards commonly report total unawareness of any attraction to prepubertal girls prior to their offense. Its initial occurrence was usually impulsive, in response to an unexpected opportunity, such as a female child wrestling with them in their pool, sharing a bath,

TABLE 8.1
Comparison of Heterosexual and Homosexual Pedophiles

Heterosexual Pedophiles	Homosexual Pedophiles
Few victims	Many victims (up to hundreds)
Victims known to offender	Victims unknown to offender
Offenses repeated with same victim for months/years	Offenses usually occur only once with same victim
Mean age of victim 8 years	Mean age of victim 10 years
Offender attracted to adult women	Offender not sexually attracted to adults of either sex
Offender commonly married	Offender single
Behavior commenced in adulthood	Behavior commenced in adolescence
Often low socioec class, unemployed, alcoholic, low IQ, psychopathic	Stable/employed, average IQ but "immature", prefers company of children, not interested in friendships with adults

or cuddling with them. This usually occurred when the subjects were adult, and the majority appeared deeply guilty and did not repeat the offense; however, some continued to take advantage of further opportunities, and the behavior became compulsive.

Freund, McKnight, Langevin, and Cibiri (1972) investigated the penile volume responses of 40 young adult men to still and moving full-figure pictures of nude males and females aged approximately 5 to 8, 9 to 11, 12 to 14, and 19 to 26 years, and to slides of the face, the chest, the pubic region, the legs, and the buttocks of the same subjects, except that the youngest age group was excluded. The subjects' mean penile reactions to females of all age groups were significantly greater than to males of any age groups. There was a relatively high reaction to the buttocks of the prepubescent boy and the pubic region of the female child, though these were significantly less than the reaction to the pubic region of the pubescent girl and to the pubic and chest regions of the adult woman. The results suggested to Freund and his colleagues that for the nondeviant adult male, the female child—at least from her sixth year—is biologically a more appropriate surrogate sexual object than a male person, and that many heterosexual pedophilic offenses may be carried out by men who are not truly pedophilic in their sexual preferences. If men can be encouraged to accept rather than repress awareness of their potential for sexual arousal to female children, it is likely that most could control it without excessive fear and guilt when they found themselves in situations which elicited such arousal. Fear and guilt, in my experience, lead to poorer rather than better control.

Fixated and Regressed Pedophiles

Groth and Birnbaum (1978) did not classify pedophiles as homosexual and heterosexual, but as fixated or regressed. Fixated pedophiles were sexually attracted primarily or exclusively to significantly younger persons from adolescence. Regressed offenders did not show evidence of sexual attraction to significantly younger persons until adulthood. In my experience, some men who offend against both boys and girls could be described as fixated in the sense employed by Groth and Birnbaum, usually because they were intellectually dull and unable to establish relationships with peers. Apart from these subjects, men who gave a history of offending against girl children could all be considered as regressed, and homosexual pedophiles and hebephiles as fixated.

Classification of pedophiles as heterosexual or homosexual, rather than regressed or fixated, is descriptive and has no etiological significance; to use Pavlov's phrase, it does not imply an hypothesis. Also, it encourages awareness in investigations of the need to examine heterosexual and homosexual pedophiles separately; studies that fail to distinguish the two groups can ignore meaningful associations in the data. Segal and Marshall (1985) investigating child molesters as a group, concluded they showed greater heterosexual inadequacy than did rapists. This would be expected, as most homosexual pedophiles show no interest in heterosexual interactions. The study did not investigate the possibility that it was only the homosexual and not the heterosexual pedophiles who showed greater heterosexual inadequacy than rapists, leaving the significance of the finding unclear. In treatment outcome studies it would also seem necessary to distinguish the two groups: Consistent with my experience, it appears generally accepted that homosexual as compared to heterosexual pedophiles are more likely to reoffend (Freund, Heasman, & Roper, 1982; Marshall & Barbaree, 1990b; Quinsey, 1986).

Sexual Sadism and Masochism and the Sexually Assaultive

The criterion for sadism and masochism, as they are defined separately in DSM-III-R, is acting on or being distressed by recurrent intense sexual urges and sexually arousing fantasies, of at least 6 months' duration, involving real acts in which psychological or physical suffering is sexually exciting. The excitement is felt by the person experiencing the suffering in masochism, and by the person inflicting the suffering in sadism. Masochists may inflict suffering upon themselves, in which case perhaps they should be referred to as sadomasochists. The acts listed in DSM-III-R include dominance such that the victim is forced to crawl, kept in a cage, physically restrained, blindfolded, paddled, spanked, whipped, pinched, beaten, burnt, administered electric shocks, raped, cut, stabbed, strangled, tortured, mutilated, or killed.

Sadistic and Nonsadistic Rape

Rape or other sexual assaults, when the suffering inflicted on the victim is far in excess of that necessary for compliance and the visible pain of the victim is sexually arousing, are considered in DSM-III-R to be an expression of sexual sadism, but to be carried out by less than 10% of rapists. The statement was added that some rapists were apparently aroused sexually by forcing a person to engage in intercourse but not by the victim's suffering, which nonetheless did not impair their arousal. This was not regarded as an expression of sadism. The existence of such rapists was not supported by empirical data and may have been postulated to accommodate the inhibition theory of rape motivation (discussed subsequently).

A significant percentage of normal men appear to find a sexually coerced woman's suffering arousing. Malamuth (1989b) administered questionnaires to male college students in which they reported the likelihood of their committing various sexual acts if they could be assured that no one would know and that they could in no way be punished for engaging in them. In three studies, 36% to 44% reported some likelihood that they would force a woman to do something sexual she did not want to do, and 16% to 20% reported some likelihood of raping a woman. Those who reported some likelihood of raping a woman experienced greater mean sexual arousal (50% of maximum arousal) to stories describing the rape of a woman during which she became sexually aroused than that (38% of maximum arousal) experienced by students who reported no likelihood of rape. The students who reported no likelihood of rape, however, were equally aroused by these stories as by stories describing consenting intercourse. Both groups experienced some arousal (33%) to descriptions of the rape of a woman in which she was disgusted. When the experimenter was male, the 16 to 20% of men who reported some likelihood of raping reported greater arousal to descriptions in which the woman experienced pain compared to those in which she did not (Malamuth & Check, 1983). These subjects also showed greater aggression against women in a laboratory setting (Malamuth, 1981) and reported greater sexual arousal to stories with a sadomasochistic theme (Malamuth, Haber, & Feshbach, 1980).

Thirty-six male undergraduates who volunteered for a study of responsiveness to sexually explicit videos reported moderate levels of sexual arousal and general enjoyment to a video depicting several members of a motorcycle gang chasing, catching, and raping a young woman (Pfaus, Myronuk, & Jacobs, 1986). Nineteen of 50 single undergraduate men reported more than one episode where their dating partners had expressed dissatisfaction because the men had exceeded the sexual limits the partner preferred. Compared to the remaining students, these 19 men found women who displayed fear, anger, disgust, and sadness more sexually attractive (Heilbrun & Loftus, 1986). Most of 54 male undergraduates reported pictures of distressed women in bondage to be more sexually stimulating than those of similar women displaying positive affect (Heilbrun & Leif, 1988). The authors concluded there was a sadistic component to normal male sexuality. In Malamuth's studies (1989b) of male students, 44% to 50% reported some likelihood they would engage in bondage, and 33% to 35% some likelihood they would engage in whipping and spanking a woman. More than 30% of men reported sexual fantasies of tying up and of raping a woman, and 10% to 20% of torturing or beating up a woman (Crepault & Couture, 1980; Person et al., 1989). Bondage and domination was the commonest nonnormative imagery on the covers of heterosexual pornographic magazines, being present on 17%. Normal heterosexual activities were found on 37% of the covers (Dietz & Evans, 1982).

The fact that many men find the thought of forcing a woman to have sex and inflicting pain on her sexually arousing, even if she is not depicted as enjoying the experience, appears incompatible with a superficial reading of the DSM-III-R statement that 90% of rapists are not sexually aroused by their victims' suffering. Actually, the statement leaves open the issue of what percentage of rapists are so aroused. All nonsadistic rapists could be, given that it requires that sadistic rapists use excessive force in addition to being aroused by the victim's pain. The statement is in fact a clever compromise that largely meets the feminist view that rape is not sexually motivated and is not a disorder but normal male behavior, and the view of the biologically oriented that many rapists are sexually aroused by the use of coercion. There appears to be no empirical evidence to support the distinction between sadistic and nonsadistic rapists in relation to the use of excessive force. Knight and Prentky (1990) were unable to substantiate it, and it would seem probable that the degree of force employed varies dimensionally rather than categorically. The distinction made in the DSM-III-R between sexually coercive behavior and sadomasochism, however, would seem valid. There is no evidence from studies of self-identified sadomasochists that they show any increased likelihood of raping nonconsenting subjects.

Sadomasochism

Sadomasochistic literature and research studies indicate that typical sadistic behavior requires that it be received masochistically, that is, that the victim is cooperative and enjoys the behavior. The same person may be sadistic on one occasion and masochistic on another. Elaborate verbalized fantasies and role playing of master-slave, humiliator-humiliated, and torturer-victim relationships are commonly involved in sadomasochistic behavior, to judge from advertisements of subjects seeking partners, though this aspect does not appear to have received much attention in the research literature. Self-identified sadists and masochists are rarely sufficiently troubled by their impulses and behaviors to seek treatment.

A number of studies have investigated by questionnaire those who joined clubs for sadomasochists or who advertised for partners in magazines. In an early German study, most of these subjects were found to be male and either bisexual or homosexual; the few female subjects were paid for their services (Spengler, 1977). In recent U.S. studies (Breslow, Evans, & Langley, 1985; Moser & Levitt, 1987) 20% to 30% of the subjects were found to be female, few of whom were prostitutes. More of the women tended to be bisexual than the men, most of whom were predominantly heterosexual. The women were more likely to adopt submissive roles but were less likely to need sadomasochistic activity to have a satisfactory sexual response. Most subjects were both sadistic and masochistic. More than 50% of men and 21% of women were aware of sadomasochistic interest by age 14. Most of the men considered it natural from childhood; most of the women were introduced to it. Beating, bondage, and fetishistic practices were common, and more extreme or dangerous practices were rare. A significant minority reported self-bondage and pain infliction during masturbation. Subjects were above average in intelligence and social status, and most wished to continue sadomasochistic activities.

Gosselin and Wilson (1980) interviewed sadomasochism club members and concluded that most sadists had no wish to hurt their partners in "sex games" more than was enjoyed or at least accepted by the partners. It may be that the sexual excitement of the majority of sadists is stimulated by the victim's pleasure or arousal rather than suffering at the infliction of pain, humiliation, or states of helplessness. If so, this would explain their need for a willing partner, and why there is no evidence they are more likely to carry out sexual assaults. In view of the rarity with which practicing sadomasochists seek medical treatment, few must suffer significant physical damage, and the statement in the DSM-III-R that the severity of the sadistic acts usually increases over time requires either support or withdrawal. Sadomasochists may act out urges that are little different from those experienced in fantasy by a significant percentage of the normal population. In some classifications bondage is reported as a separate paraphilia, and certainly one sees subjects who wish to tie up their sexual partners without carrying out other sadistic activities. They at times seek treatment at the behest of their partners, whose pleasure in the activity does not seem necessary for bondage practitioners to wish to continue it.

Little information is available concerning the prevalence of typical sadomasochistic behaviors in community samples. Of 2,000 subjects who reported their sexual behavior in a U.S. national survey (M. Hunt, 1974), sexual pleasure had been obtained by 4.8% of men and 2.1% of women by inflicting pain and by 2.5% of men and 4.6% of women by receiving pain. The majority reporting these behaviors had carried them out in the past year. Person et al. (1989), in a study of university students' sexual experiences in the preceding 3 months, found those of women included being forced to submit to sexual acts in 6%; being tied/bound during sex activities or being sexually degraded in 4%; and being tortured by a partner, being whipped/beaten by a partner, or torturing a sexual partner in 1%. Equivalent figures for men were 1% forced to submit, 3% being tied/bound, 1% degraded, 0% tortured, 1% whipped/beaten, and 1% torturing. Two percent of men also reported whipping or beating a partner. The activities were described as sadomasochistic, implying that the subjects being hurt or humiliated consented to them. This was consistent with the students' reported fantasies.

Sadomasochistic Fantasies. Recent sexual fantasies reported by the women in the study by Person et al. included being forced to submit and being tied/bound during sex activity in 20%, being sexually degraded in 12%, being a prostitute in 10%, being tortured by a sex partner in 9%, being whipped/beaten by a partner in 8%, forcing a partner to submit in 5%, whipping/beating a partner in 1%, and degrading a sex partner in 1%. Comparable percentages for men were 15% forced to submit, 15% tied/bound, 5% degraded, 5% prostitute, 5% tortured, 5% whipped/beaten, 31% forcing, 7% whipping/beating, and 7% degrading. Six percent of men also reported fantasies of torturing a sex partner. Person et al. concluded that most men and women in their population did not have fantasies that supported the stereotype that male sexuality is aggressive and sadistic, and female sexuality passive and masochistic. Their data made clear that in the significant minority of subjects with sadomasochistic fantasies, however, more males reported sadistic and more females masochistic content.

In an earlier study of 141 married upper-class New York women whose median age was 32 years (Hariton & Singer, 1974), half the women reported the coital fantasy of being overpowered or forced to surrender, 14% employing it on almost every occasion of intercourse. It was the second most popular fantasy. The much higher prevalence of this fantasy in these older married women raises the possibility that the use of sexual fantasy increases with age. Price and Miller (1984) found that the same fantasy of being overpowered or forced to surrender sexually was reported significantly more commonly during masturbation and/or intercourse by black as compared to white female college students.

Sadistic Murder

The activities listed in DSM-III-R as characterizing sadomasochism may need qualification. Acts of dominance and submission by forcing the victim to crawl, be physically restrained, blindfolded, and hurt appear typical. The inclusion of acts that appear to be rarely performed by self-identified sadomasochists (e.g., rape, mutilation, and murder) encourages acceptance of what appears to be a sexual myth that there is a strong association between sadomasochism and crimes of violence. It is inconsistent with the fact that self-identified sadists and masochists wish to continue their activities, which do not seem to result in any need for medical help. The rarity of sadistic murders is masked by the widespread media attention, both national and international, that they receive (Revitch, 1980). Quinsey (1986) cited a survey of child murders which found that only 3 of the 83 victims had been killed in a sexual assault. Bourget and Bradford (1990) concluded from a review of the literature that child murder was infrequent and committed in most instances by parents.

Swigert, Farrell, and Yoels (1976) examined all cases of homicide in a jurisdiction in the northeastern United States from 1955 through 1973. Of 444 cases, 5 qualified as sexual homicides, and only 2 of these were considered cases of sexual sadism (1 heterosexual and 1 homosexual). Two occurred in consensual sex relationships (1 heterosexual and 1 homosexual), and the fifth from fear the victim of homosexual pedophilia would reveal the offense. All the murderers were from lower social classes; most had less than a high school education and worked in unskilled occupations. Swigert et al. commented that all 5 cases received front-page newspaper coverage and weeks of follow-up reporting on their legal progress. The 350 cases of homicides that occurred over the same period and resulted from altercations among friends, relatives, and acquaintances received minimal newspaper attention. The interest and horror evoked by sexual as opposed to nonsexual violence requires explanation. It is possibly related to the ability of many people, developed in their sexual fantasies, to empathize with both the aggressor and the victim.

On the basis of 20 years of experience in forensic psychiatry, Brittain (1970) described the typical sadistic murder as carefully planned and the method of killing as usually asphyxial, and more rarely by mutilating violence or multiple stabbing. Injuries were most commonly of the victim's breasts, genitalia, or rectum. Often there appeared a deliberate attempt to offend modesty by the way the victim's body was arranged. Brittain described the typical sadistic murderer as socially isolated, emotionally flattened, and "weird" in personality or at times psychotic. He might have a record of other paraphilias such as cross-dressing, peeping, and obscene telephone calls, or a history of extreme cruelty to animals or of setting fires. A surprising number worked as butchers, and not infrequently, they had an inordinate interest in weapons, guns, or knives, in Nazism, or in black magic. Brittain found that they experienced great excitement during the act of killing, and great relief of tension following its completion. In prison they were often model prisoners, a fact that he considered could mislead the unwary to believe they had fundamentally changed.

Revitch (1980) also reported a number of these features in male sadistic murderers, as well as a background of maternal overprotection, infantilization and seduction, or rejection. He commented that maternal sexual indiscretions real or fancied were common. He had earlier reviewed accounts of 9 murders and 34 violent unprovoked assaults on women (Revitch, 1965). They involved choking, inflicting multiple knife wounds or battering with a heavy object. Erection and ejaculation may or may not have accompanied the aggressive acts. Rape and attempted rape were infrequent. Revitch commented that violence served as a substitute for it and could lead to the underlying sexual dynamics being disregarded. Thirty of the perpetrators had committed previous offenses, but only 3 were sex offenses; 12 were breaking and entering, and fetishism of female underwear was elicited in 9 cases. Revitch reported the impression that the great majority of the perpetrators were overt or latent psychotics, and emphasized their common expression of hatred, contempt, or fear of women.

Findings on case files of 30 subjects selected from those identified to the National Center for the Analysis of Violent Crime (NCAVC) over 5 years as possibly sexually sadistic criminals conflicted in a few important respects with these earlier studies (Dietz, Hazelwood, & Warren, 1990). The subjects were those the three authors agreed had been sexually aroused in response to images of suffering and humiliation on two or more occasions over at least 6 months. All were male. Seventy-three percent had murdered their victim, and 56% had murdered at least three, most often by strangulation and next most often by shooting. Their crimes often involved careful planning, the selecting of strangers as victims, approaching the victim under a pretext, participation of a partner, restraining and beating victims, holding them captive, anal rape, forced fellation, vaginal rape, foreign object penetration, and keeping records of offenses and personal items of victims. Seventy-three percent victimized only females, 17% only males, and 10% members of both sexes. Fifty-three percent victimized only adults, and 17% only children.

Thirty seven percent of the subjects collected guns; 33% had military experience, and 30% were police buffs. Thirty percent had an incestuous involvement with their child, and 43% homosexual, 20% cross-dressing, and 20% exposure, peeping, or obscene telephone-calling experiences. Forty-three percent had prior arrests for nonsexual or nonsadistic sexual offenses, 50% abused drugs other than alcohol, and the authors stated that all 30 had engaged in an extensive pattern of antisocial behavior in adulthood. Nevertheless, 30% had an established reputation as solid citizens, and none were perceived as particularly odd by those who knew them well before their offenses. None were psychotic at the time of onset of the pattern of sexually sadistic behavior; one became psychotic later in life. The authors did not report how many cases were referred to NCAVC and whether (and, if so, how) they differed from the 30 selected. It is therefore not possible to determine the appropriateness of the authors' restriction of the diagnosis of sexually sadistic criminals to those selected.

Murders of homosexuals in "gay bashings" do not appear to be considered sex murders, and there appears to be little information concerning the perpetrators. From media accounts, they would seem to be mainly groups of adolescent or young adult males.

Sexual Asphyxia

Hypoxphilia, stimulation of sexual arousal by oxygen deprivation produced by a noose, ligature, plastic bag, mask, or chemical (often a volatile nitrite) or by chest compression, is included under masochism in DSM-III-R. It makes the statement, unsupported by data, that subjects report the activity to be accompanied by sexual fantasies in which they asphyxiate or harm others, others asphyxiate or harm them, or they escape near brushes with death. Presumably these fantasies were the basis for classification of the condition under masochism. Knowledge concerning sexual asphyxia has mainly been obtained from the study of resultant accidental fatalities. Hazelwood, Dietz, and Burgess (1983) reported 132 such fatalities; 37 of the victims were teenagers, and 5 were female. The authors speculated that sexual asphyxia resulted in 500 to 1,000 deaths yearly in the United States and Canada. It is distinguished from suicide by characteristics of the mode of death. The apparatus used to induce oxygen deprivation usually shows signs of regular use and of a fail-safe procedure that proved ineffective. Evidence is present of autoerotic activity, such as erotic literature, exposure of the genitals, seminal ejaculate, pain-producing devices such as nipple clamps, and at times of cross-dressing, fetishism, and bondage. Byard, Hucker, and Hazelwood (1990) in their review of the literature found this evidence more characteristic of male victims, and that female victims did not usually employ pornographic pictures and literature or unusually complex bindings and accessory props. To induce hypoxia they usually relied on a simple neck ligature tightened by lowering the body, or by pulling on an attached cord tied to the hands or legs, so that the cause of death could be difficult to distinguish from homicide or suicide.

In the case of the 132 cases discussed above, Burgess and Hazelwood (1983) found that their family and friends usually described them as in good spirits and physical health, as active, and as having a future orientation, which should lead the investigator to question suicide as a cause. Fatalities from sexual asphyxia may at times have been prevented. The subjects' contacts not infrequently had noted evidence of the behavior, such as a preoccupation with tying knots, or the presence of red marks on their necks, bloodshot eyes, or confused behavior for short periods. Usually the contacts were not aware of its significance and did not confront the subjects concerning the potential danger and need for treatment. Though at least in male practitioners an element of masochism is common, the need for partial asphyxiation, the lack of need for a partner, and the absence of the role-playing aspects of sadomasochism suggests sexual asphyxia should be classified independently, as are other deviant practices (e.g., fetishism) that are not uncommonly associated with some sadomasochistic behaviors.

Subjects who use nitrites in sexual activities usually report they do so to produce behavioral disinhibition and to enhance excitement and orgasm. They do not appear to consider that they are producing a degree of asphyxia. Those known to the author have been surprised to learn of the fantasies of asphyxiating, or of harming themselves or others, that DSM-III-R believes to accompany the use of nitrites. Classification of their use as masochistic would also seem questionable.

Fetishism

DSM-III-R restricts fetishism to a 6-month period of recurrent, intense sexual urges and fantasies involving the use of nonliving objects, usually bras, women's underpants, stockings, shoes, boots, or other wearing apparel. When the fetishes are limited to articles of female clothing with which the subject cross-dresses, the condition is termed *transvestic fetishism*. Fetishistic use of female clothes most commonly comes to attention in adolescent males caught stealing them from clotheslines or found to be using those belonging to their mother or sisters. Adolescents typically tend to deny any sexually deviant behaviors, even to themselves, and initially it can appear that these subjects only hold the clothing against their genitals as fetishes during masturbation. After sympathetic questioning, however, some admit to wearing the clothes at the time. Others deny wearing the clothes, but admit to a masturbatory fantasy of doing so. A number of both groups also admit to a tendency to think of themselves as girls during the activity. Their behavior thus appears on a continuum with the adolescent stage of transvestism.

Earlier classifications diagnosed fetishism, transvestism, and transsexualism as three separate conditions but with intermediate states, as discussed in Chapter 4. This diagnostic system matched the clinical descriptions of the conditions more appropriately than does the separation of transvestic fetishism from fetishism and the introduction in DSM-III-R of the new and cumbersome term *gender identity disorder of adolescence or adulthood, nontranssexual type*, for transvestism. Transvestic fetishism is discussed further in relation to transvestism in Chapter 4. Sexual arousal by some body part (usually the hair, feet, or hands, or a deformity or mutilation of the human body of the preferred sex) disproportionate to the arousal to secondary sexual characteristics is classified separately in DSM-III-R under "paraphilias not otherwise specified" as partialism.

Chalkley and Powell (1983) reported that 48 subjects diagnosed as suffering from fetishism presented for treatment at a psychiatric hospital over 20 years. They made up 0.8% of all adult psychiatric patients treated over this time. Ten were predominantly homosexual and only 1 was a woman, a lesbian who reported a fetish for breasts. As breasts are secondary sexual characteristics they would not usually be classified as a fetish; if they were, the sexual arousal in response to breast and penis size reported by a number of heterosexual and homosexual men could be regarded as fetishistic. Seventeen of Chalkley and Powell's subjects had only one fetish, and 22 had three or more. The most common was clothing, reported by 28, including 10 whose object was men's pants. Seven had fetishes for parts of the body, 7 for footwear, and 7 for rubber, including tubes and enemas. Some subjects report fetishes of baby items, diapers, nursery bottles and nipples. The DSM-III-R classification related the behavior of such subjects to a desire to be treated as helpless infants, and included it under masochism with the comment that it is at times termed *infantilism*.

As the DSM-III-R description pointed out, fetishists frequently masturbate while holding, rubbing, or smelling the fetish, or they may ask their sexual partners to wear it during sexual activity. The fetish-related behaviors reported by Chalkley and Powell's subjects were as follows: wearing clothes or footwear (21 subjects); stealing, mainly clothes (18); observing someone dressed in clothes or rubber items (11); gazing at the fetish (6); inserting it up the rectum (6); hoarding it (6); and more rarely, fondling, sucking, following, rolling in, burning, and cutting or snipping the fetish. I have also noted burying and digging up of clothes; rescuing, cleaning, and preserving in plastic bags of discarded gloves; and urinating and defecating into diapers or onto valued objects, such as toy trains. Chalkley and Powell stated that few of their subjects reported that they were markedly dependent on the fetish for sexual arousal. Their information was from case notes, and many of the 48 may not have been questioned concerning this. It seemed inconsistent with the fact that 38 presented for treatment for fetishism, and is contrary to the DSM-III-R description and my experience with fetishists.

Most fetishists report a strong pleasurable interest in the fetish in their childhood, the interest becoming sexually arousing at puberty. The caring and protective—or destructive—behaviors shown by some subjects in regard to the fetish suggest they feel toward it as if it were a living object. Their emotional response is reminiscent of that of children toward a special blanket or other transitional objects. In discussing similarities and differences of fetishes and transitional objects, Greenacre (1969) appeared unaware of the interest fetishists commonly show in the fetish prior to puberty. Gosselin and Wilson (1980) found that fetishistic fantasies were common in sadomasochists and vice versa, and therefore concluded that fetishists and sadomasochists were similar. This conclusion is consistent with the behavior of fetishists who request partners to stand on them in shoes, or who use rubber clothes or corsets to produce bodily constriction. Use of Nazi or of stereotyped versions of torturers' clothing and equipment is often included in depictions of sadomasochistic activities.

In Person et al.'s study (1989) of university students, 1% of men and 4% of women reported the sexual experience of dressing in the clothes of the opposite sex in the preceding 3 months; however, 14% of the men (but only 2% of the women) reported ever having sexual fantasies of cross-dressing. Sixteen percent of female students reported recent dressing in erotic garments, compared with 7% of male students. Twenty percent of the women reported recent sexual fantasies of being dressed in special costumes, compared with 4% of the men. Women's tendency to use romantic imagery and men's to use specifically sexual imagery was discussed in relation to the possible correspondence between "Mills and Boon" fiction produced for women and the pornography produced for men (see Chapter 7). In view of the rarity of fetishism and transvestism in women compared to men (Chapter 4), and the much lower percentage of female compared to male students who reported sexual fantasies of cross-dressing in the study of Person et al., it would seem possible that the 4% of women students who reported recent cross-dressing in the study experienced romantic feelings rather than the genital arousal cross-dressing produces in men. Dressing in special costumes has been noted in homosexual men, who wear cowboy clothes or uniforms to gay bars or discos.

Frotteurism

Some workers (Freund, 1990) limit the term *frotteurism* to the pressing of the subject's penis against the body of an unknown woman and use the term *toucherism* for a man's intimate touching of an unknown woman as for example touching her on the buttocks or breast. Freund stated no female counterparts of these behaviors have been described. With toucherism, the behavior can usually be clearly identified as sexual assault and the offender charged. Frotteurism is usually carried out on crowded public transport where its deliberate nature can be less clearly established and rarely results in charges of sexual assault. For this reason and because subjects with the condition do not appear to seek treatment, there is little literature concerning it. The DSM-III-R description claimed that frotteurs usually fantasize an exclusive caring relationship with the victim while engaged in the activity. No evidence was provided for this rather charming belief. Twenty-two of 139 sexually deviant males investigated by Freund, Scher, and Hucker (1983) were referred for toucherism; a further 26 who had been referred for other paraphilias, mainly exhibitionism and voyeurism, also had carried it out. Their fantasies were not reported.

Paraphilias Not Otherwise Specified

Telephone scatologia (lewdness), necrophilia (corpses), partialism (exclusive focus on a part of the body), zoophilia (animals), coprophilia (feces), klismaphilia (enemas), and urophilia (urine) are classified in DSM-III-R as paraphilias not otherwise specified. Few individuals with these conditions seek treatment, and their prevalence is not established. Eight percent of 500 women in Albuquerque reported being victims of obscene phone calls, compared with 4% who reported being victims of voyeurs, and 30% victims of exhibitionists (DiVasto et al., 1984).

MULTIPLE DIAGNOSES OF SEX OFFENDERS AND DEVIANTS

Freund and Blanchard (1986) pointed out that a number of studies found that sex offenders had committed more than one type of sex offense or deviation belonging to the group Freund termed "courtship disorders": exhibitionism, voyeurism, obscene calls, toucherism, and sadistic rape. Freund et al. (1983) investigated 139 nonpedophile heterosexual offenders to test their prediction that there would be co-occurrence of these deviations. Only 4 of the 23 rapists reported any of the other deviations, compared with 45 of the 86 exhibitionists, 11 of the 22 touchers, and 2 of the 7 voyeurs. The authors did not investigate the presence of fetishism or transvestism in their subjects; subjects reporting heterosexual pedophilia were excluded. Heterosexual pedophilia was the most common offense reported by exhibitionists in a study by Abel, Becker, Cunningham-Rathner, Mittelman, and Rouleau (1988). Abel et al. investigated 561 male sex offenders, one-third referred by mental health routes, one-third referred from forensic sources, and one-third self-referred or from other sources. They attempted to ensure that the subjects reported honestly by obtaining for them certificates of confidentiality from the federal government; these certificates protect the identity and confidentiality of research subjects to reassure the offenders that the usual requirement of mandatory reporting to authorities will not occur. At least 72% of the sex offenders and deviants other than transsexuals reported additional deviations.

It is difficult to know what significance to attach to these findings of a high degree of co-occurrence of different sex offenses and deviations. The studies did not report the frequencies with which the additional deviations were performed, so that in many subjects they may have been isolated acts. Few studies have investigated the number and variety of sexually deviant acts performed by community samples of men. When male university students completed an inventory of sexual activities performed in the last 3 months (Person et al., 1989), 4% reported exhibiting in public, 4% watching others make love, 3% being tied and bound during sexual activities, 1% dressing in clothes of the opposite sex, 1% degrading a sexual partner, and 1% being whipped or beaten by a partner. Twenty-one percent reported a lifetime prevalence of having exhibited in public. The percentage reporting lifetime prevalences for the other sexual practices were not given. If, as seems likely, they also had been carried out occasionally by a higher percentage of the subjects than those who reported performing them in the last 3 months, these findings would suggest that as many as half the male population have carried out occasional practices of this sort.

This was also suggested by a study of Templeman and Stinnett (1991). They obtained sexual histories from 60 undergraduate men aged 18 to 50, using the Clarke Sexual History Questionnaire (SHQ), a self-report instrument developed to identify sexual anomalies in sex offenders. Three of the 60, who reported homosexual contacts, were excluded. Fifty-three percent of the remaining 57 had engaged in some arrestable sexual offense (excluding frottage), and 65% in some form of sexual misconduct (including frottage). Voyeurism was the most common offense, reported by 42%; it was defined in the SHQ as secretly trying to see a man or women having sexual relations or women undressing by looking in windows or by other means. Templeman and Stinnett rejected the possibility that their subjects were reporting only acts of sexual curiosity in early adolescence, as the item was worded to exclude activities occurring before the age of 16. The methodology for collecting the information would seem comparable with that used in the studies that reported a high level of co-occurrence of sex offenses in convicted subjects.

Thirty-five percent of the undergraduates reported having committed frottage, the next most common offensive behavior reported. Eight percent had made obscene phone calls. Only 1 subject reported exhibitionism, an anomalous finding in view of its being the most common deviation in convicted sex offenders. The authors pointed out that the students investigated were raised and educated in primarily rural environments, so that the results should not be extrapolated too freely. It may be that exhibitionism is less frequently carried out in rural environments, where the possibility of being recognized would presumably be much higher than in cities. Fifty-four percent of the subjects expressed voyeuristic and 7% exhibitionistic desires; 5% desired sex with girls under 12. Two reported they had been arrested for sexual offenses, and 3 had been in trouble with authorities for sexual behaviors.

Rape was included as a co-occurring sexual deviation in the study by Abel et al.

(1988). As discussed in Chapter 7, depending on the definition used, up to 30% of the male population could be considered rapists. Only 5% of subjects investigated by Templeman and Stinnett (1991) believed that they had carried out coercive sexual acts. Two groups of subjects were investigated in the study by Abel et al. (1988) who were not classified as paraphiliacs in the DSM-III-R. Transsexuals, classified in the DSM-III-R as suffering gender identity disorder, showed the fewest DSM-III-R paraphilias, with 52% reporting none; it was not reported how many regularly took female sex hormones, which would reduce the likelihood of their carrying out sexually deviant behaviors. Seventy-five percent of ego-dystonic homosexuals reported paraphilias. This high figure, in subjects with a condition no longer recognized in the DSM-III-R classification of sexual disorders, further indicates the need for studies to establish the prevalence of sexual deviations in representative community samples of men. If it is found that, compared to the men in such samples, sex offenders and deviants carry out more deviations additional to their identified one, this may result not from their having a higher incidence of urges to carry out such acts but from a greater readiness to perform them. Having rejected social or legal proscriptions concerning their major deviation, they may be less reluctant to do so in relation to other deviant urges they experience. My clinical experience with offenders seeking treatment is that they report having carried out mainly the same deviant behavior, although a number have occasionally carried out additional ones (McConaghy, Blaszczynski, Armstrong, & Kidson, 1989). If they have been charged repeatedly, it was usually for the same form of deviation.

SEX OFFENSES

In addition to classifications of paraphilias such as that of DSM-III-R, based largely on clinical studies, classifications have been developed in a separate literature based on investigations of incarcerated sex offenders. Most of these offenders were rapists and child molesters. Henn, Herjanic, and Vanderpearl (1976) reviewed records of all subjects referred for evaluation to a mental health forensic service in St. Louis. Of 1,195 subjects, 239 were charged with sexual crimes. In 69 the charges were rape or attempted rape; in 116, child molestation; and in 43, sodomy. Few were charged with exhibitionism. This means that many incarcerated sex offenders would not be classified as paraphiliacs, as hebephiles and most rapists are not classified as such in the DSM-III-R. Rapists and child molesters who are incarcerated are unlikely to be representative of those in the total population. As discussed in Chapters 6 and 7, the majority of rapists and child molesters are not reported to authorities; those who are are frequently not incarcerated.

Beck, Borenstein, and Dreyfus (1986) investigated 924 defendants appearing consecutively before the Cambridge District Court in the summer of 1980. Twenty-nine were charged with sex-related crimes; all were male. Of the 9 charged with serious offenses—namely, alleged rape—only 1 came to trial. He was convicted. Of the 20 charged with minor crimes, mainly open and gross lewdness (i.e., exhibitionism), 19 were tried but only 5 found guilty. All 5 had prior criminal records, the nature of which were not stated. Beck et al. concluded that when rapists are charged, few are convicted, as they often are not prosecuted. Herman (1990) hypothesized that convicted sex offenders compose less than 10% of all offenders, and so must be considered a highly skewed population in which those who attack strangers, use extreme force, and lack the social skills to avoid detection are overrepresented. They are far more likely to look abnormal than undetected offenders in the normal population.

In view of the probability that incarcerated offenders are not representative of the offenders in the population, the value of classifications based on their study is uncertain. In reviewing this literature, Knight, Rosenberg, and Schneider (1985) and Bard et al. (1987) pointed out the possible bias inherent in investigating incarcerated offenders, but did not appear to attach sufficient importance to this. It should have been considered a possible reason for the findings Knight et al. (1985) believed to be most surprising: that marked similarities were present between convicted rapists and child molesters, and that the two groups were similar to the general prison population. Several studies had described both groups as deficient in social skills and accomplishments. These findings were not replicated when the offenders were compared with socioeconomically matched community controls (Stermac, Segal, & Gillis, 1990).

Other similarities found by Knight et al. (1985) included low socioeconomic status, high rate of school failure or dropout, subsequent unstable employment record of an unskilled nature, previous convictions for nonsexual offenses, and poor and alcoholic family of origin. It would seem likely that these features contributed to the detection and conviction both of incarcerated sex offenders and the rest of the prison population. Such features are less likely to characterize the majority of perpetrators whose offenses are not reported or who are charged but not convicted. This is consistent with the finding of Knight et al. that defendants referred for evaluation as possible child molesters had less extensive criminal histories than the convicted group.

Bard et al. (1987) commented concerning investigations of incarcerated offenders that the only distinction that received consistent empirical scrutiny was that between rapists and child molesters. In addition to the many features they shared, some differences were found between the two groups in the studies reviewed by Knight et al. and Bard et al. Rapists were younger than child molesters; the latter were more evenly distributed throughout the age span. U.S. Department of Justice studies were cited by Herman (1990) as consistently finding that about 25% of rapists were under 18 years of age. Knight et al. (1985) found that a number of studies reported a higher incidence of mental retardation and organic brain syndrome in child molesters. Not unexpectedly, rapists were more likely to show behavioral excesses, to err by being overassertive or explosive, and to have greater heterosexual experience. Knight et al. (1985) commented concerning the failure of MMPI studies to reveal consistent meaningful personality disturbance in incarcerated sex offenders that because it was shown that psychopaths and criminals can "fake good," it was possible that different response sets associated with different legal statuses (self-referred outpatient, defendant awaiting trial, sentenced criminal, or committed prisoner at various stages of adjustment) could have biased the results. Kalichman

(1990) criticized the studies investigating sex offenders as being primarily univariate in method. Using a multivariate approach, he reported support for Groth's classification of incarcerated rapists (discussed subsequently).

Knight et al. (1985) and Bard et al. (1987) paid no attention to the failure of the studies they reviewed to investigate the distinction between homosexual and heterosexual child molesters. This failure would not seem to be politically based on reluctance to categorize subjects by their sexual preference following the 1980s decision to exclude homosexuality from the category of sex disorders in the DSM III-R. Of eight studies of pedophiles reviewed by Araji and Finkelhor (1985), four published from 1957 to 1976 did not differentiate subjects by the sex of their victims. Bard et al. (1987) compared Massachusetts treatment center files of 107 rapists and 68 molesters of subjects under 16 years; they did not distinguish molesters whose victims were prepubertal or postpubertal, or male or female. This may have accounted for their minimal findings that there was a group of offenders for whom victim age, (i.e., above or below 16 years) was inconsequential. Clinical findings discussed earlier indicate that some homosexual child molesters prefer prepubertal victims and some prefer immediately postpubertal victims, whereas most heterosexual child molesters have little age preference. The distinction of subjects made by Bard et al. did not allow these findings to be supported or refuted.

Classifications of Incarcerated Rapists

In reviewing classifications of incarcerated rapists, Knight et al. (1985) commented that little empirical data existed concerning their reliability or validity. Gebhard et al. (1965) divided imprisoned heterosexual aggressors against adults into seven categories. "Assaultive offenders" made up about 30% of the sample; they employed violence in excess of that necessary to gratify their needs and were more likely than other offenders to have sexual dysfunctions. "Amoral delinquents," who made up about 15%, failed to heed social controls and callously disregarded the rights of others, especially women. "Double standard" rapists, who made up 10%, were less antisocial but felt that sexually lax women could justifiably be forced to have intercourse. "Explosive rapists" also made up about 10 percent. They were in other respects typically law-abiding, and offended in an unexpected departure from generally nonaggressive life-styles. The remaining groups were considered to offend secondary to drunkenness, mental deficiency, or psychosis.

A subsequent related classification also based on interviews of incarcerated rapists attracted greater attention, being compatible with the radical feminist view that rape was not primarily sexually motivated (Groth, Burgess, & Holmstrom, 1977). Groth et al. distinguished "anger" and "power" rapists. Power rapists were the more common; they did not desire to harm their victims, but to control them so that they had no say in the matter. Two subgroups of power rapists were differentiated. Power-reassurance rapists used rape to alleviate doubts about their sexual adequacy and masculinity by placing the victim in a helpless, controlled position in which she could not refuse or reject them. Power-assertive rapists' doubts were about their sense of identity and effectiveness. They used rape to display virility, mastery, and dominance. Anger rapists expressed anger, rage, contempt, and hatred for their victims by abusing them in profane language, beating them, sexually assaulting them, and forcing them to perform or submit to additional degrading acts. They used more force than was necessary simply to subdue the victim, who suffered physical violence to all parts of her body. Older or elderly women could be particular targets. Victims described a blitz style of attack or a sudden and dramatic switch in the rapist's behavior. Anger-retaliation rapists committed rape as an expression of their hostility and rage toward women. Anger-excitement rapists found pleasure, thrills, and excitation in the suffering of the victim; they were sadistic and aimed to punish, hurt, and torture the victim, so that their aggression was eroticized.

Using a multivariate approach to analyze rapists' MMPI scores, Kalichman (1990) reported support for Groth's classification, distinguishing an anger/aggressive, a power/compensatory, and a sadistic group. In addition, he found an impulsive group showing sociopathic features and difficulties with impulse control. They were more likely to commit rape during the course of another crime and were similar to general criminal offenders. Yllo and Finkelhor (1985) found Groth's distinction between power, anger, and sadism as motivations for rape helpful in classifying marital rapes. Power motivated the husbands of nonbattered wives; anger, the husbands of battered wives; and sadism, a third group who carried out obsessive rapes. The men in the last group appeared to require the use of force to become sexually aroused. The use of force in obsessive as compared to anger rape could be distinguished by the ritualistic and preoccupied way it was inflicted.

Herman (1990), in outlining her feminist perspective, was critical of psychodynamic formulations (such as those of Groth) that describe rapists as committing their crimes in efforts to combat deep-seated feelings of insecurity and vulnerability or to express wishes for virility, masculinity, and dominance. She considered such formulations resulted in the victimizer being seen as a victim, an object no longer of fear but of pity. These euphemistic reformulations of the offender's behavior detoxified rape and made it more acceptable. She felt that the would-be therapist ran the risk of credulously accepting the offender's rationalizations for his crimes, as well as supplying him with new ones.

Knight and Prentky (1990) found the distinction between nonsadistic rapists (who used no more aggression than necessary to ensure compliance) and sadistic rapists (who used excessive aggression) difficult to substantiate. Some rapists who did not inflict severe physical damage on victims nevertheless appeared motivated by sadistic or angry fantasies. Statistical analysis of the characteristics of rapists revealed four categories: opportunistic, pervasively angry, sexual, and vindictive. These were further subdivided into nine types based on differing combinations of degree of impulse control, social competence, presence of fantasies (both sexual and aggressive), feelings of sexual inadequacy, degree of planning, expression of noneroticized anger, and whether the targets were both men and women or women only. Knight and Prentky believed that their classification based on incarcerated rapists might be applicable to noninstitutionalized rapist samples. This seems unlikely in view of the differences between the two groups, incarcerated rapists being mainly blitz rapists, and the noninstitutionalized primarily confidence rapists.

Community Rapists as Delinquents

Evidence that only a fraction of rapists in the community are at risk of incarceration was provided by Ageton (1983). Ten percent of the national sample of adolescent males she interviewed over 3 years reported having forced females into sexual behavior involving contact with the sexual parts of the body. Yearly over the same 3 years, 1 adolescent male in 200 was arrested for forcible rape. Of the 10% of adolescent males who reported being sexually assaultive, one-half responded to what Ageton termed the "date rape" item that they pressured or pushed someone such as a date or friend to do more sexually than they wanted to do. A further 34% reported that they had or tried to have sexual relations with someone against their will, and 10% that they physically hurt or threatened to hurt someone to get them to have sex. Most of the assaults were typical confidence rapes described in Chapter 7. In almost all cases the victim was a girlfriend or date and the assault took place in her home, the offender's home, or an automobile. About half the offenders had been drinking or taking drugs prior to the assault. In 70% of cases, the primary pressure employed was verbal.

Ageton concluded that most of the offenders seemed to be responding to a situation that afforded an opportunity to pursue their sexual interests. Offenders viewed their own sexual excitement and the behavior and physical appearance of the victim as instrumental in causing the assault. Ageton considered their ambivalence about the experience to be indicated by the largest proportion reporting that their response included feeling satisfied, confused, guilty, and proud. About half indicated their friends knew about the assault, and that their reactions were overwhelmingly ones of approval. These reactions were predictable in the light of Ageton's further findings: Comparing the assaultive group with nonassaultive adolescents matched for age and class, she found the assaultive subjects were alienated from home and school, showed a wide variety of delinquent behaviors (including physical assaults), and had greater exposure to delinquent peers who supported delinquent and sexually aggressive behaviors. Data obtained 2 years prior to the subjects' sexually assaultive behaviors revealed that they were then more committed to a delinquent peer group than were the controls. Ageton concluded that all her results pointed to the fact that sexual assault offenders were basically delinquent youths. She suggested that research should be directed at determining differences between sexually assaultive and nonassaultive delinquents.

Adolescent Sex Offenders

As discussed earlier, apart from heterosexual pedophilia, deviant sexual behaviors are usually commenced during or, in the case of fetishism, prior to adolescence. Groth, Longo, and McFadin (1982) commented that all too frequently, sexual offenses by juveniles were dismissed as merely adolescent sexual curiosity or experimentation. On the basis of the data reported above, Ageton (1983) emphasized how rarely adolescent males are charged for the common offense of forcing adolescent girls into sexual activity. Whereas 20% to 30% of adult sex offenders seek treatment voluntarily, adolescent offenders do not (Fehrenbach, Smith, Monastersky & Deisher, 1986; McConaghy et al., 1989; Moore, Zusman, & Root, 1985).

Fehrenbach et al. (1986) reported on 305 adolescents evaluated in a juvenile sexual offender project. Eight were female, all of whom had committed indecent liberties with children 6 years old or younger. Sixty percent of the males were referred for indecent liberties, over 80% with children, half of whom they were baby-sitting. Twenty-three percent were referred for rape, mainly of children, and the rest for hands-off offenses, mainly exhibitionism. One hundred and seventy-one of the 305 adolescents had committed at least one prior sexual offense, and 129 one prior nonsexual offense. Further supporting the concept that many male adolescent perpetrators of sex offenses are delinquent, half of 58 evaluated by structured interviews received DSM-III diagnoses of conduct disorder independent of their sexual behavior (Kavoussi, Kaplan, & Becker, 1988).

Female Sex Offenders

The conclusion of Travin, Cullen, and Protter (1990) that because of sociocultural factors only the most overt acts of sexual abuse committed by women are likely to come to the attention of the justice system is strongly supported. As pointed out in Chapters 6 and 7, a much higher percentage of women are found to have molested children and coerced adults in community studies than are charged and convicted. O'Connor (1987) stated that he could find no systematic studies of female sex offenders. He reported that according to British Home Office statistics from 1975 to 1984, 1% of all sex offenses and 1.5% of acts of indecency with children were committed by women. He provided data on 81 subjects committed to a women's prison for sex offenses. The classification he used did not make it possible to determine how many of their victims were prepubertal children, but the majority were under 16 years and possibly under 14 years. Where the sex of the victims was reported, 15 were girls and 10 were boys. Two-thirds of the offenders had carried out indecent acts; half of these had a psychiatric diagnosis and a history of previous treatment. One-third of the offenders were convicted of involvement in unlawful sexual intercourse with children; few of these had psychiatric diagnoses, and almost all were convicted of aiding and abetting a male who committed the offense. In a quarter of these cases, the offender was the mother or stepmother.

O'Connor pointed out that sexual gratification was never noted in the prison records as a motivation for the women involved in sex offenses with a victim. He did not indicate whether this was attributable to inadequacy of recording. Traven et al. (1990) cited a U.S. study that 202 women, 1.65% of the total female prison population, were convicted of sex offenses. Among the offenses categorized were sexual abuse/assault or battery (49 cases), child exploitation (34 cases), child molestation (34 cases), and rape (31 cases). In most of these cases, the women were charged as the principal offenders; however, as in the British study, a number were coerced by or acted as accomplices of men.

Faller (1987) reported on a clinical sample of 40 women who had sexually abused 63 children. About three-quarters of the women sexually abused the children in polyincestuous family situations, and more than four-fifths were mothers to at least one of their victims. Faller cautioned that such intrafamilial abuse might be overrepresented as the women were referred by child protection services, which are more likely to deal with such cases; nonrelated perpetrators are more likely to be dealt with by police. The most common form of sexual activity was group sex, and the next most common was fondling. The mean age of the women was 26 years, and the children 6.4 years. Two-thirds of the victims were female. The women tended to be poor, as well as poorly educated. About half had mental problems, both retardation and psychotic illness, and more than half had a chemical dependency. In their classification of rapists, Groth and Birnbaum (1979) noted that women as opposed to men showed a lack of expressed anger and aggression, and a primacy of children as victims.

Relatives and Contacts of Sex Offenders

Little attention has been given to the consequences of disclosure of the deviant behaviors of sex offenders to their families and social and occupational contacts. In the case of the most unacceptable of these behaviors, those against children, rejection of the offenders by many members of their immediate family is common, at least as an initial response. At times, loss of employment and threats or acts of violence from neighbors force them to shift residence. In my experience the reactions of the majority of wives of pedophiles, particularly those whose victims were outside the family, were or soon became supportive. It is possible that the parents of the offenders suffer more distress, perhaps feeling themselves in some way responsible. Burgess and Hazelwood (1983) found the families and friends of victims of sexual asphyxia to be invariably stunned and shocked. Some could accept the deaths as accidental, but not that they resulted from sexual acts. A few could not accept that they were accidental and became angry that the investigators did not continue to treat them as homicides.

ETIOLOGY OF SEX OFFENSES AND DEVIATIONS

Either or both of two models are accepted by most theorists concerning the etiology of sexual deviations. The stimulus control model, in its original form, proposed that they were motivated by sexual arousal to the related deviant stimuli. Cognitive models proposed that they were motivated by attitudes and beliefs of the offender. Usually when thesis and antithesis are advanced in an area of scientific knowledge, it is finally established that an interaction of the two is involved.

The Stimulus Control Model and Its Modifications

The stimulus control model has been held at least until recently by the majority of researchers treating sex offenders in North America (Quinsey & Earls, 1990). As Barbaree (1990) pointed out, it is opposed by the radical feminist cognitive model. The stimulus control model is supported by the community belief, presumably based on people's experience of their own sexual feelings and fantasies, that sex offenses are motivated by the subjects' sexual preferences for the related deviant sexual objects or behaviors. The strongest evidence for this belief in relation to rapists and child molesters was provided by early studies demonstrating that these sex offenders showed larger penile circumference responses (PCRs) to audiotaped descriptions of their offenses than to descriptions of consenting intercourse with adult females. These studies employed small numbers of subjects; as discussed in Chapter 1, subsequent studies investigating larger numbers were unable to replicate their findings. The PCRs of rapists (Baxter et al., 1986) and child molesters (Nagayama Hall et al., 1988) were found not to differ from those of nonoffenders.

Research workers have as yet failed to agree on an interpretation of these negative findings. Some North American workers continue to defend the validity of PCR assessment of sexual arousal (McAnulty & Adams, in press). I have argued for several years that PCR assessment lacked adequate validity (McConaghy, 1977a; 1982; 1989; 1992). Acceptance of this view would require rejection of a large number of research findings of the 1970s and 1980s that relied on PCR validity, and major revision of the conclusions based on these findings. The findings provide the only evidence of the efficacy in changing sexual arousal patterns, of aversion therapy, and of masturbatory satiation and reconditioning, treatments discussed subsequently. It was therefore inevitable, given the nature of scientific politics, that researchers showed considerable reluctance to consider the evidence that PCR assessment lacked adequate validity.

Proponents of the stimulus control model who accept the validity of PCR assessment must ignore the issue of its failure to differentiate sex offenders from controls (Quinsey & Earls, 1990). Supporters of the radical feminist view of rape employed the negative finding to reject the stimulus control model. Darke (1990) pointed out that it supported the belief that sexual arousal to aggressive sexual stimuli was not an exclusive, or essential, characteristic of identified sexual aggressors, and that sexual aggression was primarily motivated by men's desire for power and control. A factor that needs to be taken into account when evaluating the failure of PCR assessment to distinguish groups of sex offenders from nonoffenders is the number of unreported sex offenses. Some subjects included in nonoffender groups must be undetected offenders; however, if the stimulus control model and PCR assessment are both valid, only some apparent nonoffenders but all offenders should show PCRs indicative of deviant arousal. As no differences were found between the PCR assessments of the total group of offenders and of nonoffenders, either the original stimulus control model or the assessment must be invalid.

Inhibition Model

Barbaree (1990) was one of the few proponents of the stimulus control model who acknowledged and attempted to account for the negative findings with PCR assessment. To continue to accept the validity of PCR assessment, he modified the stimulus control model in relation to rape, retaining the concept that rape was motivated by sexual arousal to cues, but deciding that the cues were not those related to rape but the normal cues of women's physical attributes. Rape cues, such as nonconsent on the part of the woman and her displays of pain, fear, and discomfort, as well as use of force on the part of the man, inhibited the normal sexual arousal of most men so that they would not be motivated to rape. Rapists were those who failed to acquire this inhibitory process or in whom it was temporarily disrupted. If PCR assessment of sexual arousal is valid, however, those rapists who have failed to acquire the inhibitory process should show sexual arousal to women's physical attributes in the presence of rape cues. The inclusion of these rapists who lack inhibition to rape cues should result in the PCRs of the total group of rapists to such cues being greater than those of nonoffenders. As they are not, it is necessary that the rape-cue inhibition model be further modified, withdrawing the concept that some rapists have failed to acquire the inhibition. The model would then rely on temporary disruption of the inhibition in rapists as the cause of rape.

Support for the inhibition model was sought in laboratory studies of normal subjects' PCR-assessed arousal to descriptions of rape as compared to mutually consenting sexual relationships (Barbaree, 1990). These studies demonstrated that increased PCRs to rape descriptions were produced by blaming the victim, anger, alcohol intoxication, or preexposure to aggressive pornography. The increase in PCRs was attributed to these factors disrupting the inhibitory process; how exposure to aggressive pornography could disrupt the inhibition when the rape-cue inhibition theory postulated that cues of aggression produced the inhibition was not explained. Also, normal men were reported to show the same or greater arousal to forced-sex than consenting-sex cues if they were made angry by having a female insult them (Marshall & Barbaree, 1990a). If rape cues are only inhibitory and not of themselves sexually arousing to the majority of normal men, how their disruption produced greater arousal than consenting-sex cues under this condition was also not explained.

Studies quoted earlier in relation to sadistic and nonsadistic rape found that a high percentage of men in their normal state (i.e., without disruption of any postulated inhibitory processes) reported experiencing sexual arousal and enjoyment of depictions of a woman being raped. The complexities involved in the attempt by these workers to resolve the contradictions produced by the negative findings of PCR assessment of rapists, while leaving the validity of the assessment unquestioned, appear a further example that

> any theory can, in fact, be triumphantly vindicated, given a sufficient number of ad hoc hypotheses (like the epicycles of Ptolemaic astronomy) to account for apparent exceptions, and any doctrine can be "saved," although it will of course become progressively useless as the number of cases it would seem to apply to grow smaller with each extra ad hoc hypothesis superimposed to meet some logical obstacle. (Berlin, 1990, p. 63)

Are Sexual Deviations Not Sexually Motivated?

On the basis that few exhibitionists and child molesters showed PCR evidence of sexual arousal to narratives describing their offenses, Marshall and Barbaree (1990a) rejected the stimulus control model for these deviations. They decided that the offenders did not experience sexual arousal to the offensive behaviors; this view parallels the earlier feminist view that rape was not sexually motivated. The conclusion that many sex offenders do not show sexual arousal to cues associated with the deviant behavior is significantly at variance with both everyday and clinical experience. It would seem that only political necessity could force researchers to reject the reports of deviant subjects that they experience sexual arousal to deviant cues because they do not show PCR evidence of greater sexual arousal to the cues than do controls. In view of the extensive evidence quoted earlier that a large percentage of normal subjects experience sexual arousal to fantasies of deviant sexual activity, this requires believing that sex offenders differ from normals in not being aroused by these stimuli.

Virtually all sex offenders who seek treatment report being sexually aroused by fantasies of their deviant activity, which they often use during masturbation. McGuire et al. (1965) were so convinced of this that they suggested masturbation during adolescence to deviant fantasies produced the deviant urges of sex offenders by conditioning. Quinsey and Earls (1990) cited repeated observations that offenders (including child molesters, rapists, and sadists) reported ruminating over sexual fantasies involving the types of behaviors in which they engaged. They pointed out that the clinical importance of inappropriate sexual preferences was reflected in the DSM-III-R definition of sexual deviations or paraphilias as disorders characterized by intense sexual urges or sexually arousing fantasies involving inappropriate objects or coercive sexual activities. Freund et al. (1983) found that more than 60% of exhibitionists and almost 20% of control subjects showed penile volume responses (PVRs) to verbal descriptions of exposure as large as or larger than those to descriptions of sexual tactile interactions or intercourse. Herman (1990) cited an unpublished study by Briere, Corne, Runtz, and Malamuth that young men who had committed sexual assaults differed markedly from their peers in reporting much higher sexual arousal to a fantasized rape scenario.

Support for Marshall and Barbaree's view (1990a) is found in the reports of some subjects—in particular, exhibitionists, voyeurs, and transvestites, whose sexually deviant behaviors have become habitual—that their deviant behaviors are carried out in response to generalized excitement rather than sexual arousal. Also, the fact that a significant percentage of normal subjects report arousal to fantasies of deviant activities, but do not carry them out, conflicts with the stimulus control model in its original form. The model that sex offenses are motivated by sexual arousal to deviant cues would appear to provide only a partial explanation for sexually offensive and deviant behaviors.

Behavior Completion Model

I advanced a modification of the stimulus control model that enabled it to account for the finding that many habitual offenders report nonsexual arousal as a major motivation. This modification, the behavior completion model, was stimulated by sex offenders' accounts of the difficulty they experienced when they attempted to cease their deviant behaviors, as well as by their response to treatment. These led me to believe that in addition to sexual arousal, the general arousal system of the brain was involved (McConaghy, 1980, 1983). The arousal system is responsible for maintaining consciousness. Depending on its level of activation by environmental or internal cues, it produces different levels of alertness, from relaxed consciousness through increasing feelings of tension or excitement to extreme panic. The arousal system is very sensitive to novel or strong stimuli, which activate it to produce the commonly experienced startle response to such stimuli.

I had previously noted that patients with agoraphobia developed their initial attacks of high arousal or panic in situations that had a component of delay, most commonly waiting to be served in a crowded store or supermarket, or when on public transportation. I considered it unlikely to be a coincidence that in such situations many healthy subjects showed milder increases in arousal that they experienced as increased tension (McConaghy & Silove, 1989). An explanation was sought as to why many healthy people feel increased tension when delayed. As there was evidence that agoraphobics were chronically in a state of increased arousal, such an explanation would then account for their responding to delays with much higher levels of tension or anxiety than do healthy subjects.

Experimental findings of the Russian physiologists Sokolov and Anokhin led them to elaborate the Pavlovian hypothesis that conditioned or learned linkages set up in the brains of animals and people an internal reflection or representation of reality (McConaghy, 1987b). They concluded that these brain or neuronal models of reality not only reflected the subjects' total sensory environment, but also incorporated the totality of their habitual motor responses to the stimuli in that environment. This meant that all habitual behaviors, from the initial cues stimulating the behaviors through to their completion, were represented in subjects' brain models. When a subject encountered a situation where he or she had regularly carried out a particular behavior, the cues of that situation activated that part of the brain model representing that behavior. The activated representation then monitored incoming stimuli that indicated whether the behavior was being completed. If the subject delayed completing the habitual behavior, the incoming stimuli failed to match its neuronal representation. The failure of matching caused the neuronal representation to stimulate the arousal system, leading to the subject experiencing increased tension and excitement. These feelings could be sufficiently aversive that he or she felt driven to complete the behavior. That is to say, the neuronal representation of the behavior functioned as a behavior completion mechanism (BCM). It was suggested that there would be an evolutionary advantage in the development of such neuronal mechanisms to motivate animals and people to continue behaviors their past experience has established as rewarding.

If the BCM hypothesis is correct, when subjects who had repeatedly carried out sexual behaviors found themselves in situations where they had carried out the behaviors in the past, or when they thought of carrying out the behaviors, the BCMs for those behaviors would be activated. If the subjects then attempted not to complete the behaviors, the BCMs produced increased arousal, forcing many of the subjects to complete the behaviors against their will. To bring the model within the normal experience of many readers, it accounts for the otherwise puzzling fact that a number of people, when called to dinner, allow their meal to grow cold and risk the annoyance of the caller rather than temporarily leave unfinished an unimportant behavior in which they are engaged. Others when driving, though not in a hurry, find their tension increased when they are temporarily held up at traffic lights or are requested to stop at a roadside food stall. Sexual behaviors, which are intrinsically much more exciting, would be expected to produce much higher levels of arousal if they are provoked but not carried out.

The BCM hypothesis was initially advanced to account for the report of men who sought treatment to control homosexual behaviors. Those treated with aversive procedures reported that following treatment, they were able to control the behaviors they had experienced as compulsive. Their enjoyment of homosexual behaviors they did not wish to control was unchanged, however, as was their sexual arousal to films of nude men and women as measured by PVR assessment (McConaghy, 1976). Evidence supporting the validity of PVR assessment of sexual orientation was discussed in Chapter 1. This apparently paradoxical finding that the treated subjects were able to control unacceptable homosexual behaviors without change in their homosexual arousal led me to seek a nonsexual form of arousal that was reduced. The BCM hypothesis of motivation postulated that the homosexual behaviors were initially motivated by homosexual arousal to the relevant stimuli. After the behaviors had been repeatedly carried out, changing life circumstances in some subjects—for example, marriage or fear of HIV infection—caused them to wish to cease some or all of the behaviors. By this stage, however, BCMs for the homosexual behaviors were established by their previous regular performance in reality and fantasy. When the subjects tried to cease the behaviors, they had to combat not only sexual urges but the increased tension or excitement produced by the BCMs activating the arousal system, so that they were compelled to complete the behaviors against their will. Aversive therapy inhibited the BCMs for the activity while not modifying the subjects' basic pattern of sexual arousal, so that they could continue acceptable behaviors while being able to cease the unacceptable ones.

The same model was applied to sex offenses and deviant practices, sexual interest in which appears to be present in a significant percentage of the normal population. As the evidence of Templeman and Stinnett (1991) discussed earlier indicated, adolescent males appear to seek out a variety of sexual experiences. These would be expected to include the deviant behaviors that commonly arouse men in fantasy. Adolescents with reduced ethical values and/or who are sensation seekers because of genetically determined personality factors and/or social learning would be the most prone to carry out these behaviors. As sexuality in women is expressed much more within emotional relationships than in sexual acts carried out alone, markedly fewer adolescent girls than boys would be expected to carry out deviant sex behaviors repeatedly. For the sexually adventurous male adolescent, chance opportunities for exhibitionism or voyeurism—or sought opportunities for experientially or genetically determined interest in homosexual pedophilia, fetishism, or sexual aggression—would determine the initial act. Fortuitous discovery of the excitement produced by bondage or activities producing sexual asphyxia was considered to initiate these behaviors in some subjects (Hazelwood et al., 1983). Enjoyment of the excitement produced by the activities would encourage a percentage of adolescents to repeat them both in fantasy and reality. If with developing maturity they wished to cease these activities after repeating them for a period, the BCMs now established for the activities would render this impossible for some. They would at this stage in late adolescence or early adulthood experience them as compulsive.

A similar mechanism would operate in the rarer offenders whose behavior commenced in adulthood. It would be expected, however, that chance opportunities and factors decreasing the subject's control—depression, alcoholism, intellectual deterioration, drug taking, or increased stress leading to heightened general arousal—would play a greater role in offenses that developed in adulthood. As discussed earlier, a number of workers have noted the presence of markedly increased nonsexual arousal, tension, or excitement in sex offenders prior to the commission of the offense. Many exhibitionists do not have an erection or masturbate while exposing, suggesting that in adulthood sexual gratification is not a major motivation. This is consistent with their statements that they do not find the behavior sexually gratifying, but that it relieves the tension experienced immediately beforehand. This is also true of adult transvestites as discussed in Chapter 4. The BCM hypothesis also explains the finding of Groth and Burgess (1977) of a high incidence of sexual dysfunctions in men carrying out sexual assaults, in that this would result from the heightened anxiety associated with increased arousal. Of 101 convicted men who attempted penetration, 27 reported impotence, 5 premature ejaculation, and 26 retarded ejaculation.

It would appear that the compulsive element is strongest in exhibitionism and voyeurism. As discussed subsequently, untreated exhibitionists are more likely than other sex offenders to reoffend. Yet in my experience, they show a better response than other offenders to alternative behavior completion treatment aimed at giving them control over the compulsive aspect of their deviant behavior.

Addiction Model

An alternative to the BCM hypothesis that also accounted for the observation that the behaviors of sex offenders appeared compulsive was that sex offenders were addicts (Herman, 1990). As addictions are commonly seen as under stimulus control, this model (like the BCM model) accepts a role for such control, but it is neurophysiologically less explicit than the BCM model and hence does not have the same implications for treatment. The addiction model regards sex offenders as similar to alcoholics and other addicts in that they behave as though their primary attachment is to the mood-altering addictive activity. Herman considered that like addicts, sex offenders sacrifice or manipulate all their other relationships in the service of their sexual activity. An unhappy childhood, stormy marriage, or frustrating job provide the justification and the excuse for the addiction; the rapist's cry and the alcoholic's are one and the same: "She drove me to it." Herman's acceptance of this model seems somewhat inconsistent with her belief that "the most striking characteristic of sex offenders, from a diagnostic standpoint, is their apparent normality" (p. 180), a comment few would make of alcoholics or other addicts. No evidence was advanced that the emotional relationships of the majority of sex offenders resembled those of drug addicts, rather than those of nonsexual offenders or of socioeconomically matched normals. Compulsive sexual deviations appear much more responsive to treatment than do addictions to drugs.

Courtship Disorders Model

Freund (1990; Freund et al., 1983), from an ethological perspective, considered a number of deviant sex behaviors to be courtship disorders. He stated that he adopted the term from students of birds, who used it for precopulatory reproductive activities. Presumably, Freund believed the sex behaviors were biologically determined. He identified four phases of human sexual interactions, each with an anomalous pattern in which the phase was markedly intensified and distorted. Voyeurism was the anomaly of the phase of location and appraisal of the partner; exhibitionism, the anomaly of the phase of pretactile interaction (i.e., looking, smiling, posturing, and talking); toucherism or frotteurism, the anomaly of the phase of tactile interaction; and preferential rape, the anomaly of the phase of genital union. This meant that exhibitionists, unlike normal subjects, would experience sexual arousal typical of the later phase of courtship without having experienced the earlier phases. This was supported by evidence that normal subjects showed penile volume response (PVR) evidence of arousal to films of a woman pointing to her exposed genitals only after they viewed a preliminary stimulus of a film of the woman dressed and showing coy erotic signaling behavior; exhibitionists showed arousal to the former stimulus without the preliminary stimulation (Kolarsky & Madlafousek, 1983). The normal subjects were soldiers whose mean age was 20 years; the exhibitionists' mean age was 27 years. Difference in the sexual experiences of the two groups, including that of repeated exhibitionism, could have accounted for the less inhibited response of exhibitionists. Freund and Blanchard (1986) reported that exhibitionists did not differ from normals in their PVRs to audiotaped narratives of the four phases of normal sexual interaction. They did not regard this finding as incompatible with the courtship disorder model, but concluded it to refute the hypothesis that exhibitionism resulted from a disinclination toward intercourse.

Freund and Blanchard (1986) argued that the fact that different courtship disorders were not uncommonly committed by the same offender supported the model. In addition, they reported evidence that offenders who did not acknowledge carrying out courtship disorders other than the type with which they were charged showed PVR evidence of sexual arousal to narratives describing the other courtship disorders. Freund (1990) interpreted findings that courtship disorders showed some likelihood of being present in combination with transvestism and sadism as suggesting a relationship between the three conditions. If this is so, the concept of courtship disorder would appear in danger of becoming so broad that it could be used to account for all deviant sex behaviors and offenses, thus becoming more a classification than an explanation. The ease with which most exhibitionists and voyeurs appear to respond to behavioral treatment and the frequently reported normality of their sexual interactions with their sexual partners makes somewhat implausible the hypothesis that their condition is attributable to a strong and persistent biologically based disturbance of their courting behaviors. It would also seem incompatible with the finding of Freund et al. (1983), cited earlier, that almost 20% of control subjects showed penile volume responses to verbal descriptions of exposure as large as or larger than those to descriptions of sexual tactile interactions or intercourse.

Cognitive Models

The BCM stimulus control model of deviant sexual behaviors suggested that chance events arousing deviant urges, as well as personality features, determined which subjects initiated them. The BCMs for the behaviors then made them compulsive. The concept of personality (i.e., of innate individual differences in behavioral patterns that could be in part genetically determined), however, was not accepted in behavioral theory in the United States (Chapter 1). Individual differences were seen as temporary, caused by exposure to different environmental contigencies, and hence readily modifiable by changing the contingencies. More recently, cognitive factors reflecting social experience have been awarded major significance in determining individual differences. The cognitive model therefore treats sexual deviations as resulting from socially induced cognitions that encourage their performance.

The best-known of the cognitive models is that based on a feminist perspective. Discussed in Chapter 7, this model in its radical form considered all men to be potential victimizers of women and children and ignored the sexually coercive behavior of women. It therefore had no need to provide an explanation as to why only some men and women offended. It also proposed that rape and possibly all sexual offenses were motivated by wishes to dominate and express hostility, not sexual arousal. The detailed criticism by Palmer (1988) should have made this view untenable, particularly in combination with the evidence, discussed subsequently, of the response of male sex offenders to chemical treatment that reduced their serum levels of testosterone. It would seem plausible that some rapists are motivated by aggressive as well as sexual urges, however, though such aggression may be in part attributable to biological factors and to learning from individual experiences rather than entirely determined by politically influenced cognitions concerning the roles of women and men.

The cognitive models of sex offenses adopted by most workers modified the feminist concept by accepting that the offenses were motivated by sexual arousal and rejecting the belief that all men held equivalent cognitions supportive of sexual offending. Burt (1980) provided evidence that both men and women varied in the extent to which they held such cognitions or "rape myths," as is detailed in Chapter 7. The extent also correlated with their degree of acceptance of interpersonal violence, of sex-role stereotyping, and of the belief that the sexual interactions of men and women were adversarial. The degree to which individual men held these related cognitions was considered to determine the likelihood of their sexually victimizing women and children. Ageton (1983) investigated this hypothesis in the sexually assaultive offenders identified from the national sample of adolescents she studied. Though the offenders differed markedly from controls in evidence of delinquency, they did not differ in their beliefs concerning sex roles or their attitudes toward sexual assault. Ageton concluded that though cognitions may influence sexual acts, her data did not indicate they played a major role in predicting sexual assault.

The cognitive model has also been tested in a number of studies of college men, but it has received only weak support. Koss, Leonard, Beezley, and Oros (1985) classified male university students into four groups—sexually nonaggressive, coercive, abusive and assaultive—on the basis of their responses to the Koss and Oros (1982) questionnaire of sexual behaviors. The students' attitudes toward relationships with women and sexual aggression were assessed by a number of additional questionnaires, one of which was based on Burt's scales (1980). The statistical technique of stepwise discriminant analysis demonstrated that the students' attitudes, along with their number of sexual partners, discriminated the four groups only slightly better than chance.

In two studies of university students, Malamuth investigated the relationship between three of Burt's attitudinal measures (rape myth acceptance, acceptance of interpersonal violence against women, and adversarial sex beliefs) and measures of male students' sexually aggressive behaviors. The measure used in one study was the students' responses on the Koss and Oros questionnaire (Malamuth, 1988), and in the second, their statements that they had forced a woman to do something sexual she did not want to do (Malamuth, 1989a). Correlations were weak, accounting for at most 4% of the variance of the measures of cognitions and sexual aggression. Correlations were stronger between rape-supportive cognitions and students' reports of the likelihood of their forcing a woman into unwanted actions or of raping her if they could be assured that no one would know and that they could not be punished (Malamuth, 1989a, 1989b). Students' reports of the likelihood of their carrying out these acts have been shown to correlate to some extent with their reports of having actually been sexually aggressive, the strength of the correlations varying from $r = 0.15$ ($p < 0.005$; Malamuth, 1988) to $r = 0.5$ ($p < 0.001$; McConaghy & Zamir, 1992b). It does not seem strong evidence for the cognitive hypothesis that cognitions supportive of sexual aggression to women correlated more strongly with reported likelihood of such aggression than with its actual performance.

Koss and Dinero (1988) investigated an approximately representative national sample of 2,972 male students at 32 U.S. institutions of higher education. Though the subjects' cognitions supportive of sexual aggression correlated with their reported sexually aggressive behaviors, Koss and Dinero found that the subjects' early exposure to family violence, childhood sexual abuse, and early age of sexual initiation, predicted their later sexually aggressive behaviors equally well, suggesting that the cognitions were not causing the sexual aggression but, like the aggression, were secondary to the childhood experiences or variables associated with these experiences (perhaps including genetic determinants).

In regard to the cognitions of convicted rapists, Stermac et al. (1990) pointed out that though many investigators reported the clinical impression that the rapists showed attitudes of hostility toward women, attempts to validate this by comparing rapists to other sex offenders or men from similar socioeconomic groups found no difference between the two groups. Some studies reported that rapists showed more positive attitudes toward women and less endorsement of rape myths. Stermac et al. questioned the validity of these findings, arguing that it was easy for subjects to select the socially acceptable responses on the instruments used and that, despite assurances of confidentiality, it was unlikely that incarcerated rapists would report hostile or negative feelings they might have about women or sexuality.

Stermac et al. found little research investigating the cognitions of child molesters. They quoted an in-press study by Stermac and Segal in which subjects rated vignettes of sexual offenses against children on a number of scales, including perception of harm versus benefit to the child, child complicity, and adult responsibility. Child molesters, as compared to other offenders and nonoffenders, were more supportive of permissive attitudes toward sexual contact with children and of beliefs that children were the property of adults. Howells (1978) found that the cognitions concerning adults and children of heterosexual pedophiles, as compared with non-pedophiles, involved a dimension of dominance in which adults were seen as overbearing and threatening. Children were regarded as nondominant, nonthreatening, and easier to relate to. The cognitions of the heterosexual pedophiles concerning children were not exclusively sexual but tended to be idealistic, concerning their simplicity and innocence. As homosexual pedophiles and hebephiles compared to heterosexual pedophiles show marked preference for the company of children socially as well as sexually, they may hold different or more intense cognitions concerning them.

If the cognitions of sex offenders are consistently shown to differ from those of nonoffenders, it would be necessary to establish that they play a causal role in determining sexually offensive behaviors and are not secondary to other variables, as Koss and Dinero's findings (1988) indicated. From my knowledge of human behavior, it is highly likely that a percentage of people who carry out socially unacceptable behaviors would subsequently attempt to minimize their severity and attribute responsibility to others, including the victim, thus secondarily developing cognitions considered supportive of victimization. Possibly the most convincing evidence of a causal role for cognitions would be demonstration that treatment aimed solely at altering offenders' cognitions reduced the likelihood of their offending in comparison to treatments that did not directly attempt this.

Pornography

In relation to both stimulus control and cognitive models of motivation of sex offenses, pornography has been suggested to play a role by encouraging rape-supportive cognitions and/or by increasing offenders' sexual arousal to deviant cues. Evidence that male university students reported greater sexual arousal to depictions of rape than to those of consenting intercourse following exposure to aggressive pornography was discussed earlier. Social learning theory would suggest that with regular exposure to pornographic rape depictions, any learned negative feelings the subject experienced to rape cues would be desensitized, particularly if such depictions were sexually arousing. As pointed out in Chapter 7, virtually no attention has been given to the possible effects of the "Mills and Boon" form of soft-core pornography for women. Koss and Dinero (1988) found that male college students who reported being sexually aggressive also reported higher current use of pornography; however, both behaviors were predicted by childhood exposure to violence and early sexual experience. Consistent with this finding, Murrin and Laws (1990) in their review of studies investigating the influence of pornography on sexual crimes concluded that the increased exposure to pornography in childhood reported by sex offenders as compared to nonoffenders appeared to be attributable to the differences in the home lives of the two groups.

A number of studies found similar patterns of use by sex offenders and nonoffenders in adolescence, with both reporting masturbating to pornography. In adulthood the latter activity was more common in sex offenders; they also owned more pornography. One-third of rapists and child molesters reported that the use of pornography incited them to offend (Marshall and Barbaree, 1990a). The fact that the significant differences in use of pornography by sex offenders compared to controls was found in adulthood, whereas sexually deviant behavior appears to be established in adolescence, suggests that the use of pornography is a consequence of the deviance and its associated life-style rather than a cause. The belief of sex offenders that their acts were incited by pornography could be a false attribution. The possibility would need to be excluded that when sexually aroused they first employed pornography, but that on the occasions when this was insufficient to relieve their arousal, they proceeded to carry out the offense. This could lead to their impression that the use of pornography incited the offense. Murrin and Laws (1990) concluded that exposure to pornography of itself did not have an influence on the incidence of sexual crimes, but rather on the nature of the person being exposed to and the existing cultural milieu in which the exposure occurred.

Psychiatric-Psychopathological Model

Bart (1979) and Scully and Marolla (1985), in advancing feminist and sociological cognitive models of rape, contrasted them with the earlier psychiatric-psychopathological model in which rapists were regarded as driven by irresistible sexual impulses, as psychologically disordered, or as acting under the influence of alcohol, and victims were considered in part to have precipitated the offense. The feminist perspective was that this model removed rape from the realm of the everyday or normal world; however, the model does appear to have significant empirical support. Evidence was reviewed in Chapter 7 supporting the concept of victim vulnerability, though this should not be interpreted as suggesting that the victims precipitated the offenses. Women involved in delinquent behaviors and with delinquent peers in adolescence, who abused alcohol and drugs, who had antisocial personalities, who had liberal sexual attitudes, and who reported sexual activity with more partners in adulthood were found more likely to be sexually assaulted. As discussed earlier, some investigators from a feminist as well as a biological perspective have accepted the irresistible nature of the impulses motivating rape and other sex offenses, though not necessarily agreeing that the impulses are sexual. Herman supported an addiction model, and I advanced a physiological behavior completion model, to account for the irresistible nature of impulses to carry out sexually deviant behaviors. The success of treatment in giving subjects control over the impulses (reported subsequently) supports the concept that they were previously irresistible. The presence of psychological disorders in sex offenders has been investigated in relation to a number of hypotheses now discussed.

Lack of Social Skills

The consistently reported clinical impression that sex offenders lacked the social skills to form acceptable social and sexual relationships with women was criticized on the basis that the clinicians failed to compare sex offenders with nonoffenders or socioeconomically equivalent subjects in the community (Stermac et al., 1990). Studies that used appropriate controls and reported negative findings, however, have also been criticized. McFall (1990) argued from an information-processing perspective that social skills rely on underlying components that could be largely independent: decoding (the interpretation of social cues), decision skills (selecting the best response option), and enactment skills (carrying out the response and monitoring its effects). McFall suggested that the studies of sex offenders that used appropriate controls employed self-report and role-play measures that assessed only decision skills. He believed decoding skills could be more relevant; the acceptance of rape myths reported to characterize rapists and rape-prone students would encourage them to focus on and misinterpret ambiguous social cues from women as come-ons and to perceive women as desiring and obtaining gratification from sexual assault. This could result in inability of these subjects to discriminate between consensual and coercive sex in sexual interactions. Based on his analysis, McFall developed the Test of Reading Affective Cues, with which he demonstrated differences between incarcerated non-sexual offenders and rapists.

Childhood Sexual Abuse

The hypothesis that subjects who are sexually abused in their childhood become sex offenders through "identification with the aggressor" was criticized by Herman (1990) as unable to explain the virtual male monopoly of sex offenses. As discussed in Chapter 7, though, this belief in a male monopoly can only be sustained by ignoring the incidence of sexual coercion by women in community studies. Herman's other criticism of the theory rested on firmer grounds. She pointed out that the evidence was based on retrospective reports of identified offenders, who were not representative of the much larger undetected population of offenders. Also, most studies supporting the theory lacked appropriate comparison groups and employed vague definitions of childhood sexual abuse. It has also been argued that sex offenders, and particularly child molesters, report being victimized in childhood to obtain the sympathy of the interviewer or more lenient legal treatment, or that they unconsciously exaggerate remembered events to reduce feelings of guilt (Freund, Watson, & Dickey, 1990). Herman considered that histories of sexual abuse did appear unusually common in men who sexually molested boys or raped men, and she concluded that childhood sexual abuse may be necessary to direct male sexual aggression against other males but not against females, stating that normal male socialization was sufficient for this. If it is established that more men who molest males as compared to controls are victims of childhood sexual abuse, however, the abuse may not have caused them to become sexual offenders. The possibility would have to be excluded that some men who molest males showed features in childhood (e.g., sissy behaviors) that caused them to be selected for victimization. Sissy behaviors in childhood are associated with the later development of homosexual impulses (see Chapter 3). Presence of a homosexual component in male medical students was significantly correlated with sissy behaviors in childhood and with their both having coerced and having been coerced by males into sexual activity (McConaghy & Zamir, 1992c).

Childhood Relationships

Marshall and Barbaree (1990a) reviewed the evidence that poor socialization and, in particular, exposure to parental violence in the offender's childhood facilitated his use of aggression, as well as cut him off in adolescence from access to more appropriate sociosexual interactions. Marshall and Barbaree found that the family backgrounds of sex offenders were similar to those of people with antisocial personalities. As antisocial personality is in part inherited (Schulsinger, 1972), before it can be accepted that the disturbed childhood relationships produced the later behavior of the offender, the possibility would need to be excluded that genetic factors determined both.

Antisocial Personality

The most consistently reported finding in relation to personality differences in sex offenders, particularly the sexually aggressive, is that a high percentage show behaviors typical of antisocial or psychopathic personality disorder. Ageton (1983) reviewed evidence that from 20% to 43% of men arrested for rape and sexual assault had previous convictions for other offenses against the person. Knight et al. (1985) found that both convicted rapists and child molesters had previous convictions for nonsexual offenses. Henn et al. (1976) and Bard et al. (1987) investigated subjects referred for evaluation for sexual crimes and found that rapists had from adolescence shown more antisocial behavior and a higher incidence of victim-involved crimes as compared to child molesters. As stated above, the greater exposure to parental violence found in the childhood of sex offenders was similar to that of people with antisocial personalities (Marshall & Barbaree, 1990a). Dietz et al. (1990) noted that the 30 sexually sadistic criminals they investigated had all engaged in an extensive pattern of antisocial behavior in adulthood. Herman (1990) concluded that many convicted sex offenders met the diagnostic criteria for sociopathic, schizoid, paranoid, and narcissistic personality disorders. She was not convinced that these disorders were any more common in them than in other prisoners, and stated incorrectly that there was no evidence that these disorders were more common in undetected sexually aggressive males than in the total male population.

Ageton (1983), in her study of a representative sample of adolescents, found that those males who reported having committed sexual assaults as compared with the remainder were basically delinquent youths. In a discriminant analysis, the only variable that contributed to the discrimination of the two groups was involvement with delinquent peers, which correctly classified 76% of the cases. Koss and Dinero (1988) found in their approximately representative national sample of 2,972 male students that exposure to family violence in childhood predicted their later sexual aggression. The more serious their sexual aggression, the greater their use of alcohol and their involvement in peer groups that reinforced highly sexualized views of women. These features are consistent with the presence of antisocial personality traits.

Psychological tests investigating the presence of antisocial personality in male students who reported a likelihood of carrying out or having carried out sexually assaultive behaviors have produced inconsistent results. Malamuth (1989b) found it to be present in a number of studies, employing the Psychoticism scale of the Eysenck Personality Questionnaire; Koss et al. (1986) using the Psychopathic Deviate scale of the MMPI, did not. In view of the consistency of findings of antisocial behavior in convicted rapists and sexually assaultive male students, these results could be attributable to the low validity of the psychological tests used to assess antisocial personality.

Alcohol and Drug Abuse

In discussing the model that sex offenders were addicted, Herman (1990) regarded offenders as similar to alcoholics but was critical of studies (Knight et al., 1985) investigating convicted sex offenders that reported that from 25% to 50% were alcohol abusers. She argued that these lacked appropriate comparison groups of nonsexual offenders and demographically matched normals. Herman cited Vaillant as stating that between 11% and 60% of a large group of working-class men could be described as alcohol abusers, depending upon the definition employed. As stated above, however, Koss and Dinero (1988) found that sexually aggressive as compared to nonaggressive students reported a higher frequency of alcohol use and intoxication.

Though rejecting the association between alcohol use and propensity to rape, Herman (1990) acknowledged that alcohol could serve as an aid to overcome inhibitions in those with this propensity. Certainly the evidence is substantial that alcohol plays a role in the initiation of sexual assaults. One study of reported rapes found that the police and victims confirmed alcohol intoxication in 70% of the rapists (Marshall & Barbaree, 1990a). In contrasting the more common confidence rapes and the rarer blitz rapes, Bowie et al. (1990) found that prior to confidence rapes the assailants and victims were much more likely to have spent time together consuming alcohol or other drugs. In Ageton's study (1983) of adolescents, about half the males who reported carrying out sexual assaults stated they had been drinking or taking drugs prior to the event. Victims considered the offender being drunk to be a major factor precipitating the assault. The finding that victims of sexual assault compared to controls showed a higher use of alcohol prior to the assault (Burnam et al., 1988; Koss & Dinero, 1989) is consistent with the characteristic of confidence (as opposed to blitz) rapes that the victim spent some time drinking with the man who later assaulted her (Chapter 7).

Levels of Sex Hormones and Sexual Interest

No replicated differences of sex hormone levels have as yet been found in male sex offenders (Hucker & Bain, 1990), and no studies appear to have been carried out in women. McConaghy and Zamir (1992b, c), investigated medical students using a modified version of the Koss and Oros (1982) questionnaire that allowed women to report sexual experiences in which they were the aggressors as well as victims, and the Bem (1974) measures of masculinity and femininity. They found that reported sexual aggression in both men and women correlated positively with degree of masculinity in two studies, and negatively in men with degree of femininity in one. Consistent with this finding, women's masculinity scores correlated with their degree of opposite-sex-linked behaviors of tomboyish play and expression of physical aggression (McConaghy & Zamir, 1992a). These behaviors have been shown to be significantly increased by exposure to high levels of opposite sex hormones in utero (Ehrhardt & Baker, 1974). It is possible that in utero but not current hormone levels are of importance in contributing to the nature and intensity of sexual and related feelings.

Some sex offenders may have higher levels of sexual interest than nonoffenders. In studies quoted previously, number of sexual partners (Koss et al., 1985) and early age of sexual initiation (Koss & Dinero, 1988) predicted later reported sexually aggressive behaviors in male university students. Kanin (1985) found that self-disclosed date-rapist university students reported an average of 1.5 orgasms in heterosexual activities per week, compared with 0.8 per month for students who had not used force in sexual activities. Dopaminergic drugs have been found to increase sexual urges; following treatment with these drugs, two men put into practice masochistic fantasies they had previously not expressed (Quinn, Toone, Lang, Marsden, & Parkes, 1983). The behaviors ceased with withdrawal of the drugs and returned with their reintroduction.

Brain Damage

Clinical studies of sex offenders seeking treatment have suggested that subjects with evidence of congenital or acquired brain damage are overrepresented (Berlin & Meinecke, 1981; McConaghy et al., 1988). Clinicians have also noted the appearance of sexually anomalous behaviors such as fetishism, exhibitionism, pedophilia, and gender disorders following brain damage from accidents, surgery, epilepsy, and toxic substances (Langevin, 1990). Langevin reviewed a number of studies that suggested a link between temporal lobe impairment and sexually anomalous behaviors. He concluded the link was independent of criminality and learning disabilities, was not a function of alcohol abuse, and might be unrelated to general violence and drug abuse. There was some suggestion that sadists showed structural anomalies in the right brain lobe, whereas pedophiles showed anomalies in the left.

Kolarsky et al. (1967) found a higher incidence of sexual anomalies in subjects with epilepsy originating in the temporal lobe compared with other brain sites. They were unable to confirm the commonly reported clinical impression that there was a particular association between temporal lobe epilepsy and fetishism and transvestism. Hendricks et al. (1988) reported that compared to controls, child molesters had thinner and less dense skulls and lower regional cerebral blood flow. If an association is established between brain damage and sexually deviant behavior, it could be attributable to the brain damage weakening subjects' control of deviant urges already present, rather than producing the urges.

Genetic Factors

It is widely accepted in the United States that deviant sex practices and offenses are learned behaviors and that it is not necessary to exclude the possibility that genetic factors are involved (McConaghy, 1987a). Evidence supporting this possibility would have to be extremely convincing to be given credence; learning theories only have to be plausible to be accepted. Deviant behaviors are commonly stated to be learned by conditioning, and the theory advanced by McGuire et al. (1965) is often cited. These workers considered that an initial deviant sexual experience provided the basis for subsequent fantasies used to accompany masturbation. The stimulus value of the deviant form of sexual expression was reinforced, and the response to normal sexual stimuli extinguished. This theory does not account for the initiation of fetishistic and transvestic behaviors, which usually commence well prior to puberty, or for the presence of deviant urges in a high percentage of subjects with normal sexual responses.

Sex researchers have ignored the evidence that genetic factors in part determine antisocial personality disorder (Schulsinger, 1972), which, as stated above, appears to be a significant determinant of sexually assaultive behaviors. Workers who accept the importance of sexually stereotyped cognitions and behaviors in sexually aggressive men unquestioningly accept that they are learned. Wheller (1985), in advancing a feminist perspective on pornography and rape, stated that child socialization in the home, church, and school produced stereotyped gender behavior. Opposite-sex-linked behaviors and cognitions in men, however, have been consistently shown to correlate with degree of homosexual orientation, which is in part under genetic control (see Chapter 3). Twelve men with the chromosomal abnormality XYY, identified from 4,139 men tested, reported significantly more unconventional sexual experiences than matched normal chromosomal XY male controls (Schiavi et al., 1988). They did not differ in frequency of homosexual behavior, and the nature of the experiences was not specified. It was stated that the latter were mainly in the realm of sexual imagery, and that none of the subjects had been convicted for deviant sexual acts.

The reluctance to consider the possibility that genetic or other biological factors contribute to deviant sex behaviors and sex offenses would appear to reflect more than the political bias of North American theorists toward believing that human behavior is entirely determined by social influences. Marshall and Barbaree (1990a), when discussing the possibility that aggressive sexual tendencies in humans have a biological basis, found it necessary to point out that this did not mean that the display of these behaviors should be accepted as inevitable, nor did it in any way excuse someone for engaging in particular behaviors. They believed that failure to stress these facts by workers who supported a biological understanding of aggressive behavior was responsible for the opposition to this understanding.

Marshall and Barbaree considered that biological factors contributed to the initial learning of sexual offenses—possibly at puberty, when hormonal changes were marked—but that the contribution was minimal once the learning was established. This hypothesis is in part consistent with my own that behavior completion mechanisms increasingly motivate sexually offensive behaviors and render them compulsive as they are repeated. The response of the behaviors to chemicals that reduce testosterone levels indicate that biologically driven sexual urges continue to make some contribution to their motivation. The response of sex offenders, particularly exhibitionists and voyeurs, to behavioral treatment alone suggests that learned factors play a major role in maintaining their deviant behaviors. The intermediate response of fetishists and transvestites and the poorer response of homosexual pedophiles and hebephiles to behavioral treatments suggest that their behaviors are more strongly motivated by biological factors, which could be genetically determined and/or caused by exposure to an environmentally determined variation in the sex hormone levels to which they were exposed in utero.

Assessment of Sex Offenders

Despite the evidence reviewed in Chapter 1 that demonstrated the inability of penile circumference response (PCR) assessment to distinguish individual sex offenders from nonoffenders, the technique remains central to their assessment in most treatment programs in North America (Quinsey & Earls, 1990). Some expression of disquiet, however, is emerging. Quinsey and Earls pointed out that normal men with no history of child molestation show sizable PCRs to slides of pubescent females, and that uncertainty existed concerning the ratio of subjects' PCRs to descriptions of coercive (as opposed to consenting) sexual activity that identified individual rapists from nonrapists. Marshall and Barbaree (1990b) reported failure of posttreatment PCR assessments of child molesters to predict outcome. They commented that "if behaviorists are to maintain [their] exaggerated faith in erectile measurements, they must solve the experimental riddle of demonstrating the relevance of changing such indices to the maintenance of offensive behavior and, particularly, to the issue of treatment benefits" (p. 382).

The most valid information concerning the feelings and behaviors of sex offenders remains their self-reports, supplemented where possible by information from their social contacts and victims and their records of past offenses. As also discussed in Chapter 1, the marked distrust of self-report in favor of behavioral observation, which accompanied the development of behavioral modification in North America, has largely disappeared. Significant correlations of treated sex offenders' self-reported reduction in deviant urges and behaviors with measures of general tension (McConaghy et al., 1985) and state anxiety (McConaghy et al., 1988) provided evidence of the reliability of their self-reports. The significant correlation between their self-reported reduction in deviant urges and the reduction in their blood testosterone levels produced by medroxyprogesterone demonstrated the validity of such self-reports (McConaghy et al., 1988).

My assessment of sex offenders or deviants is based on a fairly standard psychiatric interview, except that I obtain more details concerning their daily activities than most psychiatrists seek. I first review the available data from other sources concerning the subjects' offenses, legal charges, and convictions, both sexual and nonsexual. I then interview them, first nondirectively and then directively, to obtain the relevant information concerning their sexual interest, deviant behaviors, masturbatory fantasies, and sexual and aggressive behaviors. Details of their occupational and social life, use of alcohol and other drugs, and leisure time are then obtained. On the basis of this information and the subjects' verbal expressions and body language, their overt and covert attitudes toward their sex offenses are determined. This procedure allows the assessment not only of their sexual behaviors and attitudes concerning these behaviors, but also of their personality, intelligence, habits, and relationships, as well as the stresses they are subjected to at and away from work and the sources of their enjoyment of life.

TREATMENT OF SEX OFFENSES AND DEVIATIONS

Behavioral programs for sex offenses, and the rarer nonoffensive deviations for which treatment was sought, were introduced in the 1960s and 1970s, based on the stimulus control model that sex offenses were motivated by sexual arousal to deviant stimuli. Conditioning procedures were employed with the aim of modifying the subjects' deviant sexual preferences and increasing their ability to be sexually responsive to adult heterosexual partners. PCR assessment was commonly used in single-case designs to determine that changes had occurred. As it was recognized that at least some sex offenders lacked social skills, other behavioral techniques (e.g., social skills or assertiveness training) were added. In the 1980s, with the acceptance by North American behaviorists that attention needed to be paid to subjects' cognitions as well as their behaviors, most programs added cognitive therapies.

The emerging disquiet of some therapists concerning failure of recent studies of PCR assessment to discriminate sex offenders from nonoffenders, and to predict treatment outcome, has influenced therapeutic procedures. Quinscy and Earls (1990) considered that offenders who show minimal PCRs to deviant cues were less often targeted for interventions aimed at modifying deviant preferences, at least partly because any changes that were produced by treatment would be difficult to detect. Marshall and Barbaree (1990a, b) however, advised that aversive and other procedures originally meant to change deviant arousal patterns should be used with offenders whose patterns of sexual arousal are normal, as their behaviors were nevertheless elicited by features of the environment. At the same time, they suggested it may not be necessary to direct treatment at sexual preferences even when they appeared to be deviant, as deviant preferences might be a result rather than a cause of the deviant sexual behaviors. Despite these indications of change, Quinsey and Earls (1990) concluded that the modification of inappropriate sexual preferences remains of central concern in many of the treatment programs in North America, and that some form of aversive therapy is the method most commonly used to reduce inappropriate sexual interest.

Single Therapies

Aversive Therapies

Aversive therapies were based on the classical conditioning procedure discovered by Pavlov (1927). As discussed in Chapter 1, he presented a dog with a stimulus (e.g., an auditory tone) that produced no specific response and followed the stimulus with food, which produced the specific response of salivation. After a number of these linked presentations, the dog salivated to the stimulus. The learned response of salivation was termed in English a *conditioned response*. In the application of conditioning in aversive therapy, cues producing deviant sexual arousal were followed by an aversive stimulus. The aim was to produce a conditioned aversive response to the deviant cues that would generalize to the deviant cues in the subjects' real experience. The aversive stimulus usually employed was the lowest level of electric shock the patient found unpleasant but not emotionally upsetting. Cues for approved forms of sexual behavior not followed by the aversive event were usually also incorporated, with the expectation that their presentation without punishment would increase the offender's interest in the approved behavior. For example, a heterosexual pedophile offender would be shown a slide of a nude female child. This could be immediately followed by the electric shock, or the shock might be administered only if the offender showed a predetermined level of PCR to the slide. At times during the procedure, the slide of a nude adult woman would be presented and not followed by a shock.

In the 1980s, covert sensitization has been frequently employed in preference to electric-shock aversive therapy (Marshall et al., 1983). With covert sensitization, the subject is first trained to relax. Then, while relaxed, he is instructed to visualize carrying out the deviant behavior, and then to visualize the behavior being followed by an aversive event. For example, he visualizes exposing to an adolescent girl and then visualizes a policeman suddenly appearing to arrest him, or he visualizes sexually assaulting a woman when he becomes nauseated and physically ill. Some workers added a physically nauseating odor to assist the offender's visualization of nausea (Maletzky, 1973).

PCR Evidence of Modification of Sexual Preference. The evidence commonly quoted to support the belief that sexual preferences can be modified by aversive procedures was obtained in studies carried out in the 1960s and 1970s. These studies employed the single-case design (discussed in Chapter 1) to investigate small numbers of homosexual subjects seeking treatment to become heterosexual. At that time, homosexuality was regarded as a sexual disorder. In determining whether change in the subjects' sexual orientation had occurred following treatment, more weight was attached to their PCRs than to the sexual feelings and behaviors they reported. I reviewed these studies in some detail (McConaghy, 1977b). They took maximal advantage of a methodological weakness of single-case design, namely, that the treatment under investigation could be introduced and withdrawn according to the subject's PCRs rather than to a predetermined schedule. When this is done, an apparent relationship can be produced between the introduction of the treatment and PCRs indicating greater heterosexuality, and between withdrawal of the treatment and PCRs indicating greater homosexuality. A second weakness of the studies was that the PCR assessment of the subjects' heterosexual and homosexual arousal employed as stimuli male and female nudes. Subsequent research revealed that this procedure could not validly assess heterosexual and homosexual arousal, as PCRs to these stimuli did not distinguish individual heterosexuals from homosexuals (see Chapter 1). These criticisms, though repeated (McConaghy, 1977a, 1982, 1989, 1990c), have not led to reevaluation and rejection of the conclusions of these single-case studies that aversive therapy reduced homosexual and increased heterosexual arousability.

As discussed earlier in relation to the behavior completion model of deviant sexual practices, I conducted a series of studies investigating the response of homosexual subjects to aversive procedures. These studies used a group design to compare the responses of a number of subjects randomly allocated to different procedures. The valid penile volume response (PVR) assessment of homosexual and heterosexual arousal was employed. It was found that aversive therapies, as compared to a placebo procedure, did not modify the treated subjects' sexual preferences as assessed by PVRs (McConaghy, 1975). Consistent with this finding, the subjects reported that following treatment they did not experience any aversion to the homosexual stimuli that had been paired with the aversive stimuli, and in their everyday experience they continued to be as aware of attraction to males at the time of seeing them as they were before treatment. These findings reinforced the earlier conclusion that there was no evidence of a conditioned aversive response following aversive therapy (McConaghy, 1969).

A valuable change, however, was produced by aversive therapy. Subjects reported that if they wished, they could control homosexual behaviors that prior to treatment they had experienced as compulsive. For example, some married subjects sought treatment because they were spending considerable amounts of time in public lavatories or cruising beats for transient homosexual contacts they often found unsatisfactory, yet they could not discontinue the behaviors, even though they wished to do so. Following treatment, they had no difficulty ceasing them. Other treated subjects reported they could continue homosexual activities they found acceptable, such as relationships with known partners, while ceasing behaviors they found unacceptable but had previously experienced as compulsive, such as seeking casual contacts on beats. Those subjects who had experienced homosexual fantasies as preoccupying and guilt-inducing because of their religious beliefs could easily dismiss these fantasies following treatment. Though they were still as aware of being attracted to men they encountered as they were before treatment, once these men passed from their field of vision they did not continue to have uncontrollable fantasies concerning them.

As there was no evidence of an aversive response following aversive therapy, it was concluded that the procedure did not act by conditioning. To support this conclusion, a study was conducted comparing aversive therapy administered in both forward and backward conditioning paradigms (McConaghy & Barr, 1973). With forward conditioning, aversive stimuli are administered after the homosexual cues; with backward conditioning, the order is reversed. Backward conditioning is considerably less effective in producing conditioned responses (Pavlov, 1927). It was found that equal reduction in compulsive homosexual urges was produced by the two procedures, establishing it was not attributable to the treatments acting by conditioning.

Alternative Behavior Completion: Control, Not Modification of Deviant Urges

The behavioral completion model of compulsive sexuality was advanced (McConaghy, 1980, 1983) to account for the paradoxical findings that aversive therapy did not act by conditioning, and that following it homosexual subjects' sexual orientation as assessed physiologically was unchanged, yet they were able to control homosexual urges they could not control prior to treatment. To test the BCM model and possibly produce an alternative to aversive therapy in the treatment of compulsive sexual and other behaviors, the parallel of these compulsive disorders and agoraphobia (discussed in relation to the development of the model) was followed up. A review of studies evaluating systematic desensitization in the treatment of agoraphobia showed it to be specific for this condition (McConaghy, 1970). With systematic desensitization, relaxed subjects are exposed in imagination to the cues that provoke their heightened tension and panic (Wolpe, 1958). If increased arousal produced by delay in completing behaviors was a major factor in producing the heightened tension in both agoraphobia and impulse disorders, systematic desensitization should also be effective in giving subjects control over impulse disorders.

The study to test the hypothesis was carried out at a time when academic behavior therapists were still markedly distrustful of treated subjects' self-reports (Chapter 1). As it had been shown that homosexual subjects' PVRs to pictures of male and female nudes did not alter following treatment, and as contacts of sex offenders were often not aware of their deviant activity, it was necessary to rely on sex offenders' self-reports as the major method of assessing change in their compulsive sexual behaviors. It was realized, however, that this would not be acceptable to editors of journals publishing behavior therapy research. The hypothesis was tested initially in compulsive gamblers, most of whom had social contacts who were aware of the gamblers' levels of debts and hence could confirm their reports as to whether or not they were continuing to gamble following treatment. The study showed that a form of treatment modified from systematic desensitization was significantly more effective than electric-shock aversive therapy in giving treated subjects control over compulsive gambling (McConaghy, Armstrong, Blaszczynski, & Allcock, 1983). My attempts to meet the requirements of behavior therapy journals were unsuccessful, and the study was rejected by a number before being accepted by a psychiatry journal. My criticisms of the single-case studies carried out by many of the reviewers for behavior therapy journals had been published at this time (McConaghy, 1977b, 1982).

The modified treatment used in the study was termed *imaginal desensitization;* however, this term is employed for other forms of systematic desensitization, all of which involve desensitization to stimuli in imagination. With systematic desensitization, patients are asked to visualize in a relaxed state the situations in which they experience anxiety. The situations are presented in order of intensity, commencing with those in which the patients experience minimal anxiety. When they can visualize these without anxiety, they progress to imagining those in which they experience somewhat greater anxiety. With the modified procedure used to treat gamblers and subsequently sex offenders, guided by the BCM model, no attempt was made to determine an order of intensity of the stimuli presented. Subjects were asked to describe four situations in which they commonly carried out the compulsive activities or thought of doing so.

Influenced by previous experience in treating phobic patients with systematic desensitization, I considered that the necessary information concerning these situations could be obtained from the patients within a few minutes, and detailed analyses of the compulsive behaviors were not required. Descriptions of four typical situations the subjects provided were altered so that they did not feel impelled to carry out the compulsive behaviors and left the situation in a relaxed state without having done so. A typical scenario for an exhibitionist would be as follows: "You are walking along a quiet street and see a teenaged girl walking towards you. As she approaches, the thought of exposing yourself comes into your mind. You realize the urge is not strong and you can control it. You walk past her without exposing." To emphasize this major aspect of the modified therapy—that the subject, in imagination and while relaxed, completes an alternative ending to the compulsive behavior—the therapy is now termed *alternative behavior completion.*

With systematic desensitization, patients were initially trained over several hours in a progressive muscular relaxation procedure (Wolpe, 1958). As discussed in Chapter 5, I along with many therapists found from clinical experience that this training could be markedly curtailed without apparent loss of therapeutic efficacy. With alternative behavior completion, the patient lies comfortably on a couch in a darkened room, with his arms by his sides and his eyes closed. He is then asked to clench his fists and to concentrate on the tension in them. After about 20 seconds, he is asked to relax them and to concentrate on the sensation of his hands feeling limp and heavy. He is then asked similarly to tense and then relax progressively his arms, legs, stomach, neck, and facial muscles while concentrating on the accompanying feeling of tension or relaxation. He is finally asked to tense further any muscle groups that feel tense and then to relax them and to signal by raising the index finger visible to the therapist when he feels relaxed. This procedure is carried out within 5 minutes, with the therapist conveying complete conviction that the patient will be relaxed at its termination. It is extremely rare for patients not to signal they are.

When the patient signals he is relaxed, the therapist instructs the patient to visualize performing the first behavior of one of the scenarios and to signal when he is doing so and is relaxed. Once he does so, after a few seconds the therapist instructs him to visualize performing the next behavior in the scenario and to signal when he is doing so and is relaxed, and so on until the patient signals he is visualizing leaving the situation without having carried out the compulsive behavior and is feeling relaxed. The four scenarios are presented in this manner in a treatment session lasting 15 to 20 minutes. Patients were admitted to a psychiatric unit for 5 days to receive two sessions of treatment the first day and three on the subsequent 4 days, with intervals of a few hours between the treatment sessions administered on the same day.

More recently, when it was not possible to admit subjects to the unit, I have audiotaped the initial treatment session and instructed the subjects to listen to the tape daily at home. At assessment a week later, a further session was taped with scenarios modified as indicated by the subjects' reported responses. The subjects' use of the tape was made less frequent over the following weeks. My impression that this method is equally effective as the inpatient administration has not yet been evaluated in a controlled comparison.

In an earlier study, electric-shock aversive therapy and covert sensitization had been shown to be equally effective in treating compulsive homosexuality (McConaghy et al., 1981). Following the demonstrated superiority of alternative behavior completion to electric-shock aversive therapy in compulsive gambling (McConaghy et al., 1983), it was shown to be superior to covert sensitization in treatment of 5 homosexual subjects and 15 sex offenders, all of whom reported difficulty in controlling sexual behaviors (McConaghy et al., 1985). They were randomly allocated so that 10 received covert sensitization and 10 alternative behavior completion.

Quinsey and Earls (1990) considered it disturbing that the literature concerning electrical aversive therapy appears to have dried up since 1983. They found no controlled studies of electrical aversion that investigated its effectiveness in reducing inappropriate sexual arousal. They also commented that the evidence for the efficacy of covert sensitization was not overwhelming and that a variety of techniques had been shown to reduce PCR evidence of sexual arousal, but it was not yet known which were most efficacious or what procedural details were the most important. I find this latter finding much more disturbing. Comparison studies would provide valuable information concerning the relative cost-effectiveness of the various techniques presently in use; however, in the current research climate, such studies may be a waste of resources. No North American workers have attempted to replicate the findings of the comparison studies of myself and my colleagues (McConaghy et al., 1981, 1983, 1985) demonstrating the superiority of the nonaversive alternative behavior completion to electric-shock and covert sensitization aversive therapies. The two forms of aversive therapy remain the major methods used to modify sexually offensive behaviors in North America.

After demonstrating that aversive therapy gave homosexual men control over their unacceptable compulsive behaviors without altering their sexual preference, I accepted that sexual preferences could not be changed and shifted the aim of treatment to give subjects control of preferences they experienced as compulsive (McConaghy, 1975, 1976). This shift in treatment aim appears to be gaining ground. Herman (1990) cited an experienced therapist as stating as follows:

> We only talk about controlling sexual deviances, about reducing them to minimal levels. Our long-range goal is to eliminate them, but we don't expect realistically to meet that goal. . . . We talk about sex offenders who do not offend any more. The conditioning patterns are ingrained in adult clients. We try to educate them to be aware of that, that it is really going to be a lifelong process. (p. 187)

Satiation Therapy

An alternative technique to aversive therapy that is also considered to reduce deviant sexual arousal is satiation. With satiation, the subject is instructed to fantasize the deviant activity for a prolonged period, usually while masturbating. As used by Marshall, Earls, Segal, and Darke (1983), the offender was instructed to masturbate continuously for 1 hour whether or not he ejaculated, while he verbalized aloud every variation he could think of concerning his deviant fantasies. As employed by Quinsey and Earls (1990), the offender fantasized aloud about sexually appropriate themes prior to ejaculation, after which he switched to deviant fantasies. Marshall et al. (1984) cited Abel and Annon as employing a self-managed version in which the subject carried out the procedure at home, recording his verbalized fantasies on a tape recorder for the therapist to check his compliance. Quinsey (1984) had earlier used a form of satiation in which the subject extensively rehearsed his deviant fantasies in a nonaroused state. No comparison of these different procedures appears to have been carried out, nor have any been demonstrated to have a specific effect in reducing subjects' deviant urges.

Behavioral Techniques to Increase Heterosexual Arousal

In the single-case studies carried out in the 1970s aimed at reorienting homosexual men to heterosexuality, evidence was advanced that behavioral techniques could increase the ability of the subjects to be sexually aroused by women. This evidence suffered from the same methodological problems discussed in relation to the single-case studies claiming that aversive therapies could modify sexual preference (i.e., exploitation of the weakness of single-case design, and use of the invalid PCR measure of homosexual and heterosexual arousal to pictures of nude men and women). At least one behavioral technique investigated in this way continues to be used. In its original form, termed *orgasmic reconditioning*, the subject was instructed to masturbate and to report when orgasm was imminent. When he did so he was shown a picture of an attractive, scantily dressed woman until he reported that he had ejaculated (Thorpe, Schmidt, & Castell, 1963). More than 10 years after its introduction, Conrad and Wincze (1976) pointed out that the evidence that the procedure was effective had not gone beyond the case-study level.

Evidence has been advanced rejecting the postulated mode of action of orgasmic reconditioning. This therapy was considered to act by classical conditioning; after a number of pairings of the heterosexual stimulus with sexual arousal produced by masturbation, the heterosexual stimulus was expected to produce sexual arousal as a conditioned response. This was shown not to occur in two studies. In one, pairing of slides of nude women with slides of nude men did not increase homosexual subjects' PVRs to pictures of nude women, although they showed strong PVRs to the slides of the males (McConaghy, 1975). The second investigated the pairing of heterosexual stimuli with sexual arousal that occurred when homosexual subjects had heterosexual intercourse. Married homosexuals who had regular intercourse with their wives did not show greater PVR evidence of heterosexual arousability than did homosexual men with no history of heterosexual intercourse (McConaghy, 1978). Again, lack of empirical evidence of the specific effectiveness of these techniques, as well as the presence of this evidence to the contrary, did not lead to any reconsideration of the use of the techniques. Marshall et al. (1983) reported that orgasmic reconditioning, also termed *masturbatory retraining*, was the most popular procedure for increasing appropriate sexual arousal and was in common use in many treatment programs in North America. At the same time, they considered that much more empirical research was required before its routine application could be accepted.

Multimodal Approaches: Cognitive-Behavioral Techniques

Since the 1970s, most treatment programs for sex offenders have added other components to the behavioral techniques aimed either to modify or to give subjects control of their sexual preferences. These include social skills training, reduction of heterosexual anxiety by systematic desensitization, and cognitive therapy to correct faulty cognitions. The resulting multimodal approaches have been termed *cognitive-behavioral techniques* (Marshall & Barbaree, 1990b).

Skills Training and Systematic Desensitization

McFall (1990) commented that social skills training was one of the more commonly prescribed treatments for rapists, pedophiles, and other sex offenders, although recent reviews had concluded that there was no general agreement as to nature of the techniques that should be used or convincing evidence of their efficacy.

As similar comments could be made of most other methods of treatment used for sex offenders, it is understandable that this situation has not discouraged the use of social skills training. McFall proposed an individualized assessment and treatment approach based on his information-processing analysis of social skills, discussed earlier. Though it had not been evaluated in comparison studies, he recommended it as more rigorous and systematic than treatments based on overly simplistic, poorly conceived, and inadequately tested models of social skills.

In my experience, though patients referred for social skills training report improvement in their social anxiety when meeting people unknown to them, they rarely significantly increase their circle of friends or sexual partners, at least in the following few years. Also, I have found that reduction in anxiety concerning adult heterosexual relations, produced by systematic desensitization in imagination to cues for these activities, rarely brings about an increase in heterosexual activity. Referral to a surrogate therapist of the sex to which the patient wishes to be attracted seems more effective in reducing anxiety concerning socializing with adults of that sex. Homosexual pedophiles and hebephiles are the offenders most in need of these therapies, in view of their disinterest in social and sexual relations with their peers; however, I have found this aspect of their condition to respond extremely rarely to a behavioral or, indeed, any psychotherapeutic approach, including prolonged individual or group psychoanalytic therapy. In the earlier studies aimed at increasing the heterosexual arousability of homosexual men, only rarely was it reported that subjects initiated heterosexual intercourse following treatment if they had not experienced it prior to treatment (McConaghy, 1982).

Cognitive Therapies

Quinsey and Earls (1990) suggested that in treating sex offenders, cognitive therapies may not require the addition of behavioral approaches. They argued that in view of the variety of behavioral treatments used to modify sexual arousal patterns, all of which appeared to be at least somewhat effective, all may act nonspecifically. Cognitive therapies such as responsibility training, development of empathy, social skills, and anger control might be equally effective. My clinical impression is that a behavioral component (aversive therapy or, preferably, alternative behavior completion) is necessary to give patients control over urges experienced as compulsive. A trial of cognitive therapy alone, behavioral therapy alone, and the two combined would resolve this issue. Such a trial appears extremely unlikely to be carried out, though, in view of the current lack of interest of therapists in empirical research findings.

W. Murphy (1990) summarized the aims of cognitive restructuring therapies with sex offenders as educating them concerning the impact of sexually offensive behaviors on the victims and the role faulty cognitions play in maintaining their sexually offensive behaviors, as well as helping them identify, explore, and challenge their specific faulty cognitions. Murphy recommended that the approach should be Socratic, following the model of Beck, rather than confrontational. He considered empathy training to be best carried out in group sessions in which victim counselors, preferably those counseling the offenders' victims, attend group sessions and discuss the impact of the victimization. Requiring offenders to read books by victims and subsequently to discuss them in groups and to write lists repeatedly of the impact of their sexual offenses on their victims were also considered of importance.

Herman (1990) stated that treatment based on the addiction model required that the offender's patterns of sexual fantasy and arousal, his modus operandi for securing access to his victims and evading detection, his preferred sexual activities, and his system of excuses and rationalizations must be painstakingly documented, and that changes must be closely monitored. She reported that some experienced therapists require that a victim impact statement describing the offender's crime be made available in the case record before any form of treatment is attempted. This should be frequently reviewed to counteract tendencies toward denial and minimization of the offense that both patient and therapist may share.

Relapse Prevention. A cognitive treatment approach termed *relapse prevention,* developed to treat addictive disorders (George & Marlatt, 1989), has been extended to treat sex offenders. George and Marlatt criticized multimodal treatment packages in common use on the basis that their aim was to produce an effect so powerful that it would not wear off. They argued that it was difficult for the patient to comply with the variety of techniques and procedures used in these packages, and that there was little recognition that maintenance might require qualitatively different analyses and interventions. Multimodal procedures were administered by the therapist, whereas maintenance procedures needed to be self-administered by the patient. In practice, relapse prevention techniques are added to multimodal packages (Laws, 1989), making the latter even more complex.

A feature of relapse prevention is the use of acronyms. The sex offender is considered to control his behavior until he encounters a high-risk situation (HRS), identified as an emotional state rather than a situation where he has previously offended; the latter HRS is the one considered important in stimulus control models. If offenders in HRSs "lapse" (i.e., willfully fantasize sexual offending), the effect of the lapse, the abstinence violation effect (AVE), will depend on the offender's cognitive attributions of the cause of the lapse and his affective reaction to this attribution. Decreased self-efficacy and pleasurable sensations associated with the lapse will increase the likelihood of "relapse" or offending. To help offenders handle HRSs, they prepare life autobiographies and self-monitor deviant urges. The therapist may need to confront offenders concerning their apparently irrelevant decisions (AIDs) or seemingly unimportant behaviors that lead to errors (SUBTLE). These are behaviors that enable the offender unconsciously to seek out HRSs; examples are pedophiles who seek jobs that involve contact with children (reporting benevolent reasons for their choice, such as their commitment to helping children) or rapists who leave home in the early morning to jog. Other avoidance strategies include recognizing and handling the PIG, the problem of immediate gratification that inches the offender closer to relapse.

R. Hall (1989) reported the use of relapse rehearsal but cautioned that it should only be employed with subjects who have made substantial behavior change in treatment. With relapse rehearsal, the offender is instructed to fantasize about a lapse occurring in a particular HRS and to imagine coping effectively with it using self-control and the coping strategies he has learned. The procedure resembles alternative behavior completion, except that the latter procedure is carried out with the patient in a state of relaxation. Skills training to recognize HRSs, PIGs, and AIDs and, where appropriate, to develop assertiveness; stress management; relaxation training; anger management; enhancement of empathy for victims; and communication skills and general social and/or dating skills are incorporated in relapse prevention, along with homework assignments to enhance self-efficacy (George & Marlatt, 1989). The final thrust is teaching the offender to achieve and maintain a balanced life-style. Positive addictions to regular exercise and substitute indulgences are encouraged.

W. Murphy (1990) pointed out that there was little literature evaluating the effect of cognitive therapies on sex offenders. He considered that treatments other than cognitive therapy, such as those for altering deviant arousal, could also produce cognitive changes.

Combined Cognitive-Behavioral, Group, and Family Approaches

Marshall and Barbaree (1990b) reported that most cognitive-behavioral programs combine individual treatment elements (e.g., procedures to change sexual preference) with group therapy components. They suggested that a group conducted by a male and female therapist provided modeling of an egalitarian male-female relationship and enabled the female's view of sexual offending to be presented. Group members provided insights into fellow patients' problems. Wolf, Conte, and Engel-Meinig (1988) followed the cognitive-behavioral treatment of sex offenders with family therapy to reintegrate the offender into the family. They videotaped the offender reenacting his deviant behavior using mannequins; while doing so, he described the behavior. The tape was replayed in the presence of his therapist to explore the offender's feelings. It could also be shown to his significant other to give her a clear idea of the reality of his behavior and to remove one more layer of secrecy from the offender. Wolf et al. stated that the significant other rarely abandoned the offender as a result of viewing these tapes. No outcome data was reported.

Herman (1990) hypothesized that as highly structured group treatment and self-help programs appeared to be the most successful modality for the social rehabilitation of addicts, this would also be true for sex offenders. She stated that such programs provide a group of peers reliably available on demand who are committed to the goal of recovery through abstinence. Through their testimony, these peers provide a constant reminder of the negative consequences of addiction and a new source of hope from their changed lives. The activities of the group provide a substitute addiction and social support. The model would appear to be that of Alcoholics Anonymous (AA), and Herman stated that most existing treatment programs have developed a group process explicitly or implicitly defining stages of recovery analogous to the 12 steps of AA. Belief in the relevance of this group process for sex offenders appears based on the theoretical identification of offenders as addicts, rather than on evidence from evaluation of its efficacy. Data concerning sex offenders against adults or female children do not suggest that they require social rehabilitation as compared to nonsexual offenders or demographically matched normals, unless knowledge of their offense has led to adverse community reaction. In this latter situation, most offenders shift to another locality. When I suggested to offenders against male children that they could benefit from learning to socialize with peers in the context of a self-help group of similar offenders, some expressed the fear that the group would function covertly to provide access to cooperative victims.

Psychodynamic Approaches

Though rarely reported, it is possible that psychodynamic approaches remain in common use to treat sex offenders. The program developed by Giarretto (1978) for treatment of families of father-daughter incest, discussed in Chapter 6, has been widely copied. Herman (1990) was critical of the use in such programs of a psychodynamic formulation of rape as an expression of the offender's insecurity and wishes for masculinity. She argued that this tended to minimize the sexual component of the offender's behavior and to reinterpret the assault as an ineffectual attempt to meet ordinary human needs, a problem more amenable to standard psychotherapy. Such treatment focused on the offender's general social attitudes and relationships or on his experiences as a victim, rather than on the concrete details of his sexual fantasies and behavior, and it failed to deal specifically with the offender's sexual desire for children.

Chemical Control, Not Chemical Castration

The use of castration in sex offenders, considered to act by reduction of their blood testosterone levels, was critically reviewed by Heim and Hursch (1979). Though it was never evaluated in appropriate comparison studies, and some offenders continued to obtain erections for many years following castration, the majority treated did not reoffend. Ethical objections to the procedure have encouraged its replacement by chemical methods of reducing offenders' sexual urges. Though little empirical research has evaluated the different chemicals employed, clinical experience has tended to favor two as combining efficacy with minimal side effects: medroxyprogesterone acetate (MPA), used mainly in North America, and cyproterone acetate (CPA), used mainly in Europe. Both reduce the offender's serum testosterone levels. Tennant (1984) reported that extensive German studies found side effects of gynecomastia in 15% to 20% and depressive reactions in 5% to 10% of subjects treated with CPA. Gagne (1981) used MPA in initial doses of 200 mg intramuscularly 2 to 3 times weekly and reduced it to 100 mg weekly to monthly as a maintenance dose. Gagne reported that the patients generally became impotent for some period of time, and all reported side effects that included fatigue, weight gain, hot and cold flashes, headaches, and insomnia.

I modified the dosage regime on the basis of a postulated mode of action derived from the behavior completion hypothesis. This was that MPA, by reducing the strength of the patients' deviant sexual urges, allowed them to control these urges in the presence of the cues that provoked them. Over a period of time, the behavior completion mechanisms for the deviant behaviors would therefore be extinguished, so that when the treatment was ceased, most patients would not experience returning deviant urges as compulsive. Other workers reported persistence of the therapeutic effect of androgen-suppressing chemicals following their withdrawal (Bradford,

1990) but did not advance a mode of action for the effect. As a standard procedure, I use 150 mg of MPA fortnightly for 2 months and then monthly for 4 months. The treatment is administered during brief outpatient visits. With this dose, subjects' testosterone levels are reduced on average to about 30% of the pretreatment levels.

In a study investigating the treatment, only 2 of the 20 subjects treated with MPA reported some degree of impotence that caused them to reduce their frequency of intercourse (McConaghy et al., 1988). The 2 subjects showed reduction of testosterone levels to 14% and 16% of their pretreatment levels, respectively; their impotence was reversed by ceasing the medication. In the study, patients were randomly allocated to MPA, to alternative behavior completion, or to both. Currently, offenders choose which of the two treatments they prefer (McConaghy, 1990b). Patients who choose MPA have their serum testosterone determined prior to the first injection. If at 1 month they still are aware of significant deviant urges, the dose is doubled. If they are experiencing partial impotence, it is temporarily ceased. In both cases, their serum testosterone level is determined again. Usually when the level is reported a few weeks later, in those subjects still aware of urges it is well above 30% of the pretreatment level; in those with partial impotence, it is reduced to below 20%. When the potency of the latter subjects returns, the MPA is recommenced at a lower dose, or they are treated with alternative behavior completion.

In this program, the only significant side effect of MPA has been reduced frequency of heterosexual activity or impotence. Both have been rare and have responded to reduction of the dose. If deviant sexual urges recur following cessation of MPA, it can be recommenced, or if the patient prefers, alternative behavior completion is used. Recurrence has been most common in homosexual pedophiles and hebephiles, presumably because of their inability to develop acceptable sexual relationships. Mentally retarded sex offenders who are unable to cooperate with alternative behavior completion commonly responded well to MPA, though some also required prolonged use.

A finding of the study by McConaghy et al. (1988) supported the theory that MPA produced its therapeutic effect by reduction in the subjects' serum testosterone levels. The degree of reduction in these levels of which both offenders and interviewer were unaware correlated strongly with the reduction of deviant sexual urges reported by the offenders. Though this reduction in urges enabled them to control their deviant behaviors, most subjects who received MPA in the dose I used maintained erections and their usual frequency of heterosexual intercourse. This treatment therefore produces chemical control, not "chemical castration" (Halleck, 1981). Subjects receiving MPA do report, however, that their sexual arousal in heterosexual relations occurs in response to physical stimulation, not to sexual cognitions. Interestingly, their penile volume responses to films of nude men and women were found to be unchanged (McConaghy & Blaszczynski, 1993), indicating, as discussed in Chapter 1, that the direction rather than the strength of sexual urges is assessed by these responses. A few of the small number of subjects who have needed to remain on MPA for some years showed a gradual return in their serum testosterone toward pretreatment levels, along with some return of deviant urges. Such patients could be expected to respond to LHRH agonists (Rousseau et al., 1988), but up to the present this therapy has been too expensive to employ in my program, the state and federal governments each considering it the other's responsibility to provide it.

Treatment in Prison and the Community

Cognitive-behavioral programs have been developed both for outpatient and incarcerated sex offenders. Duration of the programs reported varied considerably, that of one of the briefest being 4 months and of the longest 24 to 30 months in jail, followed by 3 to 6 months in a graduated release program and a further 18 months in intensive outpatient treatment (Marshall & Barbaree, 1990b). The components of the programs used in both settings do not seem to differ. Bradford (1990) suggested that the use of androgen-suppressing chemicals may not be appropriate with incarcerated subjects, whose ability to give informed consent may be compromised.

Though cognitive-behavioral approaches to the treatment of sex offenders are those most commonly reported, they may not be the most commonly employed. A nationwide survey of 553 child sexual abuse programs revealed that less than half treated offenders (Keller et al., 1989). Four percent focused on them solely, 3% on them and their families, and 35% on them, their victims, and families. The majority of the programs took a family-oriented approach, commonly based on the Giarretto model. Offenders typically were excluded if they exhibited violent behavior, psychopathology or fixated pedophilia, substance abuse, failure to accept responsibility for the abuse, and/or any of a variety of legal circumstances. Programs that provided only individual therapy focused predominantly on victims, whereas those which provided only group therapy were more likely to treat offenders.

Moore et al. (1985) concluded from a survey of Florida mental health facilities that the majority of sex offenders, of whom 41% were incest offenders, were treated in local outpatient services. They believed that this reduced stigmatization and allowed the breadwinner to maintain the family system. Many were under the supervision of the court, but 21% of the total were self-referred and 47%, the majority of whom were incest offenders, had not been convicted of any sex offense. The typical treatment of incest offenders was given in weekly sessions of 1 to 1½ hours for 10 months. Only 6 of the 48 facilities treating sex offenders provided special programs for them, 3 of which were limited to incest offenders and victims. Moore et al. pointed out that research and policy discussion of sex-offender treatment in Florida had always centered on two residential programs that served only a small proportion of treated offenders. They found that four basic approaches were used in treatment of sexual aggressors—behavioral, social skills training, psychodynamic, and organic (presumably chemical). They did not provide data on the frequency with which these treatments were employed in the facilities they surveyed.

As I believe that the compulsive aspect of sex offenses is that most susceptible to treatment and is maintained by behavior completion mechanisms activated by environmental cues for the offenses, I consider treatment needs to be carried out in the offender's usual environment. In my program, incarcerated offenders who wish to accept MPA therapy commence this a month prior to release and are then followed up as outpatients. Those who wish to receive alternative behavior completion are admitted for the week's therapy immediately following release.

EVALUATION OF TREATMENT OF SEX OFFENDERS

Marshall and Barbaree (1990b) pointed out the difficulty of evaluating the reported outcomes of treatment programs for sex offenders. They felt the ideal comparison would be with the outcome of offenders similar to those treated who were denied treatment. As discussed in Chapter 5, however, denial of treatment could cause resentment and anger, leading to a percentage reoffending. This would not occur in the group given treatment, who would therefore show a better response not attributable to the treatment. In addition, ethical requirements demand that patients accepted into treatment studies give informed consent. It would seem highly unlikely that the majority of sex offenders would agree to accept either no treatment or placebo therapy. The California Sex Offender Treatment and Evaluation Project (Laws, 1989) was apparently able to overcome this ethical problem; it was established to compare the outcome of incarcerated offenders who volunteered for 2 years of relapse prevention, including behavior therapies, with that of two untreated groups—one of treatment volunteers and one of nonvolunteers.

Evaluations of some programs have used as a basis for comparison the review of outcomes of earlier programs by Furby, Weinrott, and Blackshaw (1989). These workers, however, found the variability in outcome so great that they warned that using it for comparison purposes would allow one to conclude anything one wanted. This comment would seem equally applicable to the use of reported rates of reoffending in untreated offenders (Marshall & Barbaree, 1990b), which also varied widely. Incest offenders were found to show the lowest rates of reoffending, from 4% to 10%. Those for rapists were 7% to 35%, for nonfamilial molesters of girls, 10% to 29%, and for nonfamilial molesters of boys, 13% to 40%. Those for exhibitionists were the highest for all sex offenders, ranging from 41% to 71%.

In addition to type of offense treated, length of follow-up was of major importance in evaluating outcome. As expected, the longer the period of follow-up, the higher was the rate of reoffending. Marshall and Barbaree considered periods of less than 2 years to be inadequate. Some programs exclude offenders considered at high risk of reoffending, those who are severely brain damaged, and/or those convicted of sex offenses who deny they have a problem. Probably all exclude patients while they are actively psychotic. Some programs discharge patients who appear to be failing to respond, and others report high dropout rates. Many need to charge their clients to continue to operate and so exclude a number of offenders, yet few studies report the cost of the program. In my program, for which subjects are not charged, those who are sufficiently organized to be in stable employment (and hence could pay) show a better response.

Despite the large number of uncontrolled factors that would appear to make meaningful comparison impossible, Marshall and Barbaree concluded that existing programs varied in effectiveness in dealing with different types of offenses. Reported rates of reoffending in treated exhibitionists ranged from 7% to 48%, and some programs appeared to be more effective with homosexual and others with heterosexual child molesters. Rapists were found to be the least responsive to treatment. Marshall and Barbaree considered that therapists conducting existing programs could benefit by more closely examining the others. It seems unlikely, however, that such post hoc comparison of the outcome of unmatched groups of offenders selected by different criteria would provide useful information. Comparison by randomly allocating offenders to different programs or techniques is urgently required if cost-effective programs are to be developed to provide treatment for the large number of offenders who currently receive none. Some comparison studies are being initiated; one treating outpatient child molesters compared 20 weeks of rational-emotive cognitive therapy plus behavior therapy, followed by 20 weeks of relapse prevention, with rational-emotive therapy without behavior therapy, followed by 20 weeks of conventional follow-up. No outcome data was available when the study was reported (Laws, 1989).

In view of the need for effective programs that can treat large numbers of offenders, attempts to evaluate extremely expensive programs seem of academic rather than practical value. The California Sex Offender Treatment and Evaluation Project, referred to earlier, employed a staff of 44 to treat highly selected offenders in a 46-bed unit. It was commenced in 1985, and when reported on in 1989, only 36 treated subjects and 50 controls had been released for a mean period of 6 months or less. None had been arrested for sex crimes (Laws, 1989). A major problem with current treatment programs is that they are available to only a small percentage of offenders. It is possible that if they were readily available, more undetected offenders would seek help. My program described above, offering offenders either alternative behavior completion or a course of MPA, was developed to treat the maximum number of subjects with limited resources. Two therapists, each working for 10 hours a week, are able to treat four new offenders weekly. Active treatment of most patients is completed in 1 week with inpatient administered alternative behavior completion, or in eight outpatient visits over 6 months with outpatient administered alternative behavior completion or MPA. Follow-up interviews are conducted at monthly intervals or longer. Most offenders can meet these requirements, and so the dropout is low.

Comparison of programs utilizing minimal resources to treat a maximal number of subjects with highly resourced programs treating few subjects would appear to be an urgent requirement for effective provision of services. Such comparison would require the random allocation of offenders to the two types of programs. Even if low-resource programs produce results somewhat inferior to those of highly resourced programs, they could be more cost-effective given the large number of offenders, both detected and undetected. If 100 offenders are treated with a 70% success rate, the offending population is reduced by 70; if 10 are treated with a 90% success rate, it is reduced by 9.

Current outcome results do not indicate superiority for either type of program. In a comparison study of alternative behavior completion, MPA, and the two combined, 28 of 30 sex offenders ceased deviant behavior at 1 year following commencement of treatment. Two of the 28 had required the addition of electric-shock aversive therapy (McConaghy et al., 1988). Three relapsed in the following 2 - 5 years, but responded to the reinstitution of MPA. These results seem comparable with those of multimodal programs that required much longer periods of staff-patient contact. Of 100 sex offenders treated over a 3-year period, 8 were charged during the 3 years. The number ceasing deviant behavior was not reported (Maletzky, 1980b). Eighty-nine percent of 44 treated sex offenders contacted after 6 months and 79% of 19 contacted after 12 months reported no further deviant activity (Travin, Bluestone, Coleman, Cullen, & Melella, 1986). Marshall and Barbaree (1988) compared the outcome of 68 treated and 58 untreated child molesters. Subjects were not randomly allocated to treatment or no treatment. Five percent of the treated group reoffended in 1 to 2 years, and 25% in 4 years. The reoffense rate was significantly less than that of the untreated subjects only after 4 years, when 60% of the untreated group had reoffended.

RESPONSE TO TREATMENT OF DIFFERENT SEX OFFENSES

Insufficient numbers of treated offenders have been investigated to establish figures for the reoffense rates of different offenders. Despite the high rate of reported reoffending of untreated exhibitionists (41% to 71%), my experience is that they and voyeurs are among the least likely to relapse of the offenders treated in my program, with less than 5% reoffending. Both findings are consistent with the clinical impression that exhibitionism and voyeurism are the most compulsive of sex offenses, given that the program focuses on treating patients' compulsive urges. Kroth (1979) found that heterosexual pedophiles, particularly incest offenders, rarely reoffended following treatment, an average of 2% being reported. This could be in part attributable to reduced opportunities following detection of their offense, or because (as in the Giarretto program) they are treated when the mean age of the victim is 12 to 13 years (Kroth, 1979), close to the age when incestuous abuse usually ceases (Faller, 1989; Herman, 1985). The mean age of incest victims in population samples is well below this (Russell, 1983). In my experience, fetishists are somewhat more resistant to treatment and probably respond better to MPA than cognitive-behavioral approaches alone, consistent with the possibility that a biological factor is involved. Like other workers (Freund, Heasman, & Roper, 1982; Quinsey, 1986), I have found homosexual pedophiles least likely to change. They commonly required prolonged chemical reduction of their sexual interest. In my experience, adolescent as compared to adult offenders have required more intensive treatment, independent of the nature of their offense (McConaghy et al., 1989).

PREVENTION

As pointed out in Chapter 6, few efforts have been directed toward implementing possible strategies that could reduce men's likelihood of sexually coercing women, apart from treatment for the few who have offended, been reported, and convicted. I believe an obvious need is the inclusion in school and media educational programs of the little-acknowledged information concerning the propensity of a significant percentage of men to be sexually aroused by female children. The initial offense of many molesters of children occurs in response to an unexpected opportunity in which they experience this arousal, of which they were previously unaware they were capable. If they had been educated concerning this possibility that they could be sexually aroused by girl children, they may have avoided the opportunity or been ready to control (rather than act on) the arousal when it suddenly occurred. Burgess and Hazelwood (1983) pointed out that a number of relatives or close associates of victims of sexual asphyxia had noticed evidence of the behavior prior to the fatalities. Lacking knowledge of the condition, they failed to attach the significance to this evidence that might have led them to encourage the subjects to obtain treatment. Awareness of the prevalence of sexually offensive behaviors should encourage potential victims to adopt the strategies, discussed in Chapter 7, that would render them less at risk.

Public education concerning the nature of deviant sexual practices, the number of otherwise normal people who carry them out, and the availability of inexpensive treatment could have advantages additional to reducing the shame, and therefore increasing the motivation to seek help, of those sex offenders who wished but have been unable to cease their behaviors.

References

Abel, G. G., Barlow, D. H., Blanchard, E. B., & Guild, D. (1977). The components of rapists' sexual arousal. *Archives of General Psychiatry, 34,* 895–903.

Abel, G. G., Becker, J. V., Blanchard, E. B., & Djenderedjian, A. (1978). Differentiating sexual aggressives with penile measures. *Criminal Justice and Behavior, 5,* 315–332.

Abel, G. G., Becker, J. V., Cunningham-Rathner, J., Mittelman, M., & Rouleau, J.-L. (1988). Multiple paraphilic diagnoses among sex offenders. *Bulletin of the American Academy of Psychiatry and Law, 16,* 153–168.

Abel, G. G., Becker, J. V., Murphy, W. D., & Flanagan, F. (1981). Identifying dangerous child molesters. In R. B. Stuart (Ed.), *Violent behavior: Learning approaches to prediction, management and treatment.* New York: Brunner/Mazel.

Abramson, P. R., & Hayashi, H. (1984). Pornography in Japan: Cross-cultural and theoretical considerations. In N. M. Malamuth & E. Donnerstein (Eds.), *Pornography and sexual aggression* (pp. 173–183). New York: Academic Press.

Adamopoulos, D. A. Kampyli, S., Georgiacodis, F., Kapolla, N., & Abrahamian-Michalakis, A. (1988). Effects of antiandrogen-estrogen treatment on sexual and endocrine parameters in hirsute women. *Archives of Sexual Behavior, 17,* 421–429.

Adams, D. B., Gold, A. R., & Burt, A. D. (1978). Rise in female-initiated sexual activity at ovulation and its suppression by oral contraceptives. *New England Journal of Medicine, 299,* 1145–1150.

Adams, J. A., Ahmad, M., & Phillips, P. (1988). Anogenital findings and hymenal diameter in children referred for sexual abuse examination. *Adolescent and Pediatric Gynaecology, 1,* 123–127.

Adkins, E., & Jehu, D. (1985). Analysis of a treatment program for primary orgastic dysfunction. *Behavior Research and Therapy, 23,* 119–126.

Ageton, S. S. (1983). *Sexual assault among adolescents.* Lexington, MA: Lexington Books.

Alford, G. S., Wedding, D., & Jones, S. (1985). Faking "turn-ons" and "turn-offs." *Behavior Modification, 7,* 112–125.

Allen, D. M. (1980). Young male prostitutes: A psychosocial study. *Archives of Sexual Behavior, 9,* 399–426.

Alter-Reid, K., Gibbs, M. S., Lachenmeyer, J. R., Sigal, J., & Massoth, N. A. (1986). Sexual abuse of children: A review of the empirical findings. *Clinical Psychology Review, 6,* 249–266.

Althof, S. E., Turner, L. A., Levine, S. B., Risen, C., Kursh, E. D., Bodner, D., & Resnick, M. (1987). Intracavernosal injection in the treatment of impotence: A prospective study of sexual, psychological, and marital functioning. *Journal of Sex and Marital Therapy, 13,* 155–167.

Altshuler, K. Z. (1984). On the question of bisexuality. *American Journal of Psychotherapy, 38,* 484–493.

Alzate, H. (1984). Sexual behavior of unmarried Columbian university students: A five-year follow-up. *Archives of Sexual Behavior, 13,* 121–132.

Alzate, H. (1985). Vaginal eroticism: A replication study. *Archives of Sexual Behavior, 14,* 529–537.

Alzate, H. (1990). Vaginal erogeneity, "female ejaculation," and the "Grafenberg spot." *Archives of Sexual Behavior, 19,* 607–611.

Amberson, J. I., & Hoon, P. W. (1985). Hemodynamics of sequential orgasm. *Archives of Sexual Behavior, 14,* 351–360.

American Psychiatric Association. (1974). Position statement on homosexuality and human rights. *American Journal of Psychiatry, 131,* 497.

American Psychiatric Association. (1980). *Diagnostic and statistical manual of mental disorders* (3rd ed.). Washington, DC: Author.

American Psychiatric Association. (1987). *Diagnostic and statistical manual of mental disorders* (3rd ed., rev.). Washington, DC: Author.

Antonovosky, H. F., Kav-venaki, S., Lancet, M., Modan, B., & Shoham, I. (1980). *Adolescent sexuality.* Lexington, MA: Lexington Books.

Appel, M. A., Saab, P. G., & Holroyd, K. A. (1985). Cardiovascular disorders. In M. Hersen & A. S. Bellack (Eds.), *Handbook of clinical behavior therapy with adults* (pp. 381–416). New York: Plenum.

Araji, S., & Finkelhor, D. (1985). Explanations of pedophilia: Review of empirical research. *Bulletin of the American Academy of Psychiatry and Law, 13,* 17–37.

Aries, P. (1973). *Centuries of childhood.* Harmondsworth: Penguin.

Armsworth, M. W. (1989). Therapy of incest survivors: Abuse or support? *Child Abuse and Neglect, 13,* 549–562.

Asher, S. J. (1988). The effects of childhood sexual abuse: A review of the issues and evidence. In L. E. A. Walker (Ed.), *Handbook on sexual abuse of children* (pp. 3–18). New York: Springer.

Atkinson, J. H., Jr., Grant, I., Kennedy, C. J., Richman, D. D., Spector, S. A., & McCutchan, J. A. (1988). Prevalence of psychiatric disorders among men infected with human immunodeficiency virus: A controlled study. *Archives of General Psychiatry, 45,* 859–864.

AuBuchon, P. G., & Calhoun, K. S. (1985). Menstrual cycle symptomatology: The role of social expectancy and experimental demand characteristics. *Psychosomatic Medicine, 47,* 35–45.

Avery-Clark, C. A., & Laws, D. R. (1984). Differential erection response patterns of sexual child abusers to stimuli describing activities with children. *Behavior Therapy, 15,* 71–83.

Bakwin, H. (1960). Transvestism in children. *Journal of Pediatrics, 56,* 294–298.

Bakwin, H. (1968). Deviant gender-role in children: Relation to homosexuality. *Pediatrics, 41,* 620–629.

Bakwin, H., & Bakwin, R. M. (1953). Homosexual behavior in children. *Journal of Pediatrics, 43,* 108–111.

Baldwin, J. D., & Baldwin, J. I. (1989). The socialization of homosexuality and heterosexuality in a non-Western society. *Archives of Sexual Behavior, 18,* 13–29.

Bancroft, J. (1971). The application of psychophysiological measures to the assessment and modification of sexual behavior. *Behavior Research and Therapy, 9,* 119–130.

Bancroft, J., & Wu, F. C. W. (1983). Changes in erectile responsiveness during androgen replacement therapy. *Archives of Sexual Behavior, 12,* 59–66.

Bancroft, J., Jones, H. C., & Pullan, B. P. (1966). A simple transducer for measuring penile erections with comments of its use in the treatment of sexual disorders. *Behavior Research and Therapy, 4,* 239–241.

Barbaree, H. E. (1990). Stimulus control of sexual arousal. In W. L. Marshall, D. R. Laws, & H. E. Barbaree (Eds.), *Handbook of sexual assault* (pp. 115–142). New York: Plenum.

Barbaree, H. E., Marshall, W. L., & Lanthier, R. D. (1979). Deviant sexual arousal in rapists. *Behavior Research and Therapy, 17,* 215–222.

Bard, L. A., Carter, D. L., Cerce, D. D., Knight, R. A., Rosenberg, R., & Schneider, B. (1987). A descriptive study of rapists and child molesters: Developmental, clinical, and criminal characteristics. *Behavioral Sciences and the Law, 5,* 203–220.

Barker, J. C. (1966). Transsexualism and transvestism. *Journal of the American Medical Association, 198,* 254.

Barlow, D. H. (1973). Increasing heterosexual responsiveness in the treatment of sexual deviation: A review of the clinical and experimental evidence. *Behavior Therapy, 4,* 655–671.

Barlow, D. H., Abel, G. G., & Blanchard, E. B. (1977). Gender identity change in a transsexual: An exorcism. *Archives of Sexual Behavior, 6,* 387–395.

Barlow, D. H., Abel, G. G., & Blanchard, E. B. (1979). Gender identity change in transsexuals. *Archives of General Psychiatry, 36,* 1001–1007.

Barlow, D. H., & Agras, W. S. (1973). Fading to increase heterosexual responsiveness in homosexuals. *Journal of Applied Behavior Analysis, 6,* 355–366.

Barlow, D. H., Reynolds, E. J., & Agras, W. S. (1973). Gender identity change in a transsexual. *Archives of General Psychiatry, 28,* 560–576.

Barr, R. F., & McConaghy, N. (1971). Penile volume responses to appetitive and aversive stimuli in relation to sexual orientation and conditioning performance. *British Journal of Psychiatry, 119*, 377–383.

Barrett, F. M. (1980). Sexual experience, birth control usage, and sex education of unmarried Canadian university students: Changes between 1968–1978. *Archives of Sexual Behavior, 9*, 367–390.

Bart, P. B. (1979). Rape as a paradigm of sexism in society—victimization and its discontents. *Women's Studies International Quarterly, 2*, 347–357.

Bart, P. B. (1981). A study of women who both were raped and avoided rape. *Journal of Social Issues, 37*, 123–137.

Bart, P. B., & O'Brien, P. H. (1984). Stopping rape: Effective avoidance strategies. *Signs: Journal of Women in Culture and Society, 10*, 83–101.

Bates, J. E., Bentler, P. M., & Thompson, S. K. (1973). Measurement of deviant gender development in boys. *Child Development, 44*, 591–598.

Baxter, D. J., Barbaree, H. E., & Marshall, W. L. (1986). Sexual responses to consenting and forced sex in a large sample of rapists and non-rapists. *Behavior Research and Therapy, 24*, 513–520.

Baxter, D. J., Marshall, W. L., Barbaree, H. E., Davidson, P. R., & Malcolm, P. B. (1984). Deviant sexual behavior: Differentiating sex offenders by criminal and personal history, psychometric measures, and sexual response. *Criminal Justice and Behavior, 11*, 477–501.

Baylis, M. G., & Myers, A. M. (1990). Combating sexual assault: An evaluation of a prevention program. *Canadian Journal of Public Health, 81*, 341–344.

Beck, J. C., Borenstein, N., & Dreyfus, J. (1986). The relationship between verdict, defendant characteristics, and type of crime in sex-related criminal cases. *Bulletin of the American Academy of Psychiatry and Law, 13*, 141–146.

Beck, J. G., & Davies, D. K. (1987). Teen contraception: A review of perspectives on compliance. *Archives of Sexual Behavior, 16*, 337–368.

Becker, J. V., Skinner, L. J., Abel, G. G., Axelrod, R., & Treacy, E. C. (1984). Depressive symptoms associated with sexual assault. *Journal of Sex and Marital Therapy, 10*, 185–192.

Becker, J. V., Skinner, L. J., Abel, G. G., & Treacy, E. C. (1982). Incidence and types of sexual dysfunctions in rape and incest victims. *Journal of Sex and Marital Therapy, 8*, 65–74.

Becker, M. H., & Joseph, J. G. (1988). AIDS and behavioral change to reduce risk: A review. *American Journal of Public Health, 78*, 394–410.

Bell, A. P., & Weinberg, M. S. (1978). *Homosexualities: A study of diversity among men and women.* New York: Macmillan.

Bellack, A. S., & Hersen, M. (1985). General considerations. In A. S. Bellack & M. Hersen (Eds.), *Handbook of clinical behavior therapy with adults* (pp. 3–19). New York: Plenum.

Bellack, A. S., & Hersen, M. (1988). Future directions of behavioral assessment. In A. S. Bellack & M. Hersen (Eds.), *Behavioral assessment* (3rd ed., pp. 610–615). New York: Pergamon.

Bellack, A. S., Hersen, M., & Lamparaski, D. (1979). Role-play tests for assessing social skills: Are they valid? Are they useful? *Journal of Consulting and Clinical Psychology, 47*, 335–342.

Bem, S. L. (1974). The measurement of psychological androgyny. *Journal of Consulting and Clinical Psychology, 42*, 155–162.

Bem, S. L. (1981). Gender schema theory: A cognitive account of sex typing. *Psychological Review, 88*, 354–364.

Bender, L., & Blau, A. (1937). The reaction of children to sexual relations with adults. *American Journal of Orthopsychiatry, 7*, 500–518.

Bender, L., & Paster, S. (1941). Homosexual trends in children. *American Journal of Orthopsychiatry, 11*, 730–743.

Bene, E. (1965a). On the genesis of male homosexuality: An attempt to clarify the role of the patients. *British Journal of Psychiatry, 111*, 803–813.

Bene, E. (1965b). On the genesis of female homosexuality. *British Journal of Psychiatry, 111*, 815–821.

Benedik, E. P., & Schetky, D. H. (1987). Problems in validating allegations of sexual abuse. Part 1: Factors affecting perception and recall of events. *Journal of the American Academy of Child and Adolescent Psychiatry, 26*, 912–915.

Benjamin, H. (1954). Transsexualism and transvestism as psychosomatic and somatopsychic syndromes. *American Journal of Psychotherapy, 8*, 219–230.

Benjamin, H. (1966). *The transsexual phenomenon.* New York: Julian.

Bennett, G., Chapman, S., & Bray, F. (1989). Sexual practices and "beats": AIDS-related sexual practices in a sample of homosexual and bisexual men in the western area of Sydney. *Medical Journal of Australia, 151,* 309–314.

Bentler, P. M. (1976). A typology of transsexualism: Gender identity theory and data. *Archives of Sexual Behavior, 5,* 567–584.

Berlin, F. S., & Meinecke, C. F. (1981). Treatment of sex offenders with antiandrogenic medication: Conceptualization, review of treatment modalities, and preliminary findings. *American Journal of Psychiatry, 138,* 601–607.

Berlin, I. (1990). Joseph de Maistre and the origins of fascism: III. *New York Review of Books, 37,* 61–65.

Berliner, L. (1985). The child and the criminal justice system. In A. W. Burgess (Ed.), *Rape and sexual assault* (pp. 199–208). New York: Garland.

Bieber, I. (1962). *Homosexuality.* New York: Basic Books.

Birk, L., Huddleston, W., Miller, E., & Cohler, B. (1971). Avoidance conditioning for homosexuality. *Archives of General Psychiatry, 25,* 623–630.

Blair, D. C., & Lanyon, R. I. (1981). Exhibitionism: Etiology and treatment. *Psychological Bulletin, 89,* 439–463.

Blake, D. J., McCartney, C. Fried, F. A., & Fehrenbaker, L. G. (1983). Psychiatric assessment of penile implant recipient. *Urology, 21,* 252–256.

Blanchard, R., & Clemmensen, L. H. (1988). A test of the DSM-III-R's implicit assumption that fetishistic arousal and gender dysphoria are mutually exclusive. *Journal of Sex Research, 25,* 426–432.

Blanchard, R., Clemmensen, L. H., & Steiner, B. W. (1987). Heterosexual and homosexual gender dysphoria. *Archives of Sexual Behavior, 16,* 139–152.

Blanchard, R., Steiner, B. W., Clemmensen, L. H., & Dickey, R. (1989). Prediction of regret in postoperative transsexuals. *Canadian Journal of Psychiatry, 34,* 43–45.

Blendon, R. J., & Donelan, K. (1988). Discrimination against people with AIDS. *New England Journal of Medicine, 319,* 1022–1026.

Blumstein, P., & Schwartz, P. (1983). *American couples.* New York: William Morris.

Bogren, L. Y. (1991). Changes in sexuality in women and men during pregnancy. *Archives of Sexual Behavior, 20,* 35–45.

Bolling, D. R. (1977). Prevalence, goals and complications of heterosexual anal intercourse in a gynecologic population. *Journal of Reproductive Medicine, 19,* 120–124.

Bolling, D. R., & Voeller, B. (1987). AIDS and heterosexual anal intercourse. *Journal of the American Medical Association, 258,* 474.

Borneman, E. (1980). Progress in empirical research on children's sexuality. *Siecus Report, 12,* 1–6.

Bourget, D., & Bradford, J. M. W. (1990). Homicidal parents. *Canadian Journal of Psychiatry, 35,* 233–238.

Bowie, S. I., Silverman, D. C., Kalick, S. M., & Edbril, S. D. (1990). Blitz rape and confidence rape: Implications for clinical intervention. *American Journal of Psychotherapy, 44,* 180–188.

Bozett, F. W. (1989). Gay fathers: A review of the literature. *Journal of Homosexuality, 8,* 137–162.

Bradford, J. M. W. (1990). The antiandrogen and hormonal treatment of sex offenders. In W. L. Marshall, D. R. Laws, & H. E. Barbaree (Eds.), *Handbook of sexual assault* (pp. 297–310). New York: Plenum.

Brassard, M. R., Tyler, A. H., & Kehle, T. J. (1983). School programs to prevent intrafamilial child sexual abuse. *Child Abuse and Neglect, 7,* 241–245.

Brecher, E. M. (1984). *Love, sex and aging.* Boston: Little, Brown.

Breslow, N., Evans, L., & Langley, J. (1985). On the prevalence and roles of females in the sadomasochistic subculture: Report of an empirical study. *Archives of Sexual Behavior, 14,* 303–319.

Bretschneider, J. G., & McCoy, N. L. (1988). Sexual interest and behavior in healthy 80- to 102-year-olds. *Archives of Sexual Behavior, 17,* 109–129.

Bridges, C. F., Critelli, J. W., & Loos, V. E. (1985). Hypnotic susceptibility, inhibitory control, and orgasmic consistency. *Archives of Sexual Behavior, 14,* 373–376.

Briere, J., Evans, D., Runtz, M., & Wall, T. (1988). Symptomatology in men who were molested as children: A comparison study. *American Journal of Orthopsychiatry, 58,* 457–461.

Brincat, M., Magos, A., Studd, J. W. W., Cardozo, L. D., O'Dowd, T., Wardle, P. J., & Cooper, D. (1984). Subcutaneous hormone implants for the control of climacteric symptoms. *Lancet, 330,* 16–18.

Brittain, R. P. (1970). The sadistic murderer. *Medicine, Science and the Law, 10,* 198–207.

Brooks-Gunn, J., Boyer, C. B., & Hein, K. (1988). Preventing HIV infection and AIDS in children and adolescents. *American Psychologist, 43,* 958–964.

Brooks-Gunn, J., & Furstenberg, F. F. (1989). Adolescent sexual behavior. *American Psychologist, 44,* 249–257.

Broverman, I. K., Vogel, S. R., Broverman, D. M., Clarkson, F. E., & Rosenkrantz, P. S. (1972). Sex-role stereotypes: A current appraisal. *Journal of Social Issues, 28,* 59–78.

Brown, G. R., & Collier, L. (1989). Transvestites' women revisited: A nonpatient sample. *Archives of Sexual Behavior, 18,* 73–83.

Brown, P. (1983). The Swedish approach to sex education and adolescent pregnancy: Some impressions. *Family Planning Perspectives, 15,* 90–95.

Brown, W. A., Monti, P. M., & Corriveau, D. P. (1978). Serum testosterone and sexual activity and interest in men. *Archives of Sexual Behavior, 7,* 97–104.

Browne, A., & Finkelhor, D. (1986). Impact of child sexual abuse: A review of the research. *Psychological Bulletin, 99,* 66–77.

Buckman, F. G. (1974). Discussion: Nontranssexual men who seek sex reassignment. *American Journal of Psychiatry, 131,* 440–441.

Buhrich, N. (1977a). *Clinical study of heterosexual male transvestism.* Sydney: University of New South Wales.

Buhrich, N. (1977b). Transvestism in history. *Journal of Nervous and Mental Disease, 165,* 64–66.

Buhrich, N., & McConaghy, N. (1976). Transvestite fiction. *Journal of Nervous and Mental Disease, 163,* 420–427.

Buhrich, N., & McConaghy, N. (1977a). Clinical comparison of transvestism and transsexualism. *Australian and New Zealand Journal of Psychiatry, 6,* 83–86.

Buhrich, N., & McConaghy, N. (1977b). The clinical syndromes of femmiphilic transvestism. *Archives of Sexual Behavior, 6,* 397–412.

Buhrich, N., & McConaghy, N. (1977c). The discrete syndromes of transvestism and transsexualism. *Archives of Sexual Behavior, 6,* 483–495.

Buhrich, N., & McConaghy, N. (1978a). Two clinically discrete syndromes of transsexualism. *British Journal of Psychiatry, 133,* 73–76.

Buhrich, N., & McConaghy, N. (1978b). Parental relationships during childhood in homosexuality, transvestism and transsexualism. *Australian and New Zealand Journal of Psychiatry, 12,* 103–108.

Buhrich, N., & McConaghy, N. (1979). Three clinically distinct categories of fetishistic transvestism. *Archives of Sexual Behavior, 8,* 151–157.

Burgess, A. W. (1985). Sexual victimization of adolescents. In A. W. Burgess (Ed.), *Rape and sexual assault* (pp. 199–208). New York: Garland.

Burgess, A. W., & Hazelwood, R. R. (1983). Autoerotic asphyxial deaths and social network response. *American Journal of Orthopsychiatry, 53,* 166–170.

Burgess, A. W., & Holmstrom, L. L. (1974). Rape trauma syndrome. *American Journal of Psychiatry, 131,* 981–986.

Burgess, A. W., & Holmstrom, L. L. (1980). Rape typology and the coping behavior of rape victims. In S. L. McCombie (Ed.), *Rape crisis intervention handbook* (pp. 27–42). New York: Plenum.

Burgess, A. W., & Holmstrom, L. L. (1985). Rape trauma syndrome and post traumatic stress response. In A. W. Burgess (Ed.), *Rape and sexual assault* (pp. 46–60). New York: Garland.

Burgess, A. W., Groth, A. N., & McCausland, M. P. (1981). Child sex initiation rings. *American Journal of Orthopsychiatry, 51,* 110–119.

Burnam, M. A., Stein, J. A., Golding, J. M., Siegel, J. M., Sorenson, S. B., Forsythe, A. B., & Telles, C. A. (1988). Sexual assault and mental disorders in a community population. *Journal of Consulting and Clinical Psychology, 56,* 843–850.

Burt, M. R. (1980). Cultural myths and support for rape. *Journal of Personality and Social Psychology, 38,* 217–230.

Burt, M. R., & Katz, B. L. (1988). Coping strategies and recovery from rape. *Annals of the New York Academy of Sciences, 528,* 345–358.

Butler, C. A. (1976). New data about female sex response. *Journal of Sex and Marital Therapy, 2,* 40–46.

Buvat, J., Lemaire, A., Buvat-Herbaut, M., Fourlinnie, J. C., Racadot, A., & Fossati, P. (1985). Hyperprolactinemia and sexual function in men. *Hormone Research, 22,* 196–203.

Buvat, J., Lemaire, A., Buvat-Herbaut, M., Guieu, J. D., Bailleul, J. P., & Fossati, P. (1985). Comparative investigations in 26 impotent and 26 nonimpotent diabetic patients. *Journal of Urology, 133,* 34–38.

Byard, R. W., Hucker, S. J., & Hazelwood, R. R. (1990). A comparison of typical death scene features in cases of fatal male and female autoerotic asphyxia with a review of the literature. *Forensic Science International, 48,* 113–121.

Byers, E. S., & Heinlein, L. (1989). Predicting initiations and refusals of sexual activity in married and cohabitating heterosexual couples. *Journal of Sex Research, 26,* 210–231.

Byrne, D. (1983). Sex without contraception. In D. Byrne & W. A. Fisher (Eds.), *Adolescents, sex and contraception* (pp. 1–31). London: Lawrence Erlbaum.

Calderone, M. S. (1979). Childhood sexuality and the pediatrician. *American Journal of Diseases of Children, 133,* 685–686.

Calderone, M. S. (1985). Adolescent sexuality: Elements and genesis. *Pediatrics, 76*(4), 699–703.

Cammaert, L. P. (1988). Nonoffending mothers: A new conceptualization. In L. E. A. Walker (Ed.), *Handbook on sexual abuse of children* (pp. 309–325). New York: Springer.

Campion, E., & Tucker, G. (1973). A note on twin studies, schizophrenia and neurological impairment. *Archives of General Psychiatry, 29,* 460–464.

Cantwell, H. B. (1981). Sexual abuse of children in Denver, 1979: Reviewed with implications for pediatric intervention and possible prevention. *Child Abuse and Neglect, 5,* 75–85.

Cantwell, H. B. (1983). Vaginal inspection as it relates to child sexual abuse in girls under thirteen. *Child Abuse and Neglect, 7,* 171–176.

Carani, C., Zini, D., Baldini, A., Della Casa, L., Ghizzani, A., & Marrama, P. (1990). Effects of androgen treatment in impotent men with normal and low levels of free testosterone. *Archives of Sexual Behavior, 19,* 223–234.

Carlson, G. A., Greeman, M., & McClellan, T. A. (1989). Management of HIV-positive psychiatric patients who fail to reduce high-risk behaviors. *Hospital and Community Psychiatry, 40,* 511–514.

Carroll, J. L., Volk, K. D., & Hyde, J. S. (1985). Differences between males and females in motives for engaging in sexual intercourse. *Archives of Sexual Behavior, 14,* 131–139.

Carver, C. M., Stalker, C., Stewart, E., & Abraham, B. (1989). The impact of group therapy for adult survivors of childhood sexual abuse. *Canadian Journal of Psychiatry, 34,* 753–758.

Catalan, J., Hawton, K., & Day, A. (1990). Couples referred to a sexual dysfunction clinic psychological and physical morbidity. *British Journal of Psychiatry, 156,* 61–67.

Catania, J. A., Pollack, L., McDermott, L. J., Qualls, S. H., & Cole, L. (1990). Help-seeking behaviors of people with sexual problems. *Archives of Sexual Behavior, 19,* 235–250.

Cavanagh Johnson, T. (1989). Female child perpetrators: Children who molest other children. *Child Abuse and Neglect, 13,* 571–585.

Chakravarti, S., Collins, W. P., Thom, M. H., & Studd, J. W. W. (1979). Relation between plasma hormone profiles, symptoms, and response to estrogen treatment in women approaching the menopause. *British Medical Journal, 1,* 983–985.

Chalkley, A. J., & Powell, G. E. (1983). The clinical description of forty-eight cases of sexual fetishism. *British Journal of Psychiatry, 142,* 292–295.

Chambers, K. C., & Phoenix, C. H. (1982). Sexual behavior in old male rhesus monkeys: Influence of familiarity and age of female partners. *Archives of Sexual Behavior, 11,* 299–308.

Chapman, J. D. (1968). Frigidity: Rapid treatment by reciprocal inhibition. *Journal of the American Osteopathic Association, 67,* 871–878.

Christopher, F. S. (1988). An initial investigation into a continuum of premarital sexual pressure. *Journal of Sex Research, 25,* 255–266.

Clark, J. P., & Tifft, L. L. (1966). Polygraph and interview validation of self-reported deviant behavior. *American Sociological Review, 31,* 516–523.

Clark, R. D., & Hatfield, E. (1989). Gender differences in receptivity to sexual offenders. *Journal of Psychology and Human Sexuality, 2,* 39–55.

Clement, U., Schmidt, G., & Kruse, M. (1984). Changes in sex differences in sexual behavior: A replication of a study on West German students (1966–1981). *Archives of Sexual Behavior, 13,* 99–120.

Clifford, R. (1978). Development of masturbation in college women. *Archives of Sexual Behavior, 7,* 559–573.

Cohn, A. H., & Daro, D. (1987). Is treatment too late? What ten years of evaluative research tell us. *Child Abuse and Neglect, 11,* 433–442.

Coles, C. D., & Shamp, M. J. (1984). Some sexual, personality, and demographic characteristics of women readers of erotic romances. *Archives of Sexual Behavior, 13,* 187–209.

Condy, S. R., Templer, D. I., Brown, R., & Veaco, L. (1987). Parameters of sexual contact of boys with women. *Archives of Sexual Behavior, 16,* 379–394.

Conrad, S. R., & Winzee, J. P. (1976). Orgasmic reconditioning: A controlled study of its effects upon the sexual arousal and behavior of adult male homosexuals. *Behavior Therapy, 7,* 155–166.

Constantine, L. L. (1981). The effects of early sexual experiences. In L. L. Constantine & F. Martinson (Eds.), *Children and sex* (pp. 217–244). Boston: Little, Brown.

Constantinople, A. (1973). Masculinity-femininity: An exception to the famous dictum? *Psychological Bulletin, 80,* 389–407.

Constantinople, A. (1979). Sex-role acquisition: In search of the elephant. *Sex Roles, 5,* 121–133.

Conte, H. R. (1983). Development and use of self-report techniques for assessing sexual functioning: A review and critique. *Archives of Sexual Behavior, 12,* 555–576.

Conte, J. R., & Berliner, L. (1988). The impact of sexual abuse on children: Empirical findings. In L. E. A. Walker (Ed.), *Handbook on sexual abuse of children* (pp. 72–93). New York: Springer.

Cook, T. D., & Campbell, D. T. (1979). *Quasi-experimentation.* Chicago: Rand McNally.

Cooper, A. J. (1969). Some personality factors in frigidity *Journal of Psychosomatic Research, 2,* 241–265.

Cooper, A. J. (1987). Preliminary experience with a vacuum constriction device (VCD) as a treatment for impotence. *Journal of Psychosomatic Research, 31,* 413–418.

Copeland, A. R. (1985). Teenage suicide—the five-year Metro Dade County experience from 1979 until 1983. *Forensic Sciences International, 28,* 27–33.

Courtois, C. A., & Sprei, J. E. (1988). Retrospective incest therapy for women. In L. E. A. Walker (Ed.), *Handbook on sexual abuse of children* (pp. 270–308). New York: Springer.

Crepault, C., & Couture, M. (1980). Men's erotic fantasies. *Archives of Sexual Behavior, 9,* 565–581.

Croughan, J. I., Saghir, M., Cohen, R., & Robins, E. (1981). A comparison of treated and untreated male cross-dressers. *Archives of Sexual Behavior, 10,* 515–528.

Curran, D., Partridge, M., & Storey, P. (1980). *Psychological medicine.* Edinburgh: Churchill Livingstone.

Cutler, W. B., Garcia, C. R., & McCoy, N. (1987). Perimenopausal sexuality. *Archives of Sexual Behavior, 16,* 225–235.

Cvetkovich, G., & Grote, B. (1983). Adolescent development and teenage fertility. In D. Byrne & W. A. Fisher (Eds.), *Adolescents, sex and contraception* (pp. 109–123). London: Lawrence Erlbaum.

D'Agostino, R. B., Burgess, A. W., Belanger, A. J., Guio, M. V., Guio, J. J., Gould, R., & Montan, C. (1985). Investigation of sex crimes against children. In A. W. Burgess (Ed.), *Rape and sexual assault* (pp. 110–122). New York: Garland.

Darke, J. L. (1990). Sexual aggression: Achieving power through humiliation. In W. L. Marshall, D. R. Laws & H. E. Barbaree (Eds.), *Handbook of sexual assault* (pp. 55–72). New York: Plenum.

Darling, C. A., & Davidson, J. K. (1986). Enhancing relationships: Understanding the feminine mystique of pretending orgasm. *Journal of Sex and Marital Therapy, 12,* 182–196.

Darling, C. A., Davidson, J. K., & Conway-Welch, C. (1990). Female ejaculation: Perceived origins, the Grafenberg spot/area, and sexual responsiveness. *Archives of Sexual Behavior, 19,* 29–48.

Davidson, J. M., Camargo, C. A., & Smith, E. R. (1979). Effects of androgen on sexual behavior in hypogonadal men. *Journal of Clinical Endocrinology and Metabolism, 48,* 955–958.

Davidson, J. M., Camargo, C., Smith, E. R., & Kwan, M. (1983). Maintenance of sexual function in a castrated man treated with ovarian steroids. *Archives of Sexual Behavior, 12,* 263–276.

Davidson, J. M., Chen, J. J., Crapo, L., Gray, G. D., Greenleaf, W. J., & Catania, J. A. (1983). Hormonal changes and sexual functioning in aging men. *Journal of Clinical Endocrinology and Metabolism, 57,* 71–77.

Davidson, J. M., Kwan, M., & Greenleaf, W. J. (1982). Hormonal replacement and sexuality in men. *Clinics in Endocrinology and Metabolism, 11,* 599–623.

Davis, K. B. (1965). From factors in the sex life of twenty-two hundred women. In A. Krich (Ed.), *The sexual revolution* (Vol. 2, pp. 1–86). New York: Dell, (Original work published in 1929)

Davison, G. C. (1977). Homosexuality and the ethics of behavioral intervention: Paper 1. *Journal of Homosexuality, 2,* 195–204.

De Amicis, L. A., Goldberg, D. C., LoPiccolo, J., Friedman, J., & Davies, L. (1985). Clinical follow-up of couples treated for sexual dysfunction. *Archives of Sexual Behavior, 14,* 467–489.

De Jong, A. H. (1988). Maternal responses to the sexual abuse of their children. *Pediatrics, 81,* 14–21.

Deisher, R., Robinson, G., & Boyer, D. (1982). The adolescent female and male prostitute. *Pediatric Annals, 11,* 819–825.

Dekker, J., Dronkers, J., & Staffeleu, J. (1985). Treatment of sexual dysfunctions in male-only groups: Predicting outcome. *Journal of Sex and Marital Therapy, 11,* 80–90.

DeMause, L. (1974). The evolution of childhood. In L. DeMause (Ed.), *The history of childhood* (pp. 1–181). New York: Psychohistory Press.

Dennerstein, L., & Burrows, G. D. (1982). Hormone replacement therapy and sexuality in women. *Clinics in Endocrinology and Metabolism, 11,* 661–679.

Dewhurst, C. J., & Gordon, R. R. (1963). Change of sex. *Lancet, 309,* 1213–1217.

Diamond, M. (1965). A critical evaluation of the ontogeny of human sexual behavior. *The Quarterly Review of Biology, 40,* 147–175.

Diamond, M. (1982). Sexual identity, monozygotic twins reared in discordant sex roles and the BBC follow-up. *Archives of Sexual Behavior, 11,* 181–186.

Dietz, P. E., & Evans, B. (1982). Pornographic imagery and prevalence of paraphilia. *American Journal of Psychiatry, 139,* 1493–1495.

Dietz, P. E., Harry, B., & Hazelwood, R. R. (1986). Detective magazines: Pornography for the sexual sadist? *Journal of Forensic Sciences, 31,* 197–211.

Dietz, P. E., Hazelwood, R. R., & Warren, J. (1990). The sexually sadistic criminal and his offenses. *Bulletin of the American Academy of Psychiatry and Law, 18,* 163–176.

DiVasto, P. V., Kaufman, L. R., Jackson, R., Christy, J., Pearson, S., & Burgett, T. (1984). The prevalence of sexually stressful events among females in the general population. *Archives of Sexual Behavior, 13,* 59–67.

Dixon, J. M., Maddever, H., Van Maasdam, J., & Edwards, P. W. (1984). Psychosocial characteristics of applicants evaluated for surgical gender reassignment. *Archives of Sexual Behavior, 13,* 269–276.

Doerner, G., Rohde, W., Stahl, F., Krell, L., & Masius, W. G. (1975). A neuroendocrine predisposition for homosexuality in men. *Archives of Sexual Behavior, 43,* 1–8.

Donovan, B. T. (1985). *Hormones and human behavior.* London: Cambridge University Press.

Dow, M. G. T., Hart, D. M., & Forrest, C. A. (1983). Hormonal treatments of sexual unresponsiveness in postmenopausal women: A comparative study. *British Journal of Obstetrics and Gynaecology, 90,* 361–366.

Duncan, D. F. (1990). Prevalence of sexual assault victimization among heterosexual and gay/lesbian university students. *Psychological Reports, 66,* 65–66.

Durant, R. H., Jay, S., & Seymore, C. (1990). Contraceptive and sexual behavior of black female adolescents. *Journal of Adolescent Health Care, 11,* 326–334.

Earls, C. M., & David, H. (1989). A psychosocial study of male prostitution. *Archives of Sexual Behavior, 18,* 401–419.

Earls, C. M., & Marshall, W. L. (1982). The simultaneous and independent measurement of penile circumference and length. *Behavior Research Methods and Instrumentation, 14,* 447–450.

Earls, C. M., Marshall, W. L., Marshall, P. G., Morales, A., & Surridege, D. H. (1983). Penile elongation: A method for screening of impotence. *Journal of Urology, 130,* 90–92.

Edwards, J. N., & Booth, A. (1976). The cessation of marital intercourse. *American Journal of Psychiatry, 113,* 1333–1336.

Edwards, L. E., Steinman, M. E., Arnold, K. A., & Hakanson, E. Y. (1980). Adolescent pregnancy prevention services in high school clinics. *Family Planning Perspectives, 12,* 6–14.

Ehrhardt, A. A., & Baker, S. W. (1974). Fetal androgens, human central nervous system differentiation, and behavior sex differences. In R. C. Friedman & R. M. Richart (Eds.), *Sex differences in behavior* (pp. 33–51). New York: Wiley.

Ehrhardt, A. A., Epstein, R., & Money, J. (1968). Fetal androgens and female gender identification in the early-treated adrenogenital syndrome. *Johns Hopkins Medical Journal, 122,* 160–167.

Ehrhardt, A. A., Meyer-Bahlburg, H. F. L., Rosen, L. R., Feldman, J. F., Veridiano, N. P., Zimmerman, I., & McEwen, B. S. (1985). Sexual orientation after prenatal exposure to exogenous estrogen. *Archives of Sexual Behavior, 14,* 57–77.

Ehrhardt, A. A., & Money, J. (1967). Progestin-induced hermaphroditism, IQ, and psychosexual identity in a study of ten girls. *Journal of Sex Research, 3,* 83–100.

Ekblad, M. (1955). Induced abortion on psychiatric grounds. *Acta Psychiatrica et Neurologica Scandanavica,* Suppl. 99, 1–238.

Eklund, P. L. E., Gooren, L. J. G., & Bezemer, P. D. (1988). Prevalence of transsexualism in the Netherlands. *British Journal of Psychiatry, 152,* 638–640.

Ellis, E. M. (1983). A review of empirical rape research: Victim reactions and response to treatment. *Clinical Psychological Review, 3,* 473–490.

Elster, A. B., & Peters, L. (1987). Judicial involvement of conduct problems of fathers of infants born to adolescent mothers. *Pediatrics, 79,* 230–234.

Ende, J., Rockwell, S., & Glasgow, M. (1984). The sexual history in general medicine practice. *Archives of Internal Medicine, 144,* 558–581.

Ertekin, C., Akyurekli, O., Gurses, A. N., & Turgut, H. (1985). The value of somatosensory-evoked potentials and bulbocavernosus reflex in patients with impotence. *Acta Neurologica Scandinavica, 71,* 48–53.

Evans, B. A., McLean, K. A., Dawson, S. G., Teece, S. A., Bond, R. A., MacRae, K. D., & Thorp, R. W. (1989). Trends in sexual behaviour and risk factors for HIV infection among homosexual men, 1984–7. *British Medical Journal, 298,* 215–218.

Evans, R. B. (1969). Childhood parental relationships of homosexual men. *Journal of Consulting and Clinical Psychology, 33,* 129–135.

Everson, M. D., & Boat, B. W. (1990). Sexualized doll play among young children: Implications for the use of anatomical dolls in sexual abuse evaluations. *Journal of the American Academy of Child and Adolescent Psychiatry, 29,* 736–742.

Fagan, P. J., Wise, T. N., Derogatis, L. R., & Schmidt, C. W. (1988). Distressed transvestites. *Journal of Nervous and Mental Disease, 176,* 626–632.

Fagot, B. I. (1977). Consequences of moderate cross-gender behavior in preschool children. *Child Development, 48,* 902–907.

Fahrner, E. M. (1987). Sexual dysfunction in male alcohol addicts: Prevalence and treatment. *Archives of Sexual Behavior, 16,* 247–257.

Faller, K. C. (1987). Women who sexually abuse children. *Violence and Victims, 2,* 263–276.

Faller, K. C. (1989). Characteristics of a clinical sample of sexually abused children: How boy and girl victims differ. *Child Abuse and Neglect, 13,* 281–291.

Farrell, R. A., & Morrione, T. J. (1974). Social interaction and stereotypic responses to homosexuals. *Archives of Sexual Behavior, 3,* 425–442.

Fay, R. E., Turner, C. F., Klassen, A. D., & Gagnon, J. H. (1989). Prevalence and patterns of same-gender sexual contact among men. *Science, 243,* 338–348.

Fehrenbach, P. A., Smith, W., Monastersky, C., & Deisher, R. W. (1986). Adolescent sexual offenders: Offender and offense characteristics. *American Journal of Orthopsychiatry, 56,* 225–233.

Feldman, M., Mallouh, K., & Lewis, D. O. (1986). Filicidal abuse in the histories of 15 condemned murderers. *Bulletin of the American Academy of Psychiatry and the Law, 14,* 345–352.

Feldman, M. P., & MacCulloch, M. J. (1971). *Homosexual behavior: Therapy and assessment.* Oxford: Pergamon.

Ferracuti, F. (1972). Incest between father and daughter. In H. L. P. Resnick & M. L. Wolfgang (Eds.), *Sexual behaviors* (pp. 169–183). Boston: Little, Brown.

Ferrando, R. L., McCorvey, E., Simon, W. A., & Stewart, D. M. (1988). Bizarre behavior following the ingestion of levo-desoxyephidrine. *Drug Intelligence and Clinical Pharmacology, 22,* 214–217.

Fichten, C. S., Libman, E., & Brender, W. (1983). Methodological issues in the study of sex therapy: Effective components in the treatment of secondary orgasmic dysfunction. *Journal of Sex and Marital Therapy, 9,* 191–202.

Finkelhor, D. (1979). *Sexually abused children.* New York: Free Press.

Finkelhor, D. (1980). Risk factors in the sexual victimization of children. *Child Abuse and Neglect, 4,* 265–273.

Finkelhor, D. (1981). Sex between siblings. In L. L. Constantine & F. M. Martinson (Eds.), *Children and sex* (pp. 129–149). Boston: Little, Brown.

Finkelhor, D. (1983). Removing the child—prosecuting the offender in cases of sexual abuse: Evidence from the national reporting system for child abuse and neglect. *Child Abuse and Neglect, 7*, 195–205.

Finkelhor, D. (1984). *Child sexual abuse: New theory and research*. New York: Free Press.

Finkelhor, D. (1985). Sexual abuse of boys. In A. W. Burgess (Ed.), *Rape and sexual assault* (pp. 97–103). New York: Garland.

Finkelhor, D., & Browne, A. (1988). Assessing the long-term impact of child sexual abuse: A review and conceptualization. In L. E. A. Walker (Ed.), *Handbook on sexual abuse of children* (pp. 55–71). New York: Springer.

Finkelhor, D., & Lewis, I. A. (1988). An epidemiologic approach to the study of child molestation. *Annals of the New York Academy of Sciences, 528*, 64–78.

Fisher, S. (1973). *The female orgasm*. New York: Basic Books.

Fleming, M., MacGowan, B., & Costos, D. (1985). The dyadic adjustment of female-to-male transsexuals. *Archives of Sexual Behavior, 14*, 47–55.

Fleming, M., Steinman, C., & Bocknek, G. (1980). Methodological problems in assessing sex-reassignment surgery: A reply to Meyer and Reter. *Archives of Sexual Behavior, 9*, 451–456.

Flick, L. H. (1986). Paths to adolescent parenthood: Implications for prevention. *Public Health Reports, 101*, 132–147.

Foley, T. S. (1985). Family response to rape and sexual assault. In A. W. Burgess (Ed), *Rape and sexual assault* (pp. 159–188). New York: Garland.

Ford, C. S., & Beach, F. A. (1951). *Patterns of sexual behavior*. New York: Harper and Row.

Frank, E., Anderson, B., & Rubinstein, D. (1978). Frequency of sexual dysfunction in "normal" couples. *New England Journal of Medicine, 299*, 111–115.

Frank, E., Anderson, B., Stewart, B. D., Dancu, C., Hughes, C., & West, D. (1988). Immediate and delayed treatment of rape victims. *Annals of the New York Academy of Sciences, 528*, 296–309.

Frank, E., Turner, S. M., Stewart, B. D., Jacob, M., & West, D. (1981). Past psychiatric symptoms and the response to sexual assault. *Comprehensive Psychiatry, 22*, 479–487.

Frank, J. D. (1959). Problems of control in psychotherapy as exemplified by the psychotherapy research project in the Phipps psychiatric clinic. *Research in Psychotherapy, 11*, 10–26.

Freud, S. (1955). The psychogenesis of a case of homosexuality in a woman. In J. Strachey (Ed.), *The standard edition of the complete psychological works of Sigmund Freud, vol. 18* (pp. 145–176). London: Hogarth. (Original work published 1920).

Freund, K. (1963). A laboratory method of diagnosing predominance of homo- or hetero-erotic interest in the male. *Behavior Research and Therapy, 12*, 355–359.

Freund, K. (1974). Male homosexuality: An analysis of the pattern. In J. A. Loraine (Ed.), *Understanding homosexuality: Its biological and psychological basis*. St. Leonardgate, England: Medical and Technical Publishing.

Freund, K. (1990). Courtship disorder. In W. L. Marshall, D. R. Laws, & H. E. Barbaree (Eds.), *Handbook of sexual assault* (pp. 195–207). New York: Plenum.

Freund, K., & Blanchard, R. (1981). Assessment of sexual dysfunction and deviation. In M. Hersen & A. S. Bellack (Eds.), *Behavioral assessment* (pp. 427–455). New York: Pergamon.

Freund, K., & Blanchard, R. (1986). The concept of courtship disorder. *Journal of Sex and Marital Therapy, 12*, 79–92.

Freund, K., McKnight, C. K., Langevin, R., & Cibiri, S. (1972). The female child as a surrogate object. *Archives of Sexual Behavior, 2*, 119–133.

Freund, K., Langevin, R., & Barlow, D. H. (1974). Comparison of two penile measures of erotic arousal. *Behavior Research and Therapy, 17*, 451–457.

Freund, K., Nagler, E., Langevin, R., Zajac, A., & Steiner, B. (1974). Measuring feminine gender identity in homosexual males. *Archives of Sexual Behavior, 3*, 249–260.

Freund, K., Heasman, G. A., & Roper, V. (1982). Results of the main studies of sexual offenses against children and pubescents (a review). *Canadian Journal of Criminology, 24*, 387–397.

Freund, K., Steiner, B. W., & Chan, S. (1982). Two types of cross-gender identity. *Archives of Sexual Behavior, 11*, 49–63.

Freund, K., Scher, H., & Hucker, S. (1983). The courtship disorder. *Archives of Sexual Behavior, 12,* 369–379.

Freund, K., Watson, R., & Dickey, R. (1990). Does sexual abuse in childhood cause pedophilia? An exploratory study. *Archives of Sexual Behavior, 19,* 557–568.

Friedman, S. (1988). A family systems approach to treatment. In L. E. A. Walker (Ed.), *Handbook on sexual abuse of children* (pp. 326–349). New York: Springer.

Friedrich, W. N., Urquiza, A. J., & Bielke, R. L. (1986). Behavior problems in sexually abused young children. *Journal of Pediatric Psychology, 11,* 47–57.

Fritz, G. S., Stoll, K., & Wagner, N. N. (1981). A comparison of males and females who were sexually molested as children. *Journal of Sex and Marital Therapy, 7,* 54–59.

Fromuth, M. E. (1986). The relationship of childhood sexual abuse with later psychological and sexual adjustment in a sample of college women. *Child Abuse and Neglect, 10,* 5–15.

Fromuth, M. E., & Burkhart, B. R. (1989). Long-term psychological correlates of childhood sexual abuse in two samples of college men. *Child Abuse and Neglect, 13,* 533–542.

Frude, N. (1985). The sexual abuse of children within the family. *Medicine and Law, 4,* 463–472.

Fullilove, M. T., Fullilove, R. E., Haynes, K., & Gross, S. (1990). Black women and AIDS prevention: A view towards understanding the gender rules. *Journal of Sex Research, 27,* 47–64.

Furby, L., Weinrott, M. R., & Blackshaw, L. (1989). Sex offender recidivism: A review. *Psychological Bulletin, 105,* 3–30.

Furness, T. (1983). Mutual influence and interlocking professional-family process in the treatment of child sexual abuse and incest. *Child Abuse and Neglect, 7,* 207–223.

Furstenberg, F. F. (1976). *Unplanned parenthood.* New York: Free Press.

Furstenberg, F. F. (1989). Adolescent sexual behavior. *American Psychologist, 44,* 249–257.

Furstenberg, F. F., Jr., Brooks-Gunn, J., & Chase-Lansdale, L. (1989). Teenaged pregnancy and childbearing. *American Psychologist, 44,* 313–320.

Futterweit, W., Weiss, R. A., & Fagerstrom, R. M. (1986). Endocrine evaluation of forty female-to-male transsexuals increased frequency of polycystic disease in female transsexualism. *Archives of Sexual Behavior, 15,* 69–78.

Gaddis, A., & Brooks-Gunn, J. (1985). The male experience of pubertal change. *Journal of Youth and Adolescence, 14,* 61–69.

Gagne, P. (1981). Treatment of sex offenders with medroxyprogesterone acetate. *American Journal of Psychiatry, 138,* 644–646.

Gagnon, J. (1965). Female child victims of sex offenses. *Social Problems, 13,* 176–192.

Gagnon, J. (1985). Attitudes and responses of parents to pre-adolescent masturbation. *Archives of Sexual Behavior, 14,* 451–466.

Gagnon, J. H., & Simon, W. (1973). *Sexual conduct.* Chicago: Aldine.

Gardner, J. J., & Cabral, D. A. (1990). Sexually abused adolescents: A distinct group among sexually abused children. *Journal of Pediatrics and Child Health, 26,* 22–24.

Gebhard, P. H. (1966). Factors in marital orgasm. *Journal of Social Issues, 22,* 88–95.

Gebhard, P. H., Gagnon, J. H., Pomeroy, W. B., & Christenson, C. V. (1965). *Sex offenders.* New York: Harper & Row.

Gebhard, P. H., & Johnson, A. B. (1979). *The Kinsey data.* Philadelphia: Saunders.

George, L. K., & Weiler, S. J. (1981). Sexuality in middle and late life. *Archives of General Psychiatry, 38,* 919–923.

George, W. H., & Marlatt, G. A. (1989). Introduction. In D. R. Laws (Ed.), *Relapse prevention with sex offenders* (pp. 1–33). New York: Guilford.

Gewertz, B. L., & Zarins, C. K. (1985). Vasculgenic impotence. In R. T. Segraves & H. W. Schoenberg (Eds.), *Diagnosis and treatment of erectile disturbances* (pp. 105–113). New York: Plenum.

Giarretto, H. (1978). Humanistic treatment of father-daughter incest. *Journal of Humanistic Psychology, 18,* 62–76.

Giarretto, H. (1981). A comprehensive child sexual abuse treatment program. In P. B. Mrazek & C. H. Kempe (Eds.), *Sexually abused children and their families* (pp. 179–197). Oxford: Pergamon.

Giarretto, H., Giarretto, A., & Sgroi, S. M. (1978). Coordinated community treatment of incest. In A. W. Burgess, A. W. Groth, L. L. Holmstrom, & S. M. Sgroi (Eds.), *Sexual assault of children and adolescents* (pp. 231–241). Toronto: Lexington Books.

Gibbens, T. C. N., Soothill, K. L., & Way, C. K. (1978). Sibling and parent-child incest offenders. *British Journal of Criminology, 18*, 40–52.

Gibson-Ainyette, I., Templer, D. I., Brown, R., & Veaco, L. (1988). Adolescent female prostitutes. *Archives of Sexual Behavior, 17*, 431–438.

Gilbert, O. P. (1926). *Men in women's guise: Some historical instances of female impersonation*. London: Bodley Head.

Gitlin, M. J., & Pasnau, R. O. (1989). Psychatric syndromes linked to reproductive function in women: A review of current knowledge. *American Journal of Psychiatry, 146*, 1413–1422.

Gittleson, N. L., Eacott, S. E., & Mehta, B. M. (1978). Victims of indecent exposure. *British Journal of Psychiatry, 132*, 61–66.

Gladue, B. A., Green, R., & Hellman, R. E. (1984). Neuroendocrine response to estrogen and sexual orientation. *Science, 225*, 1496–1499.

Glass, R. M. (1988). AIDS and suicide. *Journal of the American Medical Association, 259*, 1369–1370.

Goddard, M. (1991, April 6). In the gay killing fields. *Sydney Morning Herald*, p. 39.

Goh, H. H., & Ratnam, S. S. (1990). Effect of estrogens on prolactin secretion in transsexual subjects. *Archives of Sexual Behavior, 19*, 507–516.

Goldman, R., & Goldman, J. (1982). *Children's sexual thinking*. London: Routledge and Kegan Paul.

Golombok, S., Sketchley, J., & Rust, J. (1989). Condom failure among homosexual men. *Journal of Acquired Immune Deficiency Syndrome, 2*, 404–409.

Golombok, S., Spencer, A., & Rutter, M. (1983). Children in lesbian and single-parent households: Psychosexual and psychiatric appraisal. *Journal of Child Psychology and Psychiatry, 24*, 551–572.

Gomes-Schwartz, B., Horowitz, J. M., & Sauzier, M. (1985). Severity of emotional distress among sexually abused preschool, school-aged, and adolescent children. *Hospital and Community Psychiatry, 36*, 503–508.

Gonsiorek, J. C. (1982). Introduction: Present and future directions in gay/lesbian health. In J. C. Gonsiorek (Ed.), *Homosexuality and psychotherapy: A practitioner's handbook of affirmative models* (pp. 5–7). New York: Haworth.

Goodchilds, J. D., & Zellman, G. L. (1984). Sexual signaling and sexual aggression in adolescent relationships. In N. M. Malamuth & E. Donnerstein (Eds.), *Pornography and sexual aggression* (pp. 233–246). New York: Academic Press.

Goodman, G. S., & Helgeson, V. S. (1988). Children as witnesses: What do they remember? In L. E. A. Walker (Ed.), *Handbook on sexual abuse of children* (pp. 109–135). New York: Springer.

Gooren, L. (1986). The neuroendocrine response of luteinizing hormone to estrogen administration in heterosexual, homosexual, and transsexual subjects. *Journal of Clinical Endocrinology and Metabolism, 63*, 583–588.

Gordon, E. (1991). Transsexual healing: Medicaid funding of sex reassignment surgery. *Archives of Sexual Behavior, 20*, 61–74.

Gordon, M. (1989). The family environment of sexual abuse: A comparison of natal and stepfather abuse. *Child Abuse and Neglect, 13*, 121–130.

Gorzynski, G., & Katz, J. L. (1977). The polycystic ovary syndrome: Psychosexual correlates. *Archives of Sexual Behavior, 6*, 215–222.

Gosselin, C., & Wilson, G. (1980). *Sexual variations*. London: Faber and Faber.

Green, R., Newman, L. E., & Stoller, R. J. (1972). Treatment of boyhood "transsexualism." *Archives of General Psychiatry, 26*, 213–217.

Green, R. (1978). Sexual identity of 37 children raised by homosexual or transsexual parents. *American Journal of Psychiatry, 135*, 692–697.

Green, R. (1985). Gender identity in childhood and later sexual orientation: Follow-up of 78 males. *American Journal of Psychiatry, 142*, 399–341.

Green, R. (1987). *The "sissy boy syndrome" and the development of homosexuality*. New Haven, CT: Yale University Press.

Green, R., & Money, J. (1961). Effeminacy in prepubertal boys. *Pediatrics, 27*, 286–291.

Green, R., & Money, J. (1969). Preface. In R. Green & J. Money (Eds.), *Transsexualism and sex reassignment* (p. xv). Baltimore: Johns Hopkins University Press.

Greenacre, P. (1969). The fetish and the transitional object. *Psychoanalytic Study of the Child, 24*, 144–164.

Greenson, R. R. (1966). A transvestite boy and a hypothesis. *International Journal of Psychoanalysis, 47,* 396–403.

Greydanus, D. E., & Geller, B. (1980). Masturbation: Historic perspective. *New York State Journal of Medicine,* 1982–1986.

Grob, C. S. (1985). Female exhibitionism. *Journal of Nervous and Mental Disease, 173,* 253–256.

Groth, A. N. (1977). The adolescent sex offender and his prey. *International Journal of Offender Therapy and Comparative Criminology, 21,* 249–254.

Groth, A. N., & Birnbaum, H. J. (1978). Adult sexual orientation and attraction to underage persons. *Archives of Sexual Behavior, 7,* 175–181.

Groth, A. N., & Birnbaum, H. J. (1979). *Men who rape: The psychology of the offender.* New York: Plenum.

Groth, A. N., & Burgess, A. W. (1977). Sexual dysfunction during rape. *New England Journal of Medicine, 297,* 764–766.

Groth, A. N., & Burgess, A. W. (1980). Male rape: Offenders and victims. *American Journal of Psychiatry, 137,* 806–810.

Groth, A. N., Burgess, A. W., & Holmstrom, L. L. (1977). Rape: Power, anger and sexuality. *American Journal of Psychiatry, 134,* 1239–1243.

Groth, A. N., Longo, R. E., & McFadin, J. B. (1982). Undetected recidivism among rapists and child molesters. *Crime and Delinquency, 28,* 450–458.

Grudzinskas, J. G., & Atkinson, L. (1984). Sexual function in the puerperium. *Archives of Sexual Behavior, 13,* 85–92.

Gutheil, T. G. (1989). Borderline personality disorder, boundary violations, and patient-therapist sex: Medicological pitfalls. *American Journal of Psychiatry, 146,* 597–602.

Hacker, A. (1987). American apartheid. *New York Review of Books, 37,* 26–33.

Hagstad, A , & Janson, P. O. (1984). Sexuality among Swedish women around forty. An epidemiological survey. *Journal of Psychosomatic Obstetrics and Gynaecology, 3,* 191–203.

Hale, K. S., Binik, Y., & DiTomasso, E. (1985). Concordance between physiological and subjective measures of sexual arousal. *Behavior Research and Therapy, 23,* 297–303.

Hall, R. L. (1989). Relapse rehearsal. In D. R. Laws (Ed.), *Relapse prevention with sex offenders* (pp. 197–206). New York: Guilford Press.

Halleck, S. L. (1981). The ethics of antiandrogen therapy. *American Journal of Psychiatry, 138,* 642–643.

Hallstrom, T. (1979). Sexuality of women in middle age: The Goteberg study. *Journal of Biosocial Science* (Suppl. 6), 165–175.

Hallstrom, T., & Samuelsson, S. (1990). Changes in women's sexual desire in middle life: The longitudinal study of women in Gothenburg. *Archives of Sexual Behavior, 19,* 259–268.

Halperin, M. E. (1982). Teenage pregnancy—myths and facts. In B. N. Barwin & S. Belisle (Eds.), *Adolescent gynecology and sexuality* (pp. 107–111). New York: Masson.

Halpern, S. (1990). The fight over teen-age abortion. *New York Review of Books, 37,* 30–32.

Hamburg, D. A., & Lunde, D. T. (1967). Sex hormones in the development of sex differences in human behavior. In E. E. Maccoby (Ed.), *The development of sex differences* (pp. 9–38). London: Tavistock.

Hamburger, C., Sturup, G. K., & Dahl-Iversen, E. (1953). Transvestism. *Journal of the American Medical Association, 152,* 391–396.

Hammersmith, S. K. (1988). A sociological approach to counseling homosexual clients and their families. In E. Coleman (Ed.), *Psychotherapy with homosexual men and women* (pp. 173–190). New York: Haworth.

Handsfield, H. H., & Schwebke, J. (1990). Trends in sexually transmitted diseases in homosexually active men in King County, Washington, 1980–1990. *Sexually Transmitted Diseases, 17,* 211–215.

Hariton, E. B., & Singer, J. L. (1974). Women's fantasies during sexual intercourse. *Journal of Consulting and Clinical Psychology, 42,* 313–322, 1974.

Harlow, H. (1965). Sexual behavior of the rhesus monkey. In F. A. Beach (Ed.), *Sexual behavior* (pp. 69–91). New York: Wiley.

Harrison, W. M., Rabkin, J. G., & Ehrhardt, A. A. (1986). Effects of antidepressant medication on sexual function: A controlled study. *Journal of Clinical Pharmacology, 6,* 144–149.

Harry, J. (1983). Defeminization and adult psychological well-being among male homosexuals. *Archives of Sexual Behavior, 12,* 1–19.

Harry, J. (1989). Parental physical abuse and sexual orientation in males. *Archives of Sexual Behavior, 18,* 251–261.

Hart, M., Roback, H., Tittler, B., Weitz, L., Walston, B., & McKee, E. (1978). Psychological adjustment of nonpatient homosexuals: Critical review of the research literature. *Journal of Clinical Psychology, 39,* 604–608.

Haseltine, B., & Miltenberger, R. G. (1990). Teaching self-protection skills to persons with mental retardation. *American Journal of Mental Retardation, 95,* 188–197.

Hatch, J. P. (1981). Psychophysiological aspects of sexual dysfunction. *Archives of Sexual Behavior, 10,* 49–64.

Haugaard, J. J., & Tilly, C. (1988). Characteristics predicting children's responses to sexual encounters with other children. *Child Abuse and Neglect, 12,* 209–218.

Hawton, K., Catalan, J., Martin, P., & Fagg, J. (1986). Long-term outcome of sex therapy. *Behavior Research and Therapy, 24,* 665–675.

Hazelwood, R. R., Dietz, P. E., & Burgess, A. W. (1983). *Autoerotic fatalities.* Lexington, MA: Lexington Books.

Hegeler, S., & Mortensen, M. (1978). Sexuality and aging. *British Journal of Sexual Medicine, 16–19.*

Heilbrun, A. B., & Leif, D. T. (1988). Erotic value of female distress in sexual explicit photographs. *Journal of Sex Research, 24,* 47–57.

Heilbrun, A. B., & Loftus, M. P. (1986). The role of sadism and peer pressure in the sexual aggression of male college students. *Journal of Sex Research, 22,* 320–332.

Heilbrun, A. B., & Thompson, N. L., Jr. (1977). Sex-role identity and male and female homosexuality. *Sex Roles, 3,* 65–79.

Heim, N., & Hursch, C. J. (1979). Castration of sex offenders: Treatment or punishment? A review and critique of recent European literature. *Archives of Sexual Behavior, 8,* 281–304.

Heiman, J. R., Gladue, B. A., Roberts, C. W., & LoPiccolo, J. (1986). Historical and current factors discriminating sexually functional from sexually dysfunctional married couples. *Journal of Marital and Family Therapy, 121,* 163–174.

Helzer, J. E., Robins, L.N., McEvoy, L.T., Spitznagel, E. L., Stoltzman, R. K., Farmer, A., & Brockington, I. F. (1985). A comparison of clinical and Diagnostic Interview Schedule diagnoses. *Archives of General Psychiatry, 42,* 657–666.

Hendricks, S. E., Fitzpatrick, D. F., Hartmann, K., Quaife, M. A., Stratbucker, R. A., & Graber, B. (1988). Brain structure and function in sexual molesters of children and adolescents. *Journal of Clinical Psychiatry, 49,* 108–112.

Henn, F. A., Herjanic, M., & Vanderpearl, R. H. (1976). Forensic psychiatry: Profiles of two types of sex offenders. *American Journal of Psychiatry, 133,* 694–696.

Herdt, G. H., & Davidson, J. (1988). The Sambia "turnim-man": Sociocultural and clinical aspects of gender formation in male pseudohermaphrodites with 5-alpha-reductase deficiency in Papua New Guinea. *Archives of Sexual Behavior, 17,* 1–31.

Herman, J. L. (1981). *Father-daughter incest.* Boston: Harvard University Press.

Herman, J. L. (1985). Father-daughter incest. In A. W. Burgess (Ed.), *Rape and sexual assault* (pp. 83–96). New York: Garland.

Herman, J. L. (1990). Sex offenders: A feminist perspective. In W. L. Marshall, D. R. Laws, & H. E. Barbaree (Eds.), *Handbook of sexual assault* (pp. 177–193). New York: Plenum.

Hersen, M. (1973). Self-assessment of fear. *Behavior Therapy, 4,* 241–257.

Heston, L. L., & Shields, J. (1968). Homosexuality in twins. *Archives of General Psychiatry, 18,* 149–160.

Hibbard, R. A., & Hartman, G. L. (1990). Emotional indicators in human figure drawings of sexually victimized and nonabused children. *Journal of Clinical Psychology, 46,* 211–219.

Hillman, R. J., O'Mara, N., Taylor-Robinson, D., & Harris, J. R. W. (1990). Medical and social aspects of sexual assault of males: A survey of 100 victims. *British Journal of General Practice, 40,* 502–504.

Hobbs, C. J., & Wynne, J. M. (1989). Sexual abuse of English boys and girls: The importance of anal examination. *Child Abuse and Neglect, 13,* 195–210.

Hochbaum, S. R. (1987). The evaluation and treatment of the sexually assaulted patient. *Emergency Medical Clinics of North America, 5,* 601–622.

Hoenig, J., Kenna, J., & Youd, A. (1970). Social and economic aspects of transsexualism. *British Journal of Psychiatry, 117,* 163–172.

Holeman, R. E., & Winokur, G. (1965). Effeminate homosexuality: A disease of childhood. *American Journal of Orthopsychiatry, 35,* 48–56.

Holmbeck, G. N. (1989). Masculinity, femininity, and multiple regression: Comment on Zeldow, Daugherty, and Clark's "Masculinity, femininity, and psychosocial adjustment in medical students: A 2-year follow-up." *Journal of Personality Assessment, 53,* 583–599.

Holmstrom, L. L. (1985). The criminal justice system's response to the rape victim. In A. W. Burgess (Ed.), *Rape and sexual assault* (pp. 189–198). New York: Garland.

Hooker, E. (1957). The adjustment of the male overt homosexual. *Journal of Projective Techniques, 21,* 18–31.

Hopkins, J. R. (1977). Sexual behavior in adolescence. *Journal of Social Issues, 33,* 67–85.

Houck, E. L., & Abramson, P. R. (1986). Masturbatory guilt and the psychological consequences of sexually transmitted diseases among women. *Journal of Research in Personality, 20,* 267–275.

Howard, M. (1985). Postponing sexual involvement among adolescents. *Journal of Adolescent Health Care, 6,* 271–277.

Howells, K. (1978). Some meanings of children for pedophiles. In M. Cook & G. Wilson (Eds.), *Love and attraction* (pp. 57–82). London: Pergamon.

Hucker, S. J., & Bain, J. (1990). Androgenic hormones and sexual assault. In W. L. Marshall, D. R. Laws, & H. E. Barbaree (Eds.), *Handbook of sexual assault* (pp. 193–202). New York: Plenum.

Huey, C. J., Kline-Graber, G., & Graber, B. (1981). Time factors and orgasmic response. *Archives of Sexual Behavior, 10,* 111–118.

Humphries, L. (1970). *Tearoom trade.* Chicago: Aldine.

Hunt, D. D., Carr, J. E., & Hampson, J. L. (1981). Cognitive correlates of biologic sex and gender identity in transsexualism. *Archives of Sexual Behavior, 10,* 65–77.

Hunt, M. (1974). *Sexual behavior in the 1970's.* New York: Dell.

Hunter, M. S. (1990). Somatic experience of the menopause. A prospective study. *Psychosomatic Medicine, 52,* 357–367.

Hutt, C. (1972). *Males and females.* Harmondsworth, UK: Penguin.

Illsley, R., & Hall, M. H. (1976). Psychological aspects of abortion. *Bulletin of the World Health Organization, 53,* 83–106.

Imperato-McGinley, J., Peterson, R. E., Gautier, T., & Sturla, E. (1979). Androgens and the evolution of male-gender identity among male pseudohermaphrodites with 5-alpha-reductase deficiency. *New England Journal of Medicine, 300,* 1233–1237.

Ingram, M. (1979). The participating victim: A study of sexual offenses against pre-pubertal boys. In M. Cook & G. Wilson (Eds.), *Love and attraction* (pp. 511–518). Oxford: Pergamon.

Jackson, J. L., Calhoun, K. S., Amick, A. E., Maddever, H. M., & Habif, V. L. (1990). Young adult women who report childhood intrafamilial sexual abuse: Subsequent adjustment. *Archives of Sexual Behavior, 19,* 211–221.

Jacobson, N. S., Follette, W. C., & Revenstorf, D. (1984). Psychotherapy outcome research: Methods for reporting variability and evaluating clinical significance. *Behavior Therapy, 15,* 336–352.

James, S. (1978). Treatment of homosexuality: II. Superiority of desensitization arousal as compared with anticipatory avoidance conditioning: Results of a controlled trial. *Behavior Therapy, 9,* 28–36.

James, S., Orwin, A., & Turner, R. K. (1977). Treatment of homosexuality: I. Analysis of failure following a trial of anticipatory avoidance conditioning: The development of an alternative treatment system. *Behavior Therapy, 8,* 840–848.

James, W. H. (1981). The honeymoon effect on marital coitus. *Journal of Sex Research, 17,* 114–123.

Jensen, S. B. (1981). Diabetic sexual dysfunction: A comparative study of 160 insulin-treated diabetic men and women and an age-matched control group. *Archives of Sexual Behavior, 10,* 493–504.

Jensen, S. B. (1986). Sexual dysfunction in insulin-treated diabetics: A six-year follow-up study of 101 patients. *Archives of Sexual Behavior, 15,* 271–283.

Johnson, A. M., & Gill, O. N. (1989). Evidence for recent changes in sexual behaviour in homosexual men in England and Wales. *Philosophical Transactions of the Royal Society of London, 325,* 153–161.

Johnson, R. L., & Shrier, D. (1987). Past sexual victimization by females of male patients in an adolescent medicine clinic population. *American Journal of Psychiatry, 144,* 650–652.

Johnston, C. M., & Deisher, R. W. (1973). Contemporary communal child rearing. *Pediatrics, 52,* 319–326.

Jones, E. F., Forrest, J. D., Goldman, N., Henshaw, S. K., Lincoln, R., Rosoff, J. I., Westoff, C. F., & Wulf, D. (1985). Teenage pregnancy in developed countries: Determinants and policy implications. *Family Planning Perspectives, 17,* 53–63.

Jones, T. M. (1985). Hormonal considerations in the evaluation and treatment of erectile dysfunction. In R. T. Segraves & H. W. Schoenberg (Eds.), *Diagnosis and treatment of erectile disturbances* (pp. 115–158). New York: Plenum.

Kagan, J., & Moss, H. A. (1962). *Birth to maturity.* New York: Wiley.

Kalichman, S. C. (1990). Affective and personality characteristics of MMPI profile subgroups of incarcerated rapists. *Archives of Sexual Behavior, 19,* 443–459.

Kalichman, S. C., Craig, M. E., & Follingstad, D. R. (1988). Mental health professionals and suspected cases of child abuse: An investigation of factors influencing reporting. *Community Mental Health Journal, 23,* 43–51.

Kallmann, F. J. (1952). Comparative twin study on the genetic aspects of male homosexuality. *Journal of Nervous and Mental Disease, 115,* 283–298.

Kanin, E. J. (1959). Male aggression in dating-courtship relations. *American Journal of Sociology, 63,* 197–204.

Kanin, E. J. (1985). Date rapists: Differential sexual socialization and relative deprivation. *Archives of Sexual Behavior, 14,* 219–231.

Kanin, E. J., & Parcell, S. R. (1977). Sexual aggression: A second look at the offended female. *Archives of Sexual Behavior, 6,* 67–76.

Kaplan, H. S. (1974). *The new sex therapy.* New York: Brunner/Mazel.

Kaplan, H. S. (1977). Hypoactive sexual desire. *Journal of Sex and Marital Therapy, 3,* 3–9.

Kaplan, H. S. (1979). *Disorders of sexual desire.* New York: Brunner/Mazel.

Kaplan, H. S. (1990). Children don't always tell the truth. *Journal of Forensic Sciences, 35,* 661–667.

Karacan, I. (1978). Advances in the psychophysiological evaluation of male erectile impotence. In J. LoPiccolo & L. LoPiccolo (Eds.), *Handbook of sex therapy* (pp. 137–145). New York: Plenum.

Katchadourian, H. A., Lunde, D. T., & Trotter, R. (1979). *Human sexuality.* New York: Holt, Rinehart & Winston.

Kaufman, A., DiVasto, P., Jackson, R., Voorhees, D., & Christy, J. (1980). Male rape victims: Noninstitutionalized assault. *American Journal of Psychiatry, 137,* 221–223.

Kavoussi, R. J., Kaplan, M., & Becker, J. V. (1988). Psychiatric diagnoses in adolescent sex offenders. *Journal of the American Academy of Child and Adolescent Psychiatry, 27,* 241–243.

Keating, S. M., Higgs, D. F., Willot, G. M., & Stedman, L. R. (1990). Sexual assault patterns. *Journal of the Forensic Science Society, 30,* 71–88.

Keller, R. A., Cicchinelli, L. F., & Gardner, D. M. (1989). Characteristics of child sexual abuse treatment programs. *Child Abuse and Neglect, 13,* 361–368.

Kelly, M. P., Strassberg, D. S., & Kircher, J. R. (1990). Attitudinal and experiential correlates of anorgasmia. *Archives of Sexual Behavior, 19,* 165–177.

Kerlinger, F. N. (1973). *Foundations of behavioral research.* New York: Holt, Rinehart & Winston.

Kidd, G. S., Glass, A. R., & Vigersky, R. A. (1979). The hypothalamic-pituitary-testicular axis in thyrotoxicosis. *Journal of Clinical Endocrinology and Metabolism, 48,* 798–802.

Kilmann, P. R., Wanlass, R. L., Sabalis, R. F., & Sullivan, B. (1981). Sex education: A review of its effects. *Archives of Sexual Behavior, 10,* 177–205.

Kilpatrick, D. G., & Best, C. L. (1984). Some cautionary remarks on treating sexual assault victims with implosion. *Behavior Therapy, 15,* 421–423.

Kilpatrick, D. G., Best, C. L., Saunders, B. E., & Veronen, L. J. (1988). Rape in marriage and in dating relationships: How bad is it for mental health? *Annals of the New York Academy of Sciences, 528,* 335–344.

Kimmel, D. C. (1979–1980). Life-history interviews of aging gay men. *International Journal of Aging and Human Development, 10,* 239–248.

Kingsley, L. A., Rinaldo, C. R., Jr., Lyter, D. W., Valdiserri, R. O., Belle, S. H., & Ho, M. (1990). Sexual transmission efficiency of hepatitis B virus and human immunodeficiency virus among homosexual men. *Journal of the American Medical Association, 264,* 230–234.

Kinsey, A. C., Pomeroy, W. B., & Martin, C. E. (1948). *Sexual behavior in the human male.* Philadelphia: Saunders.

Kinsey, A. C., Pomeroy, W. B., Martin, C. E., & Gebhard, P. H. (1953). *Sexual behavior in the human female*. Philadelphia: Saunders.

Kirkpatrick, M. (1988). Clinical implications of lesbian mother studies. In E. Coleman (Ed.), *Psychotherapy with homosexual men and women* (pp. 201–211). New York: Haworth.

Kitchur, M., & Bell, R. (1989). Group psychotherapy with preadolescent sexual abuse victims: Literature review and description of an inner-city group. *International Journal of Group Psychotherapy, 39,* 285–310.

Klassen, A. D., Williams, C. J., & Levitt, E. E. (1989). *Sex and morality in the U.S.* Middletown, CT: Wesleyen University Press.

Klassen, A. D., & Wilsnack, S. C. (1986). Sexual experiences and drinking among women in a U.S. national survey. *Archives of Sexual Behavior, 15,* 363–392.

Kleber, D. J., Howell, R. J., & Tibbits-Kleber, A. L. (1986). The impact of parental homosexuality in child custody cases: A review of the literature. *Bulletin of the American Academy of Psychiatry and Law, 13,* 81–87.

Klein, S. J., & Fletcher, W., III. (1986). Gay grief: An examination of its uniqueness brought to light by the AIDS crisis. *Journal of Psychosocial Oncology, 4,* 15–25.

Knight, R. A., & Prentky, R. A. (1990). Classifying sexual offenders. In W. L. Marshall, D. R. Laws & H. E. Barbaree (Eds.), *Handbook of sexual assault* (pp. 23–52). New York: Plenum.

Knight, R. A., Rosenberg, R., & Schneider, B. A. (1985). Classification of sexual offenders: Perspectives, methods, and validation. In A. W. Burgess (Ed.), *Rape and sexual assault* (pp. 222–293). New York: Garland.

Knoth, R., Boyd, K., & Singer, B. (1988). Empirical tests of sexual selection theory: Predictions of sex differences in onset, intensity, and time course of sexual arousal. *Journal of Sex Research, 24,* 73–89.

Knussman, R., Christiansen, K., & Couwenbergs, C. (1986). Relations between sex hormone levels and sexual behavior in men. *Archives of Sexual Behavior, 15,* 429–445.

Kockott, G., & Fahrner, E. M. (1987). Transsexuals who have not undergone surgery: A follow-up study. *Archives of Sexual Behavior, 16,* 511–522.

Kockott, G., & Fahrner, E. M. (1988). Male-to-female and female-to-male transsexuals: A comparison. *Archives of Sexual Behavior, 17,* 539–546.

Kolarsky, A., Freund, K., Machek, J., & Polak, O. (1967). Male sexual deviation: Association with early temporal lobe damage. *Archives of General Psychiatry, 17,* 735–743.

Kolarsky, A., & Madlafousek, J. (1983). The inverse role of preparatory erotic stimulation in exhibitionists: Phallometric studies. *Archives of Sexual Behavior, 12,* 123–148.

Kosky, R. J. (1987). Gender-disordered children: Does inpatient treatment help? *Medical Journal of Australia, 146,* 565–569.

Koss, M. P. (1985). The hidden rape victim: Personality, attitudinal, and situational characteristics. *Psychology of Women Quarterly, 9,* 193–212.

Koss, M. P., & Dinero, T. E. (1988). Predictors of sexual aggression among a national sample of male college students. *Annals of the New York Academy of Sciences, 528,* 133–147.

Koss, M. P., & Dinero, T. E. (1989). Discriminant analysis of risk factors for sexual victimization among a national sample of college women. *Journal of Consulting and Clinical Psychology, 57,* 242–250.

Koss, M. P., Leonard, K. F., Beezley, D. A., & Oros, C. J. (1985). Nonstranger sexual aggression: A discriminant analysis of the psychological characteristics of undetected offenders. *Sex Roles, 12,* 981–992.

Koss, M. P., & Oros, C. J. (1982). Sexual experiences survey: A research instrument investigating sexual aggression and victimization. *Journal of Consulting and Clinical Psychology, 50,* 455–457.

Kraemer, H. C., Becker, H. B., Brodie, H. K. H., Doering, C. H., Moos, R. H., & Hamburg, D. A. (1976). Orgasmic frequency and plasma testosterone levels in normal human males. *Archives of Sexual Behavior, 5,* 125–132.

Kroth, J. A. (1979). Family therapy impact on intrafamilial child sexual abuse. *Child Abuse and Neglect, 3,* 297–302.

Krug, R. S. (1989). Adult male report of childhood sexual abuse by mothers: Case descriptions, motivations and long-term consequences. *Child Abuse and Neglect, 13,* 111–119.

Krysiewicz, S., & Mellinger, B. C. (1989). The role of imaging in the diagnostic evaluation of impotence. *American Journal of Roentgenology, 153,* 1133–1139.

Kuiper, B., & Cohen-Kettenis, P. (1988). Sex reassignment surgery: A study of 141 Dutch transsexuals. *Archives of Sexual Behavior, 17,* 439–457.

Kulig, J. W. (1985). Adolescent contraception: An update. *Pediatrics, 76,* 675–680.

Kuriansky, J. B., Sharpe, L., & O'Connor, D. (1982). The treatment of anorgasmia: Long-term effectiveness of a short-term behavioral group therapy. *Journal of Sex and Marital Therapy, 8,* 29–42.

Kutchinsky, B. (1991). Pornography and rape: Theory and practice? Evidence from crime data in four countries where pornography is easily available. *International Journal of Law and Psychiatry, 14,* 47–64.

Kwan, M., VanMaasdam, J., & Davidson, J. M. (1985). Effects of estrogen treatment on sexual behavior in male-to-female transsexuals: Experimental and clinical observations. *Archives of Sexual Behavior, 14,* 29–40.

LaBarbera, J. D., Martin, J. E., & Dozier, J. E. (1980). Child psychiatrists' view of father-daughter incest. *Child Abuse and Neglect, 4,* 147–151.

Lahr, J. (1986). *The Orton diaries.* London: Methuen.

Landis, J. (1956). Experiences of 500 children with adult sexual deviants. *Psychiatric Quarterly Supplement, 30,* 91–109.

Lang, P. J., & Lazovik, A. D. (1963). Experimental desensitization of a phobia. *Journal of Abnormal and Social Psychology, 66,* 519–525.

Langevin, R. (1990). Sexual anomalies and the brain. In W. L. Marshall, D. R. Laws & H. E. Barbaree (Eds.), *Handbook of sexual assault* (pp. 103–113). New York: Plenum.

Langevin, R., & Lang, R. A. (1987). The courtship disorders. In G. D. Wilson (Ed.), *Variant sexuality: Research and theory* (pp. 202–228). London: Croom Helm.

Langfeldt, T. (1981). Sexual development in children. In M. Cook & K. Howells (Eds.), *Adult sexual interest in children.* New York: Academic Press.

Laws, D. R. (1977). A comparison of the measurement characteristics of two circumferential penile transducers. *Archives of Sexual Behavior, 6,* 45–51.

Laws, D. R. (Ed.) (1989). *Relapse prevention with sex offenders.* New York: Guilford.

Laws, D. R., & Rubin, H. H. (1969). Instructional control of an autonomic sexual response. *Journal of Applied Behavioral Analysis, 2,* 93–99.

Leff, J. J., & Israel, M. (1983). The relationship between mode of female masturbation and achievement of orgasm in coitus. *Archives of Sexual Behavior, 12,* 227–236.

Leiblum, S., Bachmann, G., Kemmann, E., Colburn, D., & Swartzman, L. (1983). Vaginal atrophy in the postmenopausal woman. *Journal of the American Medical Association, 249,* 2195–2198.

Leitenberg, H., Greenwald, E., & Tarran, M. J. (1989). The relation between sexual activity among children during preadolescence and/or early adolescence and sexual behavior and sexual adjustment in young adulthood. *Archives of Sexual Behavior, 18,* 299–243.

Lenney, E. (1979). Androgyny: Some audacious assertions toward its coming of age. *Sex Roles, 5,* 703–719.

Levin, R. J., & Wagner, G. (1985). Orgasm in women in the laboratory-quantitative studies of duration, intensity, latency, and vaginal blood flow. *Archives of Sexual Behavior, 14,* 439–449.

Lewin, B. (1982). The adolescent boy and girl: First and other experiences with intercourse from a representative sample of Swedish school adolescents. *Archives of Sexual Behavior, 11,* 417–428.

Lewis, R. J., & Janda, L. H. (1988). The relationship between adult sexual adjustment and childhood experiences regarding exposure to nudity, sleeping in the parental bed, and parental attitudes toward sexuality. *Archives of Sexual Behavior, 17,* 349–362.

Leymarie, P., Roger, M., Castanier, M., & Scholler, R. (1974). Circadian variations of plasma testosterone and estrogens in normal men: A study by frequent sampling. *Journal of Steroid Biochemistry, 5,* 167–171.

Libman, E., Fichten, C. S., & Brender, W. (1985). The role of therapeutic format in the treatment of sexual dysfunction: A review. *Clinical Psychology Review, 5,* 103–117.

Lick, J. R., & Unger, T. E. (1977). The external validity of behavioral fear assessment. *Behavior Modification, 1,* 283–306.

Lightfoot-Klein, H. (1989). The sexual experience and marital adjustment of genitally circumcised and infibulated females in the Sudan. *Journal of Sex Research, 26,* 375–392.

Lindemalm, G., Korlin, D., & Uddenberg, N. (1986). Long-term follow-up of "sex change" in 13 male-to-female transsexuals. *Archives of Sexual Behavior, 15,* 187–210.

Linehan, M. H. (1977). Issues in behavioral interviewing. In J. D. Cone & R. P. Hawkins (Eds.), *Behavioral assessment: New directions in clinical psychology* (pp. 30–51). New York: Brunner/Mazel.

Linn, L. S., Spiegel, J. S., Mathews, W. C., Leake, B., Lien, R., & Brooks, S. (1989). Recent sexual behaviors among homosexual men seeking primary medical care. *Archives of International Medicine, 149,* 2685–2690.

Lipman, R. S., Cole, J. O., Park, L. C., & Rickels, K. (1965). Sensitivity of symptom and nonsymptom-focused criteria of outpatient drug efficacy. *American Journal of Psychiatry, 122,* 24–27.

Lobitz, W. C., & Baker, E. L., Jr. (1979). Group treatment of single males with erectile dysfunction. *Archives of Sexual Behavior, 8,* 127–138.

Loney, J. (1972). Background factors, sexual experiences, and attitudes toward treatment in two "normal" homosexual samples. *Journal of Consulting and Clinical Psychology, 38,* 57–65.

LoPiccolo, J. (1978). The professionalization of sex therapy: Issues and problems. In J. LoPiccolo & L. LoPiccolo (Eds.), *Handbook of sex therapy* (pp. 511–526). New York: Plenum.

LoPiccolo, J. (1982). Book review. *Archives of Sexual Behavior, 11,* 277–279.

LoPiccolo, J. (1990). Sexual dysfunction. In A. S. Bellack, M. Hersen, & A. E. Kazdin (Eds.), *International handbook of behavior therapy and modification* (2nd ed., pp. 547–564). New York: Plenum.

LoPiccolo, J., Heiman, J. R., Hogan, D. R., & Roberts, C. W. (1985). Effectiveness of single therapists versus cotherapy teams in sex therapy. *Journal of Consulting and Clinical Psychology, 53,* 287–294.

LoPiccolo, J., & Steger, J. C. (1974). The sexual interaction inventory: A new instrument for assessment of sexual dysfunction. *Archives of Sexual Behavior, 3,* 585–595.

LoPiccolo, J., & Stock, W. E. (1986). Treatment of sexual dysfunction. *Journal of Consulting and Clinical Psychology, 54,* 158–167.

Lo Presto, C. T., Sherman, M. G., & Sherman, N. C. (1985). The effects of a masturbation seminar on high school males' attitudes, false beliefs, guilt, and behavior. *Journal of Sex Research, 21,* 142–156.

Lorenz, K. (1937). The companion in the bird's world. *Aak, 54,* 245–273.

Lorian, V. (1988). AIDS, anal sex, and heterosexuals. *Lancet, 334,* 1111.

Lothstein, L. M. (1980). The postsurgical transsexual. Empirical and theoretical considerations. *Archives of Sexual Behavior, 9,* 547–564.

Lothstein, L. M., & Levine, S. B. (1981). Expressive psychotherapy with gender dysphoric patients. *Archives of General Psychiatry, 38,* 924–929.

Lothstein, L. M., & Roback, H. (1984). Black female transsexuals and schizophrenia: A serendipitous finding. *Archives of Sexual Behavior, 13,* 371–390.

Lubinski, D., Tellegen, A., & Butcher, J. N. (1981). The relationship between androgyny and subjective indicators of emotional well-being. *Journal of Personality and Social Psychology, 40,* 722–730.

Lukianowicz, N. (1972). Incest: I. Paternal incest. II. Other types of incest. *British Journal of Psychiatry, 120,* 301–313.

Lunde, I., & Ortmann, J. (1990). Prevalence and sequelae of sexual torture. *Lancet, 336,* 289–291.

Maccoby, E. E. (1980). *Social development.* New York: Harcourt, Brace, Jovanovich.

Maccoby, E. E. (1987). The varied meanings of "masculine" and "feminine." In J. M. Reinisch, L. A. Rosenblum, & S. A. Sanders (Eds.), *Masculinity/femininity basic perspectives* (pp. 227–239). New York: Oxford University Press.

Maccoby, E. E., & Jacklin, C. N. (1974). *The psychology of sex differences.* Stanford, CA: Stanford University Press.

MacFarlane, D. F. (1984). Transsexual prostitution in New Zealand: Predominance of persons of Maori extraction. *Archives of Sexual Behavior, 13,* 301–309.

MacKenzie, K. R. (1978). Gender dysphoria syndrome: Towards standardized diagnostic criteria. *Archives of Sexual Behavior, 7,* 251–262.

Mahoney, M. J. (1977). Reflections on the cognitive-learning trend in psychotherapy. *American Psychologist, 32,* 5–13.

Malamuth, N. M. (1981). Rape proclivity among males. *Journal of Social Issues, 37,* 138–157.

Malamuth, N. M. (1985). The mass media and aggression against women: Research findings and prevention. In A. W. Burgess (Ed.), *Rape and sexual assault* (pp. 392–412). New York: Garland.

Malamuth, N. M. (1988). A multidimensional approach to sexual aggression: Combining measures of past behavior and present likelihood. *Annals of the New York Academy of Sciences, 528,* 123–132.

Malamuth, N. M. (1989a). The Attraction to Sexual Aggression scale: Part one. *Journal of Sex Research, 26,* 26–49.

Malamuth, N. M. (1989b). The Attraction to Sexual Aggression scale: Part two. *Journal of Sex Research, 26,* 324–354.

Malamuth, N. M., & Check, J. V. P. (1983). Sexual arousal to rape depictions: Individual differences. *Journal of Abnormal Psychology, 92,* 55–67.

Malamuth, N. M., & Donnerstein, E. (Eds.). (1984). *Pornography and sexual aggression.* New York: Academic Press.

Malamuth, N. M., Haber, S., & Feshbach, S. (1980). Testing hypotheses regarding rape: Exposure to sexual violence, sex differences, and the "normality" of rapists. *Journal of Research in Personality, 14,* 121–137.

Malcolm, J. (1984). *In the Freud archives.* Glasgow: William Collins.

Maletzky, B. M. (1973). "Assisted" covert sensitization: A preliminary report. *Behavior Therapy, 4,* 117–119.

Maletzky, B. M. (1980a). Assisted covert sensitization. In D. J. Cox & R. J. Daitzman (Eds.), *Exhibitionism: Description, assessment, and treatment* (pp. 289–293). New York: Garland.

Maletzky, B. M. (1980b). Self-referred versus court-referred sexually deviant patients: Success with assisted covert sensitization. *Behavior Therapy, 11,* 306–314.

Mancall, E. L., Alonso, R. J., & Marlowe, W. B. (1985). Sexual dysfunction in neurological disease. In R. T. Segraves & H. W. Schoenberg (Eds.), *Diagnosis and treatment of erectile disturbances* (pp. 65–85). New York: Plenum.

Mancini, J. A., & Orthner, D. K. (1978). Recreational sexuality preferences among middle-class husbands and wives. *Journal of Sex Research, 14,* 96–106.

Mann, E. M. (1981). Self-reported stresses of adolescent rape victims. *Journal of Adolescent Health Care, 2,* 29–33.

Margolin, L. (1990). Gender and the stolen kiss: Social support of male and female to violate a partner's sexual consent in a noncoercive situation. *Archives of Sexual Behavior, 19,* 281–291.

Margolin, L., Moran, P. B., & Miller, M. (1989). Social approval for violations of sexual consent in marriage and dating. *Violence and Victims, 4,* 45–55.

Marks, I., Gelder, M., & Bancroft, J. (1970). Sexual deviants two years after electric aversion. *British Journal of Psychiatry, 117,* 173–185.

Marquis, J. N. (1970). Orgasmic reconditioning: Changing sexual object choice through controlling masturbation fantasies. *Journal of Behavior Therapy and Experimental Psychiatry, 1,* 263–271.

Marshall, W. L. (1988). The use of sexually explicit stimuli by rapists, child molesters, and nonoffenders. *Journal of Sex Research, 25,* 267–288.

Marshall, W. L., & Barbaree, H. E. (1988). The long-term evaluation of a behavioral treatment program for child molesters. *Behavior Research and Therapy, 26,* 499–511.

Marshall, W. L., & Barbaree, H. E. (1990a). An integrated theory of the etiology of sexual offending. In W. L. Marshall, D. R. Laws & H. E. Barbaree (Eds.), *Handbook of sexual assault* (pp. 257–275). New York: Plenum.

Marshall, W. L., & Barbaree, H. E. (1990b). Outcome of comprehensive cognitive-behavioral treatment programs. In W. L. Marshall, D. R. Laws & H. E. Barbaree (Eds.), *Handbook of sexual assault* (pp. 363–385). New York: Plenum.

Marshall, W. L., Earls, C. M., Segal, Z., & Darke, J. (1983). A behavioral program for the assessment and treatment of sexual aggressors. In K. D. Craig & R. J. McMahon (Eds.), *Advances in clinical behavior therapy* (pp. 148–174). New York: Brunner/Mazel.

Marshall, W. L., Barbaree, H. E., & Christophe, D. (1986). Sexual offenders against female children: Sexual preferences for age of victims and type of behaviour. *Canadian Journal of Behavioral Science, 18,* 424–439.

Martin, A. D. (1982). Learning to hide: The socialization of the gay adolescent. *Adolescent Psychiatry, 10,* 52–65.

Martin, C. E. (1981). Factors affecting sexual functioning in 60–79-year-old married males. *Archives of Sexual Behavior, 10,* 399–420.

Martinson, F. M. (1976). Eroticism in infancy and childhood. *Journal of Sex Research, 12,* 251–262.

Martinson, F. M. (1981). Eroticism in infancy and childhood. In L. L. Constantine & F. Martinson (Eds.), *Children and sex* (pp. 23–35). Boston: Little, Brown.

Marzuk, P. M., Tierney, H., Tardiff, K., Gross, E. M., Morgan, E. B., Hsu, M. A., & Mann, J. J. (1988). Increased risk of suicide in persons with AIDS. *Journal of the American Medical Association, 259,* 1333–1337.

Mascola, L., Albritton, W. L., Cates, W., & Reynolds, G. H. (1983). Gonorrhea in American teenagers, 1960–1981. *Pediatric Infectious Disease, 2,* 302–303.

Masters, W. H., & Johnson, V. E. (1966). *Human sexual response.* Boston: Little, Brown.

Masters, W. H., & Johnson, V. E. (1970). *Human sexual inadequacy.* Boston: Little, Brown.

Masters, W. H., & Johnson, V. E. (1979). *Homosexuality in perspective.* Boston: Little, Brown.

Matarazzo, J. D. (1983). The reliability of psychiatric and psychological diagnosis. *Clinical Psychology Review, 3,* 103–145.

Mavissakalian, M., Blanchard, E. B., Abel, G. G., & Barlow, D. H. (1975). Responses to complex erotic stimuli in homosexual and heterosexual males. *British Journal of Psychiatry, 126,* 252–257.

McAnulty, R. D., & Adams, H. E. (1992). Validity and ethics of penile circumference measures of sexual arousal: A reply to McConaghy. *Archives of Sexual Behavior, 21,* 177–186.

McCann, J., Voris, J., Simon, M., & Wells, R. (1989). Perianal findings in prepubertal children selected for nonabuse: A descriptive study. *Child Abuse and Neglect, 13,* 179–193.

McCarthy, B. W. (1986). A cognitive-behavioral approach to understanding and treating sexual trauma. *Journal of Sex and Marital Therapy, 12,* 322–329.

McCombie, S. L., & Arons, J. H. (1980). Counseling rape victims. In S. L. McCombie (Ed.), *The rape crisis intervention handbook* (pp. 145–171). New York: Plenum.

McConaghy, N. (1960). Modes of abstract thinking and psychosis. *American Journal of Psychiatry, 117,* 106–110.

McConaghy, N. (1961). The measurement of an inhibitory process in human higher nervous activity: Its relation to allusive thinking and fatigue. *American Journal of Psychiatry, 118,* 125–132.

McConaghy, N. (1967). Penile volume change to moving pictures of male and female nudes in heterosexual and homosexual males. *Behavior Research and Therapy, 5,* 43–48.

McConaghy, N. (1969). Subjective and penile plethysmograph responses following aversion-relief and apomorphine therapy for homosexual impulses. *British Journal of Psychiatry, 115,* 723–730.

McConaghy, N. (1970). Results of systematic desensitization with phobias re-examined. *British Journal of Psychiatry, 117,* 89–92.

McConaghy, N. (1974). Measurements of change in penile dimensions. *Archives of Sexual Behavior, 3,* 381–388.

McConaghy, N. (1975). Aversive and positive conditioning treatments of homosexuality. *Behaviour Research and Therapy, 13,* 309–319.

McConaghy, N. (1976). Is a homosexual orientation irreversible? *British Journal of Psychiatry, 129,* 556–563.

McConaghy, N. (1977a). Behavioral intervention in homosexuality. *Journal of Homosexuality, 2,* 221–227.

McConaghy, N. (1977b). Behavioral treatment in homosexuality. In M. Hersen, R. M. Eisler, & P. M. Miller (Eds.), *Progress in behavior modification, vol. 5,* (pp. 309–380). New York: Academic Press.

McConaghy, N. (1978). Heterosexual experience, marital status and orientation of homosexual males. *Archives of Sexual Behavior, 7,* 575–581.

McConaghy, N. (1979). Maternal deprivation: Can its ghost be laid? *Australian and New Zealand Journal of Psychiatry, 13,* 209–217.

McConaghy, N. (1980). Behavior completion mechanisms rather than primary drives maintain behavioral patterns. *Activitas Nervosa Superior, 22,* 138–151.

McConaghy, N. (1982). Sexual deviation. In A. S. Bellack, M. Hersen, & A. E. Kazdin (Eds.), *International handbook of behavior therapy and modification* (pp. 683–716). New York: Plenum.

McConaghy, N. (1983). Agoraphobia, compulsive behaviors and behavior completion mechanisms. *Australian and New Zealand Journal of Psychiatry, 17,* 170–179.

McConaghy, N. (1984). Psychosexual disorders. In S. M. Turner & M. Hersen (Eds.), *Adult psychopathology and diagnosis* (pp. 370–405). New York: Wiley.

McConaghy, N. (1985). Psychosexual dysfunction. In M. Hersen & A. S. Bellack (Eds.), *Handbook of clinical behavior therapy with adults* (pp. 659–692). New York: Plenum.

McConaghy, N. (1987a). Heterosexuality/homosexuality: Dichotomy or continuum. *Archives of Sexual Behavior, 16,* 411–424.

McConaghy, N. (1987b). A learning approach. In J. H. Geer & W. T. O'Donohue (Eds.), *Theories of human sexuality* (pp. 287–333). New York: Plenum.

McConaghy, N. (1988a). Sexual dysfunction and deviation. In A. S. Bellack & M. Hersen (Eds.), *Behavioral assessment* (3rd ed., pp. 490–541). New York: Pergamon.

McConaghy, N. (1988b). Sex-linked behaviors questionnaire. In C. M. Davis, W. L. Yarber, & S. L. Davis (Eds.), *Sexuality-related measures: A compendium* (pp. 171–176). Lake Mills, IA: Graphic Publishing.

McConaghy, N. (1988c). Assessment and management of pathological gambling. *British Journal of Hospital Medicine, 40,* 131–135.

McConaghy, N. (1989). Validity and ethics of penile circumference measures of sexual arousal: A critical review. *Archives of Sexual Behavior, 18,* 357–369.

McConaghy, N. (1990a). Can reliance be placed on a single meta-analysis? *Australian and New Zealand Journal of Psychiatry, 24,* 405–415.

McConaghy, N. (1990b). Assessment and management of sex offenders: The Prince of Wales Program. *Australian and New Zealand Journal of Psychiatry, 24,* 175–181.

McConaghy, N. (1990c). Sexual deviation. In A. S. Bellack, M. Hersen, & A. E. Kazdin (Eds.), *International handbook of behavior therapy and modification* (2nd ed., pp. 565–580). New York: Plenum.

McConaghy, N. (1992). Validity and ethics of penile circumference measures of sexual arousal: A response. *Archives of Sexual Behavior, 21,* 187–195.

McConaghy, N., & Armstrong, M. S. (1983). Sexual orientation and consistency of sexual identity. *Archives of Sexual Behavior, 12,* 317–327.

McConaghy, N., Armstrong, M. S., Birrell, P. C., & Buhrich, N. (1979). The incidence of bisexual feelings and opposite sex behavior in medical students. *Journal of Nervous and Mental Disease, 167,* 685–688.

McConaghy, N., Armstrong, M. S., & Blaszczynski, A. (1981). Controlled comparisons of aversive therapy and covert sensitization in compulsive homosexuality. *Behaviour Research and Therapy, 19,* 425–434.

McConaghy, N., Armstrong, M. S., & Blaszczynski, A. (1985). Expectancy, covert sensitization and imaginal desensitization in compulsive sexuality. *Acta Psychiatrica Scandinavica, 72,* 1176–1187.

McConaghy, N., Armstrong, M. S., Blaszczynski, A., & Allcock, C. (1983). Controlled comparison of aversive therapy and imaginal desensitization in compulsive gambling. *British Journal of Psychiatry, 142,* 366–372.

McConaghy, N., & Barr, R. F. (1973). Classical, avoidance and backward conditioning treatments of homosexuality. *British Journal of Psychiatry, 122,* 151–162.

McConaghy, N., & Blaszczynski, A. (1980). A pair of monozygotic twins discordant for homosexuality: Sex-dimorphic behavior and penile volume responses. *Archives of Sexual Behavior, 9,* 123–131.

McConaghy, N., & Blaszczynski, A. (1988). Imaginal desensitization: A cost-effective treatment in two shop-lifters and a binge-eater resistant to previous therapy. *Australian and New Zealand Journal of Psychiatry, 22,* 78–82.

McConaghy, N., & Blaszczynksi, A. (1991). Initial stages of validation by penile volume assessment that sexual orientation is distributed dimensionally. *Comprehensive Psychiatry, 32,* 52–58.

McConaghy, N., & Blaszczynski, A. (1993). Effect of medroxyprogesterone on penile volume responses. Manuscript submitted for publication.

McConaghy, N., Blaszczynski, A., Armstrong, M. S., & Kidson, W. (1989). Resistance to treatment of adolescent sexual offenders. *Archives of Sexual Behavior, 18,* 97–107.

McConaghy, N., Blaszczynski, A., & Kidson, W. (1988). Treatment of sex offenders with imaginal desensitization and/or medroxyprogesterone. *Acta Psychiatrica Scandinavica, 77,* 199–206.

McConaghy, N., Buhrich, N., & Silove, D. (1993). *Opposite-sex-linked behaviours and homosexual feelings in predominantly heterosexual twins.* Manuscript submitted for publication.

McConaghy, N., & Lovibond, S. H. (1967). Methodological formalism in psychiatric research. *Journal of Nervous and Mental Disease, 144,* 117–123.

McConaghy, N., & Silove, D. (1991). Opposite sex behaviours correlate with degree of homosexual feelings in the predominantly heterosexual. *Australian and New Zealand Journal of Psychiatry, 25,* 77–83.

McConaghy, N., & Silove, D. (1992). Do sex-linked behaviors in children influence their relationships with their parents? *Archives of Sexual Behavior, 21,* 469–479.

McConaghy, N., Silove, D., & Hall, W. (1989). Behaviour completion mechanisms, anxiety and agoraphobia. *Australian and New Zealand Journal of Psychiatry, 23,* 373–378.

McConaghy, N., & Zamir, R. (1992a). *Sissiiness, tomboyism, sex role, identity and orientation.* Manuscript submitted for publication.

McConaghy, N., & Zamir, R. (1992b). *Non-sexist sexual experiences survey and attraction to sexual aggression scale.* Manuscript submitted for publication.

McConaghy, N., & Zamir, R. (1992c). *Heterosexual and homosexual coercion, sexual orientation and sexual roles.* Manuscript submitted for publication.

McCoy, N., Cutler, W., & Davidson, J. M. (1985). Relationships among sexual behavior, hot flashes, and hormone levels in perimenopausal women. *Archives of Sexual Behavior, 14,* 385–394.

McCoy, N. L., & Davidson, J. M. (1985). A longitudinal study of the effects of menopause on sexuality. *Maturitas, 7,* 203–210.

McCusker, J., Hill, E. M., & Mayer, K. H. (1990). Awareness and use of hepatitis B vaccine among homosexual male clients of a Boston community health center. *Public Health Report, 105,* 59–64.

McFall, R. M. (1990). The enhancement of social skills. In W. L. Marshall, D. R. Laws, & H. E. Barbaree (Eds.), *Handbook of sexual assault* (pp. 311–330). New York: Plenum.

McGrady, R. E. (1973). A forward-fading technique for increasing heterosexual responsiveness in male homosexuals. *Journal of Behavior Therapy and Experimental Psychiatry, 4,* 257–261.

McGrory, A. (1990). Menarche: Responses of early adolescent females. *Adolescence, 25,* 265–270.

McGuire, R. J., Carlisle, J. M., & Young, B. G. (1965). Sexual deviations as conditioned behavior: A hypothesis. *Behavior Research and Therapy, 2,* 185–190.

McLaws, M. L., Cooper, D., Leeder, S., & Chapman, S. (1988). AIDS quiz results: Knowledge and risk practices of women attending 24-hour clinics. *Medical Journal of Australia, 148,* 154.

Mead, M. (1950). *Male and female.* London: Gollancz.

Meisler, A. W., & Carey, M. P. (1990). A critical reevaluation of nocturnal penile tumescence monitoring in the diagnosis of erectile dysfunction. *Journal of Nervous and Mental Disease, 178,* 78–89.

Metz, P., & Bengtsson, J. (1984). Penile blood pressure. *Scandinavian Journal of Urology and Nephrology, 15,* 161–164.

Meyer, J. K. (1974). Clinical variants among applicants for sex reassignment. *Archives of Sexual Behavior, 3,* 527–558.

Meyer, J. K., Knorr, N. J., & Blumer, D. (1971). Characterization of a self-designated transsexual population. *Archives of Sexual Behavior, 1,* 219–230.

Meyer, J. K., & Reter, D. J. (1979). Sex reassignment. *Archives of General Psychiatry, 36,* 1010–1015.

Meyer, W. J., III, Finkelstein, J. W., Stuart, C. A., Webb, A., Smith, E. R., Payer, A. F., & Walker, P. A. (1981). Physical and hormonal evaluation of transsexual patients during hormonal therapy. *Archives of Sexual Behavior, 10,* 347–356.

Meyer, W. J., III, Webb, A., Stuart, C. A., Finkelstein, J. W., Lawrence, B., & Walker, P. A. (1986). Physical and hormonal evaluation of transsexual patients: A longitudinal study. *Archives of Sexual Behavior, 15,* 121–138.

Meyer-Bahlburg, H. F. L. (1979). Sex hormones and female homosexuality: A critical examination. *Archives of Sexual Behavior, 8,* 101–119.

Meyer-Bahlburg, H. F. L., Grisanti, G. C., & Ehrhardt, A. A. (1977). Prenatal effects of sex hormones on human male behavior: Medroxyprogesterone acetate. *Psychoneuroendocrinology, 2,* 383–390.

Mezey, G. C., & Taylor, P. A. J. (1988). Psychological reactions of women who have been raped. *British Journal of Psychiatry, 152,* 330–339.

Milan, R. J., Kilmann, P. R., & Boland, J. P. (1988). Treatment outcome of secondary orgasmic dysfunction: A two- to six-year follow-up. *Archives of Sexual Behavior, 17,* 463–480.

Miller, W. R., Williams, A. M., & Bernstein, M. H. (1982). The effects of rape on marital and sexual adjustment. *American Journal of Family Therapy, 10,* 51–58.

Money, J. (1970). Critique of Dr. Zuger's manuscript. *Psychosomatic Medicine, 32,* 463–465.

Money, J., Hampson, J. G., & Hampson, J. L. (1955). An examination of some basic concepts: The evidence of human hermaphroditism. *Johns Hopkins Hospital Bulletin, 97,* 301–319.

Money, J., Hampson, J. G., & Hampson, J. L. (1957). Imprinting and the establishment of gender role. *Archives of Neurology and Psychiatry, 77,* 333–336.

Money, J., & Pollitt, E. (1964). Cytogenic and psychosexual ambiguity. *Archives of General Psychology, 11,* 589–595.

Money, J., & Russo, A. J. (1979). Homosexual outcome of discordant gender identity/role in childhood: Longitudinal follow-up. *Journal of Pediatric Psychology, 4,* 29–41.

Money, J., Schwartz, M., & Lewis, V. G. (1984). Adult erotosexual status and fetal hormonal masculinization and demasculinization: 46, XX congenital virilizing adrenal hyperplasia and 465, XY androgen-insensitivity syndrome compared. *Psychoneuroendocrinology, 9,* 405–414.

Moore, H. A., Zusman, J., & Root, G. C. (1985). Noninstitutional treatment of sex offenders in Florida. *American Journal of Psychiatry, 142,* 964–967.

Morgan, A. J. (1978). Psychotherapy for transsexual candidates screened out of surgery. *Archives of Sexual Behavior, 7,* 273–283.

Morgenstern, F. S., Pearce, J. F., & Rees, W. L. (1965). Predicting the outcome of behavior therapy to psychological tests. *Behavior Research and Therapy, 2,* 191–200.

Morokoff, P. (1978). Determinants of female orgasm. In J. LoPiccolo & L. LoPiccolo (Eds.), *Handbook of sex therapy* (pp. 147–165). New York: Plenum.

Morris, N. M., Udry, J. R., Khan-Dawood, F., & Dawood, M. Y. (1987). Marital sex frequency and midcycle female testosterone. *Archives of Sexual Behavior, 16,* 27–37.

Moser, C., & Levitt, E. E. (1987). An exploratory-descriptive study of a sadomasochistically oriented sample. *Journal of Sex Research, 23,* 322–337.

Moss, M., Frank, E., & Anderson, B. (1990). The effects of marital status and partner support on rape trauma. *American Journal of Orthopsychiatry, 60,* 379–391.

Mrazek, P. J., Lynch, M. A., & Bentovim, A. (1983). Sexual abuse of children in the United Kingdom. *Child Abuse and Neglect, 7,* 147–153.

Mrazek, P. B., & Mrazek, D. A. (1981). The effects of child sexual abuse: Methodological considerations. In P. B. Mrazek & C. H. Kempe (Eds.), *Sexually abused children and their families* (pp. 235–245). Oxford: Pergamon.

Muehlenhard, C. L., & Cook, S. W. (1988). Men's self-reports of unwanted sexual activity. *Journal of Sex Research, 24,* 58–72.

Mullaly, P. (1970). *Psychoanalysis and interpersonal psychiatry.* New York: Science House.

Mullen, P. E., Romans-Clarkson, S. E., Walton, V. A., & Herbison, G. P. (1988). Impact of sexual and physical abuse on women's mental health. *Lancet, 334,* 841–845.

Mulligan, T., & Katz, P. G. (1989). Why aged men become impotent. *Archives of Internal Medicine, 149,* 1365–1366.

Mulligan, T., & Moss, C. R. (1991). Sexuality and aging in male veterans: A cross-sectional study of interest, ability, and activity. *Archives of Sexual Behavior, 20,* 17–25.

Munjack, D., Cristol, A., Goldstein, A., Phillips, D., Goldberg, A., Whipple, K., Staples, F., & Kanno, P. (1976). Behavioral treatment of orgasmic dysfunction: A controlled study. *British Journal of Psychiatry, 129,* 497–502.

Munjack, D. J., & Kanno, P. H. (1979). Retarded ejaculation: A review. *Archives of Sexual Behavior, 8,* 139–150.

Murphy, P. J., III. (1980). The police investigation. In S. L. McCombie (Ed.), *Rape crisis intervention handbook* (pp. 69–78). New York: Plenum.

Murphy, W. D. (1990). Assessment and modification of cognitive distortions in sex offenders. In W. L. Marshall, D. R. Laws, & H. E. Barbaree (Eds.), *Handbook of sexual assault* (pp. 331–342). New York: Plenum.

Murphy, W. D., Haynes, M. R., Stalgaitis, S. J., & Flanagan, B. (1986). Differential sexual responding among four groups of sexual offenders against children. *Journal of Psychopathology and Behavioral Assessment, 8,* 339–353.

Murphy, W. D., Krisar, J., Stalgaitis, S., & Anderson, K. (1984). The use of penile tumescence measures with incarcerated rapists: Further validity issues. *Archives of Sexual Behavior, 13,* 545–554.

Murrin, M. R., & Laws, D. R. (1990). The influence of pornography on sexual crimes. In W. L. Marshall, D. R. Laws, & H. E. Barbaree (Eds.), *Handbook of sexual assault* (pp. 73–91). New York: Plenum.

Mussen, P. H. (1971). Some antecedents and consequents of masculine sex-typing in adolescent boys. In M. C. Jones, N. Bayley, J. W. Macfarlane, & M. P. Honzik (Eds.), *The course of human development* (pp. 350–356). Waltham, MA: Xerox College Publishing.

Myers, L. S., & Morokoff, P. J. (1986). Physiological and subjective sexual arousal in pre- and postmenopausal women and postmenopausal women taking replacement therapy. *Psychophysiology, 23,* 283–292.

Myrick, R. O. (1970). The counselor consultant and the effeminate boy. *Personnel and Guidance Journal, 48,* 355 361.

Nadelson, C. C., Notman, M. T., Zackson, H., & Gornick, J. (1982). A follow-up study of rape victims. *American Journal of Psychiatry, 139,* 1266–1270.

Nagayama Hall, G. C., Proctor, W. C., & Nelson, G. M. (1988). Validity of physiological measures of pedophilic sexual arousal in a sexual offender population. *Journal of Consulting and Clinical Psychology, 56,* 118–122.

Nelson, J. A. (1986). Incest self-report findings from a nonclinical sample. *Journal of Sex Research, 22,* 463–477.

Nelson, R. O., & Hayes, S. C. (1981). Nature of behavioral assessment. In A. S. Bellack & M. Hersen (Eds.), *Behavioral assessment* (2nd ed., pp. 3–37). New York: Pergamon.

Nettelbladt, P., & Uddenberg, N. (1979). Sexual dysfunction and sexual satisfaction in 58 married Swedish men. *Journal of Psychosomatic Research, 23,* 141–147.

Nicholls, J. B., Licht, B. G., & Pearl, R. A. (1982). Some dangers of using personality questionnaires to study personality. *Psychological Bulletin, 92,* 572–580.

Norris, J., & Feldman-Summers, S. (1981). Factors related to the psychological impacts of rape on the victim. *Journal of Abnormal Psychology, 90,* 562–567.

Nutter, D. E., & Condron, M. K. (1985). Sexual fantasy and activity patterns of males with inhibited sexual desire and males with erectile dysfunction versus normal controls. *Journal of Sex and Marital Therapy, 11,* 91–98.

O'Carroll, R., & Bancroft, J. (1984). Testosterone therapy for low sexual interest and erectile dysfunction in men: A controlled study. *British Journal of Psychiatry, 145,* 146–151.

O'Connor, A. A. (1987). Female sex offenders. *British Journal of Psychiatry, 150,* 615–620.

Open Forum. (1978). *Archives of Sexual Behavior, 7,* 387–415.

Osborn, M., Hawton, K., & Gath, D. (1988). Sexual dysfunctions among middle age women in the community. *British Medical Journal, 296,* 959–962.

Ostow, M. (1953). Transvestism. *Journal of the American Medical Association, 152,* 1553.

Otterbein, K. F. (1979). A cross-cultural study of rape. *Aggressive Behavior, 5,* 425–435.

Ozer, E. M., & Bandura, A. (1990). Mechanisms governing empowerment effects: A self-efficacy analysis. *Journal of Personality and Social Psychology, 58,* 472–486.

Padian, N., Marquis, L., Francis, D. P., Anderson, R. E., Rutherford, G. W., O'Malley, P. M., & Winkelstein, W. (1987). Male-to-female transmission of human immunodeficiency virus. *Journal of the American Medical Association, 258,* 788–790.

Palmer, C. T. (1988). Twelve reasons why rape is not sexually motivated: A skeptical examination. *Journal of Sex Research, 25,* 512–530.

Palmer, R. L. (1990). Childhood sexual experiences with adults reported by women with eating disorders. *British Journal of Psychiatry, 156,* 699–703.

Parcel, G. S. (1977). Sex and the preschooler. *Texas Medicine, 73,* 37–41.

Paredes, A., Baumgold, J., Pugh, L. A., & Ragland, R. (1966). Clinical judgment in the assessment of psychopharmacological effects. *Journal of Nervous and Mental Disease, 142,* 153–160.

Pauly, I. B. (1974). Female transsexualism: Parts I, II. *Archives of Sexual Behavior, 3,* 487–526.

Pauly, I. B., & Edgerton, M. T. (1986). The gender identity movement: A growing surgical-psychiatric liaison. *Archives of Sexual Behavior, 15,* 315–329.

Pavlov, I. (1927). *Conditioned reflexes* (C. V. Anrep, Jr., Ed.). Oxford: Oxford University Press.

Perry, S., Jacobsberg, L., & Fishman, B. (1990). Suicidal ideation and HIV testing. *Journal of the American Medical Association, 263,* 679–682.

Person, E. S., & Ovesey, L. (1974). The psychodynamics of male transsexualism. In R. C. Friedman & R. M. Richart (Eds.), *Sex differences in behavior* (pp. 315–325). New York: Wiley.

Person, E. S., & Ovesey, L. (1984). Homosexual cross-dressers. *Journal of the American Academy of Psychoanalysis, 12,* 167–186.

Person, E. S., Terestman, N., Myers, W. A., Goldberg, E. L., & Salvadori, C. (1989). Gender differences in sexual behaviors and fantasies in a college population. *Journal of Sex and Marital Therapy, 15,* 187–198.

Peters, H. (1989). The epidemiology of sexually transmitted diseases. In R. Richmond & D. Wakefield (Eds.), *AIDS and other sexually transmitted diseases.* Sydney: Harcourt Brace Jovanovich.

Petrovich, M., & Templer, D. I. (1984). Heterosexual molestation of children who later became rapists. *Psychological Reports, 54,* 810.

Pfaus, J. G., Myronuk, L. D. S., & Jacobs, W. J. (1986). Soundtrack contents and depicted sexual violence. *Archives of Sexual Behavior, 15,* 231–237.

Pfeiffer, E., & Davis, G. C. (1972). Determinants of sexual behavior in middle and old age. *Journal of the American Geriatrics Society, 20,* 151–158.

Pfeiffer, E., Verwoerdt, A., & Davis, G. C. (1972). Sexual behavior in middle life. *American Journal of Psychiatry, 128,* 1262–1267.

Pleak, R. R., & Meyer-Bahlburg, H. F. L. (1990). Sexual behavior and AIDS knowledge of young male prostitutes in Manhattan. *Journal of Sex Research, 27,* 557–587.

Pleak, R. R., Meyer-Bahlburg, H. F. L., O'Brien, J. D., Bowen, H. A., & Morganstein, A. (1989). Cross-gender behavior and psychopathology in boy psychiatric outpatients. *Journal of the American Academy of Child and Adolescent Psychiatry, 28,* 385–393.

Pleck, J. H. (1981). *The myth of masculinity.* Cambridge: MIT Press.

Plomin, R., De Fries, J. C., & McClearn, G. E. (1980). *Behavioral genetics: A primer.* San Francisco: Freeman.

Plummer, K. (1979). Images of pedophilia. In M. Cook & G. Wilson (Eds.), *Love and attraction* (pp. 537–540). Oxford: Pergamon.

Plummer, K. (1981). Pedophilia: Constructing a sociological baseline. In M. Cook & K. Howells (Eds.), *Adult sexual interest in children* (pp. 221–250). Oxford: Pergamon.

Pomeroy, W. B. (1967). A report on the sexual histories of twenty-five transsexuals. *Transactions of the New York Academy of Sciences, 29,* 444–447.

Porteous, M. A. (1985). Developmental aspects of adolescent problem disclosure in England and Ireland. *Journal of Child Psychology and Psychiatry, 26,* 465–478.

Potterat, J. J., Woodhouse, D. E., Muth, J. B., & Muth, S. Q. (1990). Estimating the prevalence and career longevity of prostitute women. *Journal of Sex Research, 27,* 233–245.

Price, J. H. (1982). High school students' attitudes toward homosexuality. *The Journal of School Health, 52,* 469–474.

Price, J. H., & Miller, P. A. (1984). Sexual fantasies of black and of white college students. *Psychological Reports, 54,* 1007–1014.

Primov, G., & Kieffer, C. (1977). The Peruvian brothel as sexual dispensary and social arena. *Archives of Sexual Behavior, 6,* 245–253.

Prince, V., & Bentler, P. M. (1972). Survey of 504 cases of transvestism. *Psychological Reports, 32,* 903–917.

Quinn, N. P., Toone, B., Lang, A. E., Marsden, C. D., & Parkes, J. D. (1983). Dopa dose-dependent sexual deviation. *British Journal of Psychiatry, 142,* 296–298.

Quinsey, V. L. (1984). Sexual aggression: Studies of offenders against women. In D. N. Weisstub (Ed.), *Law and mental health, international perspectives, vol. 1* (pp. 86–121). New York: Pergamon.

Quinsey, V. L. (1986). Men who have sex with children. In D. N. Weisstub (Ed.), *Law and mental health, international perspectives, vol. 2* (pp. 140–172). New York: Pergamon.

Quinsey, V. L., Chaplin, T. C., & Carrigan, W. F. (1979). Sexual preference among incestuous and non-incestuous child molesters. *Behavior Therapy, 10,* 562–565.

Quinsey, V. L., & Earls, C. M. (1990). The modification of sexual preferences. In W. L. Marshall, D. R. Laws, & H. E. Barbaree (Eds.), *Handbook of sexual assault* (pp. 279–295). New York: Plenum.

Quinsey, V. L., Steinman, C. M., Bergersen, S. G., & Holmes, J. (1975). Penile circumference, skin conductance and ranking responses of child molesters and "normals" to sexual and non-sexual visual stimuli. *Behavior Therapy, 6,* 213–219.

Quinsey, V. L., & Upfold, D. (1985). Rape completion and victim injury as a function of female resistance strategy. *Canadian Journal of Behavioral Science, 17,* 40–50.

Raboch, J., & Bartak, V. (1980). Changes in the sexual life of Czechoslovak women born between 1911 and 1958. *Archives of Sexual Behavior, 9,* 495–502.

Raboch, J., Kobilkova, J., Raboch, J., & Starka, L. (1985). *Archives of Sexual Behavior, 14,* 263–277.

Randell, J. B. (1971). Indications for sex re-assignment surgery. *Archives of Sexual Behavior, 1,* 153–161.

Randolph, B. J., & Winstead, B. (1988). Sexual decision making and object relations theory. *Archives of Sexual Behavior, 17,* 389–409.

Ratzan, R. M. (1988). AIDS, autopsies, and abandonment. *Journal of the American Medical Association, 260,* 3466–3469.

Reading, A. E. (1983). A comparison of the accuracy and reactivity of methods of monitoring male sexual behavior. *Journal of Behavioral Assessment, 5,* 11–23.

Reading, A. E., & Wiest, W. M. (1984). An analysis of self-reported sexual behavior in a sample of normal males. *Archives of Sexual Behavior, 13,* 69–83.

Realmuto, G. M., Jensen, J. B., & Wescoe, S. (1990). Specificity and sensitivity of sexually anatomically correct dolls in substantiating abuse: A pilot study. *Journal of the American Academy of Child and Adolescent Psychiatry, 29,* 743–746.

Reamy, K. J., & White, S. E. (1985). Dyspareunia in pregnancy. *Journal of Psychosomatic Obstetrics and Gynecology, 4,* 263–270.

Reamy, K. J., & White, S. E. (1987). Sexuality in the puerperium: A review. *Archives of Sexual Behavior, 16,* 165–186.

Reinisch, J. (1974). Fetal hormones, the brain, and human sex differences: A heuristic, integrative review of the recent literature. *Archives of Sexual Behavior, 3,* 51–90.

Rekers, G. A., & Lovaas, O. I. (1974). Behavioral treatment of deviant sex-role behavior in a male child. *Journal of Applied Behavior Analysis, 7,* 173–190.

Remafedi, G. (1985). Adolescent homosexuality: Issues for pediatricians. *Clinical Pediatrics, 24,* 481–485.

Remafedi, G. (1987a). Homosexual youth: A challenge to contemporary society. *Journal of the American Medical Association, 258,* 222–225.

Remafedi, G. (1987b). Adolescent homosexuality: Psychosocial and medical implications. *Pediatrics, 79,* 331–377.

Renshaw, D. C. (1988). Profile of 2,376 patients treated at Loyola sex clinic between 1972 and 1987. *Sexual and Marital Therapy, 3,* 111–117.

Revitch, E. (1965). Sex murder and the potential sex murderer. *Diseases of the Nervous System, 26,* 640–648.

Revitch, E. (1980). Gynocide and unprovoked attacks on women. *Correctional and Social Psychiatry, 26,* 6–11.

Richman, J. A., Raskin, V. D., & Gaines, C. (1991). Gender roles, social support, and postpartum depressive symptomatology. *Journal of Nervous and Mental Disease, 179,* 139–147.

Rinear, E. E. (1985). Sexual assault and the handicapped victim. In A. W. Burgess (Ed.), *Rape and sexual assault* (pp. 139–145). New York: Garland.

Rio, L. M. (1991). Psychological and sociological research and the decriminalization or legalization of prostitution. *Archives of Sexual Behavior, 20,* 205–218.

Risin, L. I., & Koss, M. P. (1987). Sexual abuse of boys: Prevalence and descriptive characteristics of childhood victimization. *Journal of Interpersonal Violence, 2,* 309–319.

Robins, L. N., Helzer, J. E., Croughan, J., & Ratcliff, K. (1981). National Institute of Mental Health Diagnostic Interview Schedule: Its history, characteristics and validity. *Archives of General Psychiatry, 38,* 381–389.

Robins, L. N., Helzer, J. E., Weissman, M. M., Orvaschel, H., Gruenberg, E., Burke, J. D., & Regier, D. A. (1984). Lifetime prevalence of specific psychiatric disorders in three sites. *Archives of General Psychiatry, 41,* 949–958.

Robinson, B. E., & Barrett, R. L. (1985). Teenage fathers. *Psychology Today, 19,* 68–70.

Robson, K. M., Brant, H. A., & Kumar, R. (1981). Maternal sexuality during first pregnancy and after childbirth. *British Journal of Obstetrics and Gynaecology, 88*, 882–889.

Rodkin, L. I., Hunt, E. J., & Cowan, S. D. (1982). A men's support group for significant others of rape victims. *Journal of Marital and Family Therapy, 8*, 91–97.

Rodman, H., Lewis, S. H., & Griffith, S. B. (1984). *The sexual rights of adolescents*. New York: Columbia University Press.

Roesler, T., & Deisher, R. W. (1974). Youthful male homosexuality. *Journal of the American Medical Association, 219*, 1018–1023.

Romans-Clarkson, S. E. (1989). Psychological sequelae of induced abortion. *Australian and New Zealand Journal of Psychiatry, 23*, 555–565.

Rooth, F. G. (1973). Exhibitionism outside Europe and America. *Archives of Sexual Behavior, 2*, 351–363.

Rosen, G. M. (1987). Self-help treatment books and the commercialization of psychotherapy. *American Psychologist, 42*, 46–51.

Rosen, R. C., & Beck, J. G. (1988). *Patterns of sexual arousal*. New York: Guilford.

Rosen, R.C., & Keefe, R. J. (1978). The measurement of human penile tumescence. *Psychophysiology, 15*, 366–376.

Rosler, A., & Kohn, G. (1983). Male pseudohermaphroditism due to 17beta-hydroxysteroid dehydrogenase deficiency: Studies on the natural history of the defect and effect of androgens on gender role. *Journal of Steroid Biochemistry, 19*, 663–674.

Rousseau, L., Dupont, A., Labrie, F., & Couture, M. (1988). Sexuality changes in prostate cancer patients receiving antihormonal therapy combining the antiandrogen Flutamide with medical (LHRH agonist) or surgical castration. *Archives of Sexual Behavior, 17*, 87–98.

Rubin, R. T., Reinisch, J. M., & Haskett, R. F. (1981). Postnatal gonadal steroid effects on human behavior. *Science, 211*, 1318–1324.

Russell, D. E. H. (1982). *Rape in marriage*. New York: Macmillan.

Russell, D. E. H. (1983). The incidence and prevalence of intrafamilial and extrafamilial sexual abuse of female children. *Child Abuse and Neglect, 7*, 133–146.

Russell, D. E. H. (1984). The prevalence and seriousness of incestuous abuse: Stepfathers vs. biological fathers. *Child Abuse and Neglect, 8*, 15–22.

Russell, D. E. H. (1986). *The secret trauma: Incest in the lives of girls and women*. New York: Basic Books.

Russell, D. E. H. (1988). The incidence and prevalence of intrafamilial and extrafamilial sexual abuse of female children. In L. E. A. Walker (Ed.), *Handbook on sexual abuse of children* (pp. 19–36). New York: Springer.

Rust, J., Golombok, S., & Collier, J. (1988). Marital problems and sexual dysfunctions: Are they related? *British Journal of Psychiatry, 152*, 629–631.

Rutter, M., & Hersov, L. (1985). *Child and adolescent psychiatry*. Oxford: Blackwell.

Rychtarik, R. G., Silverman, W. K., Van Landingham, W. P., & Prue, D. M. (1984a). Treatment of an incest victim with implosion therapy: A case study. *Behavior Therapy, 15*, 410–420.

Rychtarik, R. G., Silverman, W. K., Van Landingham, W. P., & Prue, D. M. (1984b). Further considerations in treating sexual assault victims with implosion. *Behavior Therapy, 15*, 423–426.

Saghir, M., & Robins, E. (1973). *Male and female homosexuality: A comprehensive investigation*. Baltimore: Williams and Wilkins.

Sakheim, D. K., Barlow, D. H., Beck, J. G., & Abrahamson, D. J. (1985). A comparison of male heterosexual and male homosexual patterns of sexual arousal. *Journal of Sex Research, 21*, 183–198.

Salmimies, P., Kockett, G., Pirke, K. M., Vogt, H. J., & Schill, W. B. (1982). Effects of testosterone replacement on sexual behavior in hypogonadal men. *Archives of Sexual Behavior, 11*, 345–353.

Sandberg, D. E., Meyer-Bahlburg, H. F. L., Rosen, T. S., & Johnson, H. L. (1990). Effects of prenatal methadone exposure on sex-dimorphic behavior in early school-age children. *Psychoendocrinology, 15*, 77–82.

Sarrel, P. M. (1987). Sexuality in the middle years. *Obstetrics and Gynecology Clinics of North America, 14*, 49–62.

Sarrel, P., & Masters, W. (1982). Sexual molestation of men by women. *Archives of Sexual Behavior, 11*, 117–133.

Satterfield, S. (1975). Common sexual problems of children and adolescents. *Pediatric Clinics of North America, 22,* 643–652.

Saunders, J. M., & Valente, S. M. (1987). Suicide risk among gay men and lesbians: A review. *Death Studies, 11,* 1–23.

Savitz, L., & Rosen, L. (1988). The sexuality of prostitutes: Sexual enjoyment reported by "streetwalkers." *Journal of Sex Research, 24,* 200–208.

Saypol, D. C., Peterson, G. A., Howards, S. S., & Yazel, J. J. (1983). Impotence: Are the newer diagnostic methods a necessity? *Journal of Urology, 130,* 260–262.

Schaefer, S. (1977). Sociosexual behavior in male and female homosexuals: A study in sex differences. *Archives of Sexual Behavior, 6,* 355–364.

Schaffer, B., & DeBlassie, R. R. (1984). Adolescent prostitution. *Adolescence, 19,* 689–696.

Schatzberg, A. F., Westfall, M. P., Blumetti, A. B., & Birk, C. L. (1975). Effeminacy 1: A quantitative rating scale. *Archives of Sexual Behavior, 4,* 31–41.

Schiavi, R. C., Derogatis, L. R., Kuriansky, J., O'Connor, D., & Sharpe, I. (1979). The assessment of sexual function and marital interaction. *Journal of Sex and Marital Therapy, 5,* 169–224.

Schiavi, R. C., Fisher, C., White, D., Beers, P., & Szechter, R. (1984). Pituitary-gonadal function during sleep in men with erectile impotence and normal controls. *Psychosomatic Medicine, 46,* 239–254.

Schiavi, R. C., Schreiner-Engel, P., Mandeli, J., Schanzer, H., & Cohen, E. (1990). Healthy aging and male sexual function. *American Journal of Psychiatry, 147,* 766–771.

Schiavi, R. C., Schreiner-Engel, P., White, D., & Mandeli, J. (1988). Pituitary-gonadal function during sleep in men with hypoactive sexual desire and in normal controls. *Psychosomatic Medicine, 50,* 304–318.

Schiavi, R. C., Theilgaard, A., Owen, D. R., & White, D. (1988). Sex chromosome anomalies, hormones, and sexuality. *Archives of General Psychiatry, 45,* 19–24.

Schneider, S. G., Farberow, N. L., & Kruks, G. N. (1989). Suicidal behavior in adolescent and young gay men. *Suicide and Life-Threatening Behavior, 19,* 381–394.

Schofield, M. (1968). *The sexual behavior of young people.* Harmondsworth, UK: Penguin.

Schofield, M. (1973). *The sexual behavior of young adults.* London: Allen Lane.

Schover, L. R. (1989). Sex therapy for the penile prosthesis recipient. *Urology Clinics of North America, 16,* 91–98.

Schulsinger, F. (1972). Psychopathy, heredity and environment. *International Journal of Mental Health, 1,* 190–206.

Schwartz, M. F., Kolodny, R. C., & Masters, W. H. (1980). Plasma testosterone levels of sexually functional and dysfunctional men. *Archives of Sexual Behavior, 9,* 355–366.

Scott, F. B., Byrd, G. J., & Karacan, I. (1979). Erectile impotence treated with an inplantable inflatable prosthesis: Five years of clinical experience. *Journal of the American Medical Association, 241,* 2609–2612.

Scully, D., & Marolla, J. (1985). Rape and vocabularies of motive: Alternative perspectives. In A. W. Burgess (Ed.), *Rape and sexual assault* (pp. 294–312). New York: Garland.

Segal, Z. V., & Marshall, W. L. (1985). Heterosexual social skills in a population of rapists and child molesters. *Journal of Consulting and Clinical Psychology, 53,* 55–63.

Segraves, R. T., Madsen, R., Carter, C. S., & Davis, J. M. (1985). Erectile dysfunction associated with pharmacological agents. In R. T. Segraves & H. W. Schoenberg (Eds.), *Diagnosis and treatment of erectile disturbances* (pp. 23–63). New York: Plenum.

Segraves, R. T., Schoenberg, H. W., & Ivanoff, J. (1983). Serum testosterone and prolactin levels in erectile dysfunction. *Journal of Sex and Marital Therapy, 9,* 19–26.

Segraves, R. T., Schoenberg, H. W., & Segraves, K. A. B. (1985). Evaluation of the etiology of erectile failure. In R. T. Segraves & H. W. Schoenberg (Eds.), *Diagnosis and treatment of erectile disturbances* (pp. 165–195). New York: Plenum.

Segraves, R. T., Schoenberg, H. W., Zarins, C. K., Camic, P., & Knopf, J. (1981). Characteristics of erectile dysfunction as a function of medical care system entry point. *Psychosomatic Medicine, 43,* 227–234.

Segraves, K. A., Segraves, R. T., & Schoenberg, H. W. (1987). Use of sexual history to differentiate organic from psychogenic impotence. *Archives of Sexual Behavior, 16,* 125–137.

Semans, J. H. (1956). Premature ejaculation: A new approach. *Southern Medical Journal, 49,* 373–377.

Sgroi, S. M. (1975). Sexual molestation of children. *Children Today, 4,* 18–44.

Sgroi, S. M. (1978). Comprehensive examination of child sexual assault: Diagnostic, therapeutic and child protection issues. In A. W. Burgess, A. W. Groth, L. L. Holmstrom, & S. M. Sgroi (Eds.), *Sexual assault of children and adolescents* (pp. 143–157). Toronto: Lexington Books.

Shapiro, F. (1989). Efficacy of the eye movement desensitization procedure in the treatment of traumatic memories. *Archives of Traumatic Stress, 2,* 199–223.

Sherwin, B. B., & Gelfand, M. M. (1987). The role of androgen in the maintenance of sexual functioning in oophorectomized women. *Psychosomatic Medicine, 49,* 397–409.

Sherwin, B. B., Gelfand, M. M., & Brender, W. (1985). Androgen enhances sexual motivation in females: A prospective, crossover study of sex steroid administration in the surgical menopause. *Psychosomatic Medicine, 47,* 339–351.

Sholty, M. J., Ephross, P. H., Plaut, S. M., Fischman, S. H., Charnas, J. F., & Cody, C. A. (1984). Female orgasmic experience: A subjective study. *Archives of Sexual Behavior, 13,* 155–164.

Siegel, J. M., Sorenson, S. B., Golding, J. M., Burnam, M. A., & Stein, J. A. (1987). The prevalence of childhood sexual assault. *American Journal of Epidemiology, 126,* 1141–1153.

Siegel, L., & Zitrin, A. (1978). Transsexuals in the New York City welfare population: The function of illusion in transsexuality. *Archives of Sexual Behavior, 7,* 285–290.

Silverman, D. C., Kalick, S. M., Bowie, S. I., & Edbril, S. D. (1988). Blitz rape and confidence rape: A typology applied to 1,000 consecutive cases. *American Journal of Psychiatry, 145,* 1438–1441.

Silverstein, C. (1977). Homosexuality and the ethics of behavioral intervention: Paper 2. *Journal of Homosexuality, 2,* 205–211.

Silverstein, C., & White, E. (1977). *The joy of gay sex.* New York: Simon and Schuster.

Singer, J., & Singer, I. (1978). Types of female orgasm. In J. LoPiccolo & L. LoPiccolo (Eds.), *Handbook of sex therapy* (pp. 175–186). New York: Plenum.

Siraj, Q. H., Bomanji, J., & Akhtar, M. A. (1990). Quantitation of pharmacologically-induced penile erections: The value of radionuclide phallography in the objective evaluation of erectile haemodynamics. *Nuclear Medicine Communications, 11,* 445–458.

Sisley, E. L., & Harris, B. (1977). *The joy of lesbian sex.* New York: Crown.

Skakkebaek, N. E., Bancroft, J., Davidson, D. W., & Warner, P. (1981). Androgen replacement with oral testosterone undeconate in hypogonadal men: A double blind controlled study. *Clinical Endocrinology, 14,* 49–61.

Skinner, B. F. (1966). What is the experimental analysis of behavior? *Journal of the Experimental Analysis of Behavior, 9,* 213–218.

Skinner, B. F. (1972). *Cumulative record.* New York: Appleton-Century-Crofts.

Skipper, J. K., Jr., & Nass, G. (1966). Dating behavior: A framework for analysis and an illustration. *Journal of Marriage and the Family, 28,* 412–419.

Slag, M. F., Morley, J. E., Elson, M.K., Trence, D. L., Nelson, C. J., Nelson, A. E., Kinlaw, W. B., Beyer, H. S., Nuttall, F. Q., & Shafer, R. B. (1983). Impotence in medical clinic outpatients. *Journal of the American Medical Association, 249,* 1736–1740.

Smith, E. A., & Udry, J. R. (1985). Coital and non-coital behaviors of white and black adolescents. *American Journal of Public Health, 75,* 1200–1203.

Smith, R. S. (1976). Voyeurism: A review of the literature. *Archives of Sexual Behavior, 5,* 585–608.

Smith, S. R., & Meyer, R. G. (1984). Child abuse reporting laws and psychotherapy: A time for reconsideration. *International Journal of Law and Psychiatry, 7,* 351–366.

Smukler, A. J., & Schiebel, D. (1975). Personality characteristics of exhibitionism. *Diseases of the Nervous System, 36,* 600–603.

Snyder, D. K., & Berg, P. (1983a). Determinants of sexual dissatisfaction in sexually distressed couples. *Archives of Sexual Behavior, 12,* 237–246.

Snyder, D. K., & Berg, P. (1983b). Predicting couples' response to brief directive sex therapy. *Journal of Sex and Marital Therapy, 9,* 114–120.

Sobell, M. B., Wilkinson, D. A., & Sobell, L. C. (1990). Alcohol and drug problems: In A. S. Bellack, M. Hersen, & A. E. Kazdin (Eds.), *International handbook of behavior therapy and modification* (2nd ed., pp. 415–435). New York: Plenum.

Social worker scapegoated. (1990, August 5). *Weekend Australian,* p. 4.

Sohn, N., & Robilotti, S. G. (1977). The gay bowel syndrome. *American Journal of Gastroenterology, 67,* 478–484.

Sophie, J. (1988). Internalizing homophobia and lesbian identity. In E. Coleman (Ed.), *Psychotherapy with homosexual men and women* (pp. 53–65). New York: Haworth.

Sorensen, R. C. (1973). *Adolescent sexuality in contemporary America.* New York: World.

Sorenson, S. B., Stein, J. A., Siegel, J. M., Golding, J. M., & Burnam, M. A. (1987). The prevalence of adult sexual assault. *American Journal of Epidemiology, 126,* 1154–1164.

Soyinka, F. (1979). Sexual behavior among university students in Nigeria. *Archives of Sexual Behavior, 8,* 15–26.

Spark, R. F., White, R. A., & Connolly, P. B. (1980). Impotence is not always psychogenic. *Journal of the American Medical Association, 243,* 750–755.

Spector, I. P., & Carey, M. P. (1990). Incidence and prevalence of the sexual dysfunctions: A critical review of the empirical literature. *Archives of Sexual Behavior, 19,* 389–408.

Spence, J. T. (1985). Gender identity and its implications for the concepts of masculinity and femininity. In T. B. Sonderegger (Ed.), *Psychology and gender: Nebraska symposium on motivation 1984* (pp. 59–96). Lincoln: University of Nebraska Press.

Spence, J. T., Helmreich, R. L., & Holahan, C. K. (1979). Negative and positive components of psychological masculinity and femininity and their relationship to self-reports of neurotic and acting-out behaviors. *Journal of Personality and Social Psychology, 37,* 1673–1682.

Spencer, C. C., & Nicholson, M. A. (1988). Incest investigation and treatment planning by child protective services. In L. E. A. Walker (Ed.), *Handbook on sexual abuse of children* (pp. 152–174). New York: Springer.

Spengler, A. (1977). Manifest sadomasochism of males: Results of an empirical study. *Archives of Sexual Behavior, 6,* 441–456.

Spijkstra, J. J., Spinder, T., & Gooren, L. J. G. (1988). Short-term patterns of pulsatile luteinizing hormone secretion do not differ between male-to-female transsexuals and heterosexual men. *Psychoneuroendocrinology, 13,* 279–283.

Sreenivasan, U. (1985). Effeminate boys in a child psychiatric clinic: Prevalence and associated factors. *Journal of the American Academy of Child Psychiatry, 23,* 689–694.

St. Lawrence, J. S., Hood, H. V., Brasfield, T., & Kelly, J. A. (1989). Differences in gay men's AIDS risk knowledge and behavior patterns in high and low AIDS prevalence cities. *Public Health Report, 104,* 391–395.

Stall, R., & Wiley, J. (1988). A comparison of alcohol and drug use patterns of homosexual and heterosexual men: The San Francisco men's health study. *Drug and Alcohol Dependence, 22,* 63–73.

Standards of Care. (1985). The hormonal and surgical sex reassignment of gender dysphoric persons. *Archives of Sexual Behavior, 14,* 79–90.

Steege, J. F., Stout, A. L., & Carson, C. C. (1986). Patient satisfaction in Scott and Small-Carrion penile implant recipients: A study of 52 patients. *Archives of Sexual Behavior, 15,* 393–399.

Steiner, A. E. (1981). Pretending orgasm by men and women: An aspect of communication in relationships. *Dissertation Abstracts International, 42,* 2553-B.

Steketee, G., & Foa, E. B. (1987). Rape victims: Post-traumatic stress responses and their treatment. *Journal of Anxiety Disorders, 1,* 69–86.

Stermac, L. E., Segal, Z. V., & Gillis, R. (1990). Social and cultural factors in sexual assault. In W. L. Marshall, D. R. Laws, & H. E. Barbaree (Eds.), *Handbook of sexual assault* (pp. 143–159). New York: Plenum.

Stoller, R. J. (1968). *Sex and gender.* London: Hogarth.

Stoller, R. J. (1970). Psychotherapy of extremely feminine boys. *International Journal of Psychiatry, 9,* 278–282.

Stoller, R. J. (1971). The term "transvestism." *Archives of General Psychiatry, 24,* 230–237.

Stoller, R. J. (1972). Etiological factors in female transsexualism: A first approximation. *Archives of Sexual Behavior, 2,* 47–64.

Stoller, R. J. (1982). Transvestism in women. *Archives of Sexual Behavior, 11,* 99–115.

Stoller, R. J., & Herdt, G. H. (1985). Theories of origins of male homosexuality. *Archives of General Psychiatry, 42,* 399–404.

Stouthamer-Loeber, M. (1986). Lying as a problem behavior in children: A review. *Clinical Psychology Review, 6,* 267–289.

Strassberg, D. S., Mahoney, J. M., Schaugaard, M., & Hale, V. E. (1990). The role of anxiety in premature ejaculation: A psychophysiological model. *Archives of Sexual Behavior, 19,* 251–257.

Strommen, E. F. (1989). "You're a what?" Family member reactions to the disclosure of homosexuality. *Journal of Homosexuality, 18,* 37–58.

Struckman-Johnson, C. (1988). Forced sex on dates: It happens to men, too. *Journal of Sex Research, 24,* 234–241.

Stuart, F. M., Hammond, D. C., & Pett, M. A. (1987). Inhibited sexual desire in women. *Archives of Sexual Behavior, 16,* 91–106.

Sugar, M. (1984). *Adolescent parenthood.* New York: MTP Press.

Summit, R. C. (1983). The child sexual abuse accommodation syndrome. *Child Abuse and Neglect, 7,* 177–193.

Swan, G. E., & MacDonald, M. L. (1978). Behavior therapy in practice: A national survey of behavior therapists. *Behavior Therapy, 9,* 799–807.

Swanson, D. W. (1968). Adult sexual abuse of children. *Diseases of the Nervous System, 29,* 677–683.

Swift, C. F. (1985). The prevention of rape. In A. W. Burgess (Ed.), *Rape and sexual assault* (pp. 413–433). New York: Garland.

Swigert, V. L., Farrell, R. A., & Yoels, W. C. (1976). Sexual homicide: Social, psychological and legal aspects. *Archives of Sexual Behavior, 5,* 391–401.

Symonds, C. L., Mendoza, M. J., & Harrell, W. C. (1981). Forbidden sexual behavior among kin. In L. L. Constantine & F. M. Martinson (Eds.), *Children and sex* (pp. 151–162). Boston: Little, Brown.

Symonds, M. (1980). The second injury. In *Evaluation and change,* (Special issue: Services to Survivors): Minnesota Medical Research Foundation.

Szasz, G., Stevenson, R. W. D., Lee, L., & Sanders, H. D. (1987). Induction of penile erection by intracavernosal injection: A double-blind comparison of phenoxybenzamine versus papaverine-phentolamine versus saline. *Archives of Sexual Behavior, 16,* 371–378.

Takefman, J., & Brender, W. (1984). An analysis of the effectiveness of two components in the treatment of erectile dysfunction. *Archives of Sexual Behavior, 13,* 321–340.

Tanner, J. M. (1978). *Fetus to man.* Cambridge, MA: Harvard University Press.

Tartagni, D. (1978). Counselling gays in a school setting. *The School Counselor, 26,* 26–32.

Taylor, C. B., Agras, W. S., Schneider, J. A., & Allen, R. A. (1983). Adherence to instructions to practise relaxation exercises. *Journal of Consulting and Clinical Psychology, 51,* 952–953.

Taylor, M. C., & Hall, J. A. (1982). Psychological androgeny: Theories, methods, and conclusions. *Psychological Bulletin, 92,* 347–366.

Templeman, T. L., & Stinnett, R. D. (1991). Patterns of sexual arousal and history in a "normal" sample of young men. *Archives of Sexual Behavior, 20,* 137–150.

Tennant, G. (1984). Review of the research into the use of drugs and the treatment of sexual deviations with special reference to the use of cyproterone acetate (Androcur). In H. C. Stancer, P. E. Garfinkel & V. M. Rakoff (Eds.), *Guidelines for the use of psychotropic drugs* (pp. 411–426). New York: Spectrum.

Terman, L. M. (1938). *Psychological factors in marital happiness.* New York: McGraw-Hill.

Terman, L. M. (1951). Correlates of orgasm adequacy in a group of 556 wives. *Journal of Psychology, 32,* 115–172.

Terman, L. M., & Miles, C. C. (1936). *Sex and personality.* New York: McGraw-Hill.

Tharinger, D., Horton, C. B., & Millea, S. (1990). Sexual abuse and exploitation of children and adults with mental retardation. *Child Abuse and Neglect, 14,* 301–312.

Thase, M. E., Reynolds, C. F., III, & Jennings, J. R. (1988). Nocturnal penile tumescence is diminished in depressed men. *Biological Psychiatry, 24,* 33–46.

Thorpe, J. G., Schmidt, E., & Castell, D. A. (1963). A comparison of positive and negative (aversive) conditioning in the treatment of homosexuality. *Behaviour Research and Therapy, 1,* 357–362.

Tollison, C. D., Adams, H. E., & Tollison, J. W. (1979). Cognitive and physiological indices of sexual arousal in homosexual, bisexual, and heterosexual males. *Journal of Behavioral Assessment, 1,* 305–314.

Tong, L., Oates, K., & McDowell, M. (1987). Personality development following sexual abuse. *Child Abuse and Neglect, 11,* 371–383.

Townsend, J. M., & Levy, G. D. (1990). Effects of potential partners' physical attractiveness and socioeconomic status on sexuality and partner selection. *Archives of Sexual Behavior, 19,* 149–164.

Travin, S., Bluestone, H., Coleman, E., Cullen, K., & Melella, J. (1986). Pedophile types and treatment perspectives. *Journal of Forensic Sciences, 31,* 614–620.

Travin, S., Cullen, K., & Protter, B. (1990). Female sex offenders: Severe victims and victimizers. *Journal of Forensic Sciences, 35,* 140–150.

Tsai, M., Feldman-Summers, S., & Edgar, M. (1979). Childhood molestation: Variables related to differential impact on psychosexual functioning in adult women. *Journal of Abnormal Psychology, 88,* 407–417.

Tsitouras, P. D., Martin, C. E., & Harman, S. M. (1982). Relationship of serum testosterone to sexual activity in healthy elderly men. *Journal of Gerontology, 37,* 288–293.

Tsoi, W. F. (1988). The prevalence of transsexualism in Singapore. *Acta Psychiatrica Scandinavica, 78,* 501–504.

Tsoi, W. F. (1990). Developmental profile of 200 male and 100 female transsexuals in Singapore. *Archives of Sexual Behavior, 19,* 595–605.

Tucker, P. K., Rothwell, S. J., Armstrong, M. S., & McConaghy, N. (1982). Creativity, divergent and allusive thinking in students and visual artists. *Psychological Medicine, 12,* 835–841.

Turner, B. F., & Adams, C. G. (1988). Reported change in preferred sexual activity over the adult years. *Journal of Sex Research, 25,* 299–303.

Tuttle, W. B., Cook, W. L., & Fitch, E. (1964). Sexual behavior in post myocardial infarction patients. *American Journal of Cardiology, 13,* 140.

Udry, J. R. (1980). Changes in the frequency of marital intercourse from panel data. *Archives of Sexual Behavior, 9,* 319–326.

Udry, J. R., Billy, J. O. G., Morris, N. M., Groff, T. R., & Raj, H. R. (1985). Serum androgenic hormones motivate sexual behavior in adolescent boys. *Fertility and Sterility, 43,* 90–94.

Udry, J. R., & Morris, N. M. (1967). A method for validation of reported sexual data. *Journal of Marriage and the Family, 29,* 442–446.

Udry, J. R., Talbert, L. M., & Morris, N. M. (1986). Biosocial foundations for adolescent female sexuality. *Demography, 23,* 217–227.

van de Wiel, H. B. M., Jasper, J. P. M., Schultz, W. C. M., & Gal, J. (1990). Treatment of vaginismus: A review of concepts and treatment modalities. *Journal of Psychosomatic Obstetrics and Gynecology, 11,* 1–18.

van den Brink, W., Koeter, M. W. J., Ormel, J., Dijkstra, W., Giel, R., Slooff, C. J., & Wohlfarth, T. D. (1989). Psychiatric diagnosis in an outpatient population. *Archives of General Psychiatry, 46,* 369–372.

van der Holk, J. A. R., van Griensven, G. J. P., & Coutinho, R. A. (1990). Increase in unsafe homosexual behaviour. *Lancet, 336,* 179–180.

Van Gelder, L. (1982). America's gay women. *Rolling Stone, 360,* 69–75.

van Griensven, G. J., de Vroome, E. M., Tielman, R. A., & Coutinho, R. A. (1988). Failure rate of condoms during anogenital intercourse in homosexual men. *Genitourinary Medicine, 64,* 344–346.

Van Wyk, P. H., & Geist, C. S. (1984). Psychosocial development of heterosexual, bisexual, and homosexual behavior. *Archives of Sexual Behavior, 13,* 505–544.

Vance, E. B., & Wagner, N. N. (1976). Written descriptions of orgasm: A study of sex differences. *Archives of Sexual Behavior, 5,* 87–98.

Vershoor, A. M., & Poortinga, J. (1988). Psychosexual differences between Dutch male and female transsexuals. *Archives of Sexual Behavior, 17,* 173–178.

Virag, R., Bouilly, P., & Frydman, D. (1985). Is impotence an arterial disorder? *Lancet, 331,* 181–184.

Visano, L. A. (1991). The impact of age on paid sexual encounters. *Journal of Homosexuality, 20,* 207–226.

Vitulano, L. A., Lewis, M., Doran, L. D., Nordhaus, B., & Adnopoz, J. (1986). Treatment recommendation, implementation, and follow-up in child abuse. *American Journal of Orthopsychiatry, 56,* 478–480.

Wabrek, A. J., & Burchell, R. C. (1980). Male sexual dysfunction associated with coronary artery disease. *Archives of Sexual Behavior, 9,* 69–75.

Wald, M. S. (1982). State intervention on behalf of endangered children—a proposed legal response. *Child Abuse and Neglect, 6,* 3–45.

Walinder, J., Lundstrom, B., & Thuwe, I. (1978). Prognostic factors in the assessment of male transsexuals for sex reassignment. *British Journal of Psychiatry, 132,* 16–20.

Walker, L. E. A. (1988). Introduction. New techniques for assessment and evaluation of child sexual abuse victims: Using anatomically "correct" dolls and videotape procedures. In L. E. A. Walker (Ed.), *Handbook on sexual abuse of children* (pp. ix–xx, 175–197). New York: Springer.

Walker, L. E. A., & Bolkovatz, M. A. (1988). Play therapy with children who have experienced sexual assault. In L. E. A. Walker (Ed.), *Handbook on sexual abuse of children* (pp. 249–269). New York: Springer.

Walling, M., Anderson, B. L., & Johnson, S. R. (1990). Hormonal replacement therapy for postmenopausal women: A review of sexual outcomes and related gynecologic effects. *Archives of Sexual Behavior, 19,* 119–137.

Ward, I. L. (1972). Prenatal stress feminizes and demasculinizes the behavior of males. *Science, 175,* 82–84.

Ward, I. L. (1984). The prenatal stress syndrome: Current status. *Psychoneuroendocrinology, 9,* 3–11.

Wasserman, M. D., Pollak, C. P., Spielman, A. J., & Weitzman, E. D. (1980). Theoretical and technical problems in the measurement of nocturnal penile tumescence for the differential diagnosis of impotence. *Psychosomatic Medicine, 42,* 575–585.

Watson, J. B. (1914). *Behavior.* New York: Kegan Paul.

Watson, J. B. (1925). *Behaviorism.* London: Kegan Paul, Trench, Trubner.

Weeks, R. B. (1976). The sexually exploited child. *Southern Medical Journal, 69,* 848–850.

Weinberg, S. K. (1955). *Incest behavior.* New York: Citadel.

Weiner, I. (1982). *Child and adolescent psychopathology.* New York: Wiley.

Weinstock, R., & Weinstock, D. (1988). Child abuse reporting trends: An unprecedented threat to confidentiality. *Journal of Forensic Science, 33,* 418–431.

Weis, D. L. (1985). The experience of pain during women's first sexual intercourse: Cultural mythology about female sexual initiation. *Archives of Sexual Behavior, 14,* 421–439.

Weisman, R., & Hart, J. (1987). Sexual behavior in healthy married elderly men. *Archives of Sexual Behavior, 16,* 1987.

Weiss, J., Rogers, E., Darwin, M. R., & Dutton, C. E. (1955). A study of girl sex victims. *Psychiatric Quarterly, 29,* 1–27.

Weizman, R., & Hart, J. (1987). Sexual behavior in healthy married elderly men. *Archives of Sexual Behavior, 16,* 39–44.

Westney, O. E., Jenkins, R. R., Butts, J. D., & Williams, I. (1984). Sexual development and behavior in black preadolescents. *Adolescence, 19,* 557–568.

Wheller, D., & Rubin, H. B. (1987). A comparison of volumetric and circumferential measures of penile erection. *Archives of Sexual Behavior, 16,* 289–301.

Wheller, H. (1985). Pornography and rape: A feminist perspective. In A. W. Burgess (Ed.), *Rape and sexual assault* (pp. 374–391). New York: Garland.

Whitam, F. L. (1977). Childhood indicators of male homosexuality. *Archives of Sexual Behavior, 6,* 89–96.

Whitam, F. L. (1980). The prehomosexual male child in three societies: The United States, Guatemala, Brazil. *Archives of Sexual Behavior, 9,* 87–99.

Whitam, F. L. (1990). Review: Journey into sexuality; an exploratory voyage. *Archives of Sexual Behavior, 19,* 531–534.

White, C. B. (1982). Sexual interest, attitudes, knowledge, and sexual history in relation to sexual behavior in the institutionalized aged. *Archives of Sexual Behavior, 11,* 11–21.

White, J. R., Case, D. A., McWhirter, D., & Mattison, A. M. (1990). Enhanced sexual behavior in exercising men. *Archives of Sexual Behavior, 19,* 193–209.

Whitfield, M. (1989). Development of sexuality in female children and adolescents. *Canadian Journal of Psychiatry, 34,* 879–883.

Whiting, B., & Edwards, C. P. (1973). A cross-cultural analysis of sex differences in the behavior of children aged 3 through 11. *Journal of Social Psychology, 91,* 171–188.

Whitley, B. E. (1983). Sex role orientation and self-esteem: A critical meta-analytic review. *Journal of Personality and Social Psychology, 44,* 765–778.

Wild, N. J., & Wynne, J. M. (1986). Child sex rings. *British Medical Journal, 293,* 183–185.

Williams, W. (1984). Secondary premature ejaculation. *Australian and New Zealand Journal of Psychiatry, 18,* 333–340.

Williams, W. (1985). Psychogenic erectile impotence—a useful or a misleading concept? *Australian and New Zealand Journal of Psychiatry, 19,* 77–82.

Wilson, G. D. (1981). Cross-generational stability of gender differences in sexuality. *Personality and Individual Differences, 2,* 254–257.

Wilson, G. D. (1987). Male-female differences in sexual activity, enjoyment and fantasies. *Personality and Individual Differences, 8,* 125–127.

Wilson, G. D., & Cox, D. N. (1983). Personality of paedophile club members. *Personality and Individual Differences, 3,* 323–329.

Wincze, J. P., Bansal, S., & Malamud, M. (1986). Effects of medroxyprogesterone acetate on subjective arousal, arousal to erotic stimulation, and nocturnal penile tumescence in male sex offenders. *Archives of Sexual Behavior, 15,* 293–305.

Wincze, J. P., & Lange, J. P. (1981). Assessment of sexual behavior. In D. H. Barlow (Ed.), *Behavioral assessment of adult disorders* (pp. 301–328). New York: Guilford.

Wincze, J. P., & Qualls, C. B. (1984). A comparison of structural patterns of sexual arousal in male and female homosexuals. *Archives of Sexual Behavior, 13,* 361–370.

Winfield, L., George, L. K., Swartz, M., & Blazer, D. G. (1990). Sexual assault and psychiatric disorders among a community sample of women. *American Journal of Psychiatry, 147,* 335–341.

Wing, J. K., & Sturt, E. (1978). *The PSE-ID-Catego system: Supplementary manual.* London: MRC Social Psychiatry Unit.

Winokur, G., Guze, S. B., & Pfeiffer, E. (1959). Developmental and sexual factors in women: A comparison between control, neurotic and psychotic groups. *American Journal of Psychiatry, 115,* 1097–1100.

Wolf, S. C., Conte, T. R., & Engel-Meinig, M. (1988). Assessment and treatment of sex offenders in a community setting. In L. E. A. Walker (Ed.), *Handbook on sexual abuse of children* (pp. 365–383). New York: Springer.

Wolf, T. J. (1988). Group psychotherapy for bisexual men and their wives. In E. Coleman (Ed.), *Psychotherapy for homosexual men and women: Integrated identity approaches for clinical practice* (pp. 191–199). New York: Haworth.

Wolpe, J. (1958). *Psychotherapy by reciprocal inhibition.* Stanford, CA: Stanford University Press.

Worden, F. G., & Marsh, J. T. (1955). Psychological factors in men seeking sex transformation. *Journal of the American Medical Association, 157,* 1292–1298.

Wyatt, G. E. (1985). The sexual abuse of Afro-American and white American women in childhood. *Child Abuse and Neglect, 9,* 507–519.

Wyatt, G. E., & Peters, S. D. (1986a). Issues in the definition of child sexual abuse in prevalence research. *Child Abuse and Neglect, 10,* 231–240.

Wyatt, G. E., & Peters, S. D. (1986b). Methodological considerations in research on the prevalence of child sexual abuse. *Child Abuse and Neglect, 10,* 241–251.

Yalom, I. D., Green, R., & Fisk, N. (1973). Prenatal exposure to female hormones: Effect on psychosexual development in boys. *Archives of General Psychiatry, 28,* 554–561.

Yates, A. (1987). Should young children testify in cases of sexual abuse? *American Journal of Psychiatry, 144,* 476–480.

Yllo, K., & Finkelhor, D. (1985). Marital rape. In A. W. Burgess (Ed.), *Rape and sexual assault* (pp. 146–158). New York: Garland.

Zelnik, M., Kantner, J. F., & Ford, K. (1981). *Sex and pregnancy in adolescence.* Beverly Hills, CA: Sage.

Zilbergeld, B., & Evans, M. (1980). The inadequacy of Masters and Johnson. *Psychology Today, 14,* 29–43.

Zorgniotti, A. W., & Lefleur, R. S. (1985). Auto-injection of the corpus cavernosum with a vasoactive drug combination for vasculgenic impotence. *Journal of Urology, 133,* 39–41.

Zucker, K. J. (1985). Book review. *Archives of Sexual Behavior, 13,* 377–381.

Zuckerman, M. (1971). Physiological measures of sexual arousal in the human. *Psychological Bulletin, 75,* 297–329.

Zuger, B. (1966). Effeminate behavior present in boys from early childhood. I. The clinical syndrome and follow-up studies. *Journal of Pediatrics, 69,* 1098–1107.

Zuger, B. (1970). Gender role determination and rebuttal. *Psychosomatic Medicine, 3,* 449–467.

Zuger, B. (1978). Effeminate behavior present in boys from childhood: Ten additional years of follow-up. *Comprehensive Psychiatry, 19,* 363–369.

Zuger, B. (1984). Early effeminate behavior in boys: Outcome and significance for homosexuality. *Journal of Nervous and Mental Disease, 172,* 90–97.

Zuger, B. (1988). Is early homosexual behavior in boys early homosexuality? *Comprehensive Psychiatry,* *29,* 509–519.

Zuger, B., & Taylor, P. (1969). Effeminate behavior present in boys from early childhood. II. Comparison with similar symptoms in non-effeminate boys. *Pediatrics, 44,* 375–380.

Zverina, J., Lachman, M., Pondelickova, J., & Vanek, J. (1987). The occurrence of atypical sexual experience among various female patient groups. *Archives of Sexual Behavior, 16,* 321–326.

Index

Research methodology (*Cont.*)
  outcome evaluation
    problem of untreated controls, 33, 223–226, 296, 360
    post hoc analyses of data, 31, 34–35, 38
  single-case design, 11, 32–33, 348, 353
  type one errors, 33–35
  type two errors, 35
  see also Ideological influences on sexuality research; Politics of science
Retarded ejaculation. *See* Inhibited male orgasm

Sadistic murder, 316–317
  incidence, 316
  other sexual deviations and, 317
  perpetrators, 316–317, 342
  nature, 316–317
  victims
    child, 316, 317
    sex of, 317
Sadomasochism, 312–319
  club members, 314–315
  DSM-III-R criteria, 312, 315, 316, 318, 319
  fantasies, 313, 314, 315
  fetishism and, 314–315, 320
  nature of, 314–315
  prevalence, 315
    of inclination, 313
  sexual assault, rape and, 312–314
Sambia, 114–115
Script theory of behavior, 79, 292
  oral-anal activity and, 88
Self-report, 8–17, 346, 350
  bias, 14
  reactivity, 15
Sensate focusing, 220–221
Sex conversion. *See* Transvestism; Transsexualism
Sex differences. *See* Female and Male sexuality; Heterosexuality; Homosexuality
Sex education, 69–70
Sex identity, 143, 162–168
  assignment of, 163, 164–168
  biological determination of, 165–166
  core identity, 166
  dimensional nature of, 163–164, 165, 170
  DSM-III-R diagnostic criteria, 168
  etiology, 163, 164–168
  5-alpha-reductase deficiency syndrome and, 166–168
  imprinting and, 163
  see also Gender identity disorder of childhood; Hermaphroditism; Homosexuality; Transsexualism; Transvestism
Sex-linked behaviors
  biological determination of, 116–117, 122
  cultural determination of, 122, 345

Sex-linked behaviors (*Cont.*)
  dimensional nature of, 109–110
  effeminacy, 108
    attitude to, 109, 133
    families of boys with, 108, 116
    gender identity disorder of childhood and, 112
    management of, 112, 133
    observational assessment of, 18
  femininity and masculinity and, 122–123, 343–344
  homosexuality/heterosexuality and, 108–112, 114, 122–123, 145
    female-male differences, 111, 118–119, 121
  parent-child relationships and, 116, 117, 345
  prenatal sex hormone levels and, 116–118
  range of, 121
  tomboyism
    attitude to, 133
    dimensional or categorical condition, 110–111
    gender identity disorder of childhood and, 112
    homosexuality and, 110, 111, 117–119
    masculine sex-role and, 124
    prenatal hormones and, 117–118
  see also Transsexualism; Transvestism
Sex murder. *See* Sadistic murder
Sex offences, 304, 323–326
  prevention, 362–363
  see also Childhood sexual abuse; Exhibitionism; Incest; Sadistic murder; Sex offenders; Sexual assault; Sexual deviations; Voyeurism
Sex offenders
  adolescent, 327–328
  alcohol and drug abuse and, 282, 293, 310, 327, 340, 342–343
  assessment of, 346
    penile circumference assessment, 28, 330–331, 346
  brain damage in, 324, 344, 360
  characteristics of offenders, 324–325
  DSM-III-R classification and, 323
  female, 328–329
  lack of social skills, 340–341
  multiple diagnoses, 321–323, 336
  nature of offences, 323
  psychological disorders in, 340–346
  relatives and contacts of, 329
  reoffending rate of untreated, 360
  response to treatment, 360, 362
  sexual interest level of, 344
  treatment. *See* Sexual deviations
  see also Child sexual abuse, perpetrators; Exhibitionism; Incest, perpetrators; Sadistic murder; Sexual assault, perpetrators; Sexual deviations; Voyeurism